I. Gordon · S. Fischer · K. Hahn
Atlas of Bone Scintigraphy in the Pathological
Paediatric Skeleton

Springer-Verlag Berlin Heidelberg GmbH

Isky Gordon
Sibylle Fischer
Klaus Hahn

Atlas of Bone Scintigraphy in the Pathological Paediatric Skeleton

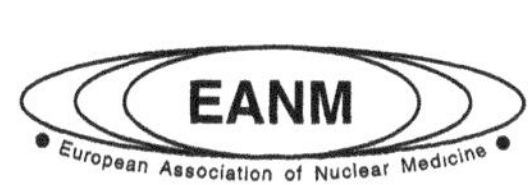

Under the Auspices of
the Paediatric Committee of the European
Association of Nuclear Medicine

Foreword by James J. Conway

With 347 Figures in 1 023 Separate Illustrations

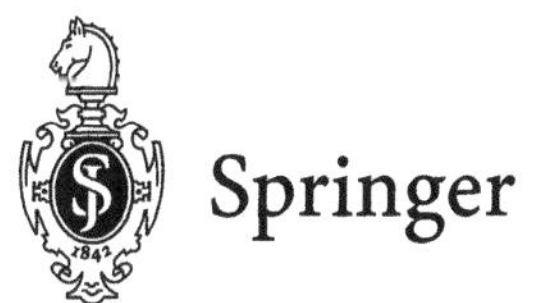

Springer

Isky Gordon, M.D.
Great Ormond Street Hospital for Children
Department of Radiology
Great Ormond Street
London WC1N 3JH, United Kingdom

Prof. Dr. med. Klaus Hahn
Sibylle Fischer
Ludwig-Maximilians-Universität München
Klinik und Poliklinik für Nuklearmedizin
Ziemssenstr. 1, D-80336 München

ISBN 978-3-642-64675-1   ISBN 978-3-642-61060-8 (eBook)
DOI 10.1007/978-3-642-61060-8

Library of Congress Cataloging-in-Publication Data
Gordon, Isky: Atlas of bone scintigraphy in the pathological paedriatic skeleton /
Isky Gordon, Sibylle Fischer, Klaus Hahn ; under the auspices of the Paedriatic
Committee of the European Association of Nuclear Medicine. p. cm.
To be used in conjunction with: Atlas of bone scintigraphy in the developing pae-
diatric skeleton / Klaus Hahn, Sibyllle Fischer, Isky Gordon. © 1993.
Includes index.

1. Bones–Radionuclide imaging–Atlases. 2. Bone diseases in children–Radio-
nuclide imaging–Atlases. 3. Human skeleton-Abnormalities–Diagnosis–
Atlases. I. Fischer, Sibylle, 1961 – II. Hahn, K. (Klaus) III. Hahn K. (Klaus)
Atlas of bone scintigraphy in the developing paedriatic skeleton. IV. Title.
[DNLM: 1. Bone Diseases–in infancy & childhood–atlases. 2. Bone Diseases–
radionuclide imaging–atlases.3. Fractures–radionuclide imaging–atlases.
WS 17 G663a 1996]
RJ482.B65H34 1996 suppl
618.92'71075745–dc20   95-52577
DNLM/DLC for Library of Congress   CIP

Typesetting: FotoSatz Pfeifer GmbH, Gräfelfing

SPIN: 10484476   21/3132 – 5 4 3 2 1 0 – Printed on acid-free paper

Foreword

The publication of a nuclear medicine atlas on musculoskeletal disorders indicates that the practice of paediatric nuclear medicine has matured. There are several general paediatric nuclear medicine text books available, but none which specifically addresses the use of radionuclides for musculoskeletal disorders. Yet, approximately one third of all paediatric nuclear medicine studies are of the musculoskeletal system. It is therefore timely that a publication specifically related to the largest organ system of the body be available to describe the rational use of paediatric bone scintigraphy and to ensure the quality of those studies.

Formal training in paediatric nuclear medicine is limited for most practitioners of nuclear medicine. As a consequence, paediatric diseases and their appearances on bone scintigraphy are familiar only to the practitioner and technologist who encounter children on a daily basis. In addition, the technical requirements for quality radionuclide imaging in children are more demanding and are less well understood. The size of children varies significantly which poses technical difficulties for those with limited training and experience in the subspecialty of paediatric nuclear medicine.

Since many children, if not a majority, are studied in nonpaedriatic imaging centers, an atlas of bone scintigraphy is valuable as a handy reference. An atlas allows a rapid search and a quick review of those conditions unfamiliar to the practitioner. Specific images of common and rare pathological conditions define the technique required for appropriate imaging and assist in the interpretation of unfamiliar disorders. Further an atlas concentrates the information into one easy access volume for busy practitioners to quickly localize the disease process or disorder and recognize its clinical significance.

The topics presented in this atlas include all of the common and rare musculoskeletal conditions encountered in children. Special emphasis on infection, arthritis simulating infection, the characteristics of benign and malignant tumours, dysplastic conditions and unusual appearances on bone scintigraphy provide a comprehensive review of musculoskeletal disorders. This atlas is an excellent companion and complement to the publication in 1993 by the same authors ("Atlas of Bone Scintigraphy in the Developing Paediatric Skeleton", Hahn et al. Springer, Berlin Heidelberg New York). The authors are internationally renowned and acknowledged as experts in paediatric nuclear medicine. The information in this volume is based on their numerous, cumulative years of experience in both the technique and the interpretation of musculoskeletal disorders in children. Both volumes should be a standard reference in the library of every nuclear medicine department where children are studied. Its regular use will repay the user in time saved, knowledge gained, and improved quality of their practice for years to come.

James J. Conway, Chicago
Children's Memorial Hospital
Chicago / USA

Preface

This atlas represents the second of two atlases. The Paediatric Committee of the European Association of Nuclear Medicine (EANM) believes that the quality of paediatric bone scintigraphy is very variable. Many poor quality bone scans have been seen by members of this committee as well as published in reputable journals. The first atlas was produced in an attempt to improve the overall quality of the bone scan images as well as give physicians the possibility to understand normal maturation of the growing skeleton. This second atlas focuses on pathological processes affecting the skeleton, but should be used in conjunction with the first atlas.

The Paediatric Committee acknowledges the requirement of both high-quality bone-seeking Technetium 99m labelled radiopharmaceuticals and gamma camera equipment providing images of the highest quality. The nuclear medicine industry has contributed so that this atlas could be produced at a price which will hopefully allow the widest possible distribution. Acknowledgement for financial support to the following companies is gratefully expressed: Amersham Healthcare, Elscint, Kodak, Mallinckrodt Medical, Picker International, Polaroid and Siemens.

I. Gordon, London
S. Fischer, Munich
K. Hahn, Munich

The authors would like to thank the Paediatric Committee of the European Association of Nuclear Medicine (EANM) for their continuing support of this project. The images used in this atlas have come from:

- Great Ormond Street Hospital for Children, Department of Radiology, London, Great Britain (Dr. Isky Gordon)
- Klinik und Poliklinik für Nuklearmedizin der Johannes-Gutenberg-Universität Mainz, Mainz, Germany (Prof. Dagmar Eißner)
- Klinik und Poliklinik für Nuklearmedizin der Ludwig-Maximilians-Universität München, München, Germany (Prof. Klaus Hahn)
- Red Cross Children's Memorial Hospital, Department of Nuclear Medicine, Cape Town, South Africa (Prof. Michael Mann)
- Hospital St. Pierre, Akademisch Zickenhuis, Department of Radiology, Brussels, Belgium (Prof. Amy Piepsz)
- Hospital General Vall d'Hebron, Department of Nuclear Medicine, Barcelona, Spain (Dr. Isabel Roca)
- Hôspital d'Enfants Armand-Trousseau, Service de Médicine Nucleaire, Paris, France (Dr. Michél Wioland)

A special thanks goes to Prof. Michael Mann and the staff of the Nuclear Medicine Department at the Red Cross Children's Memorial Hospital, Cape Town, South Africa, who have provided a large portion of the cases in the section on "Infection" as well as other cases in other chapters.

Thanks are also due to Prof. Amy Piepsz, who reviewed the entire manuscript in its penultimate format.

The high quality images produced by the photolaboratory in Mainz (head: Mrs. A. Keuchel) are greatly appreciated.

We would also like to thank Lorenzo, Natasha and Hannah for setting up the computerized nuclear medicine museum at the Great Ormond Street Hospital for Children in London.

Acknowledgements

Contents

Contents

1 Introduction

The use of radioisotopes to image the skeleton has been in practice for over two decades. With the introduction of Technetium (Tc 99m) and the use of compounds which adsorb onto the hydroxy apatite, radioisotope bone scans have been used for both benign and malignant diseases in paediatrics. The paediatric skeleton is maturing throughout childhood with growth occurring principally at the growth plates of the long bones.

Technique

The undertaking of a radioisotope bone scan in children requires a number of important considerations so that the final images will be diagnostic. The preparation of the child (including mother/father), the injection of the appropriate amount of Tc 99m bone seeking tracer and the acquisition of images (blood flow, blood pool, static, whole body, pin hole and SPECT) of the highest quality must be obtained with special care.

An adequate examination involves full participation of the child and the parents so that both come out feeling that they have helped to create high quality images. The injection of the appropriate amount of radiopharmaceutical, either based on the child's weight or body surface area should follow the recommendations of the Paediatric Task Group of the EANM (see Table 1.1). It must be undertaken with minimal discomfort for the child. There are numerous bone seeking agens which combine with Tc 99m to provide high quality images of the osteoblastic turnover in the skeleton (MDP, HDP, HMDP, DPD)

The acquisition of the appropriate images is the domain of the nuclear medicine physician/radiologist and the technologist together. Indications for blood flow and blood pool images must be understood, the use of pin hole collimators is essential for hip pathology whilst SPECT for the spine is proving useful. Not every child requires all the different imaging techniques.

Blood flow images are obtained with sequences of 1 or 2 s over a 60 to 120 s period.

Static gamma camera blood pool images are completed within 5 min of the injection The minimun acquired count rate should be 50 000–100 000 counts for the hands, feet and knees and 200 000–500 000 counts or a maximum time of 3 min for other areas. Using whole body scans, the imaging is started directly after the injection of the radioisotope with a scan speed of 30 cm/min.

The bone scan images are obtained 2–4 h after the injection of the radioisotope. The minimum count rate for images of the hands and feet is 50 000 counts and 100 000 counts for the knee joints. 200 000 counts are acquired for images of the skull. The remaining skeleton requires 250 000–500 000 counts per image.

Whole body scans are acquired with a scan speed of 8 cm/min in children up to the age of 8 years, 10 cm/min in children ranging from 8–12 years and 12 cm/min in children ranging from 12–16 years. In children beyond this age, the scan speed is 15 cm/min.

Pin hole images are obtained with an imaging time of 600–900 s.

If SPECT is required, 120 steps with an imaging time of 30 s per step is undertaken. Acquisition matrix is 64×64 or 128×128.

The use of sedation varies widely. There are however institutions who obtain high quality images but yet rarely use sedation. There should be an

1 Introduction

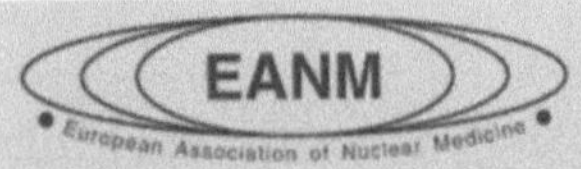

Table 1.1 Paediatric Task Group

Fraction of Adult Administered Activity		
3 kg = 0.1	22 kg = 0.50	42 kg = 0.78
4 kg = 0.14	24 kg = 0.53	44 kg = 0.80
6 kg = 0.19	26 kg = 0.56	46 kg = 0.82
8 kg = 0.23	28 kg = 0.58	48 kg = 0.85
10 kg = 0.27	30 kg = 0.62	50 kg = 0.88
12 kg = 0.32	32 kg = 0.65	52–54 kg = 0.90
14 kg = 0.36	34 kg = 0.68	56–58 kg = 0.92
16 kg = 0.40	36 kg = 0.71	60–62 kg = 0.96
18 kg = 0.44	38 kg = 0.73	64–66 kg = 0.96
20 kg = 0.46	40 kg = 0.76	68 kg = 0.99

Recommended Adult and Minimum Amounts in MBq		
Radiopharmaceutical	**Adult**	**Minimum**
Tc99m DTPA (Kidney)	200	20
Tc99m DMSA	100	15
Tc99m MAG3	70	15
Tc99m Pertechnetate (Cystography)	20	20
Tc99m MDP	500	40
Tc99m COLLOID (Liver/Spleen)	80	15
Tc99m COLLOID (Marrow)	300	20
Tc99m SPLEEN (Denatured R B C)	40	20
Tc99m R B C (Blood Pool)	800	80
Tc99m ALBUMIN (Cardiac)	800	80
Tc99m Pertechnatate (First Pass)	500	80
Tc99m MAA / Microspheres	80	10
Tc99m Pertechnetate (Ectopic Gastric)	150	20
Tc99m Colloid (Gastric Reflux)	40	10
Tc99m IDA (Biliary)	150	20
Tc99m Pertechnetate (Thyroid)	80	10
Tc99m HMPAO (Brain)	740	100
Tc99m HMPAO (W B C)	500	40
I-123 HIPPURAN	75	10
I-123 (Thyroid)	20	3
I-123 Amphetamine (Brain)	185	18
I-123 mIBG	200	35
I-123 mIBG	80	35
GALLIUM 67	80	10

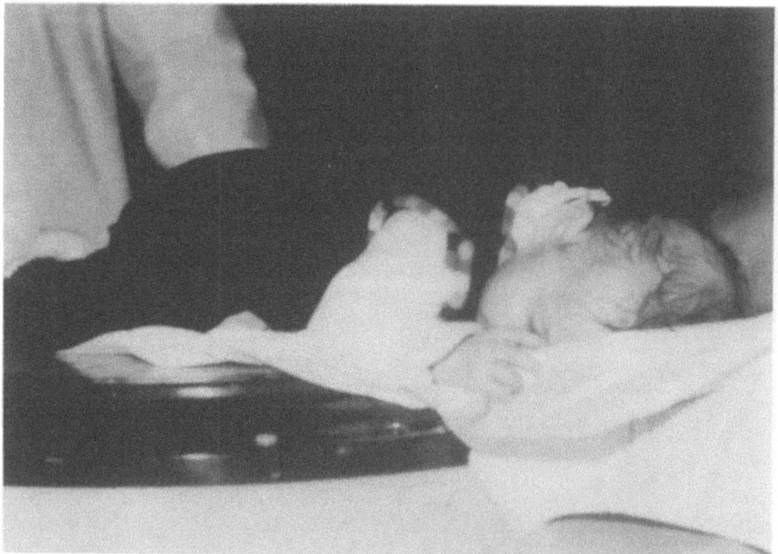

Fig. 1.1

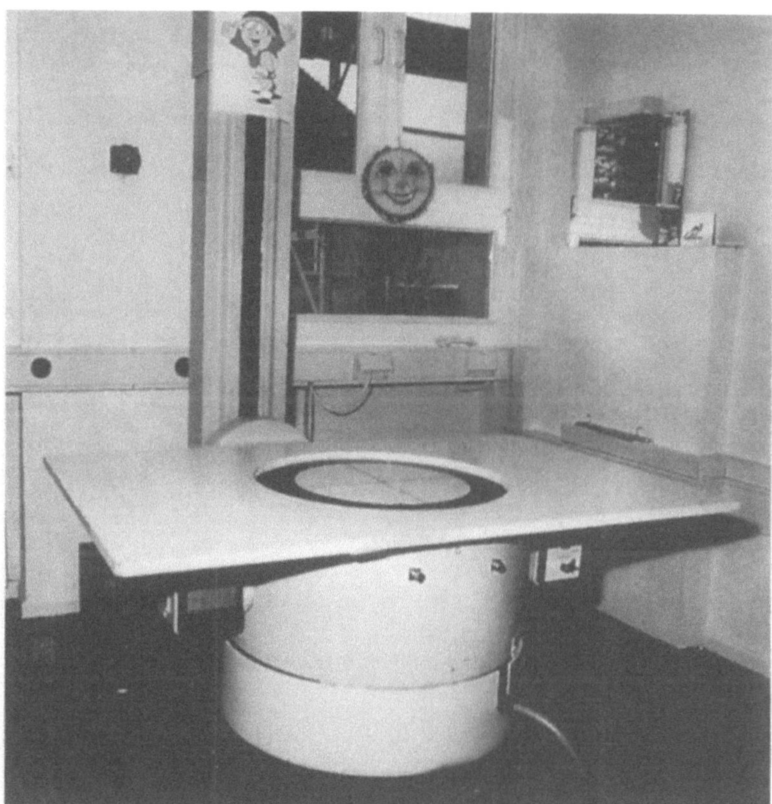

Fig. 1.2

active policy of reviewing how many children receive sedation and whether your department cannot reduce this number and maintain the highest quality images.

High quality images require the use of a high resolution collimator with the child as close to the head of the gamma camera as possible. The camera should generally be located underneath the child rather than the child squashed between the camera and imaging table (Figs. 1.1, 1.2).

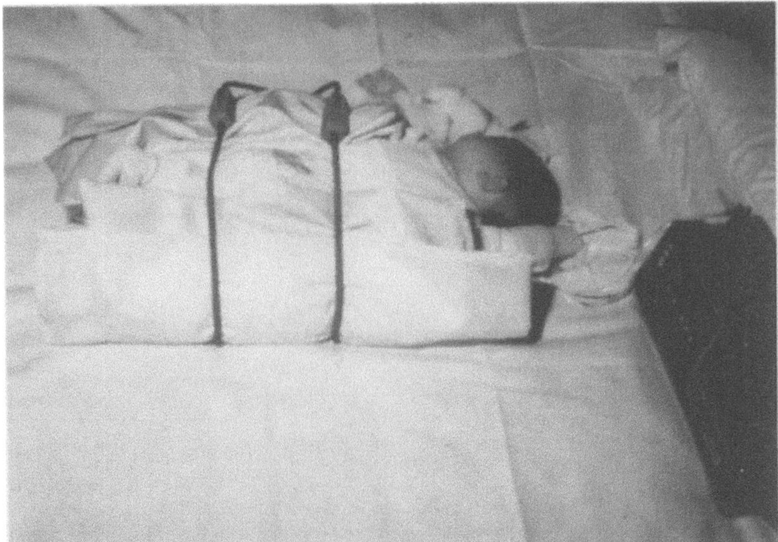

Fig. 1.3

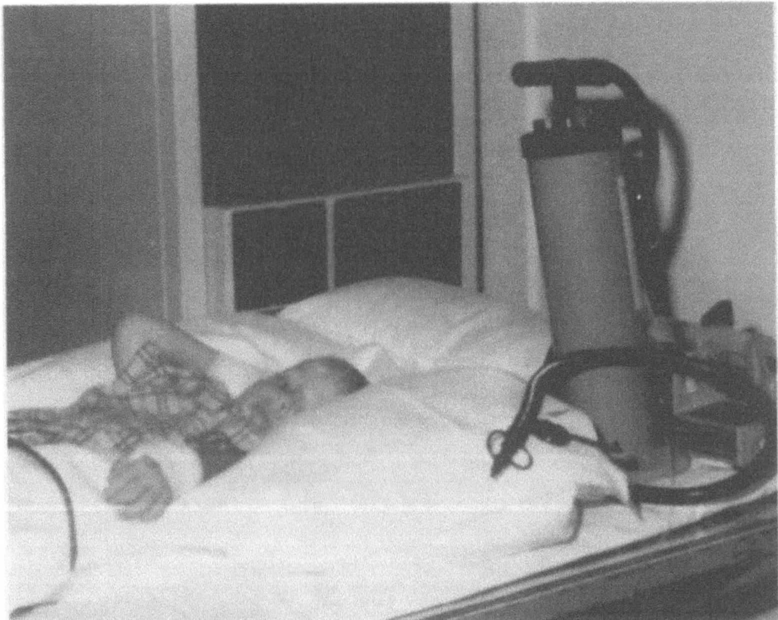

Fig. 1.4

Immobilisation is essential. This may be achieved either using velcro straps around sand bags placed on either side of the child or using a vacuum mattress (Figs. 1.3, 1.4). Simple methods of amusement of the child can be used such as a portable tape recorder with music and or nursery rhythms.

To obtain further co-operation from child and parent, the child should be encouraged to drink his/her favourite drink so that there is frequent spontaneous bladder emptying. Images of the hips and pelvis should be obtained as soon as the bladder is empty.

Recognition of Normality

The knowledge of the normal appearances of the paediatric skeleton on Tc 99m bone scans must be known. In order to achieve these aims members of the Paediatric Committee of the European Association of Nuclear Medicine have worked together to produce images of the "normal" paediatric skeleton. This resulted in the publication of the *Atlas of Bone Scintigraphy in the Developing Paediatric Skeleton – The normal skeleton, variants and pitfalls* (Springer-Verlag 1993). The activity of the members of the Paediatric Committee have continued in an attempt to produce this atlas of bone pathologies which may be seen on Tc 99m bone scans.

Indications

Indications for radioisotope bone scans include known malignant disease where staging is required, benign disease and where signs or symptoms exist and there is a strong clinical suspicion that the skeleton may be the source of the disease. This includes infection, trauma or inflammation. Occasionally the radioisotope bone scan may be carried out to assess the significance of an abnormality seen on the radiograph.

The response of the skeleton to pathology is similar i.e. bone scans have high sensitivity for increased osteoblastic activity for whatever pathology (fracture, infection, malignancy) and the Tc 99m bone scan is a test with a high sensitivity but a low specificity. In order to improve the specificity of the Tc 99m bone scan it is essential to interpret the abnormality seen in clinical context and in relation to the radiographic appearances.

Use of Atlas

The atlas has been divided into chapters based on disease processes, yet bone scans are non-specific and the clinical setting and radiology are crucial to come to a diagnosis. For this reason many illustrations in the atlas are cross referenced to point out similarities in bone scans from different pathologies.

2 Infection

In all the cases illustrated in this chapter and in the section on septic arthritis in Chap. 3, bacteriological proof of the infection was obtained either from blood culture, culture from surgical exploration or the discovery of "sterile" pus at surgery. The only exceptions to this are certain cases of spinal abnormalities in which there is controversy about the condition and in which no surgical exploration was undertaken. The same applies to the cases of sacro-ileitis (see Chap. 3).

Teaching Point

Early images (blood pool) versus late images (2–4 h after injection). When the abnormal increased uptake of isotope is more pronounced on the late images than on the early images, there is a strong probability of osteomyelitis. If the early images show increased activitiy while the late images are either normal or show only slightly increased activity, there is a probability of cellulitis with no underlying osteomyelitis. The slightly increased bone activity on the late images in such cases is due to hyperaemia (see "Non-skeletal Infection", chapter 2.4).

2.1 Typical Hot Lesions in Bone

2.1.1 Lower Limbs
(8 Cases; Figs. 2.1–2.8)

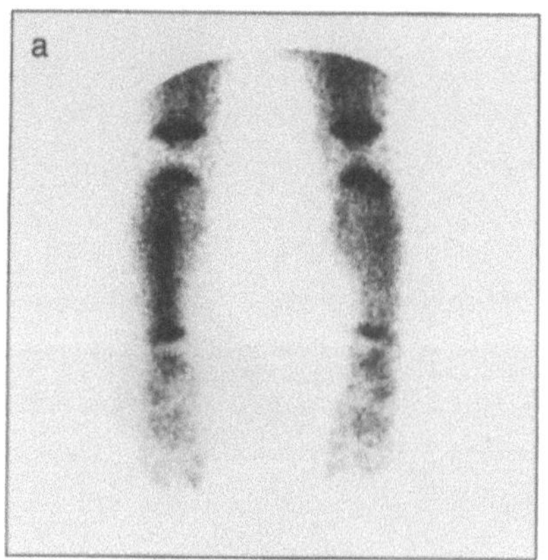

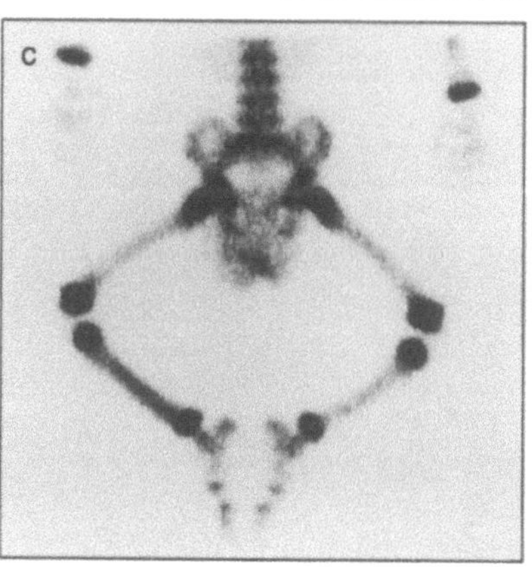

Case 2.1. A 12-month-old girl who was acutely unwell and was not moving her lower limbs. Final diagnosis was osteomyelitis of the right tibia

Fig. 2.1a. Blood pool image taken anteriorly shows diffuse increased uptake of tracer throughout the right lower limb including both bone and soft tissues

Fig. 2.1b. Anterior image of the lower limbs shows increased uptake of isotope throughout the diaphysis and metaphysis of the right tibia extending down to the distal epiphyseal plate

Fig. 2.1c. Frog lateral image of the lower limbs and anterior image of the pelvis shows increased uptake of isotope in the right tibia from the distal epiphyseal plate extending almost to the proximal epiphyseal plate

Teaching Point

1. Note the radiographic neutral position of the feet, allowing clear differentiation of the tibia from the fibula, permitting differentiation between involvement of these two bones in Fig. 2.1b. In the lateral projection (Fig. 2.1c) the tibia and fibula cannot be separated.

2. A similar bone scan appearance may be seen with a spiral fracture of the tibia (see Cases 5.19 and 5.40) and also with Ewing's sarcoma (see Case 4.31).

Case 2.2. A 9-month-old boy who was pyrexial, unwell and not moving his right leg. Final diagnosis was osteomyelitis of the right distal tibia

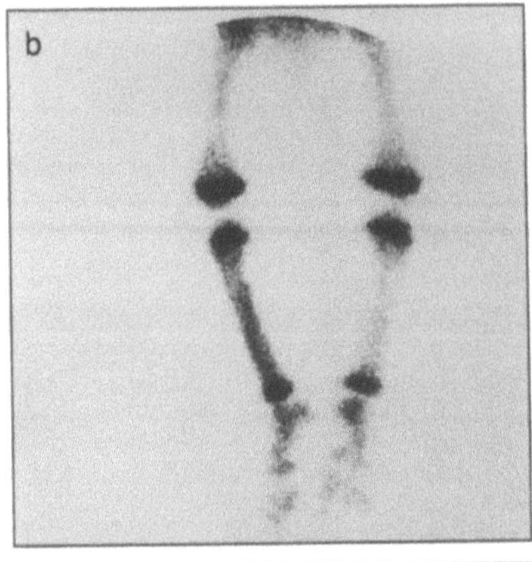

Fig. 2.2a. Blood pool anterior image of the lower limbs shows increased activity throughout the right tibia including the distal epiphyseal plate

Fig. 2.2b. Anterior image of the lower limbs shows increased activity extending from the distal metaphysis of the right tibia proximally to involve the middle and distal thirds of the tibia

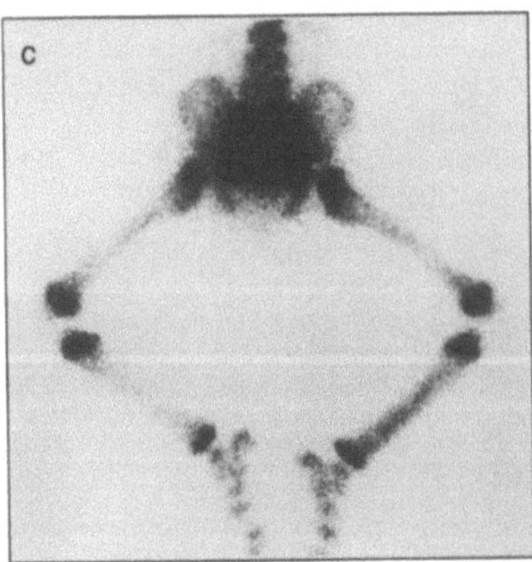

Fig. 2.2c. Frog lateral posterior view shows increased uptake in the middle and distal thirds of the right tibia

Technical Comment

Figure 2.2b shows poor positioning of the feet which precludes differentiation between the tibia and fibula. Compare this to the good positioning in the blood pool image above.

Teaching Point

Similar appearances may be seen with Ewing's sarcoma (see Case 4.31).

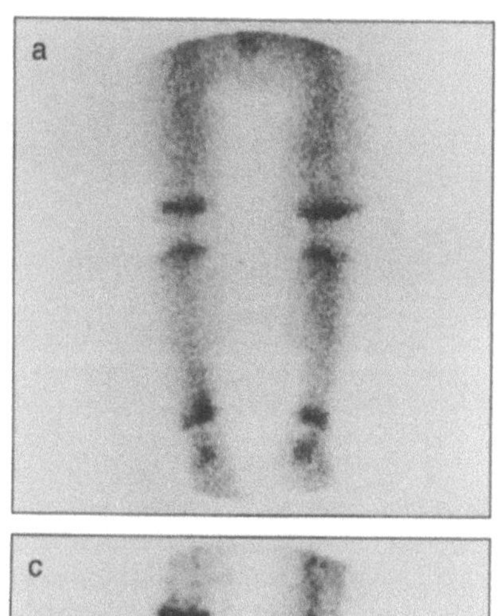

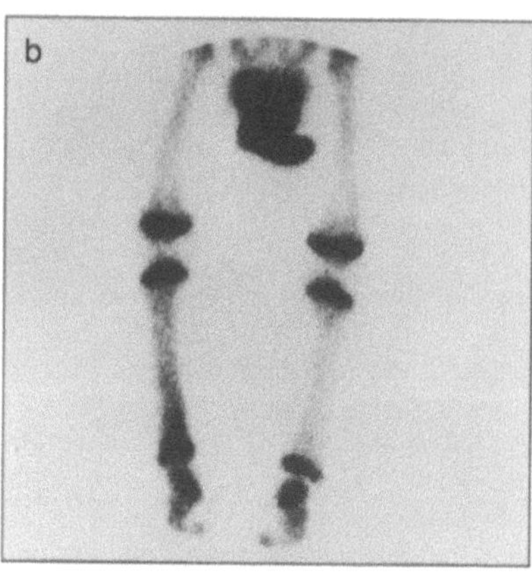

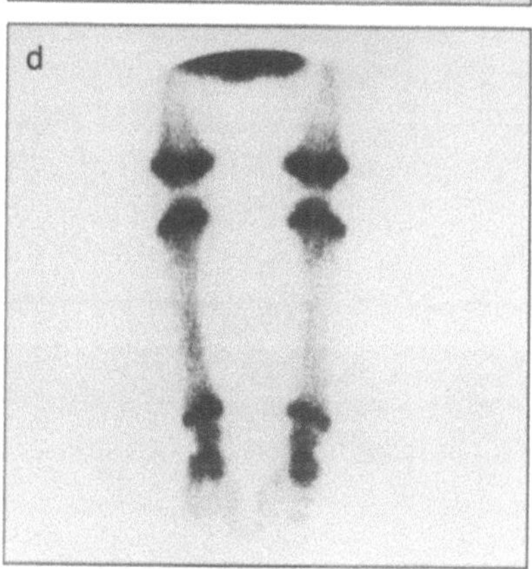

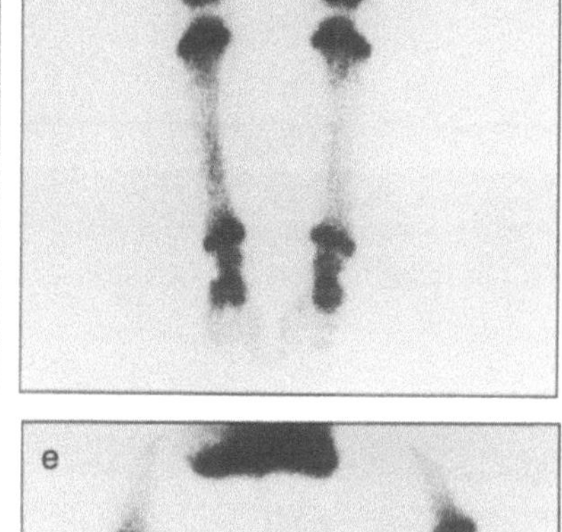

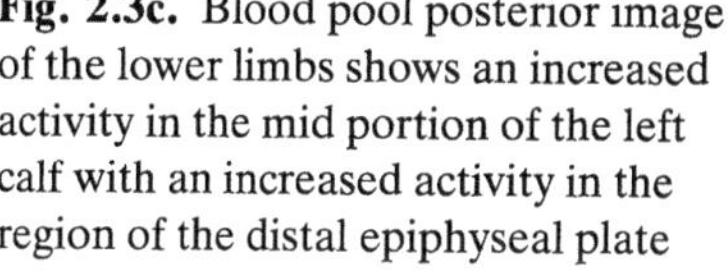

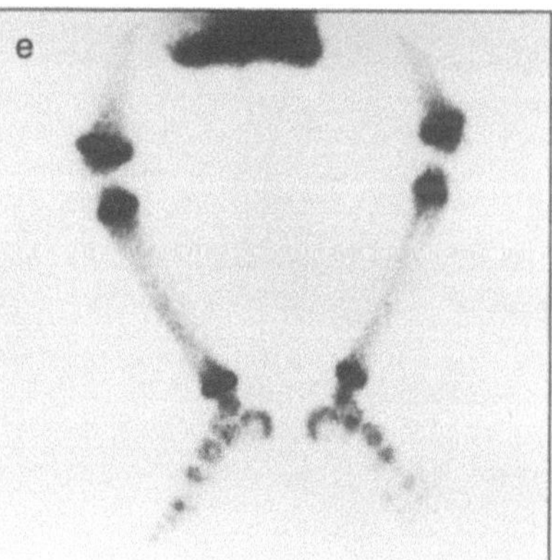

Case 2.3. A 15-month-old boy who was unwell and pyrexial with pain and hyperthermia of the left lower limb. Final diagnosis was osteomyelitis of the distal left tibia

Fig. 2.3a. Posterior blood pool image shows increased activity in the distal left tibia close to the epiphyseal plate

Fig. 2.3b. Posterior image of the lower limbs shows increased activity most marked in the distal left tibia extending from the epiphyseal plate proximally into the mid tibia.

A follow-up scan was undertaken 5 weeks later after antibiotic therapy

Fig. 2.3c. Blood pool posterior image of the lower limbs shows an increased activity in the mid portion of the left calf with an increased activity in the region of the distal epiphyseal plate

Fig. 2.3d. Posterior view of the lower limbs shows increased activity in the distal third of the left tibia extending down to the epiphyseal plate with increased activity in the metaphysis on the left to a lesser extend compared with the previous study

Fig. 2.3e. Lateral view of the lower limbs shows the increased activity in the left distal tibia

Technical Comment

Note poor positioning of the left foot in Fig. 2.3b with subsequent loss of clarity of the fibula. This was due to the infection which precluded adequate positioning.

Teaching Point

High-quality images of the epiphyseal plates are essential in order to diagnose pathology extending close to the epiphyseal plates which have normal increased activity.

Case 2.4. A 13-year-old boy with
acute pain around the right ankle.
Final diagnosis was osteomyelitis of
the distal right tibia

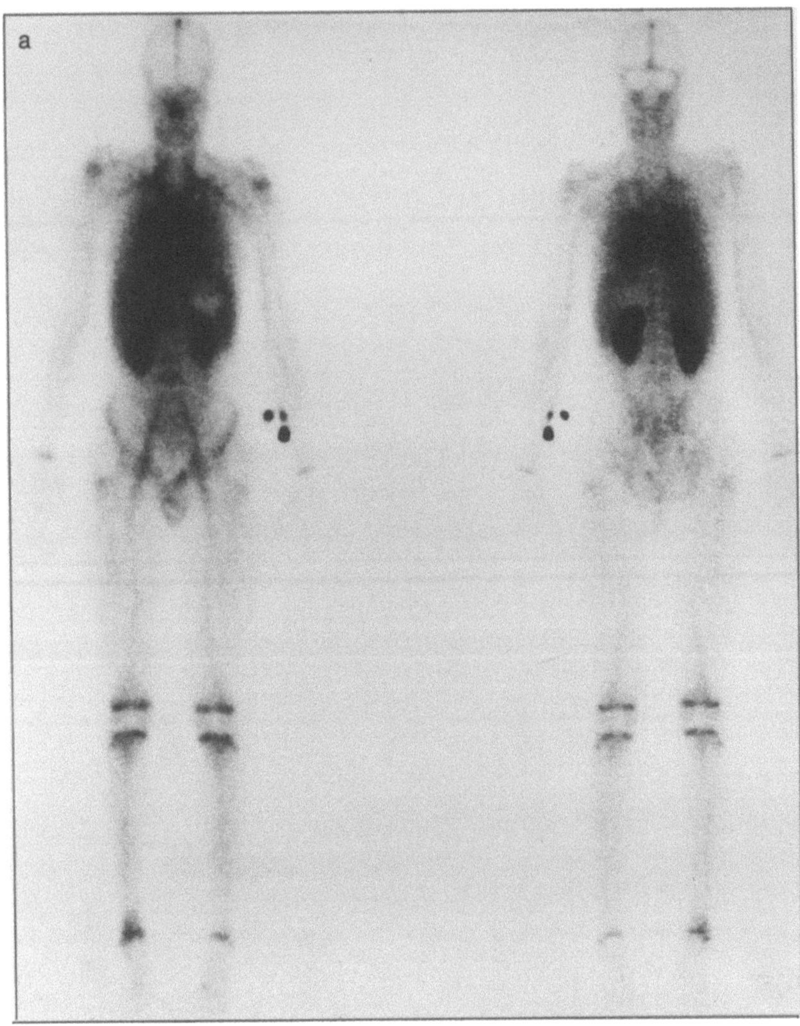

Fig. 2.4a. Whole body blood pool
images show increased activity in the
region of the distal right tibia

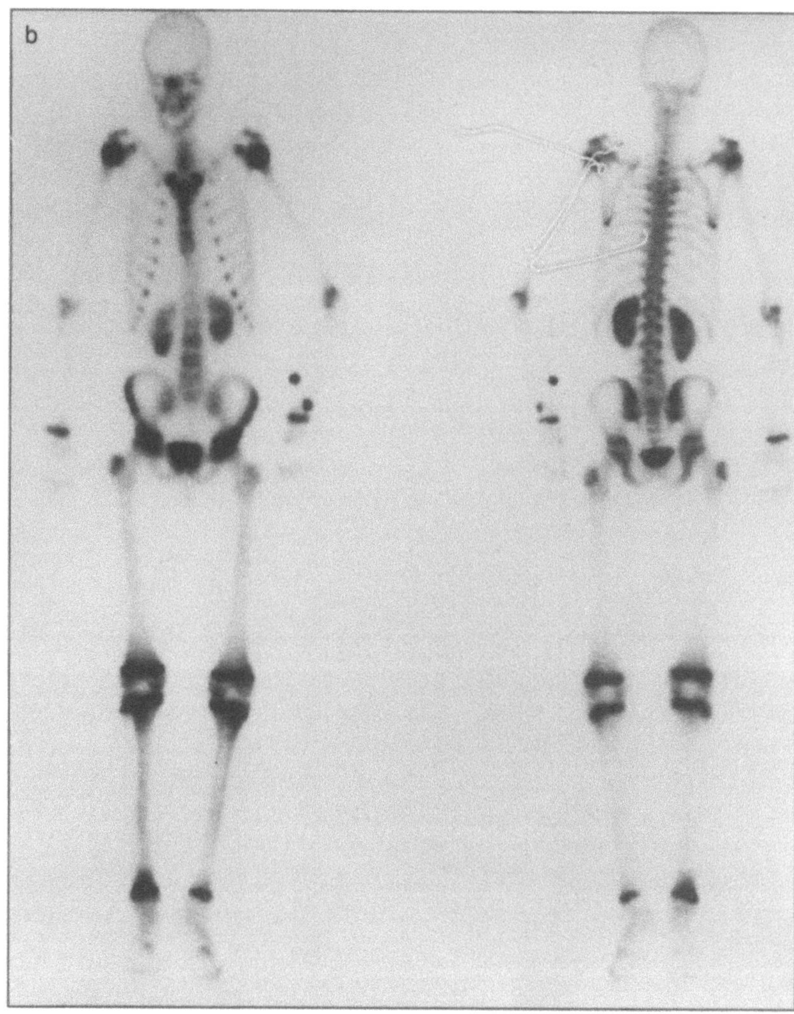

Fig. 2.4b. Whole body images show marked increased uptake of isotope from the distal right tibial epiphysis extending proximally into the diaphysis

Technical Comment

Note isotope in the left forearm, the site of the injection.

Teaching Point

1. Note increased activity in the kidneys. The reason for this is unclear but the child was septicaemic. There was no previous history of renal disease but the child was on intravenous antibiotics at the time of the scan. The significance of this latter situation is unclear.
2. Similiar appearances may be seen with benign bone cyst (see Case 4.18).

Case 2.5. A 20-year-old patient with pain in the right knee of short duration. The final diagnosis was osteomyelitis of the right tibia

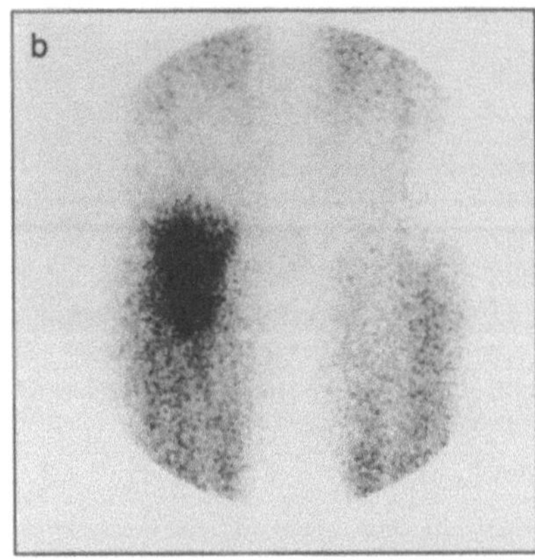

Fig. 2.5a. Blood flow anterior images of the knees show increased tracer to the right knee

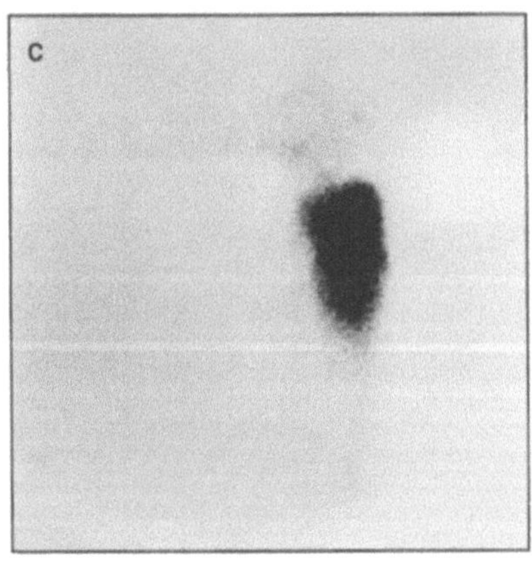

Fig. 2.5b. Blood pool anterior image of the knees shows marked increased activity in the region of the upper tibia as well as throughout the right calf

Fig. 2.5c. Lateral image of the right knee shows the increased activity extending up to and including the tibial plateau

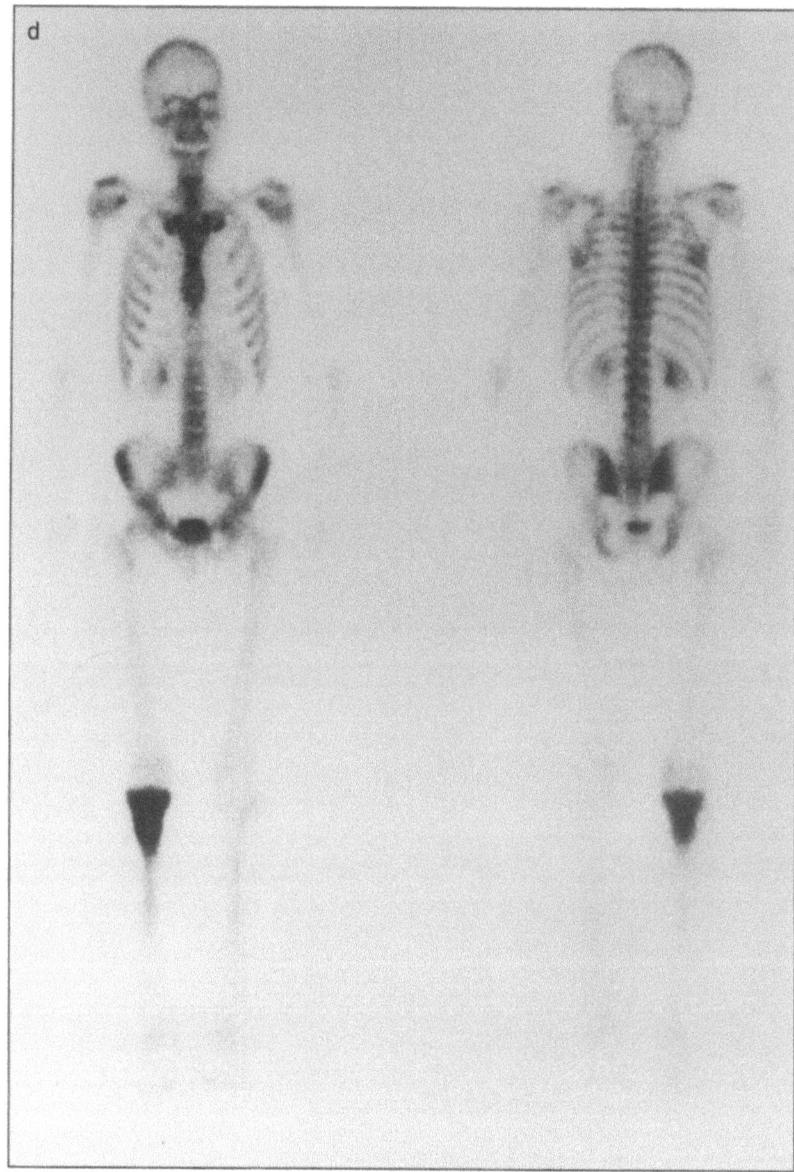

Fig. 2.5d. Whole body images show marked increased uptake of isotope throughout the upper portion of the right tibia extending into the diaphysis

Teaching Point

1. Infection usually spares the epiphyseal plate and is usually seen in the metaphysis/diaphysis of the long bones. In this case the increased activity extends to the bony confines of the joint surface. The epihyseal growth plate has fused. There was however no evidence of an arthritis.
2. Similar appearances may be seen in osteogenic sarcoma (see Case 4.49) or Langerhans' histiocytosis (see Case 4.85).

Case 2.6. A 12-year-old boy with pain for 5 days in the region of the left hip and groin. Final diagnosis was osteomyelitis of the upper femur

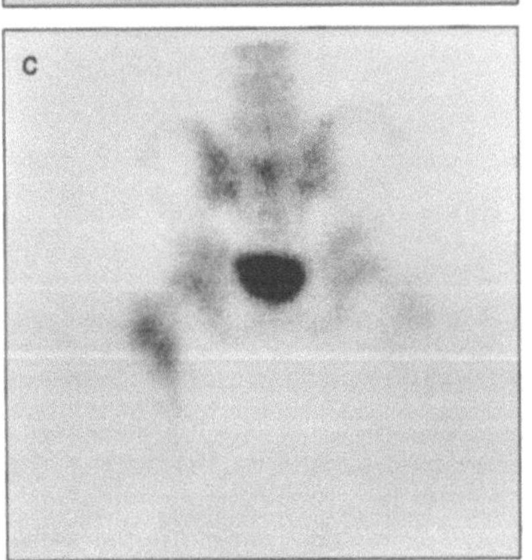

Fig. 2.6a. Whole body blood pool image posterior view shows increased uptake in the upper shaft of the left femur

Fig. 2.6b. Whole body posterior image shows increased activity extending from the greater trochanter into the shaft of the left femur

Fig. 2.6c. Posterior view of the pelvis shows increased uptake of isotope in the upper shaft of the left femur

Fig. 2.6d. Anterior view of the pelvis and upper femora shows increased activity in the left femoral shaft

Technical Comment

Note the small volume but high specific activity of isotope in the bladder due to the child refusing to drink. This detracts from the quality of the images and images with a greater total count should have been obtained.

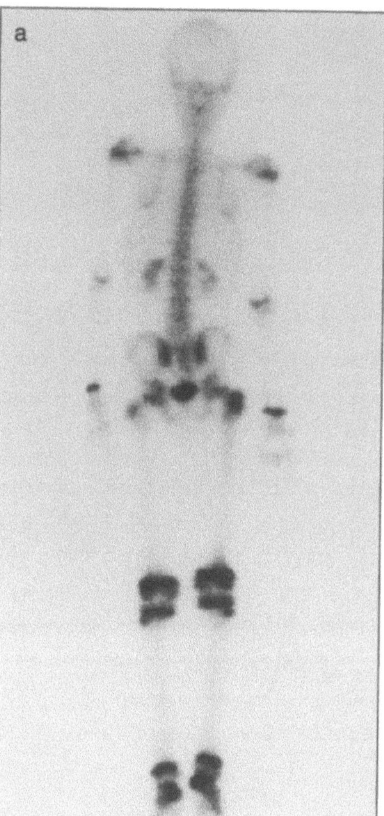

Case 2.7. An 11-year-old boy with fever and pain in the hip. Final diagnosis was osteomyelitis of the upper right femur

Fig. 2.7a. Whole body posterior image shows increased uptake of isotope in the region of the right greater trochanter

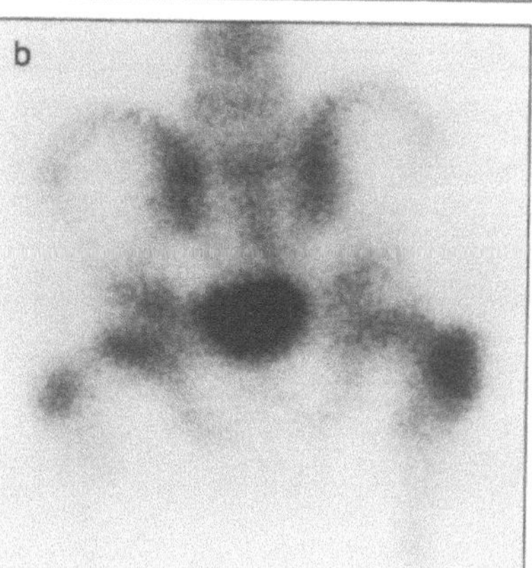

Fig. 2.7b. Posterior view of the pelvis shows increased activity in the region of the right greater trochanter extending into the neck of the femur proximally and into the shaft of the femur distally

Technical Comment

Note the loss of clarity of the epiphyseal plate of the femoral head in Fig. 2.7b due to the abnormal increased activity in the femoral neck.

Case 2.8. An 9-year-old boy with septicaemia. Final diagnosis was osteomyelitis of the distal right femur

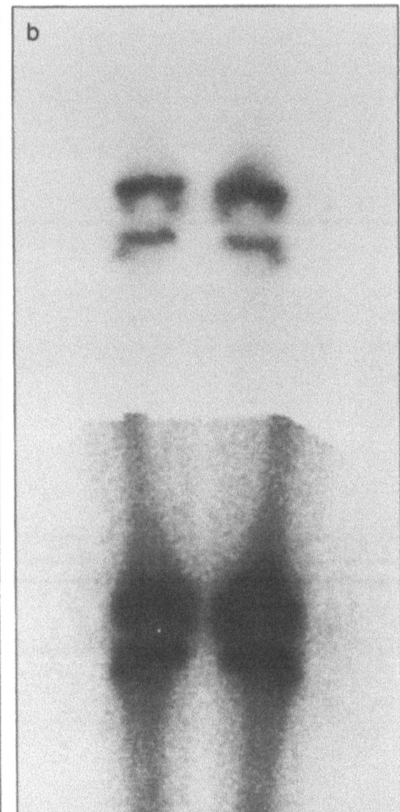

Fig. 2.8a. Whole body posterior view shows abnormal increased uptake of isotope in the distal right femur medially and in the right foot

Fig. 2.8b. Posterior view of the knees (two different exposures of the same image) shows increased uptake of isotope in the growth plate mainly medially with loss of clarity of the growth plate and abnormal activity extending up into the metaphysis on the right

Fig. 2.8c. Lateral view of the feet shows increased uptake of isotope in the epiphyseal areas of the distal tibia and fibula as well as in the distal small bones of the right foot

Fig. 2.8d. Plantar view of the feet shows abnormal increased uptake of isotope mainly in the right hind foot and ankle

Teaching Point
The infection was proved in the distal femur but no surgical exploration of the foot was undertaken. The presumption is that there was infection in the foot/ankle as well as in the distal femur since the child was septicaemic.

2.1.2 Upper Limbs
(3 Cases; Figs. 2.9–2.11)

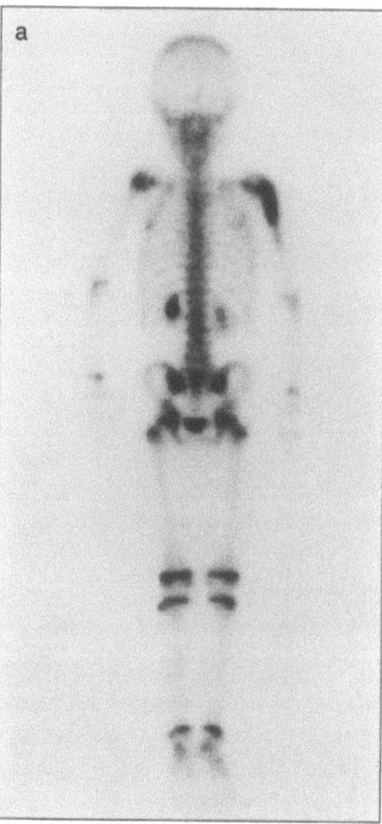

Case 2.9. A 6-year-old girl with pain for 1 month in the right shoulder, the child was pyrexial and had been treated with antibiotics. Final diagnosis was osteomyelitis of the upper right humerus

Fig. 2.9a. Whole body posterior scan shows marked increased uptake of isotope throughout the right humeral head extending into the mid shaft of the humerus

Fig. 2.9b. Posterior view of the shoulder girdle and upper limbs. The increased activity in the right humerus is seen to better advantage. There is a small area of decreased uptake of isotope in the upper right humerus surrounded by areas of intense increased uptake of isotope suggesting that the infection had been present for some time

Technical Comment

Retention of isotope is seen in both kidneys on Fig. 2.9a (child in a lying position). This improves but is still seen in the left kidney in Fig. 2.9b (sitting position).

Teaching Point

Focal areas of increased uptake of isotope on whole body scans should be followed up by static high resolution images of the abnormal areas.

Case 2.10. A 15-year-old girl with fever and pain in the right elbow. Final diagnosis was osteomyelitis of the proximal right ulna

Fig. 2.10a. Posterior image of the right arm shows intense increased uptake of isotope in the proximal right ulna extending into the diaphysis

Fig. 2.10b. Prone view of the right arm shows the extent of the increased uptake in the ulna

Fig. 2.10c. Prone view of the normal left arm

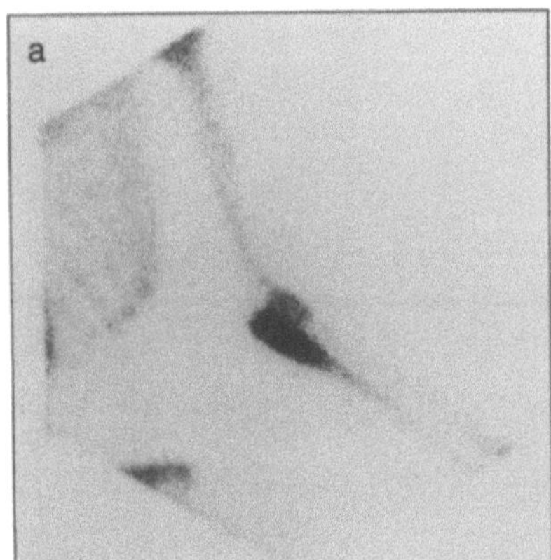

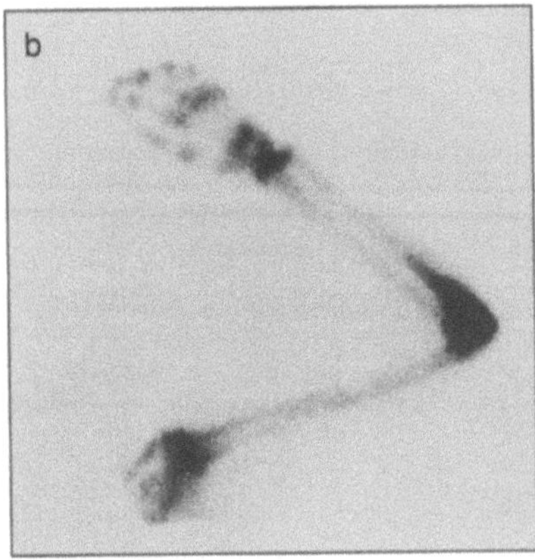

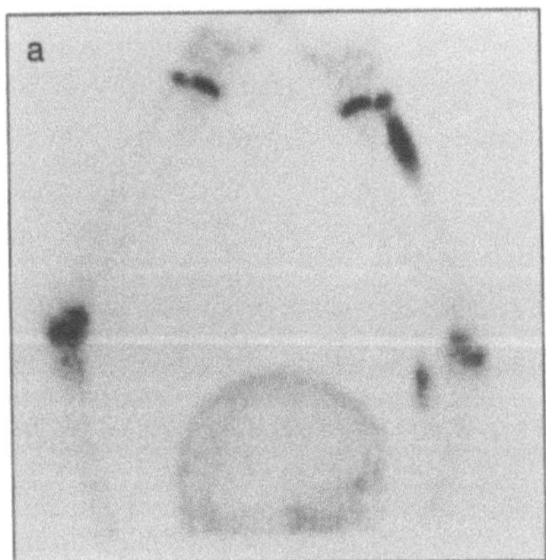

Case 2.11. A 13-year-old boy with pain in the forearm and backache as well as pyrexia. Final diagnosis was osteomyelitis of the distal right ulna, left elbow and right sacro-iliac joint

Fig. 2.11a. Posterior view of the upper limbs shows increased uptake of isotope in the distal third of the right ulna and the left elbow

Fig. 2.11b. Posterior view of the lower thorax, spine and pelvis shows increased uptake in the right sacro-iliac joint and in the left elbow

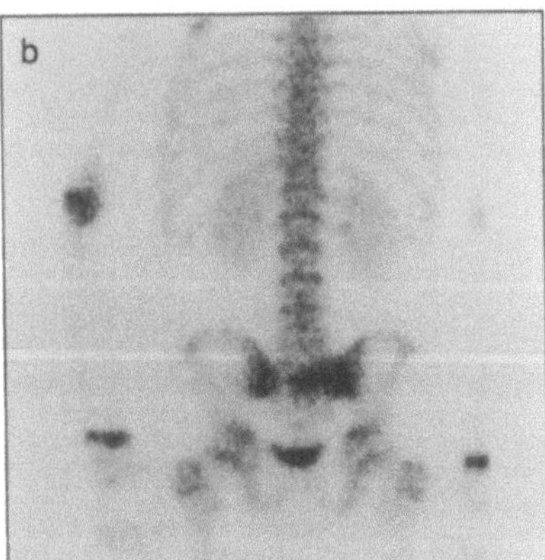

Technical Comment
1. Note extravasation of isotope in the right elbow, the site of the injection.
2. In Fig. 2.11b, the right ulna has been excluded from the field of view.

Teaching Point
Bacteriological proof of infection was only obtained from the right ulna. The abnormal uptake in the left elbow and right sacro-iliac joint was presumed to be due to infection.

2.2 Less Common Appearances

2.2.1 Normal Scan Going on to Abnormal
(1 Case; Fig. 2.12)

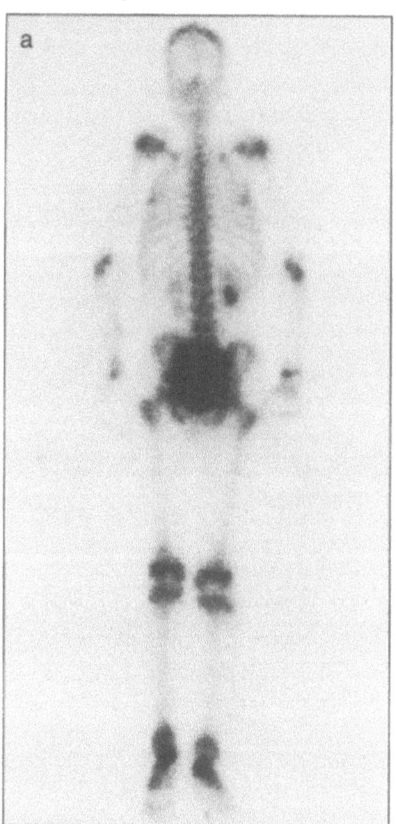

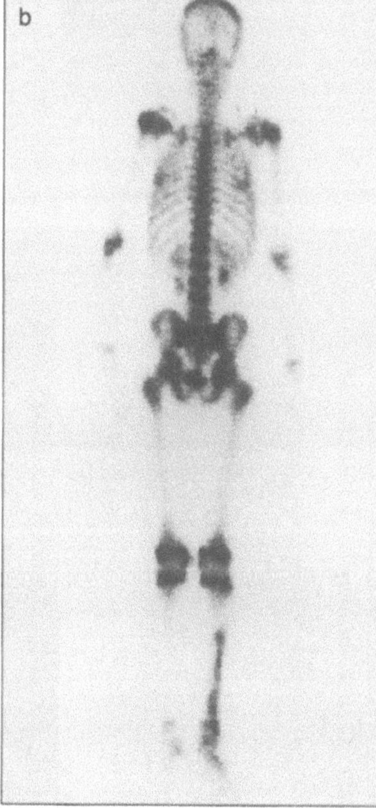

Case 2.12. A 10-year-old boy with septic osteomyelitis of the distal right tibia who presented unwell with a pyrexia and pain in the right lower limb

Fig. 2.12a. Whole body scan on the day of presentation (posterior view). The skeleton appears normal, especially the right tibia. Retention of isotope in the pelvis of the right kidney is seen. Note the full bladder since the child was too ill to co-operate

Fig. 2.12b. Whole body scan (posterior view) undertaken 3 days following the previous scan. There is extensive abnormal increased uptake of isotope in the right tibia extending from the ankle joint up to the junction of the upper and middle third of the right tibia. The retention of isotope in the pelvis of the right kidney on the earlier scan with the full bladder is not longer seen

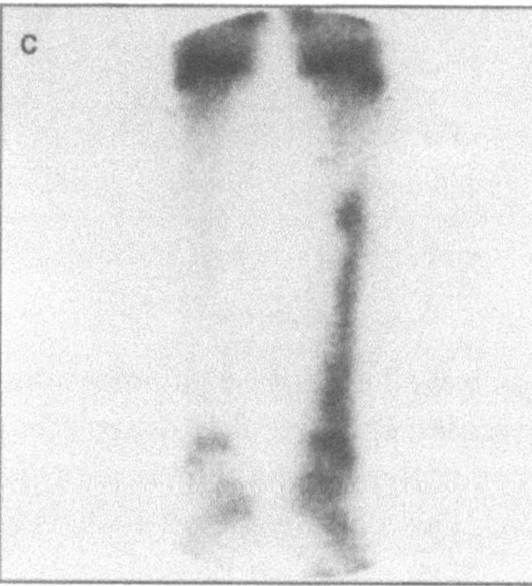

Fig. 2.12c. Posterior image of the lower limbs shows patchy abnormal increased uptake of tracer in the lower two thirds of the right tibia

Technical Comment

Note the positioning of the feet on both whole body scans with failure of internal rotation of the feet, thus making it difficult to separate the fibula from the tibia.

Teaching Point

A full bladder often prevents renal pelvic drainage (compare Fig. 2.12a to Fig. 2.12b).

2.2.2 Single Bone with Increased and Decreased Uptake

(4 Cases; Fig. 2.13–2.16)

Case 2.13. A 4-year-old boy with pain in the left leg, pyrexial and unwell. The child had osteomyelitis of the left tibia

Teaching Point

A cold lesion in acute osteomyelitis is a sign of acute vascular compression and represents an emergency.

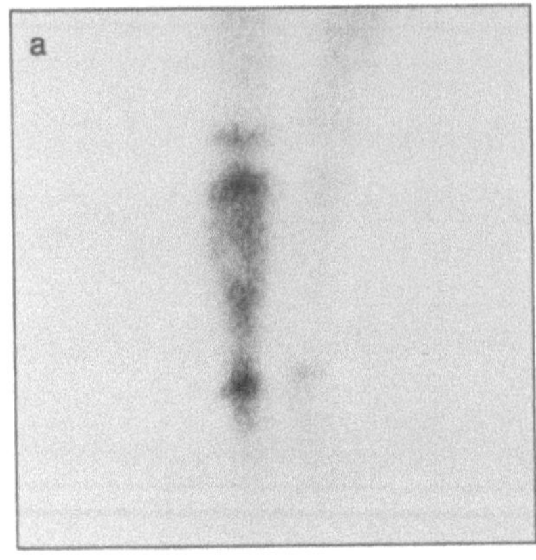

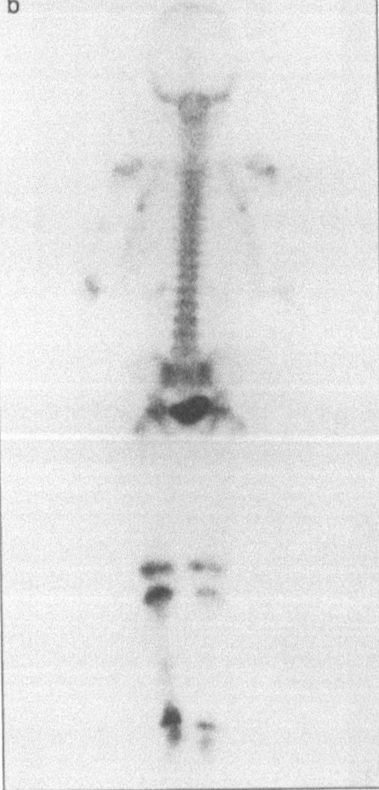

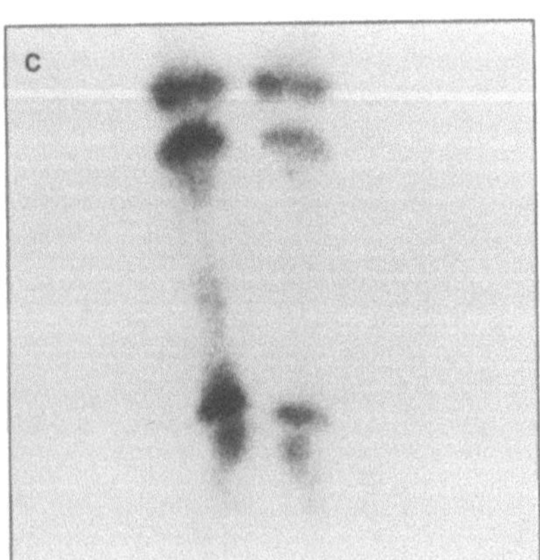

Fig. 2.13a. Posterior blood pool image of the lower limbs shows marked increased uptake of isotope in the left tibia with an area of focal decreased uptake in the mid portion of the calf. The soft tissue also shows an increased uptake of isotope as does the tibia

Fig. 2.13b. Whole body scan (posterior view). Abnormal increased uptake of isotope is noted at both ends of the left tibia

Fig. 2.13c. Posterior image of the lower limbs shows the indistinct distal epiphyseal plate with increased uptake in the proximal epiphyseal plate extending down into the shaft of the left tibia. The mid third of the tibia shows total absence of activity

Teaching Point

Combination of "hot" and "cold" lesions is well described but uncommon in acute osteomyelitis. The clearly demarcated epiphyseal growth plates of the normal right tibia show the importance of the gamma camera spot view in revealing the extent of the infection. This child went on to develop chronic osteomyelitis of the tibia.

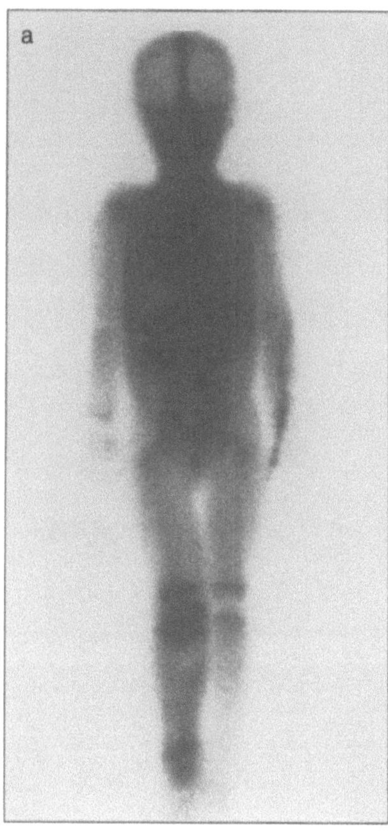
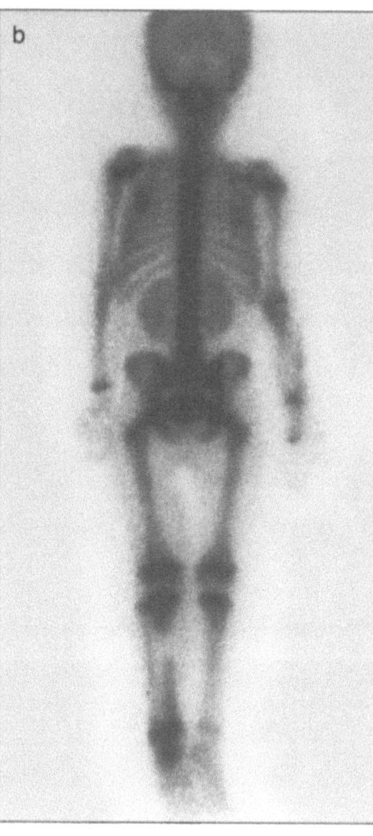

Case 2.14. A 3-year-old boy who had been treated for sepsis of the left leg. Final diagnosis was osteomyelitis of the left tibia

Fig. 2.14a. Blood pool whole body scan (posterior view) shows marked increased activity in the region of the upper left tibia as well as the soft tissues of the calf extending down to involve the ankle joint

Fig. 2.14b. Whole body scan (posterior view) shows abnormal increased uptake of isotope in the distal left tibial shaft with total absence of activity in the mid third of the tibia. Also note the marked increased activity around the ankle joint (no pus was found in the ankle joint)

Technical Comment

1. Note isotope in the veins of the right forearm, the site of the injection.
2. Note increased uptake of isotope in both kidneys; this is presumably related to the chronic sepsis and antibiotic therapy.

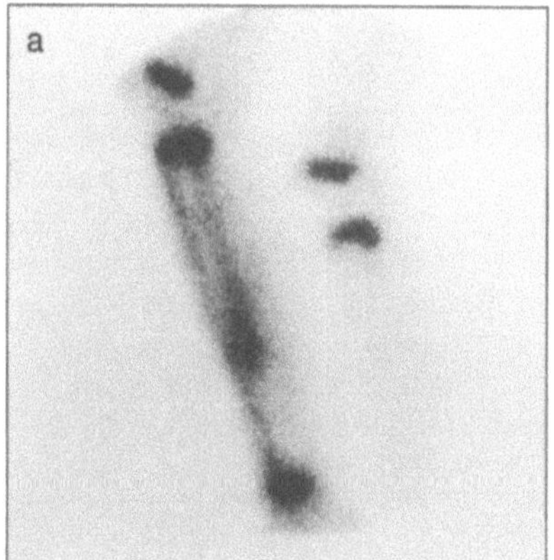
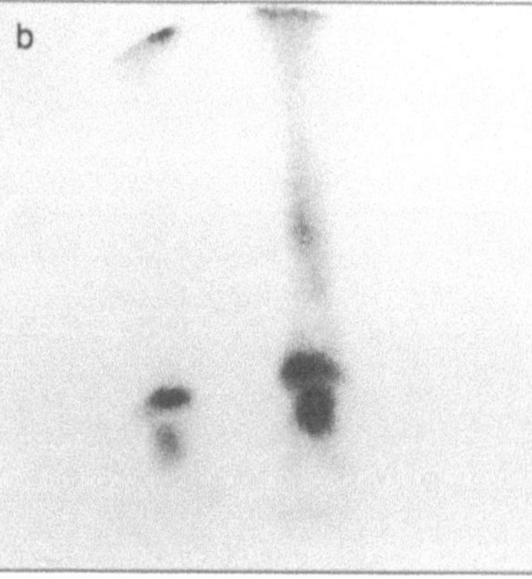

Case 2.15. A 4-year-old girl with a long history of being unwell due to osteomyelitis of the right tibia as well as septic arthritis of the right ankle

Fig. 2.15a. Lateral late blood pool image of the lower limbs shows focal increased uptake in the mid shaft of the right tibia with absent activity in the lower third of the tibia

Fig. 2.15b. Posterior image shows abnormal increased uptake of isotope in the mid portion of the right tibia with total absence of activity in the distal third. Increased uptake of isotope is noted around the ankle joint. (This is the same patient as in Case 3.20)

Case 2.16. A 12-year-old boy with acute osteomyelitis of the right upper femur

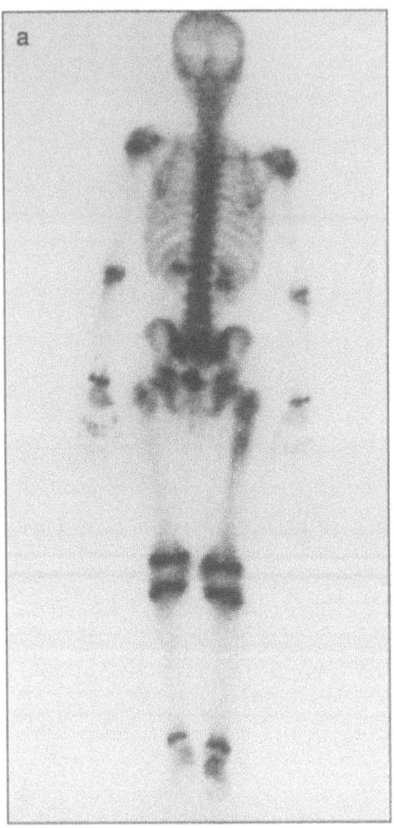

Fig. 2.16a. Whole body posterior view shows abnormal increased uptake of isotope in the right femur extending from the greater trochanter down into the mid shaft of the femur

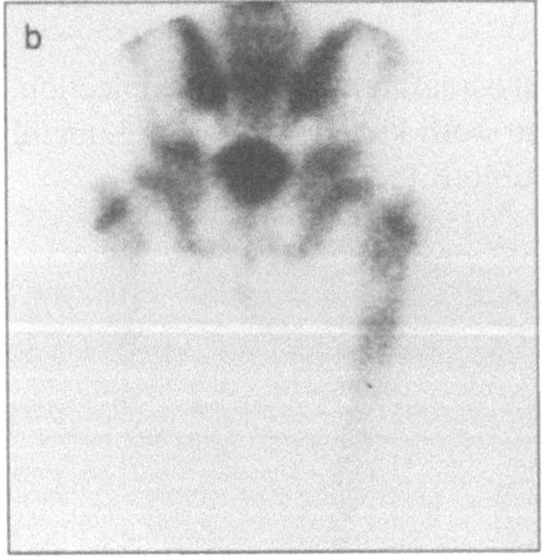

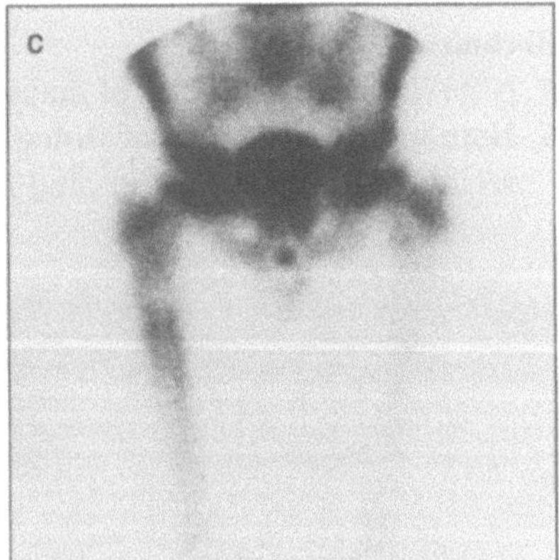

Fig. 2.16b. Posterior image of the pelvis and femora shows increased uptake of isotope in the shaft of the right femur with an area of total absence of activity in the upper third

Fig. 2.16c. Anterior image of the pelvis and upper femora shows increased activity in the upper third of the right femur. The area of decreased activity medially within the right femur is again noted

Technical Comment

Contamination with isotope is noted below the symphysis (Fig. 2.16c).

2.2.3 Acute Osteomyelitis, Cold Lesions Only
(3 Cases; Figs. 2.17–2.19)

Teaching Point

Cold lesions in acute osteomyelitis are a sign of acute vascular compression and represent an emergency.

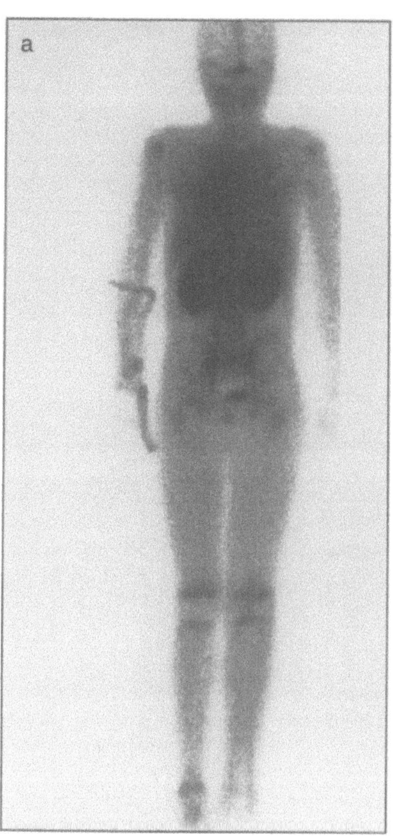

Case 2.17. A 10-year-old boy with cellulitis of the right leg and ankle on antibiotics who became toxic and pyrexial. Final diagnosis was osteomyelitis of the right tibia and ankle

Fig. 2.17a. Whole body blood pool image (posterior view) shows total absence of activity on the right in the distal tibial and fibula growth plates as well as in the foot

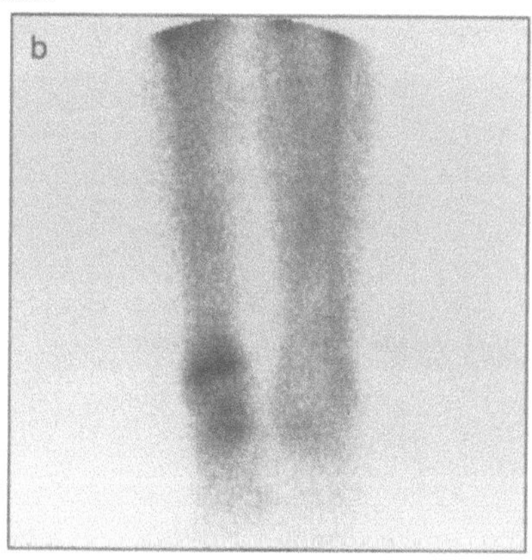

Fig. 2.17b. Blood pool posterior image of the ankles and feet shows decreased activity in the distal right tibia but, however, there is evidence of a swollen right calf. The right foot also shows decreased activity

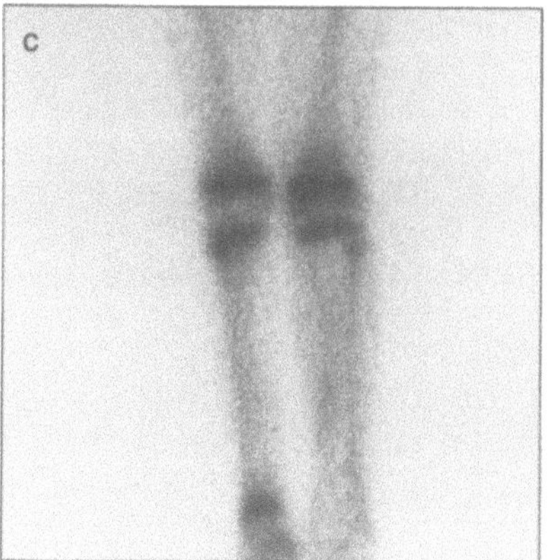

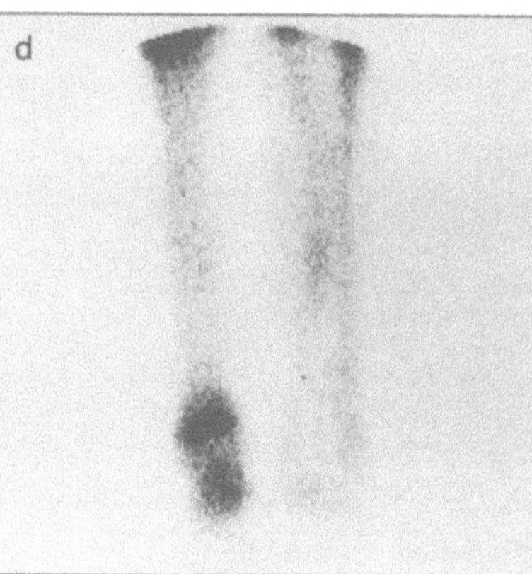

Fig. 2.17c,d. Posterior views of the lower limbs show virtually total absence of activity extending from the proximal right tibial diaphysis down to, and including, the distal tibial epiphyseal growth plate

Technical Comment

In Fig. 2.17a, isotope is noted in the intravenous infusion line overlying the left arm. The isotope was injected through this line.

Case 2.18. A 2-year-old boy with osteomyelitis of the distal left femur

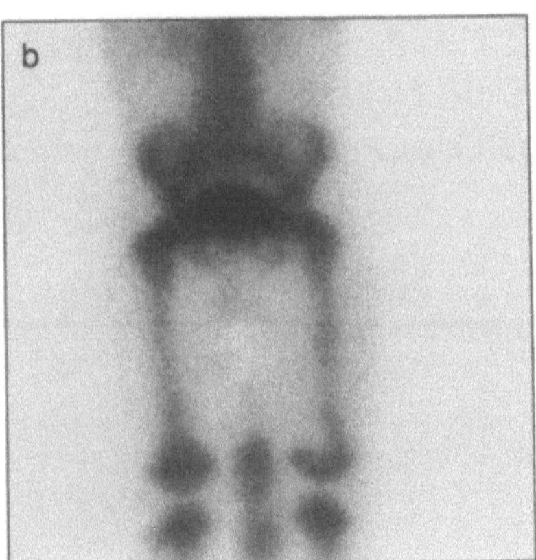

Fig. 2.18a,b. Anterior views of the pelvis, femora and knees with two different exposures show a cold lesion on the medial aspect of the left distal femoral shaft extending down to the epiphyseal plate

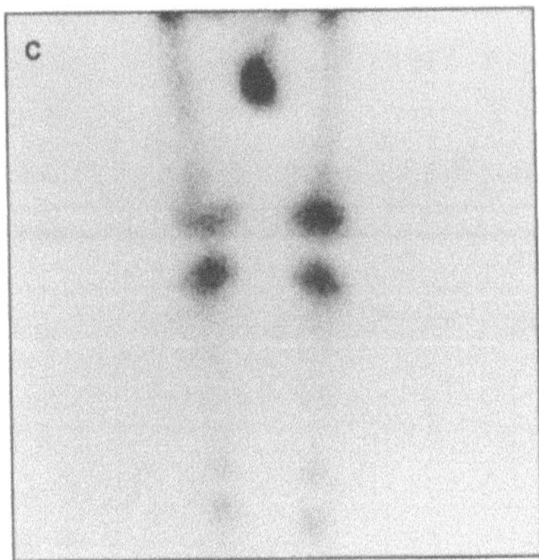

Fig. 2.18c. Posterior view of the knees shows decreased activity in the region of the distal left femoral growth plate with total absence of activity immediately above this growth plate medially

Technical Comment

Contamination of urine is noted. On Fig. 2.18a,b, this is between the knees, while on Fig. 2.18c it is within the nappy.

Teaching Point

Fig. 2.18a and Fig. 2.18b are from the same acquisition but with different exposure factors. If the bone scans are in digital format it is important to view the scan on the console where windowing of the images is possible.

Case 2.19 A 9-year-old boy with osteomyelitis of the right iliac bone

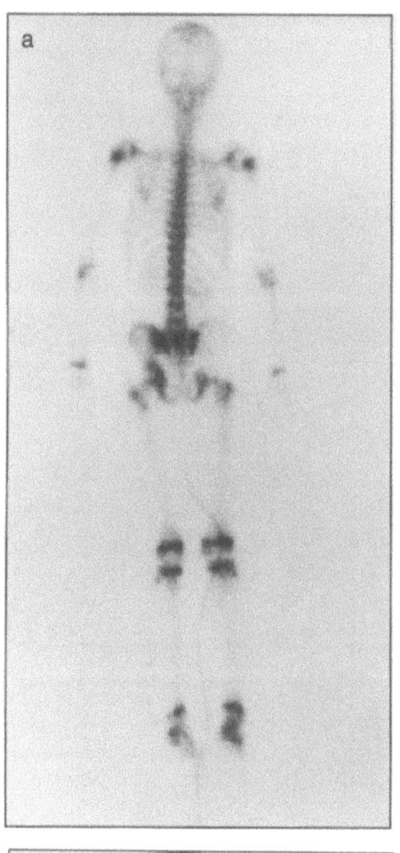

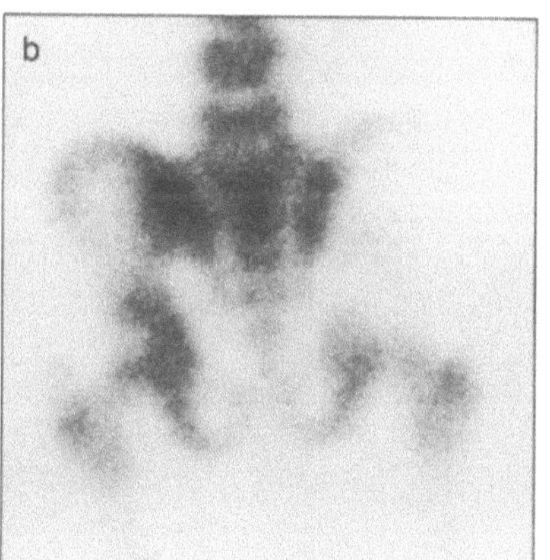

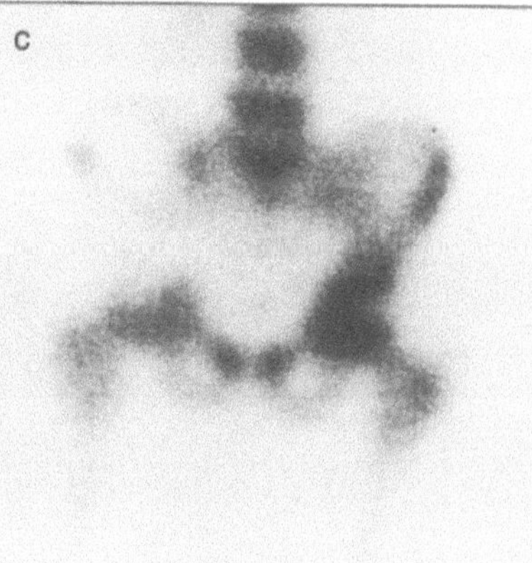

Fig. 2.19a. Posterior whole body scan. Total absence of activity is noted in the right iliac bone which includes the roof of the acetabulum

Fig. 2.19b. Posterior view of the pelvis. This shows absent activity extending from the right sacro-iliac joint involving the entire ilium

Fig. 2.19c. Anterior image of the pelvis. The absent activity in the right iliac bone is noted

Technical Comment

Note in Fig. 2.19a the activity in the catheter draining the bladder.

2.2.4 Acute Multifocal Osteomyelitis
(3 Cases; Figs. 2.20–2.22)

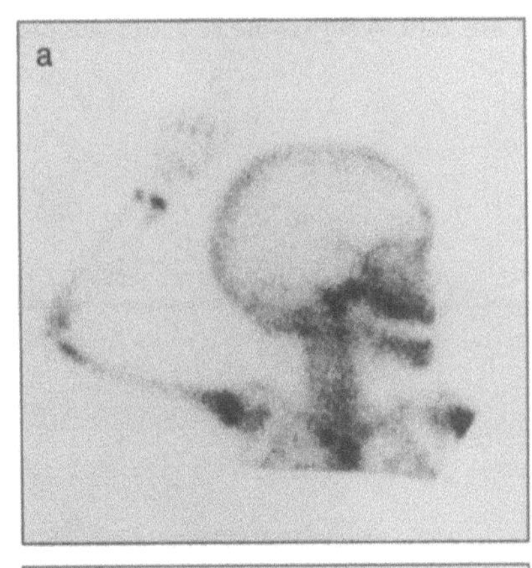

Case 2.20. A 4-year-old girl with multifocal osteomyelitis

Fig. 2.20a. Right lateral view of the skull and right arm is normal

Fig. 2.20b. Left lateral view of the skull and left arm shows focal abnormal increased uptake of isotope at two sites in the radius, one in the mid shaft and the other at the growth plate

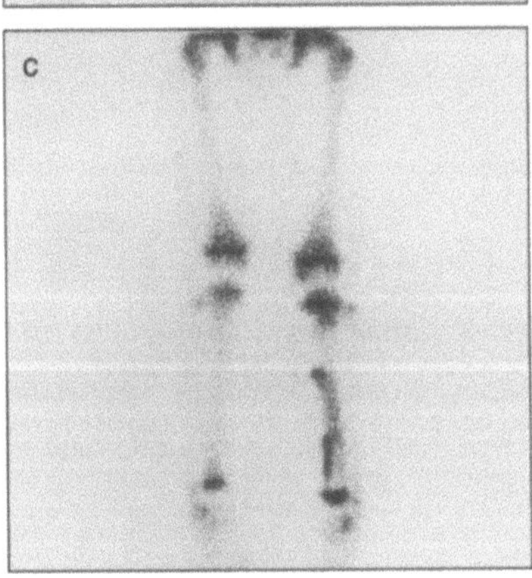

Fig. 2.20c. Posterior view of the knees shows abnormal increased uptake of isotope in the right tibia which involves the mid and distal thirds of the shaft with a skip area and involvement of the proximal tibia close to the epiphyseal plate as well

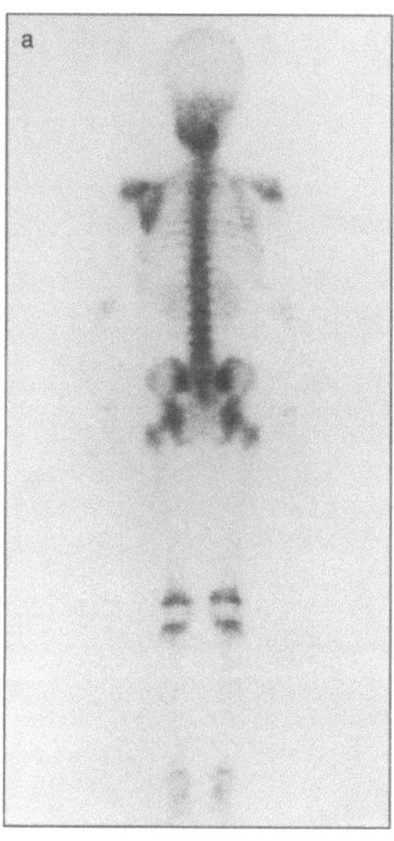

Case 2.21. A 9-year-old boy with multifocal osteomyelitis involving the mandible, left scapula and right sacro-iliac joint

Fig. 2.21a. Whole body posterior view shows abnormal increased uptake of isotope in the left scapula, mandible and right sacro-iliac joint

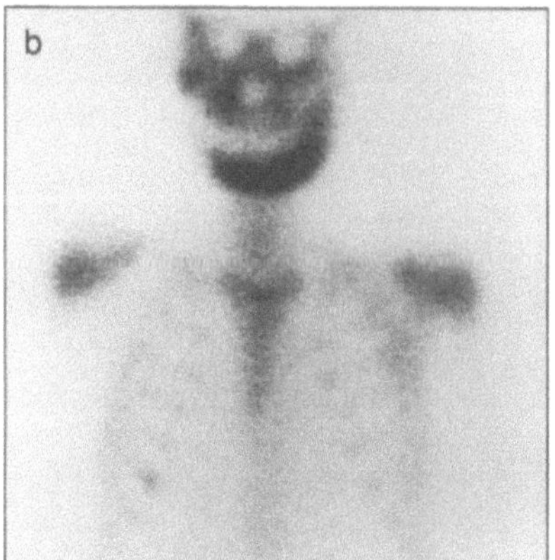

Fig. 2.21b. Anterior view of face, mandible and thorax shows the full extent of the involvement of the mandible with marked increased activity extending from the angle on the left through to the body of the mandible on the right. The angle of the mandible on the right shows total absence of activity

Fig. 2.21c. Posterior image of the thorax including the shoulders shows marked increased activity of the left scapula but also involvement of the humerus

Teaching Point

1. Bacteriological proof of the staphylococcal infection was obtained from the mandible only. The other sites of abnormal increased uptake of isotope were presumed to be infective in origin.
2. For other cases with infection of scapula, see Cases 2.36 and 2.37. Similar appearances of the mandible may be seen in Ewing's sarcoma (see Case 4.36). Similar appearances of the mandible may also be seen in germ cell tumours (see Case 4.73).

Case 2.22. **A 3-year-old girl with multifocal osteomyelitis of the left acetabulum, right sacro-iliac joint, right ileum, left fibula and right posterior rib. There are three bone studies within 3 months**

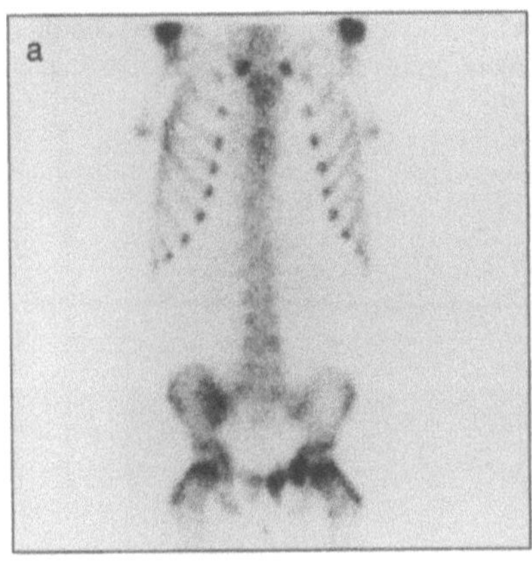 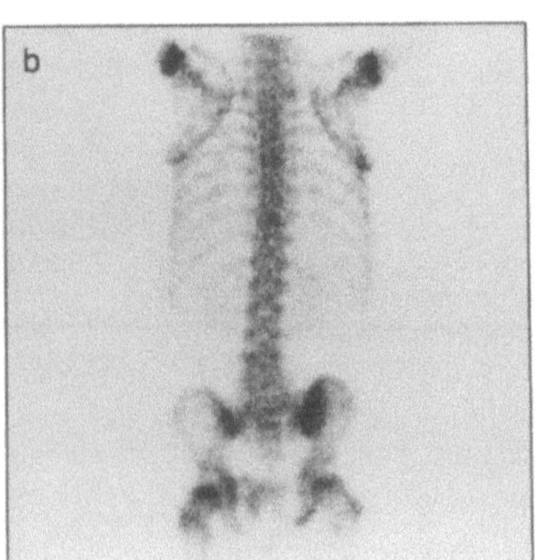

Fig. 2.22a. Anterior image of thorax and pelvis shows increased activity in the right sacro-iliac joint extending to involve most of the iliac bone. Abnormal increased uptake of isotope is also noted in the roof of the left acetabulum medially and left pubic bone

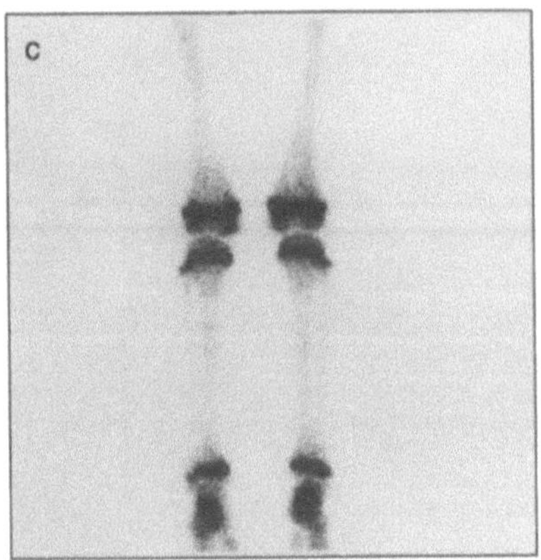

Fig. 2.22b. Posterior image of thorax, spine and pelvis. The abnormal right hemipelvis is again noted and the increased activity in the right sacro-iliac joint is better seen. The abnormal acetabular roof is better seen on the anterior view

Fig. 2.22c. Posterior view of the lower limbs; this is normal.

The child was treated with intensive antibiotics and a repeat scan was undertaken 2 months later

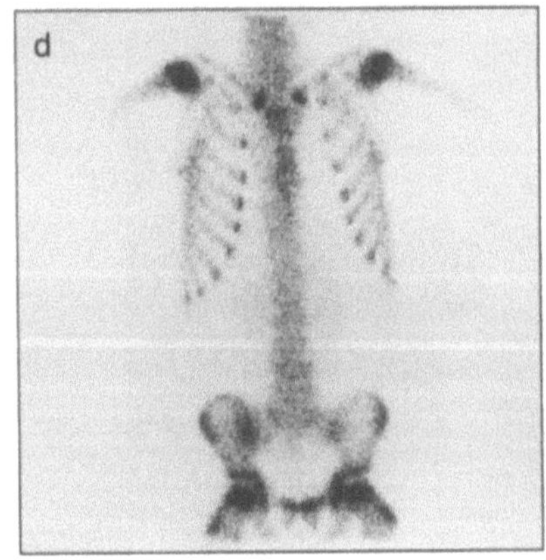 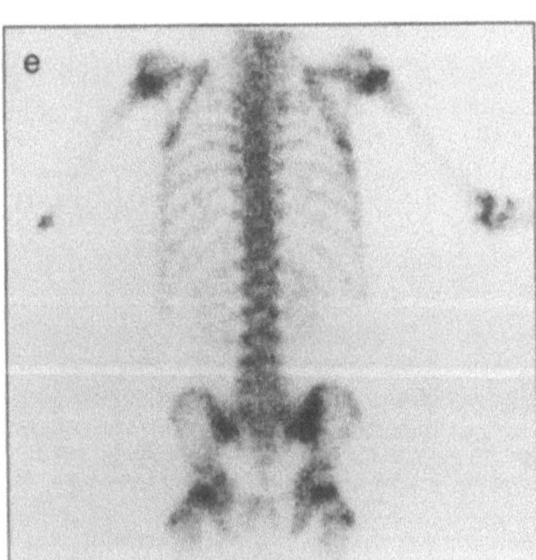

Fig. 2.22d. Anterior image of thorax and pelvis shows some improvement in the right hemipelvis and left acetabulum

Fig. 2.22e. Posterior image of thorax, spine and pelvis. No improvement in the right sacro-iliac joint is noted.

The antibiotics were stopped and the child returned symptomatic 1 month after the second scan. Therefore the third scan was undertaken

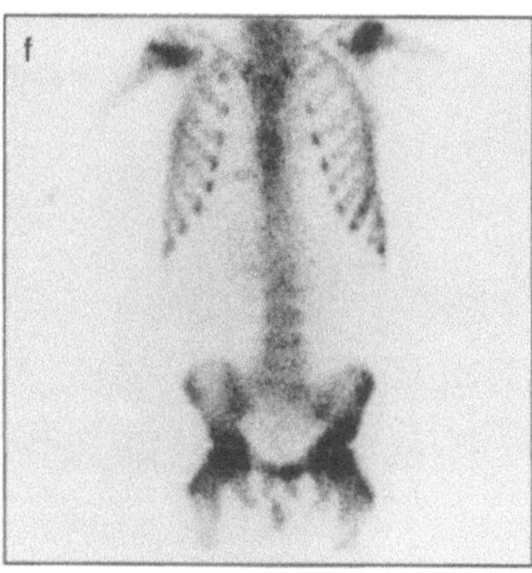

Fig. 2.22f. Anterior image of thorax and pelvis. The left hemipelvis is now abnormal with increased activity in the left iliac bone. Abnormal increased uptake of isotope is also noted in the anterior portion of the left seventh rib

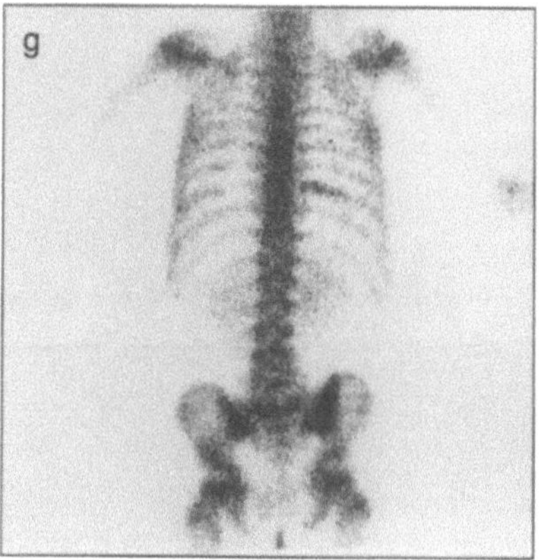

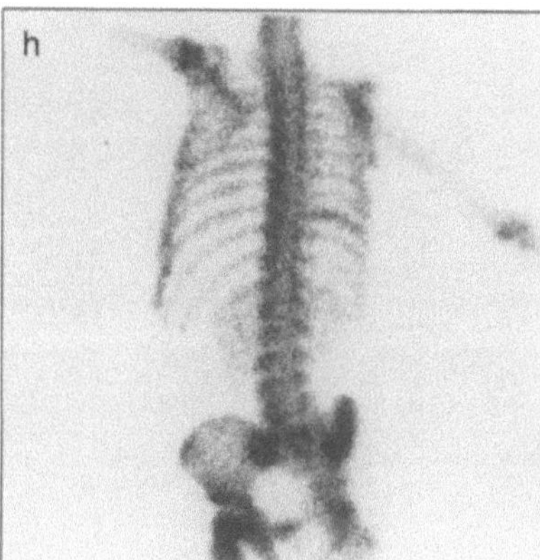

Fig. 2.22g. Posterior image of thorax, spine and pelvis shows abnormal increased uptake of isotope in the posterior aspect of the right ninth rib as well as in the right sacro-iliac joint

Fig. 2.22h. Left posterior oblique image of the thorax shows the abnormal increased uptake of isotope in the right ninth rib to better advantage; the abnormal left iliac bone is also clearly seen

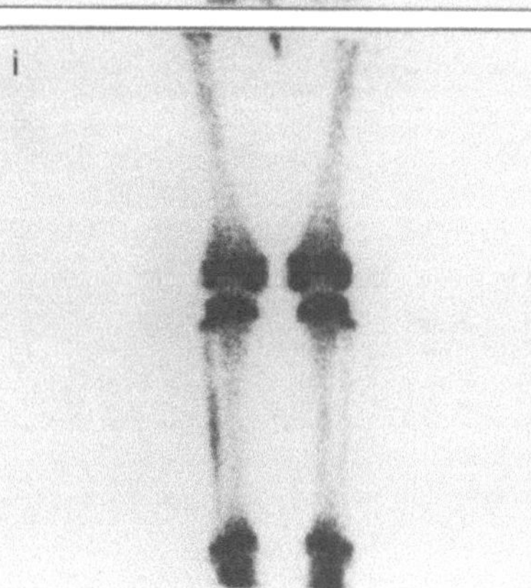

Fig. 2.22i. Posterior image of the lower limbs. Abnormal increased uptake of isotope is seen in the mid portion of the left fibula and, to a lesser extent, in the upper third of the shaft of this bone

Teaching Point

1. Routine follow-up bone scans are of little value, since residual abnormal uptake of isotope may represent the healing of the bone rather than continued infection. If, for clinical reasons, a repeat bone scan is untertaken and a new area of abnormal uptake is seen, then there is a high probability that this represents another focus of infection.
2. For infection of ribs, also see Cases 2.30, 2.34 and 2.35. Similar appearances of the ribs may be seen in children with Ewing's sarcoma (see Cases 4.28 and 4.30) and sickle cell disease (see Cases 6.16–6.18).

2.2.5 Chronic Infection, Not Tuberculosis

(5 Cases; Figs. 2.23–2.27)

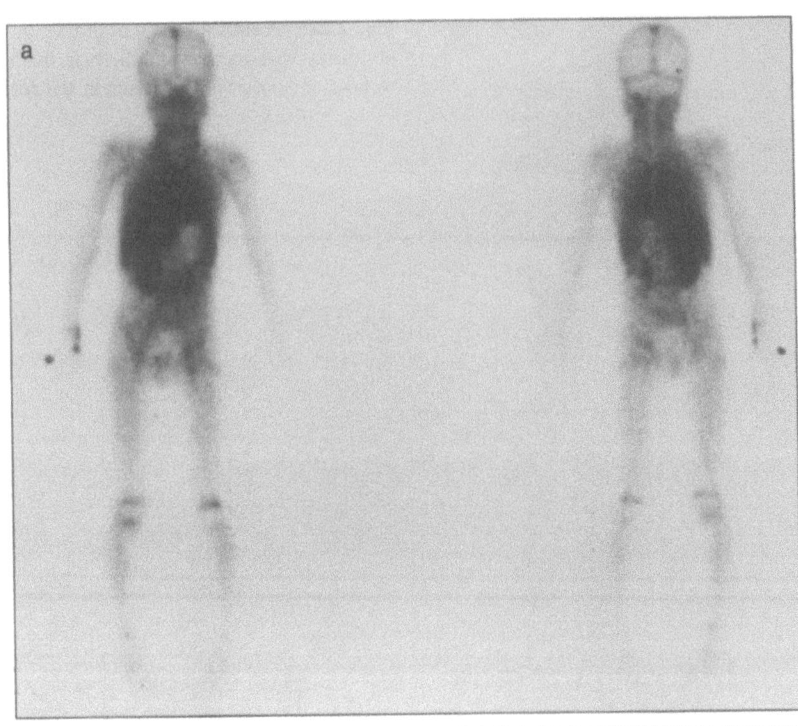

Case 2.23. A 15-year-old boy with chronic multifocal osteomyelitis

Fig. 2.23a. Blood pool images of the whole body show increased activity in both kidneys. Increased activity in the right ankle and knee and right hand is also noted

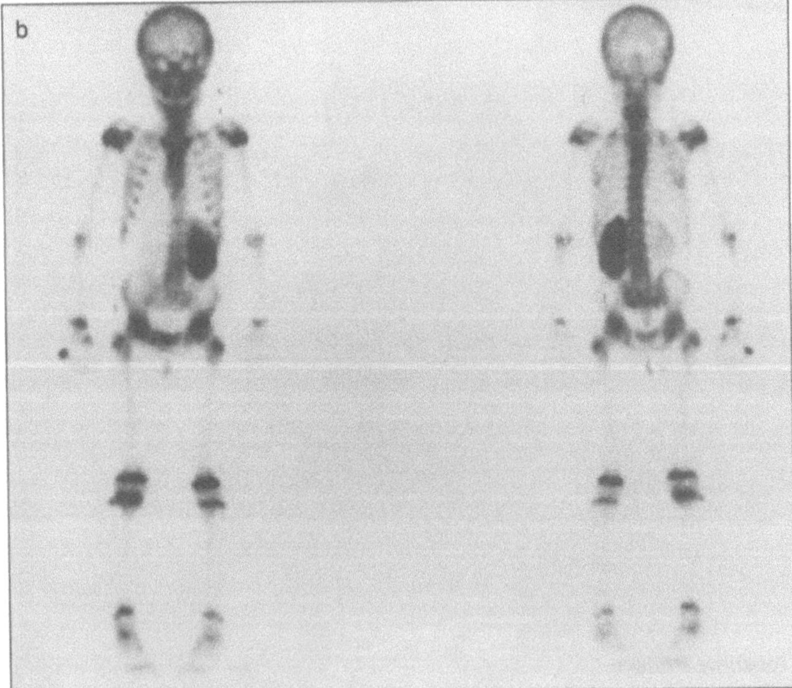

Fig. 2.23b. Whole body images. There is abnormal uptake of isotope in the cervical spine, right ankle, right knee as well as in the distal right radius. Intense increased uptake of isotope in the enlarged region of the left kidney is noted.

Technical Comment

There is extravasation of isotope at the right hand on all images.

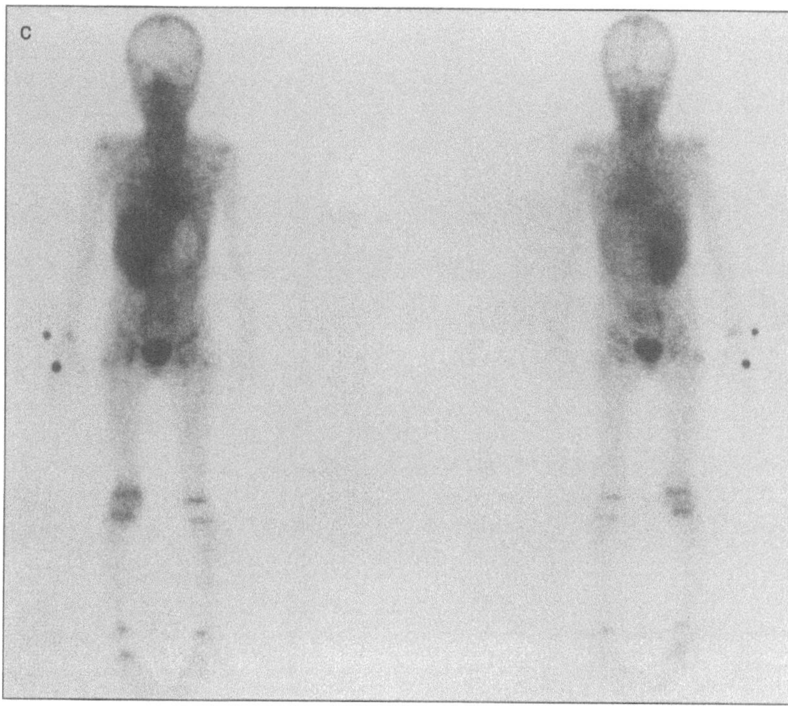

A follow-up study was undertaken 6 months later

Fig. 2.23c. Whole body blood pool images still show abnormal increased uptake of isotope in the os sacrum, the right knee, right ankle and right wrist. Only the right kidney is visualised

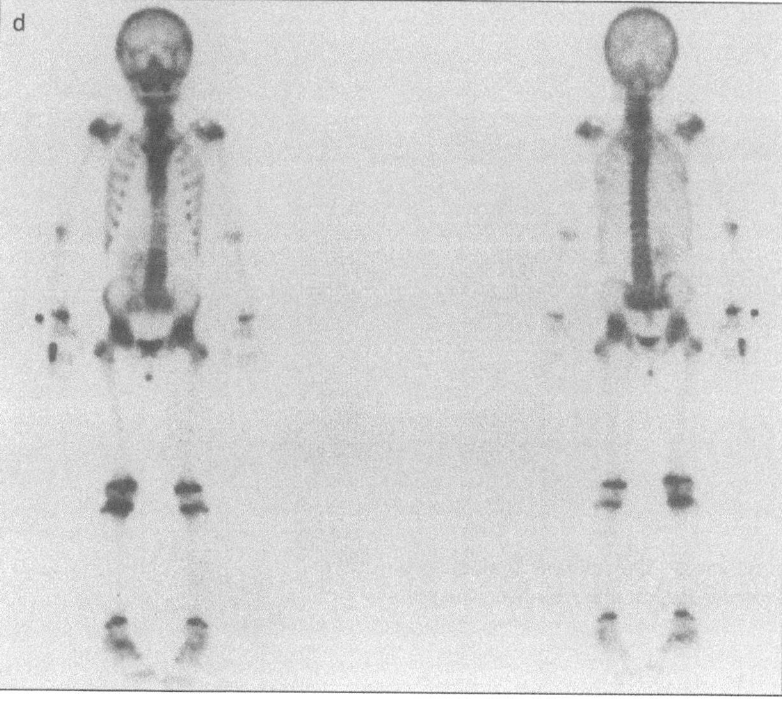

Fig. 2.23d. Whole body scans show abnormal increased uptake of isotope in the os sacrum, on both sides of the right knee joint as well as in the distal right radius. The abnormal uptake in the cervical spine is again noted as is the increased uptake of isotope in the proximal small bones of the right foot

Teaching Point

This child was found to have obstruction of the pelviureteric junction of the left kidney and underwent nephrectomy between the two bone scans. Infection of the obstructed kidney was found at the time of nephrectomy and the osteomyelitis was presumed to be secondary to the renal infection in the obstructed kidney.

Case 2.24. A 6-year-old boy with chronic osteomyelitis due to histoplasmosis

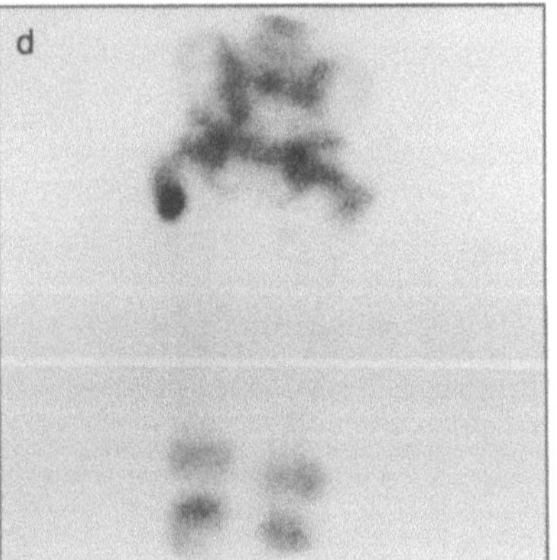

Fig. 2.24a. Blood pool posterior whole body image shows abnormal increased uptake of isotope in the upper femora as well as in the ankle joints

Fig. 2.24b. Posterior whole body scan shows abnormal hip joints. The proximal left femur shows generalised increased uptake of isotope with a focal area of intense increased uptake in the upper third of the femur. There is increased uptake of isotope in the left scapula, the entire left tibia and the distal right tibia

Fig. 2.24c. Posterior image of the thorax shows the abnormal increased activity in the left scapula

Fig. 2.24d. Posterior image of the pelvis shows both hip joints to be abnormal as well as the focal abnormal uptake of isotope in the proximal left femoral shaft

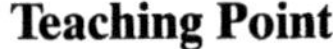

Fig. 2.24e. Anterior image of the knees and ankles. The multiple focal areas of abnormal increased uptake of isotope are noted in the left tibia; the distal and proximal right tibia is also abnormal

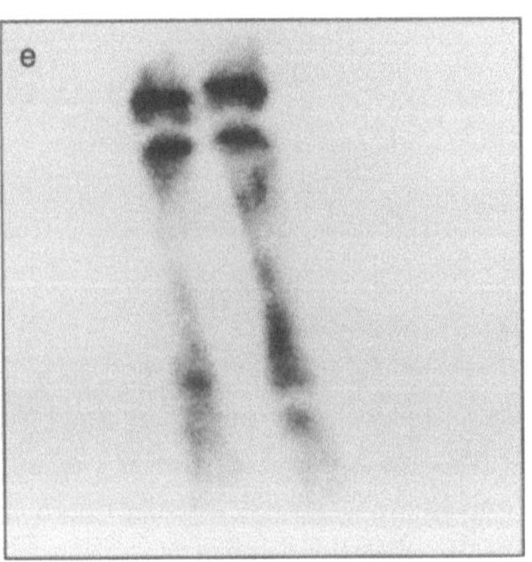

Teaching Point

The clarity of the growth plates around the hips and the ankles have been lost bilaterally. Only when recording the age of the child and the appearance of the epiphyseal plates around the knee does one realise the extent of involvement at the other joints.

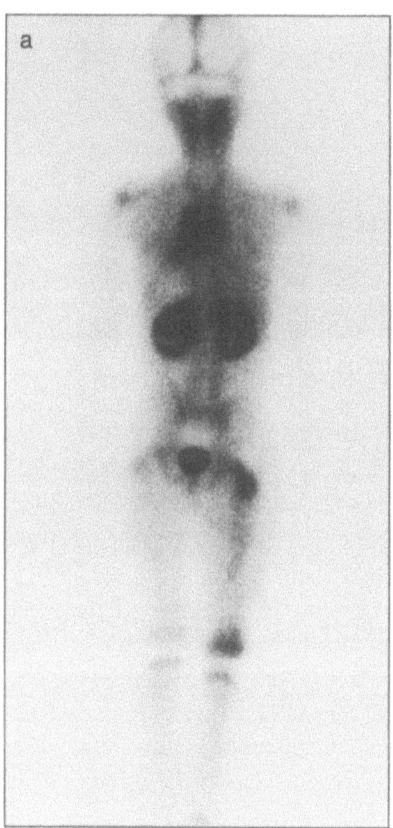

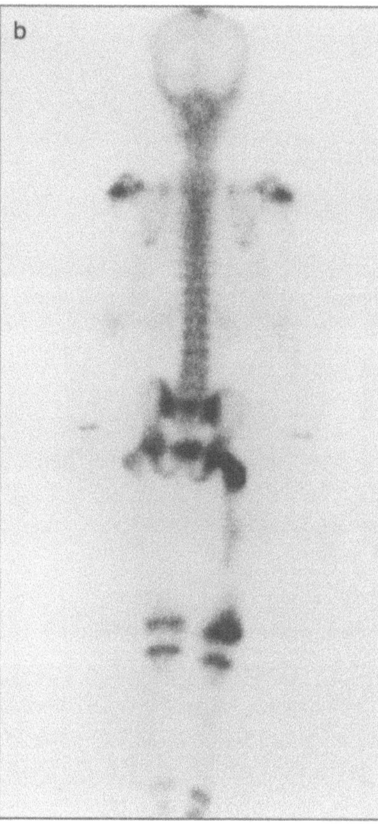

Case 2.25. A 5-year-old boy with infection of the right femur drained on two previous occasions

Fig. 2.25a. Blood pool posterior whole body scan shows abnormal increased uptake of isotope in both the proximal and distal ends of the right femur as well as in the mid shaft. The activity in the mid portion of the right thigh involves more than simply the femur

Fig. 2.25b. Whole body posterior image shows abnormal increased uptake of isotope at the proximal and distal ends of the right femur extending into the femoral shaft. The mid portion of the femur shows generalised increased activity on its medial aspect with total absence of activity on the lateral aspect

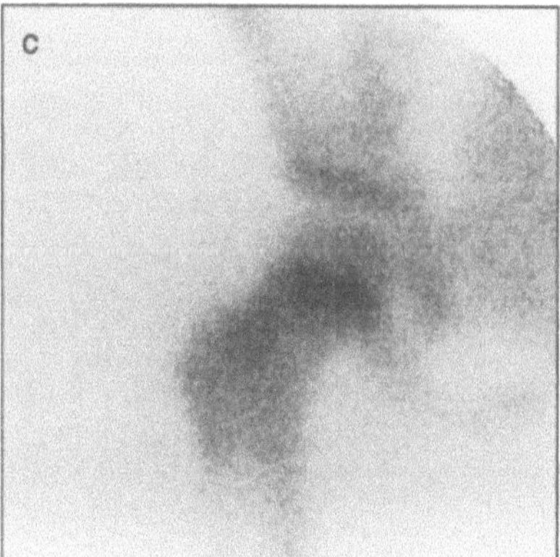

Fig. 2.25c. Pin hole view of the right hip shows that the femoral capital epiphysis appears normal and that the osteomyelitis has not threatened the femoral head

Teaching Point

The clinical question as to the viability of the right femoral capital epiphysis could not be answered on the whole body scan. The pin hole image shows the normal femoral capital epiphysis, thus proving the viability of the femoral head.

**Case 2.26. A 6-year-old child with
well established chronic osteomyelitis
of the lower right femur**

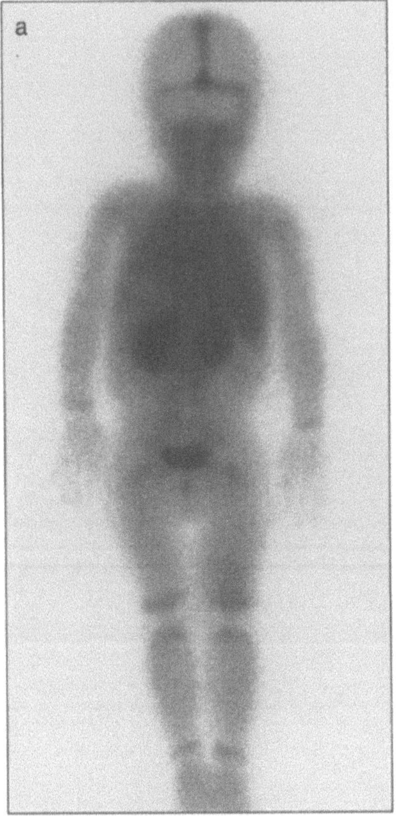

Fig. 2.26a. Blood pool whole body
image shows abnormal increased
activity in the lower third of the right
femur

Fig. 2.26b. Whole body scan posterior view shows abnormal increased
uptake in the distal right femur extending to the epiphyseal plate

Fig. 2.26c. Posterior image of the
knees shows the increased uptake of
isotope in the distal right femoral
shaft extending down to the epiphyseal plate which shows increased
uptake. There is also increased uptake
of isotope in the right distal and proximal tibial epiphyseal plates

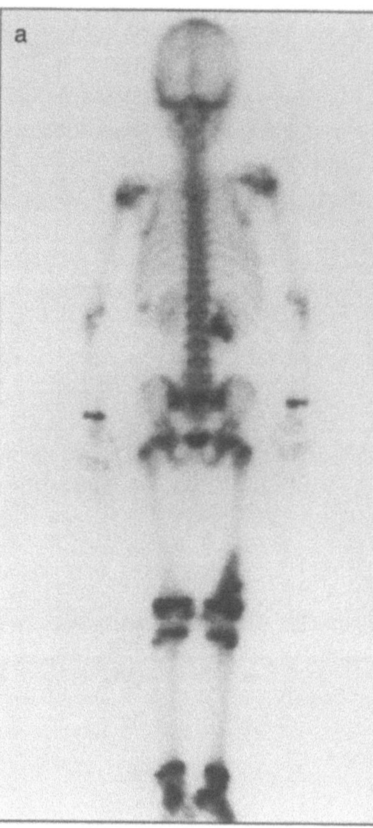

Case 2.27. Following trauma, a 5-year-old boy had pain in his right knee which was proven to be subacute osteomyelitis following the closed trauma

Fig. 2.27a. Posterior whole body scan shows abnormal increased uptake in the distal right femur which extends to involve the epiphyseal plate and also the lateral femoral condyle. The activity in the distal femoral shaft is patchy with a focal area of intense increased uptake of isotope compatible with subacute osteomyelitis. Note increased uptake of isotope in the region of the right kidney

Technical Comment

The cause for the abnormal accumulation of isotope in the region of the right kidney was not ascertained. This could have been related to the previous trauma or underlying pathology in the right kidney.

2.2.6 Tuberculosis
(4 Cases; Figs. 2.28–2.31)

Case 2.28. A 3-year-old boy being treated for pulmonary tuberculosis with a tender swelling over the right clavicle

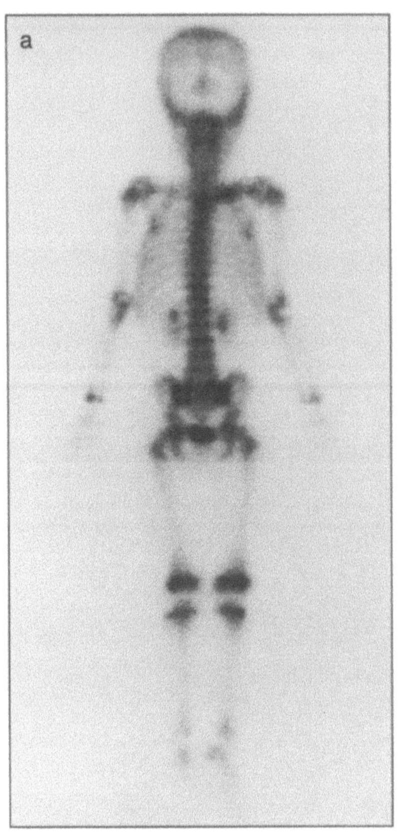
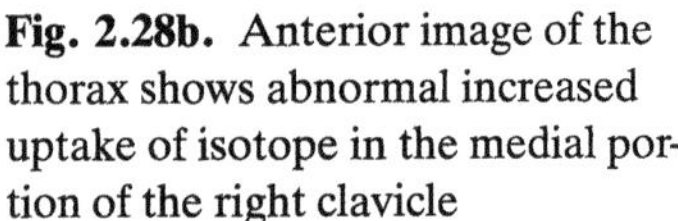

Fig. 2.28a. Whole body scan posterior view shows increased uptake of isotope in the region of the right clavicle; this is not easily seen on this posterior view

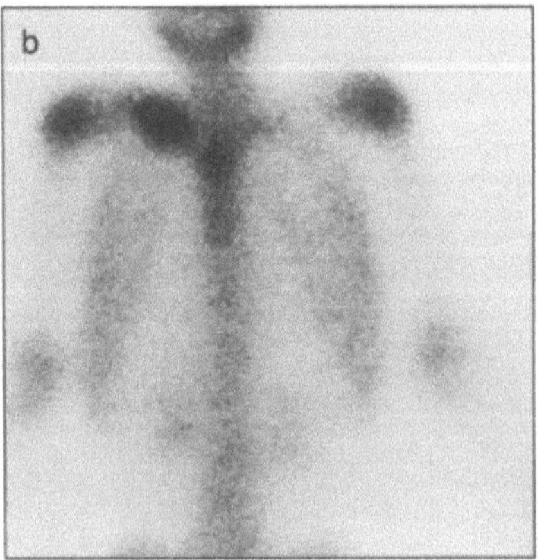
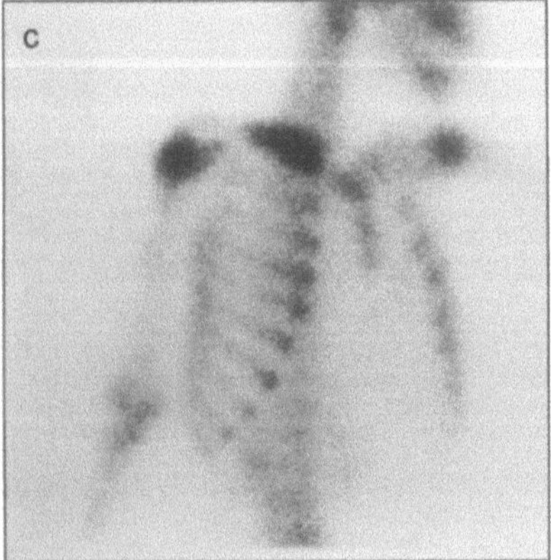

Fig. 2.28b. Anterior image of the thorax shows abnormal increased uptake of isotope in the medial portion of the right clavicle

Fig. 2.28c. Right anterior oblique image shows the abnormal increased uptake of isotope in the clavicle to better advantage

Technical Comment
Figure 2.28b (the anterior view) is of poor quality due to movement artefact.

Teaching Point
Similar appearance may be seen with Ewing's sarcoma (see Case 4.36) or trauma (see Case 5.3).

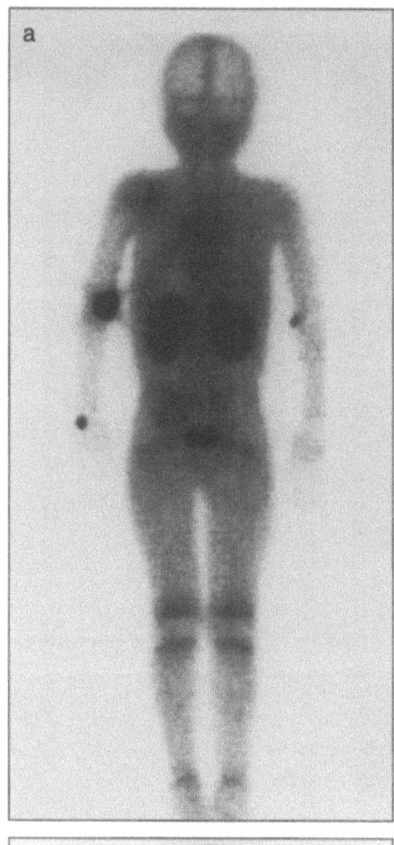

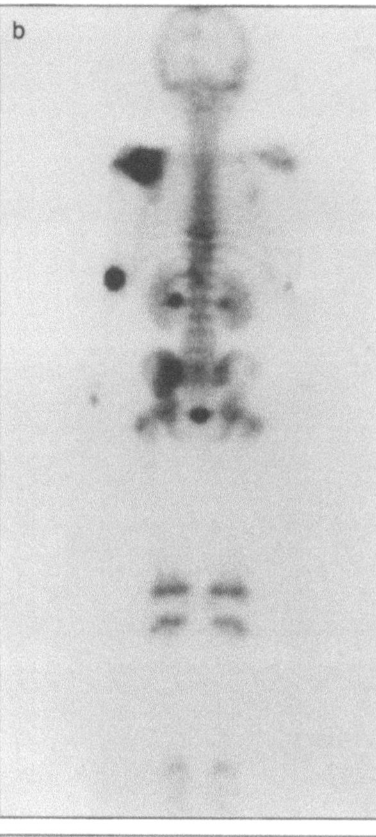

Fig. 2.29a. Blood pool posterior image shows abnormal increased uptake of isotope in the left shoulder and the left sacro-iliac joint

Fig. 2.29b. Whole body posterior scan shows abnormal increased uptake of isotope in the left shoulder, mid and lower dorsal spine as well as the left sacro-iliac joint

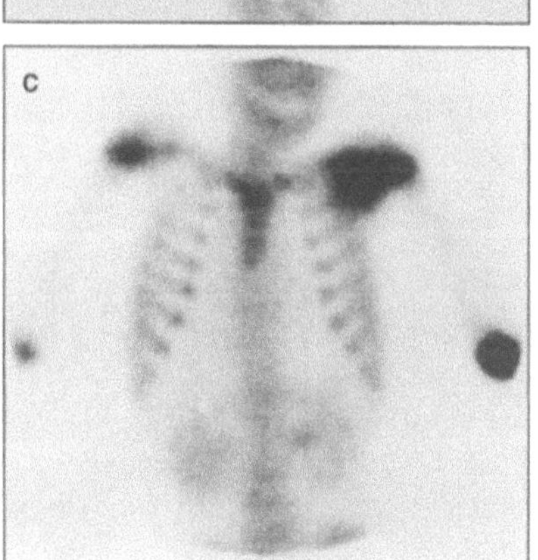

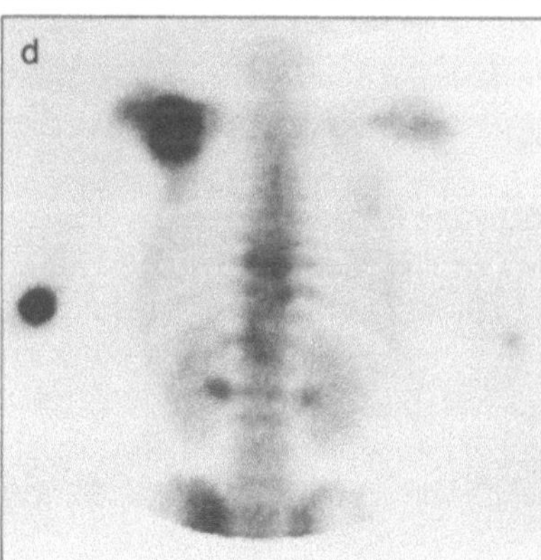

Fig. 2.29c. Anterior image of the thorax shows increased uptake of isotope in the left shoulder

Fig. 2.29d. Posterior image of the thorax and lumbar spine shows abnormal increased uptake of isotope in the left scapula, dorsal vertebrae 9–11, as well as at L1 and the left sacro-iliac joint

Technical Comment

Note extravasation of isotope in both elbows and the left hand region from the injection sites in all the images.

Case 2.30. A 13-year-old boy with tuberculosis of the left lung who had an abscess in the region of the left nipple and multifocal osteomyelitis

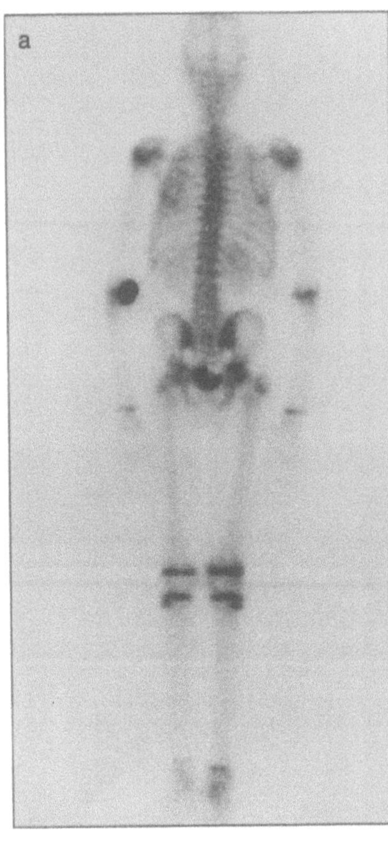

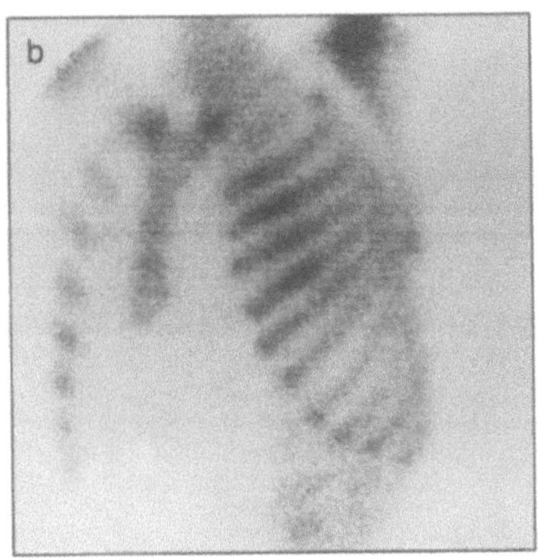

Fig. 2.30a. Posterior whole body scan shows vague abnormal increased uptake of isotope in the region of the left scapula. There is asymmetry of the pelvis and lower limbs with decreased activity in the left sacro-iliac joint. Reduced uptake of isotope is noted in the left hip, left knee and left ankle.

Fig. 2.30b. Anterior image (right oblique view) of the left thorax cage shows abnormal increased uptake of isotope in the left second, third, fourth, fifth and sixth ribs

Technical Comment
Note extravasation of isotope in the left elbow region, the site of injection.

Teaching Point
1. The cause for the asymmetry in the pelvis and lower limbs was not ascertained. This could have resulted simply from asymmetric weight-bearing over a prolonged period, but without bacteriological investigation of the sacro-iliac joint, infection as the cause could not be excluded.
2. For infection of ribs, also see cases 2.22, 2.34, 2.35. Similar appearances may be seen in Ewing's sarcoma (see Cases 4.28, 4.30) and in sickle cell disease (see Cases 6.16–6.18).

Case 2.31. A 3-year-old girl with backache who was shown on computed tomography (CT) scan to have a destructive lesion involving L4 and L5, but no soft tissue mass was seen. There was a high sedimentation rate with a positive Mantoux test. Final diagnosis: tuberculosis of the spine

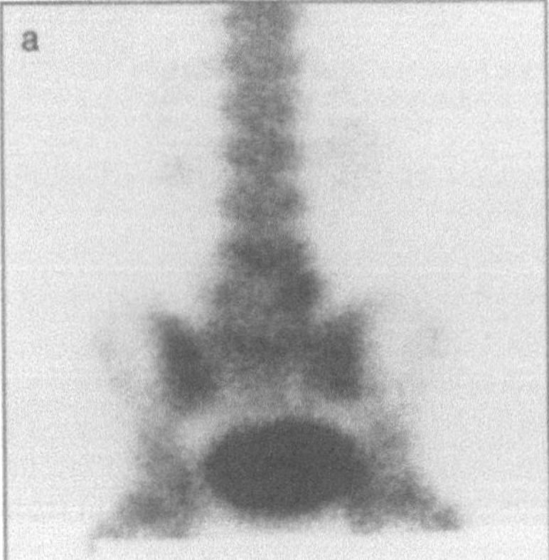

Fig. 2.31a. Posterior image of the lumbar spine and pelvis. Focal abnormal uptake of isotope is noted at L4 and at L5. This is not particularly intense and shows the need for high-quality spot views of the appropriate area

Technical Comment
When high resolution of the spine is required, single photon emission computed tomography (SPECT) is preferable.

Teaching Point
Also see Chap. 5.2.3, "Spondylolisthesis".

2.3 Unusual Sites, Excluding the Long Bones

2.3.1 Skull
(2 Cases; Figs. 2.32, 2.33)

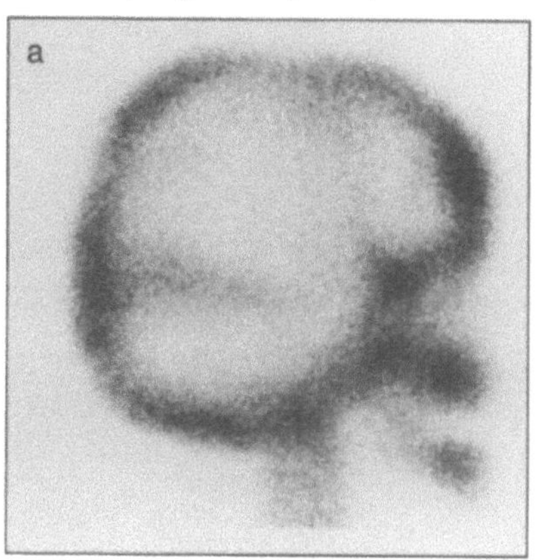

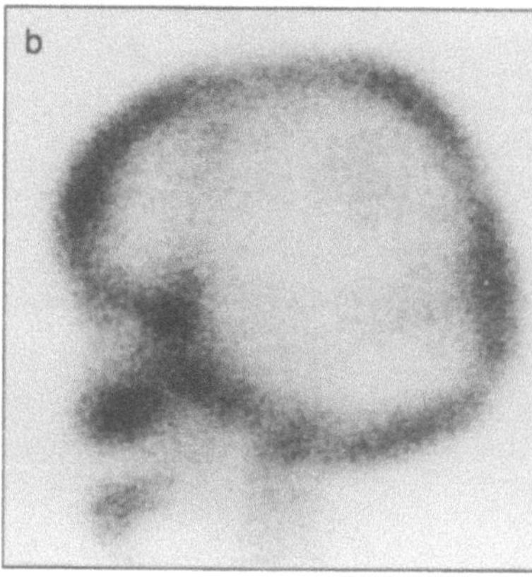

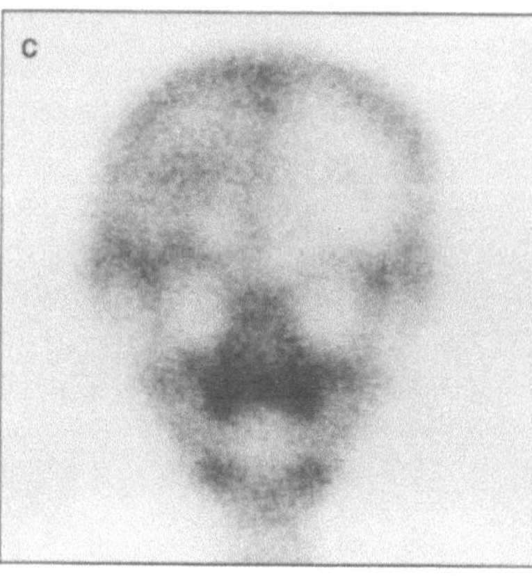

Case 2.32. A 3-year-old boy who presented acutely unwell with cellulitis extending from the right orbit over the vertex. Final diagnosis was osteomyelitis of the frontal bone

Fig. 2.32a. Right lateral view of the skull shows abnormal increased uptake of isotope in the frontal bone; this is more intense in the mid portion

Fig. 2.32b. Left lateral view of the skull shows diffuse increased uptake of isotope in the frontal bone

Fig. 2.32c. Anterior view of the skull shows the extent of the abnormal increased uptake of isotope in the right frontal bone extending posteriorly.

Following antibiotics, a follow-up scan 2 months later was completely normal (not shown)

Case 2.33. A 14-year-old boy who had undergone craniotomy and presented with swelling in the region of the surgery due to osteomyelitis in the vault adjacent to the surgery

Fig. 2.33a. Blood pool image of the skull (right lateral position) shows abnormal increased uptake of isotope in the parietal bone extending towards the occipital bone

Fig. 2.33b. Blood pool image of the skull left lateral view is normal

Fig. 2.33c. Posterior blood pool image of the skull shows marked abnormal increased uptake of isotope on the right side. The deformity of the skull vault is also noted

Fig. 2.33d. Anterior blood pool image confirms the generalised increased uptake of isotope in the parietal bone on the right

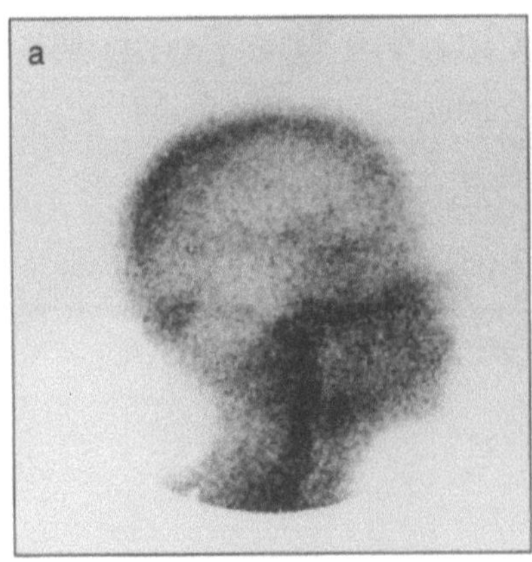
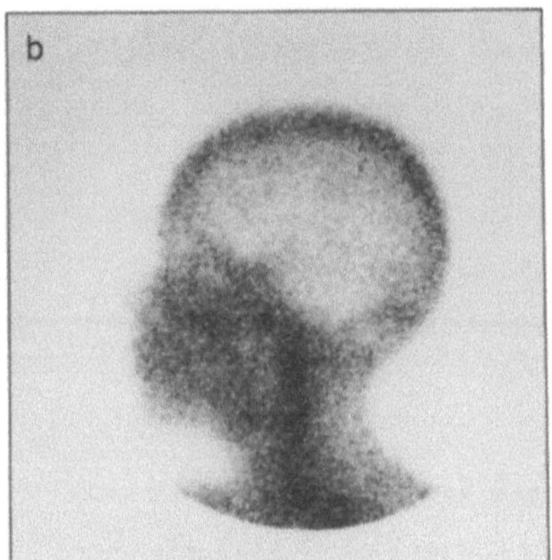
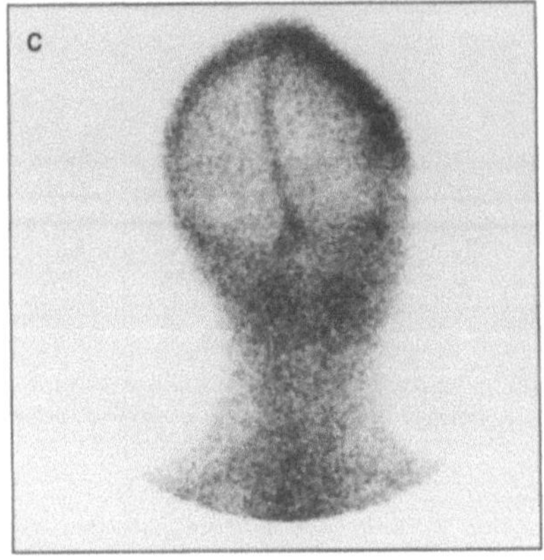
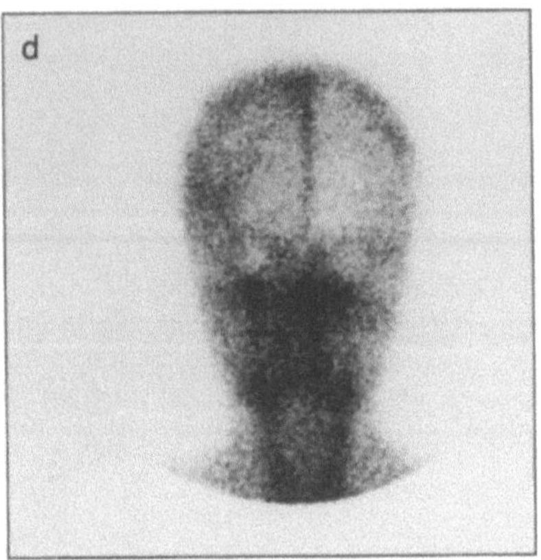

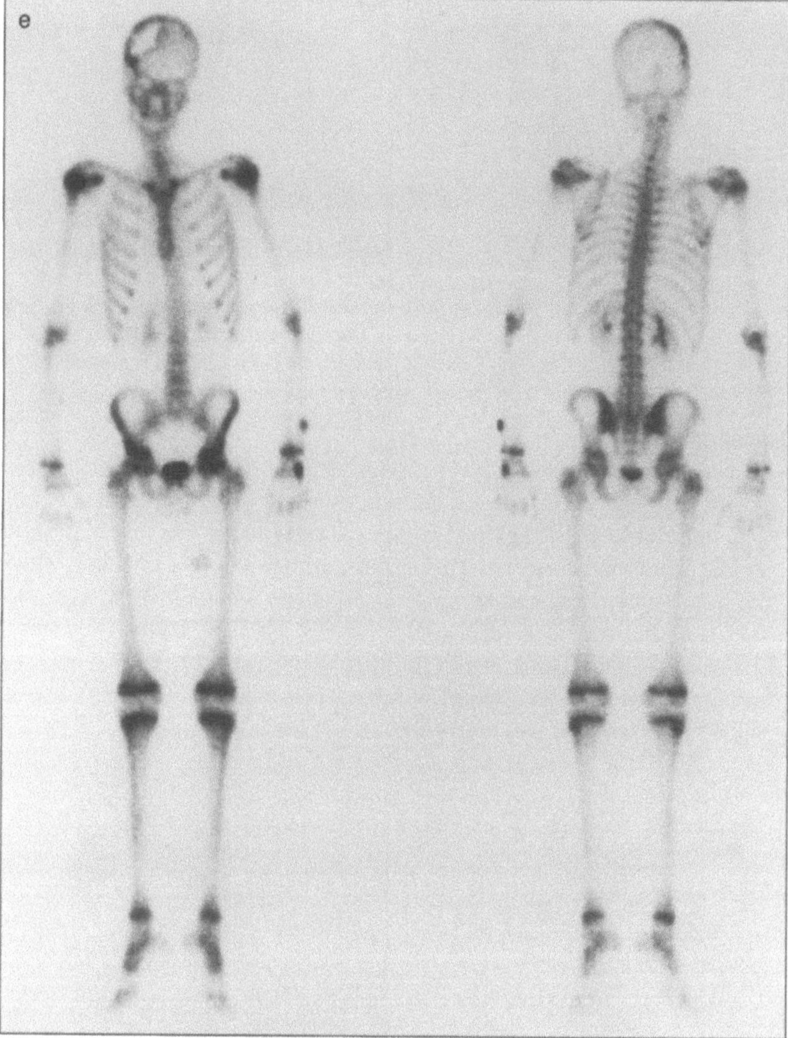

Fig. 2.33e. Whole body scans. These show a large photon-deficient area in the right temporo-parietal region with abnormal increased uptake of isotope around the edges of the photon-deficient area

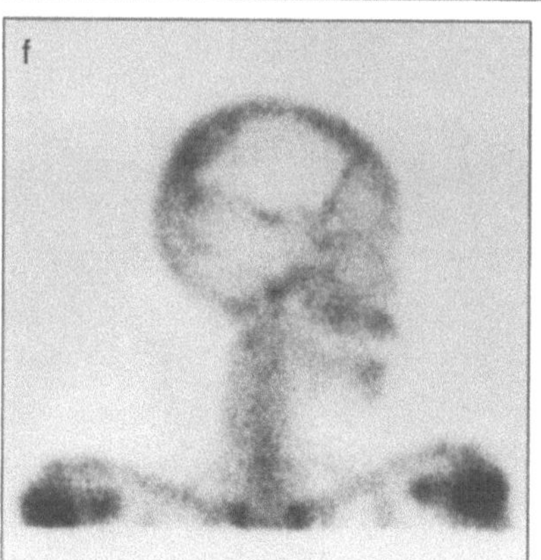

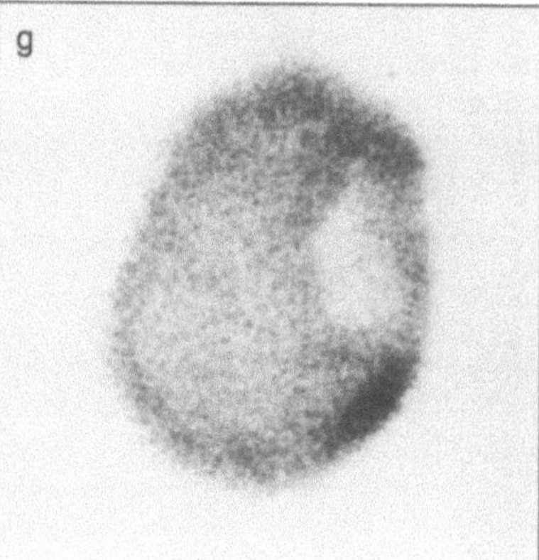

Fig. 2.33f. Right lateral view of the skull shows the photon-deficient area extending from the frontal into the parietal bone and also involving the temporal bone. There is abnormal increased uptake of isotope in the parietal bone

Fig. 2.33g. Vertex view shows to better advantage the focal abnormal accumulation of isotope posterior to the bony defect

Technical Comment

Note increased uptake of isotope in Fig. 2.33e over the left wrist and the left distal ulna; this was due to extravasation at the injection sites.

2.3.2 Thorax
(4 Cases; Figs. 2.34–2.37)

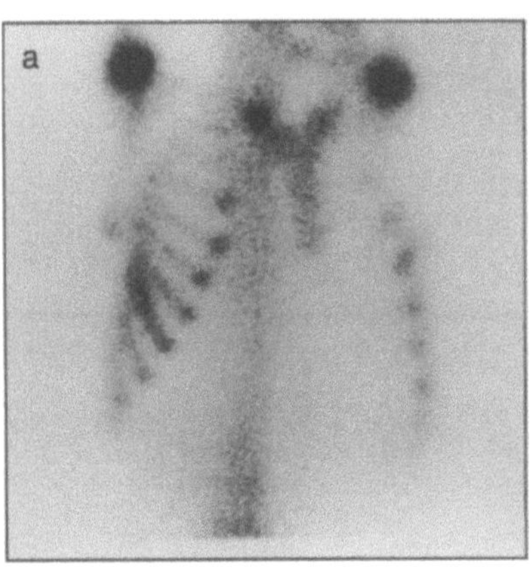

Case 2.34. A 5-year-old boy who had empyema of the chest which was drained but the infection continued with a sinus developing. Osteomyelitis of the ribs was confirmed following the bone scan

Fig. 2.34a. Right anterior oblique view of the chest shows abnormal increased uptake of isotope in the anterior portion of the right sixth and seventh rib. The seventh rib is involved to a greater extent than the sixth rib

Teaching Point

1. Compare this case to the child with tuberculosis (Case 2.30). With bacterial infection of the thoracic cage, one rib is involved to a greater extent than the remaining ribs, whilst in tuberculosis, all the ribs involved show almost equal involvement. This is not pathognomonic, but does allow the bone scan to suggest an unusual organism when all the ribs are involved to the same degree.

2. For other cases of infection in the ribs, see Case 2.22. Similar appearances may be seen in Ewing's sarcoma (see Cases 4.28, 4.30) and in sickle cell disease (Cases 6.16–6.18).

Case 2.35. A 16-year-old boy who remained unwell with a pyrexia following drainage of an empyema of the left chest. Osteomyelitis of the ribs was proven following the bone scan

Fig. 2.35a. Anterior view of thorax shows multiple areas of increased uptake of isotope in the anterior portion of the left ribs involving the third to seventh rib

Fig. 2.35b. Left anterior oblique view of the ribs shows to better advantage the abnormalities

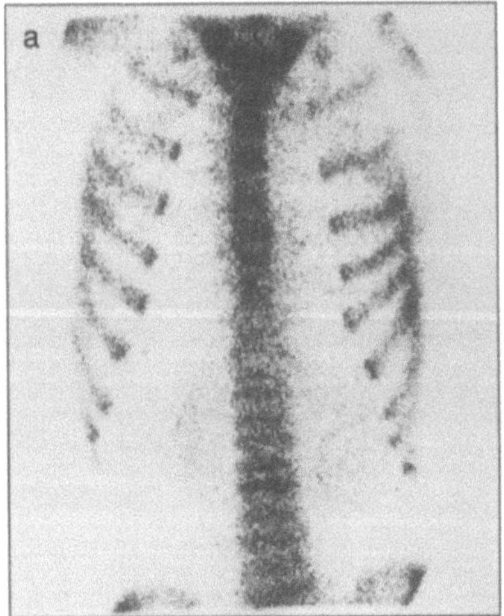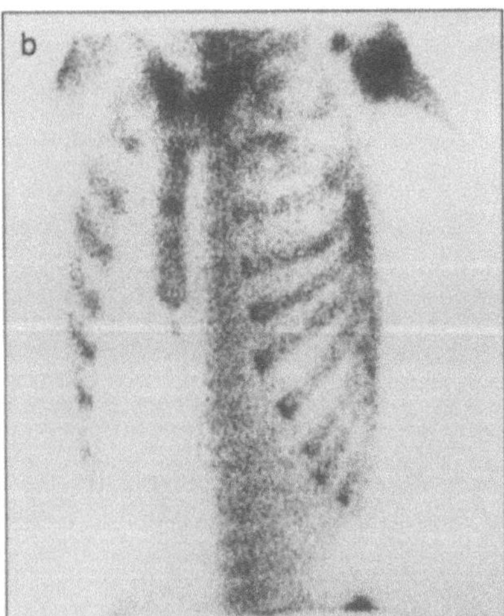

Teaching Point

For other cases of infection in the ribs, see Cases 2.22 and 2.30. Similar appearances may be seen in Ewing's sarcoma (see Cases 4.28, 4.30) and in sickle cell disease (see Cases 6.16–6.18).

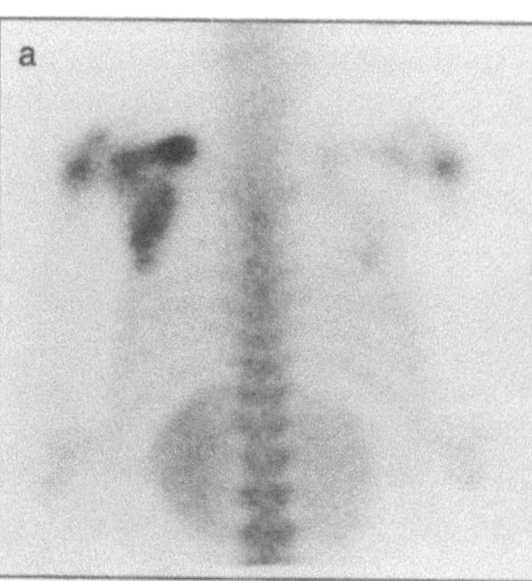

Case 2.36. A 4-year-old boy, acutely unwell with fever and pain in the left shoulder. Final diagnosis was osteomyelitis of the left scapula with possible involvement of the humerus

Fig. 2.36a. Posterior view of the thorax shows abnormal increased uptake of isotope in the left scapula. The epiphysis of the proximal portion of the humerus also shows increased uptake of isotope but this may well be secondary simply to hyperaemia. The kidneys are well seen

Teaching Point

1. The cause for the retention of isotope in the kidneys is uncertain; this is however a frequent observation in children who have septicaemia.
2. For other cases with infection of the scapula, see Case 2.21. Similar appearances may be seen in Ewing's sarcoma (see Case 4.29).

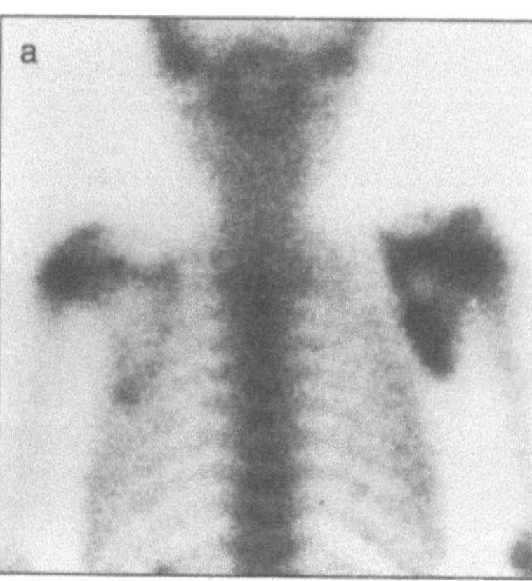

Case 2.37. A 5-year-old boy with pain and fever. Final diagnosis was osteomyelitis of the right scapula involving the inferior portion only

Fig. 2.37a. Posterior view of thorax and shoulder girdle shows abnormal increased uptake of isotope in the angle of the scapula extending up in the body but not involving the entire scapula. The scapula is displaced laterally

Teaching Point

For other cases with infection of the scapula, see Case 2.21. Similar appearances may be seen in Ewing's sarcoma (see Case 4.29).

2.3.3 Spine
(8 Cases; Figs. 2.38–2.45)

Case 2.38. An 8-year-old girl with backache who was found to have osteomyelitis of the spine

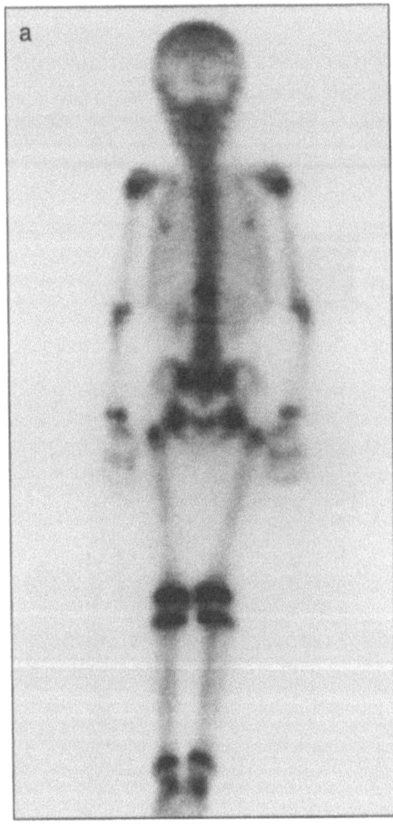
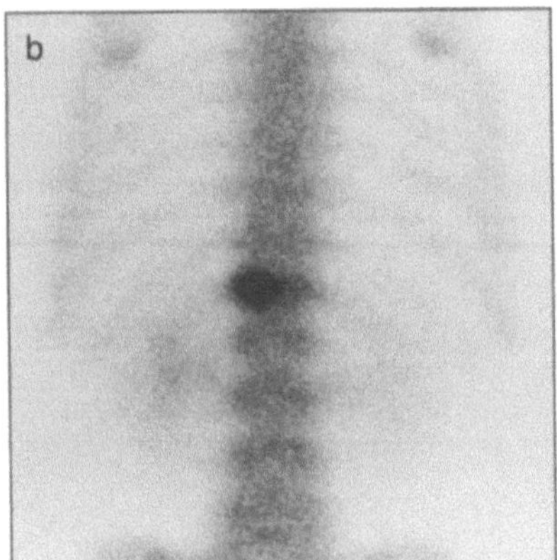

Fig. 2.38a. Whole body posterior image. There is abnormal increased uptake of isotope in the lower dorsal spine

Fig. 2.38b. Posterior view of the lower dorsal and upper lumbar spine. Focal abnormal uptake of isotope is noted on the left side of the body of D12 with only minimal involvement of the remainder of the body

Technical Comment
Note the importance of the spot image in order to increase the resolution of abnormality shown on the whole body image. SPECT of the spine may also be useful.

Teaching Point
The appearances on bone scan are non-specific and similar appearances could be due to a primary benign bone tumor, e.g. osteoid osteoma or osteoblastoma (see Cases 4.9, 4.10, 4.12, 4.13), to aneurysmal bone cyst (Case 4.24) or trauma (see Case 5.13).

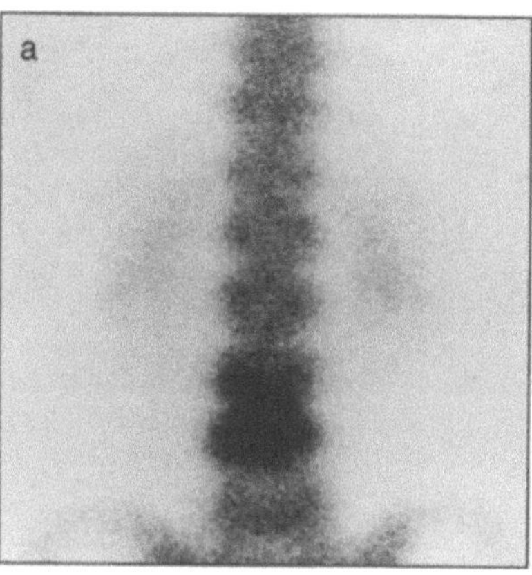

Case 2.39. A 6-year-old boy with a 2-week history of backache. Following the bone scan, CT confirmed osteomyelitis of the spine and the associated soft tissue mass, which was due to infection

Fig. 2.39a. Posterior view of the lumbar spine shows diffuse abnormal increased uptake of isotope in the body of L4 with less marked changes on the left side of the body of L3 extending across the mid line

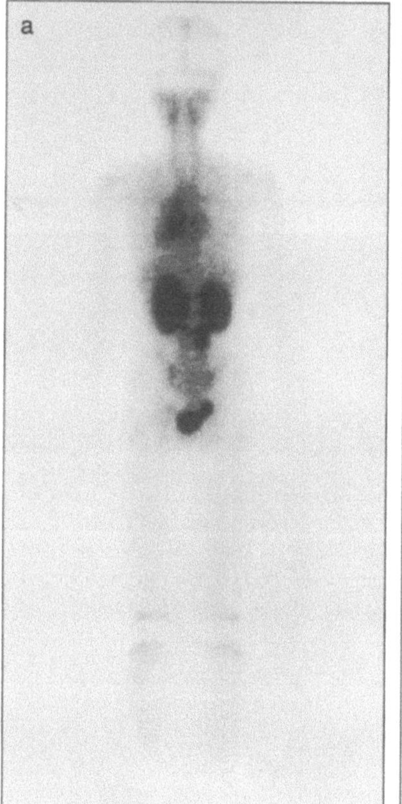

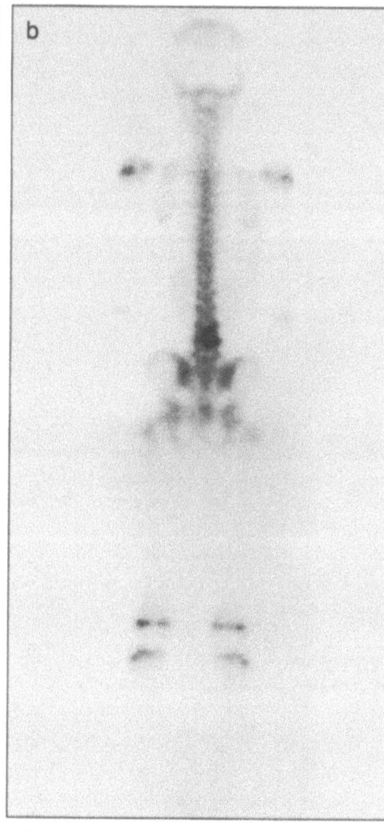

Case 2.40. A 9-year-old girl with backache and a high sedimentation rate (ESR). The final diagnosis was osteomyelitis of the spine

Fig. 2.40a. Blood pool whole body image shows abnormal increased uptake of isotope in the mid lumbar spine immediately below the level of the kidneys

Fig. 2.40b. Whole body scan shows abnormal increased uptake of isotope in the lower lumbar spine involving two vertebral bodies

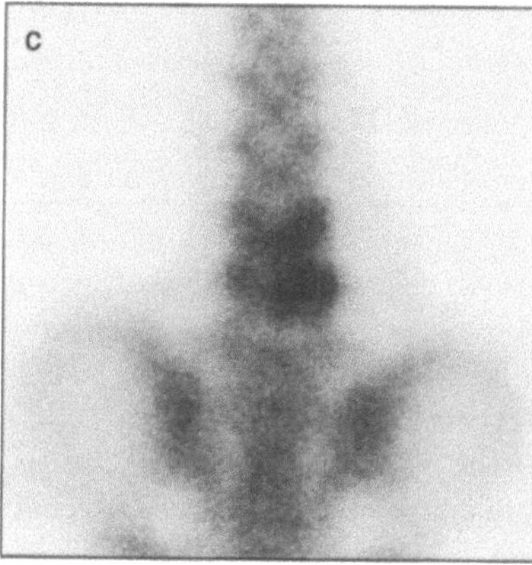

Fig. 2.40c. Posterior view of the lumbar spine and part of the pelvis shows that the abnormal increased uptake of isotope is more marked on the right side of the vertebral bodies of L3 and L4 but extends across to the left side of the vertebral bodies

Case 2.41. An 8-year-old girl with backache. The final diagnosis was discitis; no organism was found. The radiographs were normal

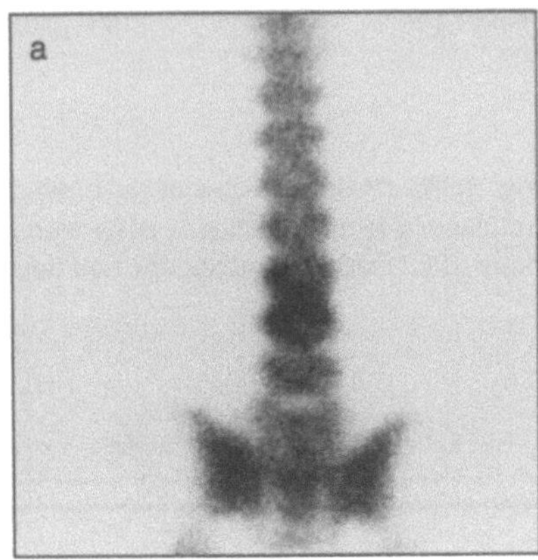

Fig. 2.41a. Posterior view shows abnormal increased uptake of isotope in the body of L3 and, to a lesser extent, the left side of the body of L2

Case 2.42. A 5-year-old girl with a stiff painful back for 1 month; the radiographs were normal at time of the scan, but subsequently became abnormal with features typical of "discitis". Final diagnosis was that of discitis

Fig. 2.42a. Posterior blood pool image of the lumbar spine and pelvis fails to reveal any abnormality

Fig. 2.42b. Posterior image of the lumbar spine shows generalised increased uptake of isotope at the L3 and L4 level

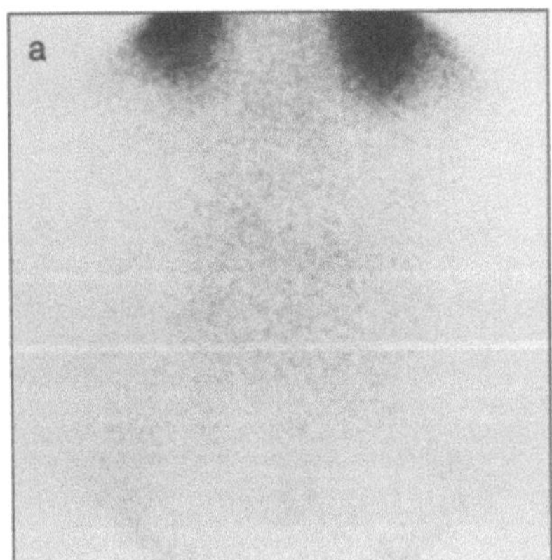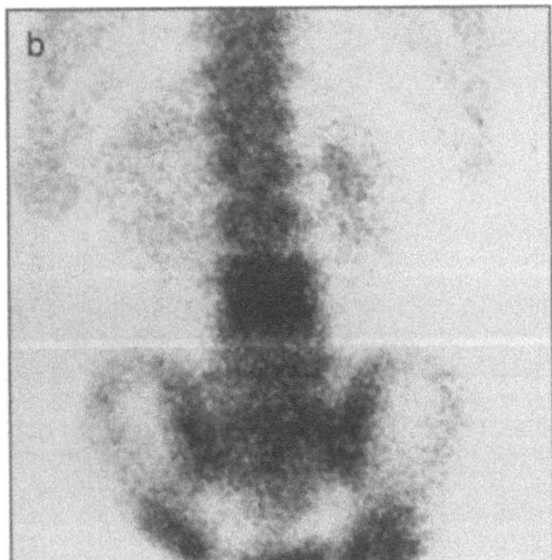

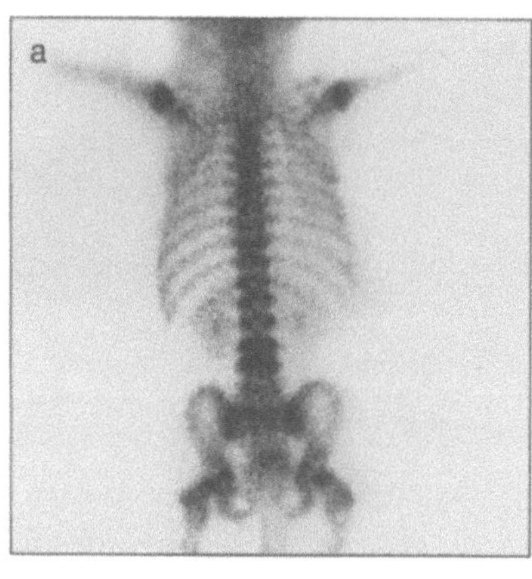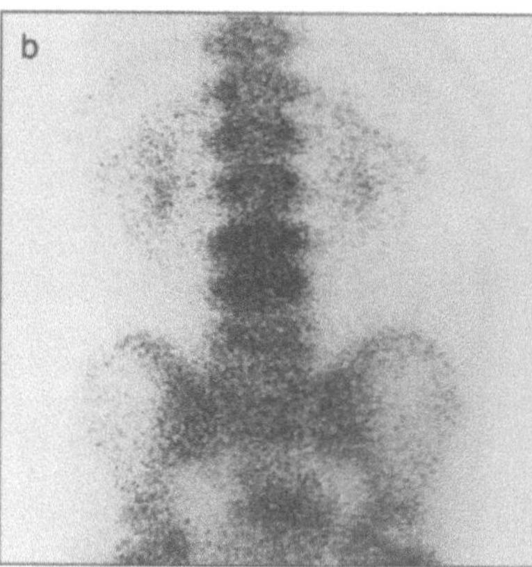

Case 2.43. A 2-year-old girl with back-ache. The radiographs were normal but later went on to show disc space narrowing. The final diagnosis was that of discitis

Fig. 2.43a. Posterior image of the dorsal and lumbar spine and pelvis. Abnormal increased uptake of isotope was noted in the lower lumbar spine

Fig. 2.43b. Posterior magnification image of the lumbar spine shows abnormal increased uptake of isotope at L3 and L4

Technical Comment

Figure 2.43b was acquired in the zoom mode. Magnification post-acquisition is of limited value since there is no additional clinical information.

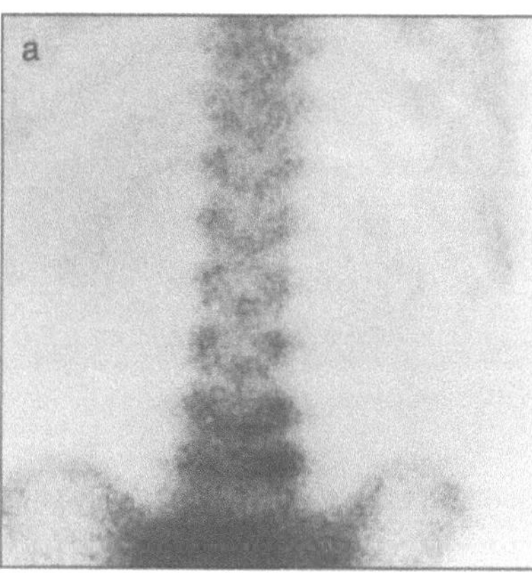

Case 2.44. A 2-year-old girl with lower backache for 1 month. Final diagnosis was that of discitis

Fig. 2.44a. Posterior image of the lumbar spine is abnormal with increased uptake of isotope at the level of L4 and L5. This is mainly on the right side of the vertebral bodies

Teaching Point

Similar appearances may be seen in spondylolisthesis (see Chap. 5.2.3, "Spondylolisthesis").

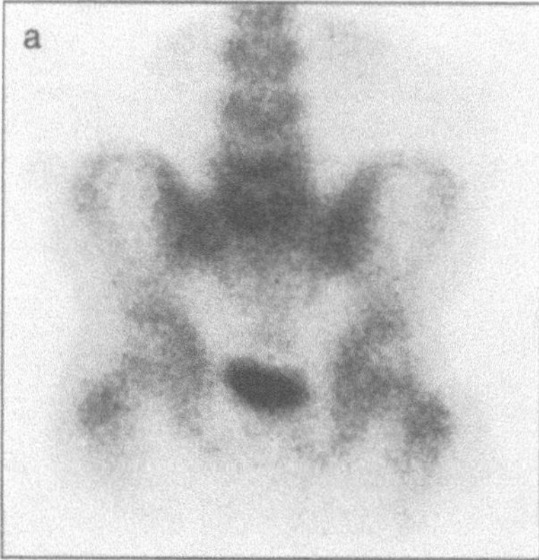

Case 2.45. A 5-year-old boy with backache for 6 months. Long-term follow-up revealed disc space narrowing radiologically. No organism was isolated and the final diagnosis was that of discitis

Fig. 2.45a. Posterior view of the lumbar spine and pelvis. There is generalised abnormal increased uptake of isotope in the body of L5

2.3.4 Pelvis
(2 Cases; Figs. 2.46, 2.47)

Case 2.46. A 10-year-old boy with acute history of pain in the right groin with a limp; the child was generally unwell. Final diagnosis was osteomyelitis of the ischial bone

Fig. 2.46a. Blood pool whole body image shows slightly increased uptake of isotope in the right ischial bone

Fig. 2.46b. Whole body posterior view shows abnormal increased uptake of isotope in the right ischial tuberosity

Fig. 2.46c. Posterior image of the pelvis. The normal right hip joint is noted, but the abnormal increased uptake of isotope can be seen throughout the right ischial tuberosity extending towards the inferior pubic ramus

Fig. 2.46d. Anterior image of the pelvis. Increased uptake of isotope between the pubic ramus and the right ischium is noted

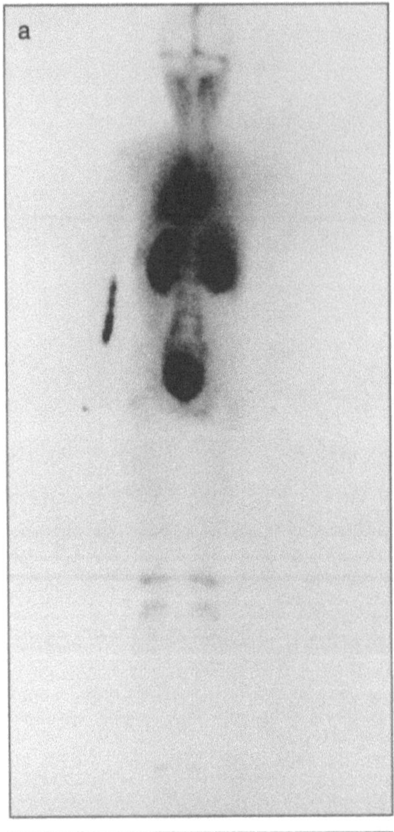

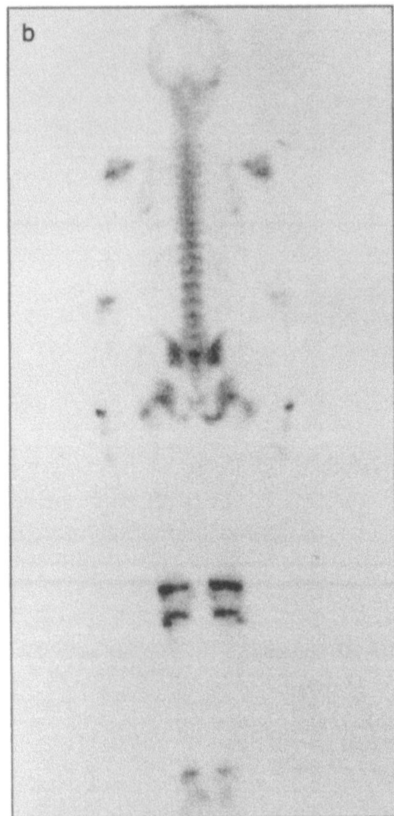

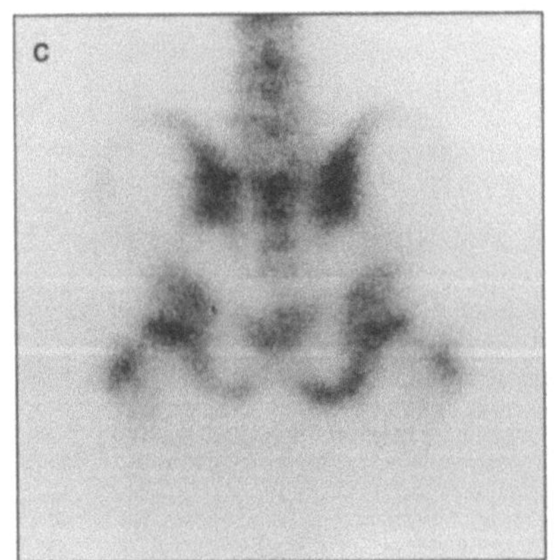

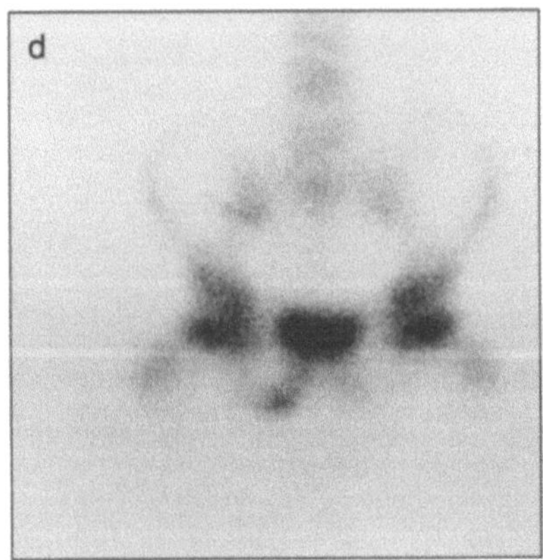

Case 2.47. An 8-year-old boy with synchondrosis on the left side. This is normal

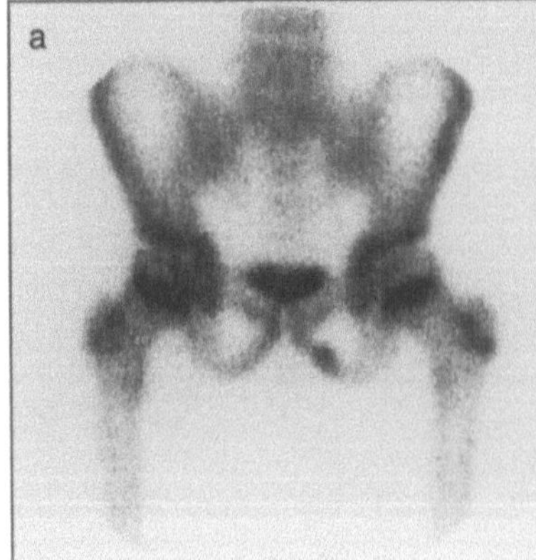

Fig. 2.47a. Anterior image of the pelvis

Teaching Point

The anterior image of the pelvis (Fig. 2.46d) shows the normal synchondrosis between the inferior pubic ramus and ischial bone. Note the asymmetry between the two sides; this should not be misinterpreted as either infection nor a fracture, since it is normal (see Case 2.47). The posterior view (Fig. 2.46c) is abnormal, since the activity is not localised to the synchondrosis.

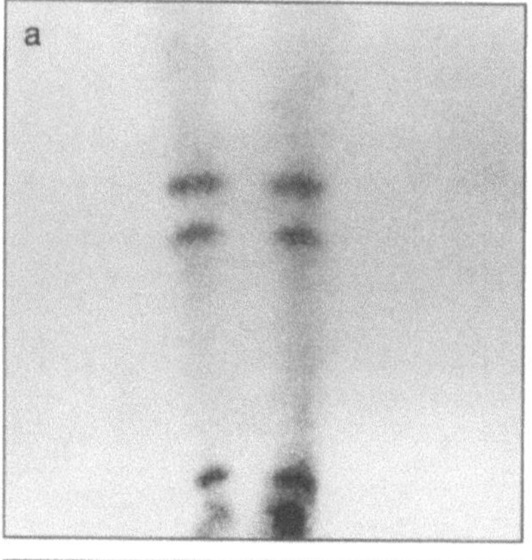

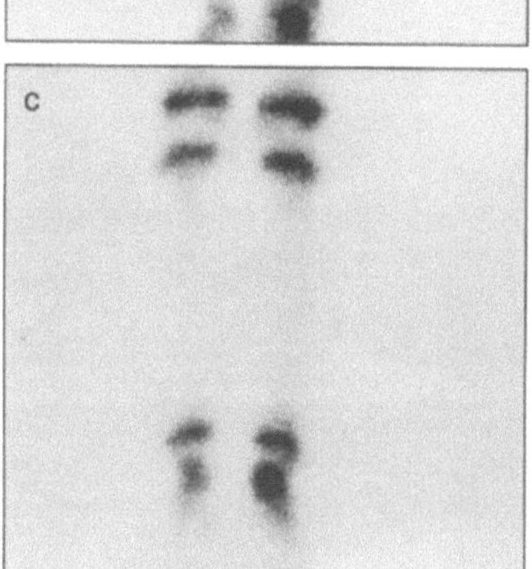

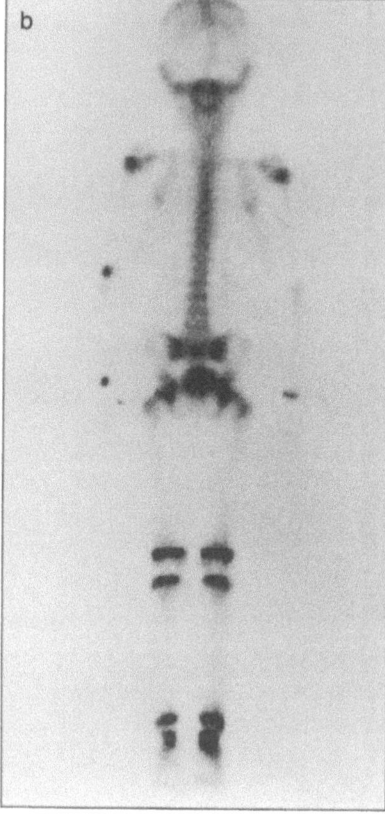

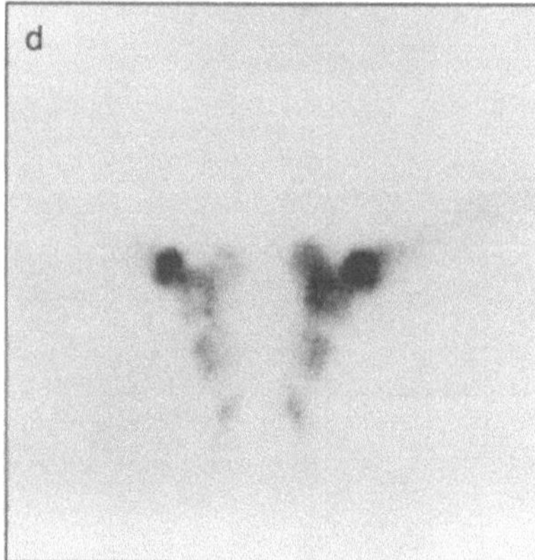

2.3.5 Feet
(4 Cases; Figs. 2.48–2.51)

Case 2.48. A 4-year-old boy with pain in the right foot, pyrexial and unwell. Final diagnosis: osteomyelitis of the right talus

Fig. 2.48a. Blood pool posterior view of the lower limbs shows diffuse increased uptake of isotope throughout the region of the right calf, the distal tibial epiphysis as well as intense increased uptake in the region of the talus

Fig. 2.48b. Posterior whole body scan shows marked increased uptake of isotope in the right hind foot with only slight increased uptake of isotope in the distal tibial and fibula epiphyses compared to the left

Fig. 2.48c. Posterior view of the lower limbs and feet shows intense increased uptake of isotope in the region of the right talus

Fig. 2.48d. Lateral view of the feet shows abnormal increased uptake of isotope in the talus on the right. Note the generalised diffuse increased uptake in the calcaneus and also again the increased uptake in the distal tibial epiphysis

Technical Comment

Note extravasation of isotope in the whole body image on the left elbow region.

Teaching Point

The epiphyseal plates of the right lower limb are generally increased compared to that on the opposite side. This presumably reflects the increased blood flow as seen on the blood pool image.

Case 2.49. Osteomyelitis of the left calcaneus in a 7-year-old girl who presented with pain in the foot

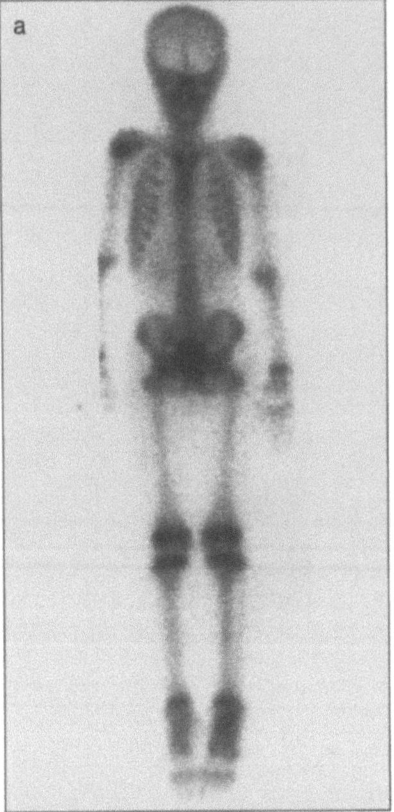

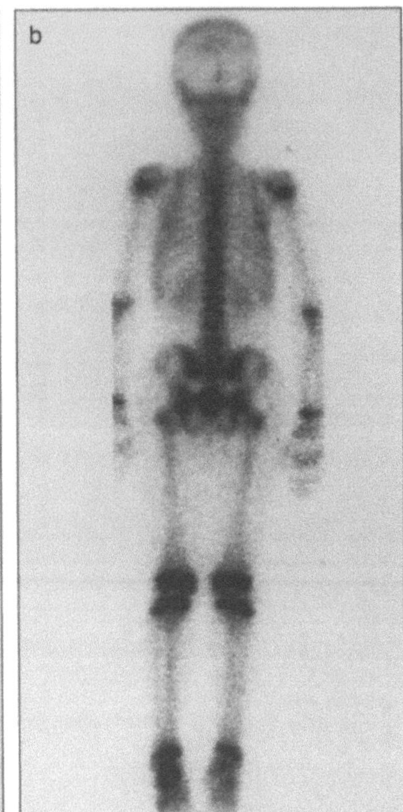

Fig. 2.49a. Whole body anterior scan shows abnormal increased uptake of isotope in the left foot

Fig. 2.49b. Whole body posterior view shows diffuse increased uptake in the left foot; in addition, there is a focal area of intense increased uptake in the hind foot

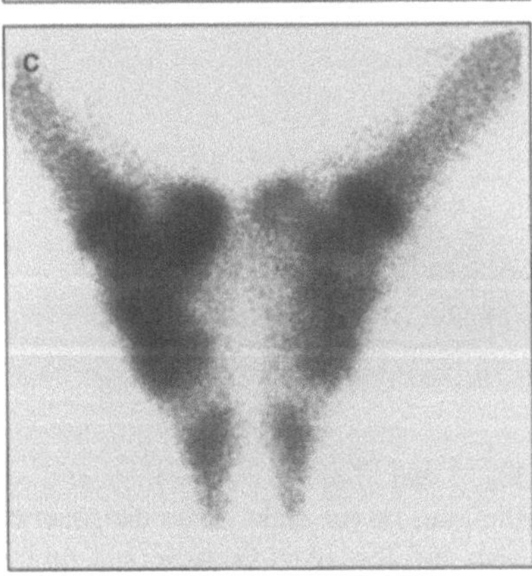

Fig. 2.49c. Lateral view of the feet shows marked abnormal increased uptake of isotope in the calcaneus with generalised increased uptake of isotope throughout the remainder of the left foot

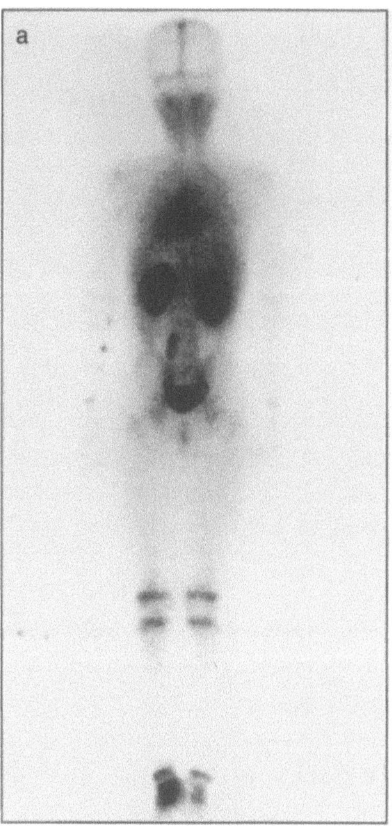

Case 2.50. A 10-year-old boy with acute pain in the left foot due to osteomyelitis of the left calcaneus

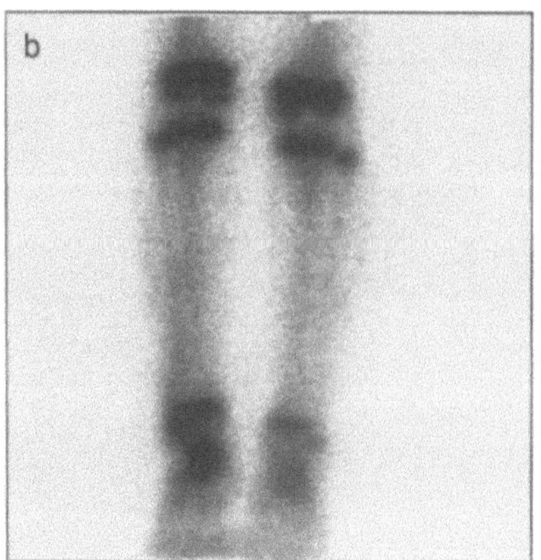

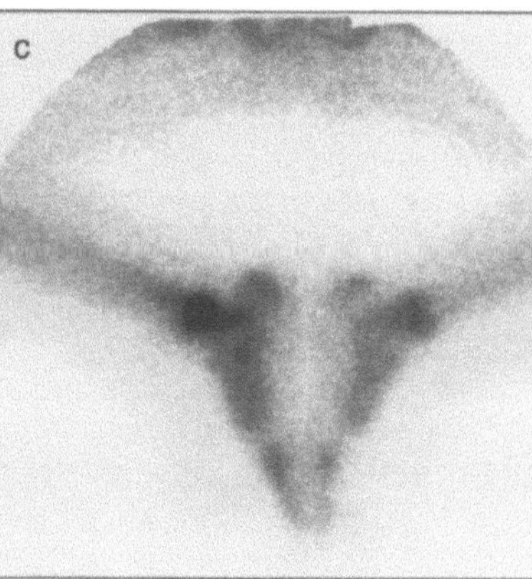

Fig. 2.50a. Blood pool whole body posterior image shows marked abnormal increased uptake of isotope in the left foot. Increased uptake of isotope in the distal left tibial epiphysis is noted

Fig. 2.50b. Posterior view of knees and ankles shows abnormal increased uptake of isotope in the calcaneus on the left. Increased uptake of isotope in the distal left tibial epiphysis is noted

Fig. 2.50c. Lateral view of the feet shows generalised increased uptake of isotope throughout the left foot with focal abnormal accumulation in the left calcaneus. Increased uptake of isotope in the distal left tibial epiphysis is noted

Teaching Point
The uptake of isotope in the distal left tibial epiphysis is probably related to the hyperaemia rather than the infection.

Case 2.51. A 6-year-old girl who had suffered penetrating trauma to the left ankle and presented 1 week later with signs of sepsis. Final diagnosis was that of osteomyelitis of the left calcaneus

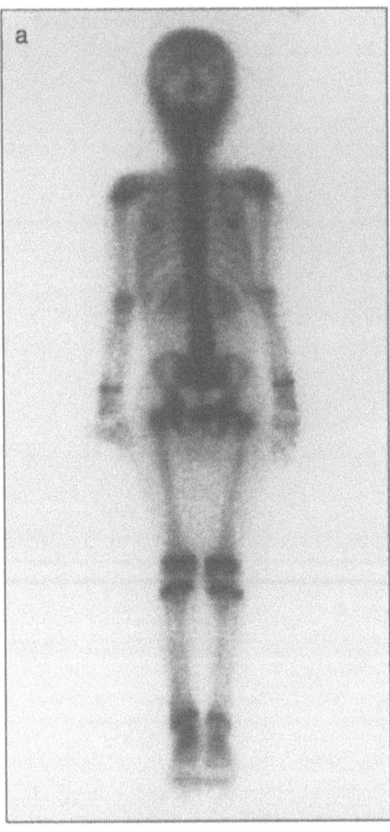

Fig. 2.51a. Whole body scan posterior view. There is increased activity in the epiphyseal plates of the left distal tibia and fibula. The left foot shows generalised increased uptake of isotope

Fig. 2.51b. Posterior view of the feet shows marked focal abnormal increased uptake of isotope in the left calcaneus

Fig. 2.51c. Lateral view of the feet shows to best advantage the involvement of the left calcaneus with generalised increased uptake in the remainder of the left foot simply reflecting the increased blood flow to the foot

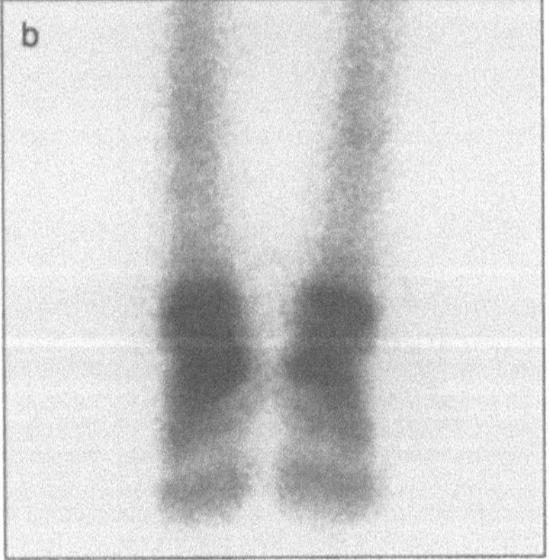

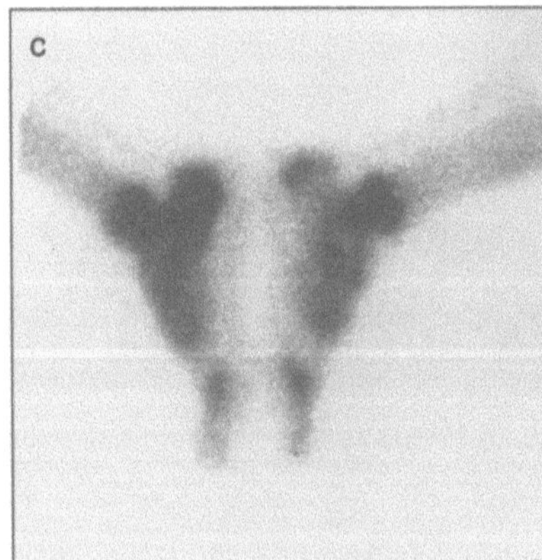

2.4 Non-skeletal Infection
(6 Cases; Figs. 2.52–2.57)

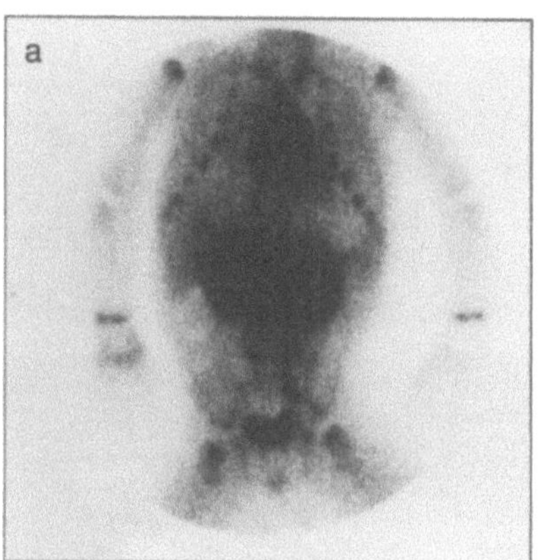

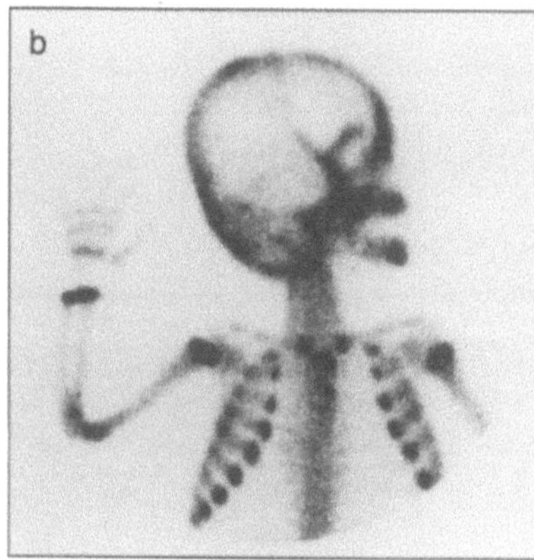

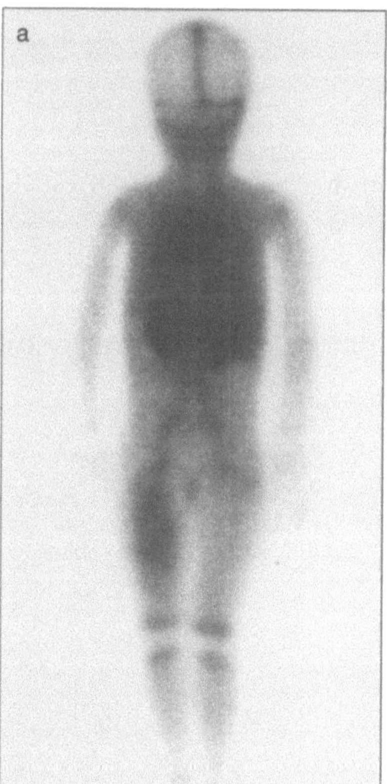

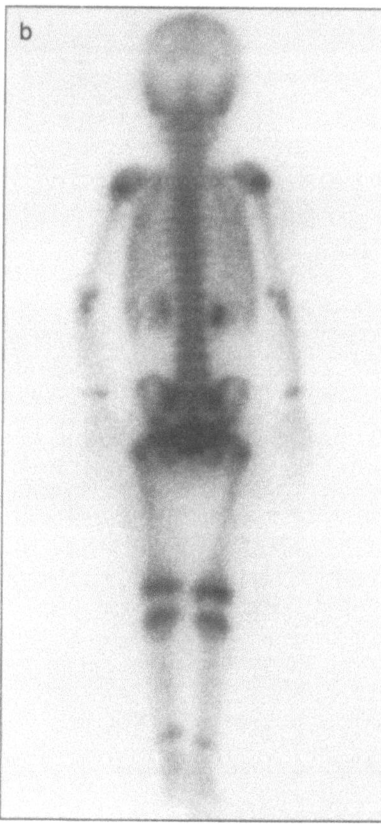

Case 2.52. Cellulitis of the right hand with hyperaemia in a 7-month-old baby boy with no underlying osteomyelitis

Fig. 2.52a. Anterior blood pool image of the thorax, abdomen, pelvis and upper limbs shows generalised increased uptake of isotope in the right hand

Fig. 2.52b. Anterior view of the thorax, right hand and right lateral skull. No abnormality is seen in the skeleton

Case 2.53. An 8-year-old girl with cellulitis of the left thigh who was quite unwell and pyrexial. There was no underlying osteomyelitis

Fig. 2.53a. Whole body blood pool posterior image shows diffuse increased activity in the region of the upper two thirds of the left thigh

Fig. 2.53b. Whole body posterior view fails to reveal any abnormality in the skeleton

Case 2.54. A 6-year-old girl with lower abdominal pain, fever and a raised ESR. Final diagnosis was that of an abscess in the right iliac fossa with no bone involvement

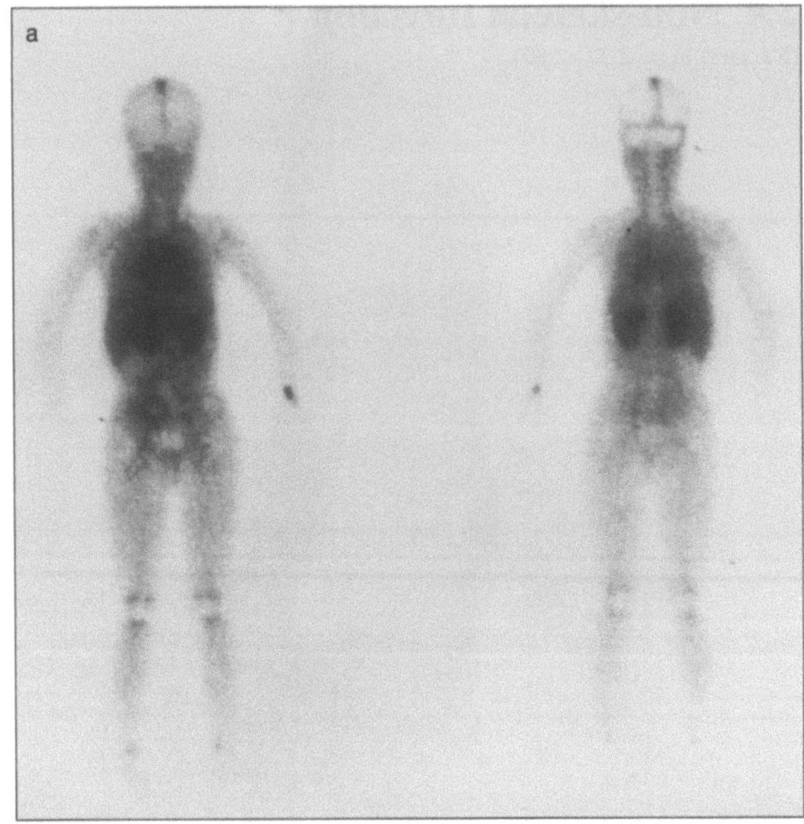

Fig. 2.54a. Whole body blood pool images show marked increased uptake of isotope in the region of the right iliac fossa best seen on the anterior view

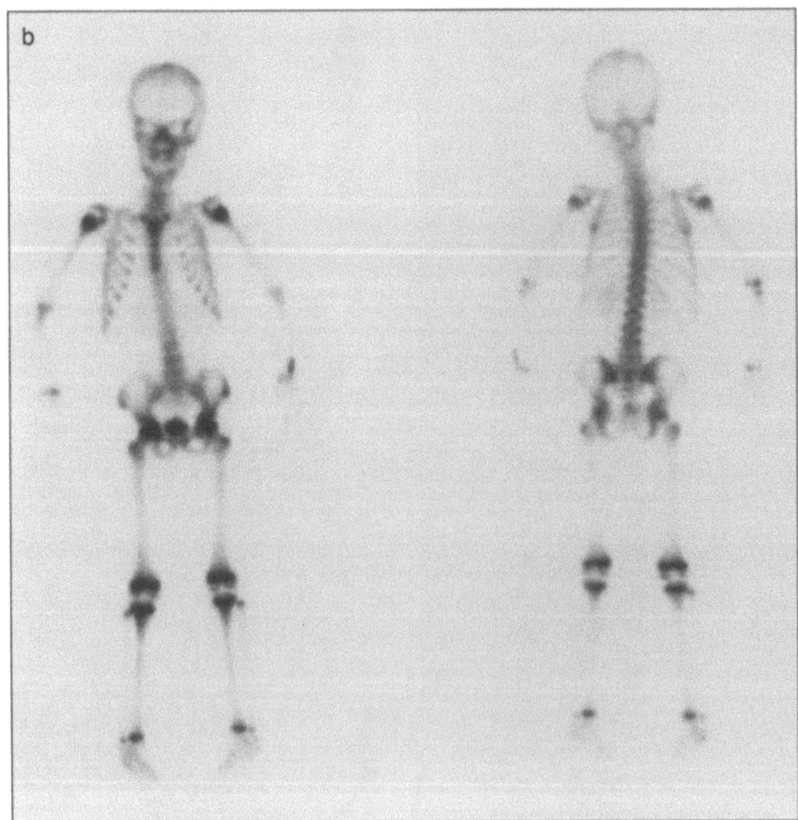

Fig. 2.54b. Whole body images are normal

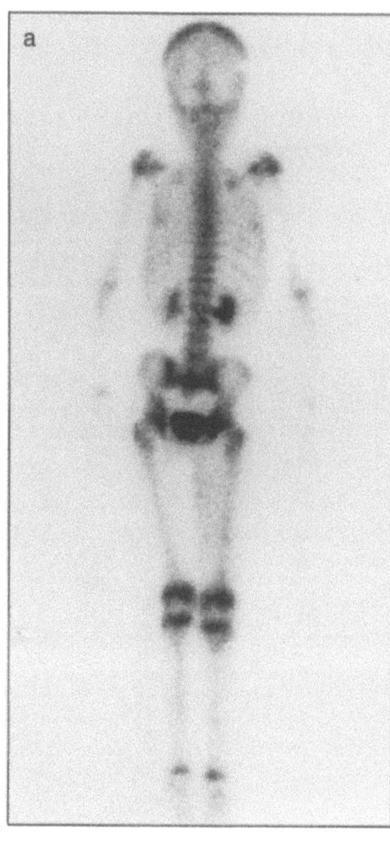

Case 2.55. A 10-year-old boy with a soft tissue infection of the thigh but no underlying osteomyelitis

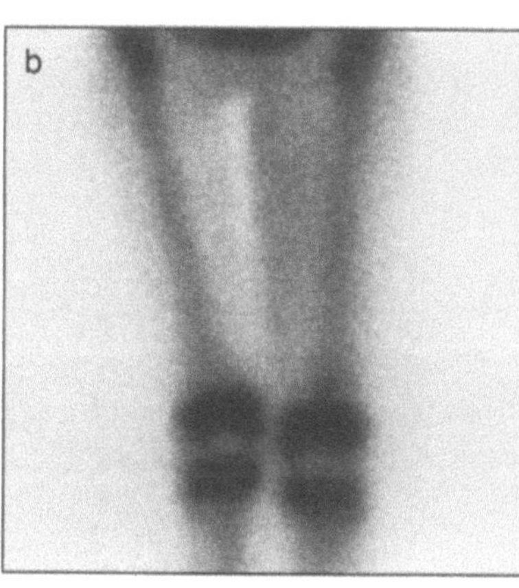

Fig. 2.55a. Whole body posterior view shows diffuse increased uptake of isotope throughout the soft tissue of the right thigh but the underlying bone appears normal

Fig. 2.55b. Posterior view of the femora shows the diffuse increased uptake of isotope throughout the soft tissue of the thigh on the right. No abnormality is seen in the femora

Technical Comment

Fig. 2.55b was set to show the mid shaft region to best advantage; this is too dark to look for pathology at the epiphyseal plates.

Case 2.56. A 2-year-old girl with pain in the left ankle and cellulitis of the ankle. No underlying osteomyelitits was found

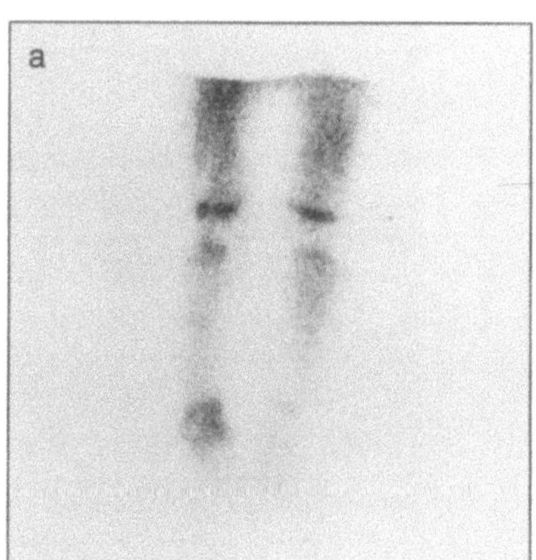

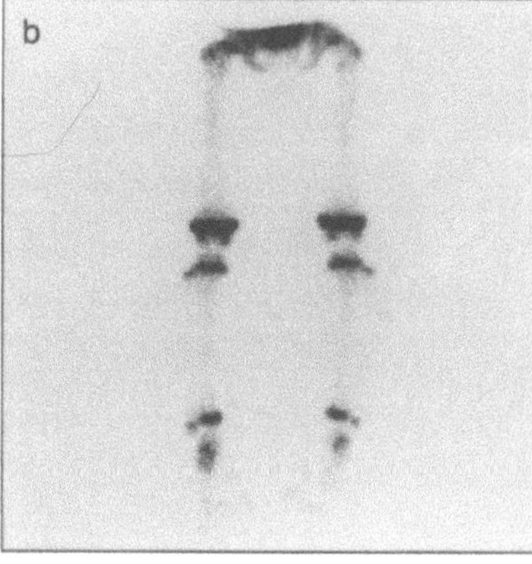

Fig. 2.56a. Blood pool posterior image of the lower limbs shows increased distribution of isotope in the left foot and, to a lesser extent, around the distal left tibia and fibula

Fig. 2.56b. Posterior image of the lower limbs shows slight increased uptake of isotope in the left hind foot compatible with the increased blood pool, but no evidence of osteomyelitis was found

Case 2.57. A 5-year-old girl with cellulitis of the right knee. The underlying bone was normal

Fig. 2.57a. Blood pool anterior image of the knees shows increased uptake of isotope in the soft tissue around the right distal femur

Fig. 2.57b. Lateral blood pool image of the right knee shows abnormal increased uptake of isotope in the posterior compartment of the distal third of the thigh

Fig. 2.57c. Whole body images. No obvious abnormality is seen

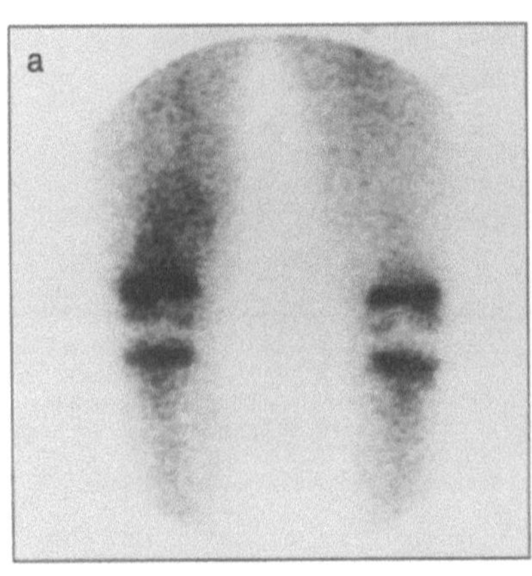
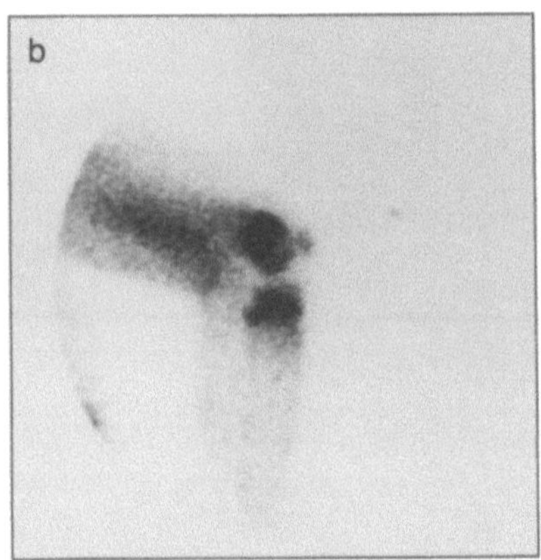
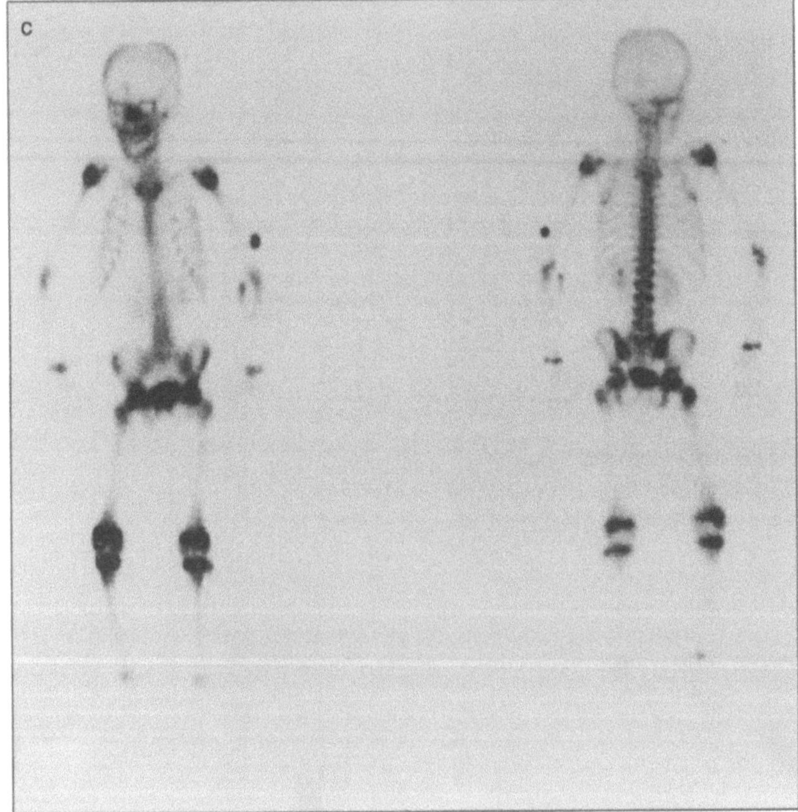

Fig. 2.57d. Anterior view of the knees shows slight increased uptake of isotope in the epiphyseal plate of the distal right femur related to the hyperaemia

Fig. 2.57e. Lateral view of the right knee fails to demonstrate any local abnormality

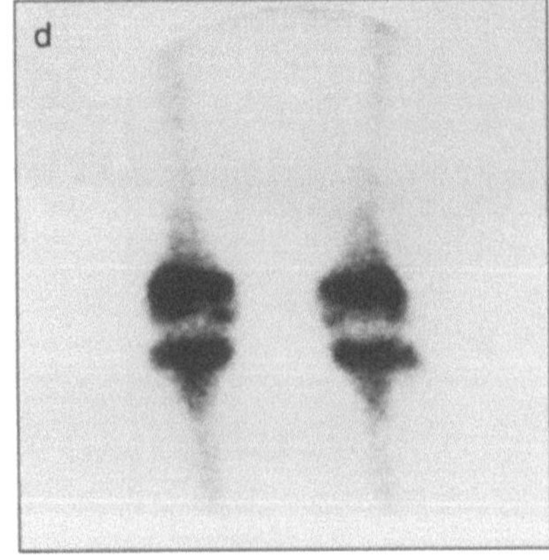
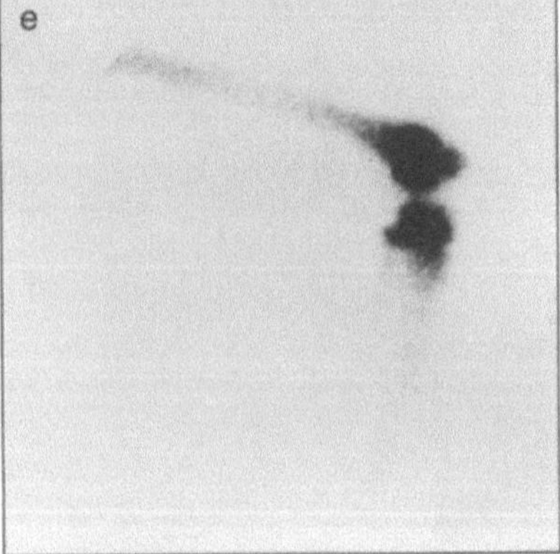

Technical Comment
1. Poor positioning of the feet in Fig. 2.57c is noted.
2. There is extravasation of isotope in the region of the left elbow, the site of injection.

2.5 Growth Arrest

(1 Case; Fig. 2.58)

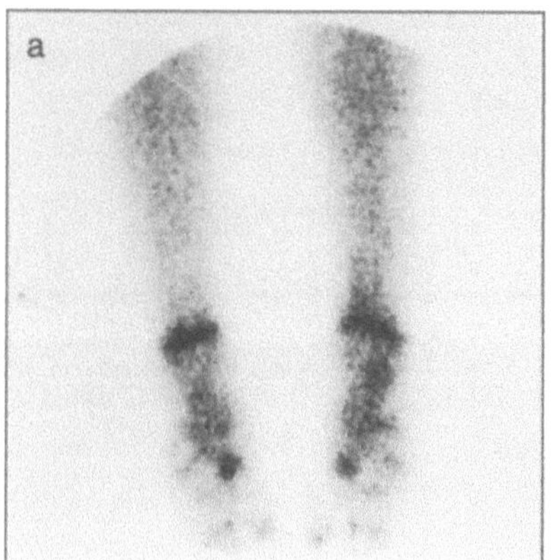

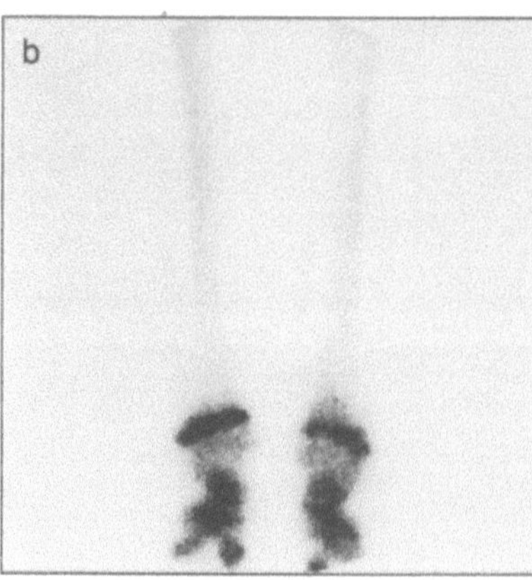

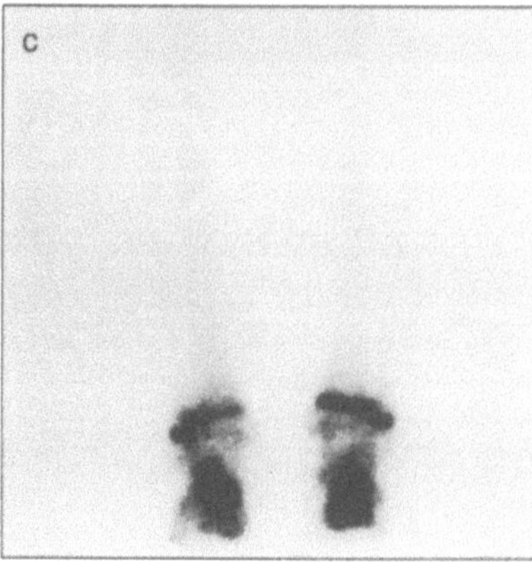

Case 2.58. An 8-year-old boy with known osteomyelitis of the left tibia who now presented with pain in the left ankle. The final diagnosis was that of partial fusion of the mid portion of the distal left tibial epiphyseal plate. This complication can occur due to damage of the epiphyseal plate for any reason, e.g. trauma.

Fig. 2.58a. Anterior blood pool image of the ankles and feet shows slight increased activity in the distal left tibia. There is decreased activity in the poorly defined left epiphyseal plate as compared to that on the right

Fig. 2.58b. Anterior view of the ankles shows generalised decreased activity in the left tibial growth plate with slight increased activity in the distal end of the left tibia

Fig. 2.58c. Posterior view of the feet shows marked difference between the two epiphyseal plates with decreased activity especially on the medial aspect of the left tibial epiphyseal plate

Teaching Point

For other Cases of growth arrest see 5.54, 7.35 and 7.36.

3 Arthritis

3.1 Septic Arthritis

Bone scans have a limited role in the diagnosis of acute septic arthritis. The reasons for this include the relative ease with which the clinician can make the diagnosis in superficial joints, e.g. the hand or ankle, and the well-recognized possibility of a normal three-phase bone scan in acute septic arthritis of the hip. The task of bone scans is to assess the presence or absence of osteomyelitis in the adjacent bone.

3.1.1 Typical Appearances
(14 Cases; Figs. 3.1–3.14)

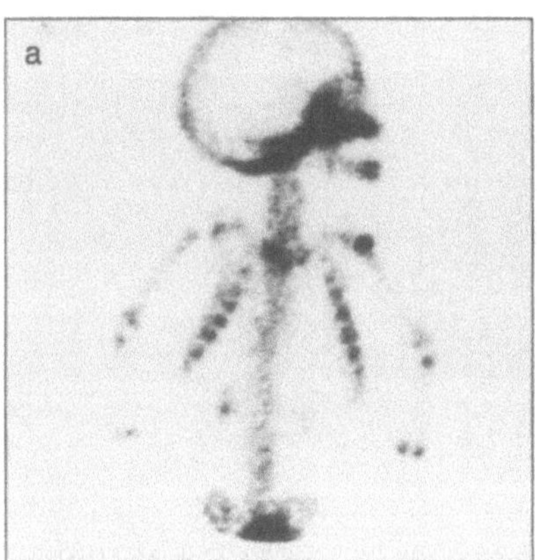
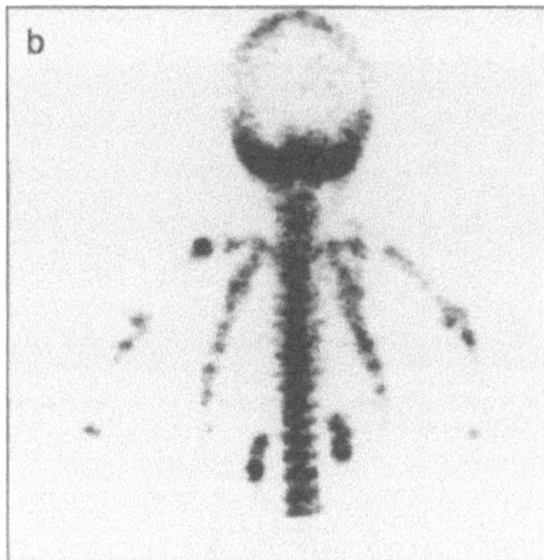

Case 3.1. A 3-week-old boy with septic arthritis of the right shoulder

Fig. 3.1a. Anterior view of the thorax shows total absence of activity in the head of the right humerus

Fig. 3.1b. The posterior view shows the same defect

Teaching Point
1. The absence of activity in the cold joint is more frequently seen in the young child or if there is an effusion with the joint, especially in the hip.
2. The reason why some infected joints show increased activity while others show a photopenic area is uncertain and may relate to the amount of fluid/pus in the joint and the associated pressure effect this may have. Note the importance of multiple views, especially of the small bones to elucidate the extent of the disease.

Case 3.2. A 10-year-old girl with soft tissue swelling around the right humerus, the child was unwell and pyrexial. The final diagnosis was septic arthritis of the right elbow.

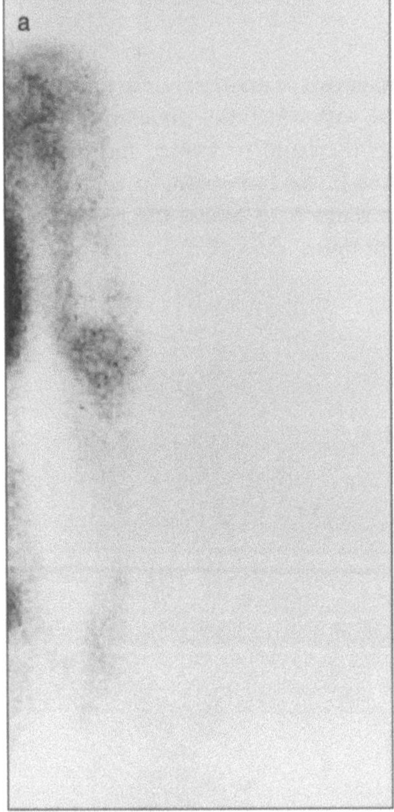

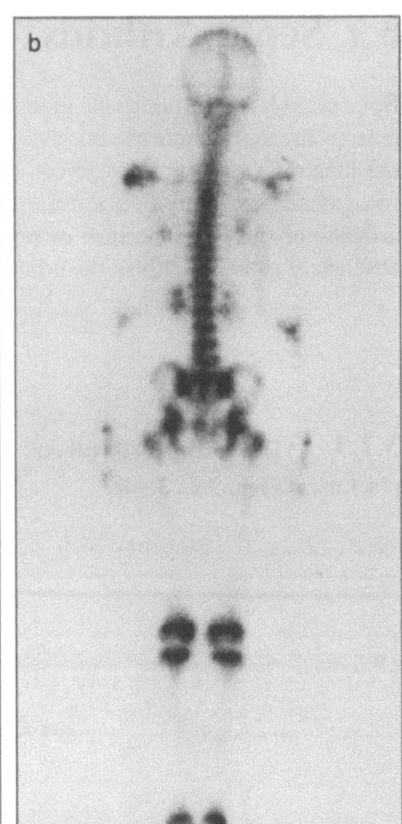

Fig. 3.2a. Blood pool posterior image of the right arm shows abnormal increased uptake of tracer in the region of the right elbow joint

Fig. 3.2b. Whole body scan posterior view. There is abnormal increased uptake of isotope around the right elbow joint. Note the decreased uptake of isotope in the proximal epiphysis of the right humerus

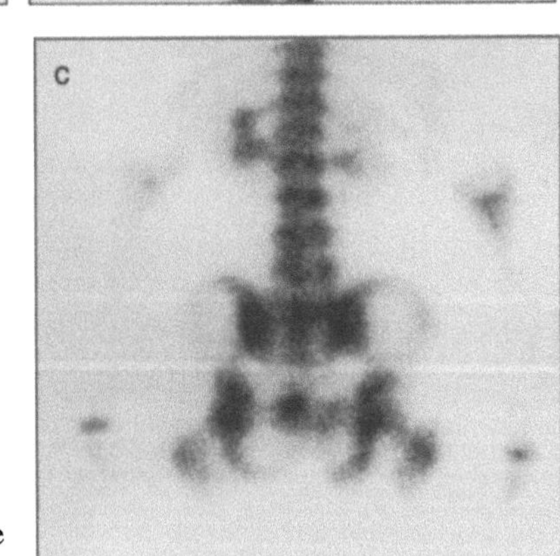

Fig. 3.2c. Posterior image of lumbar spine, pelvis and elbows. This shows that the increased uptake in the right elbow is mainly in the radius and ulna

Teaching Point
Acute disuse of the right upper limb over a week has lead to the decreased activity in the proximal right humeral epiphyseal plate since no infection was present in this joint.

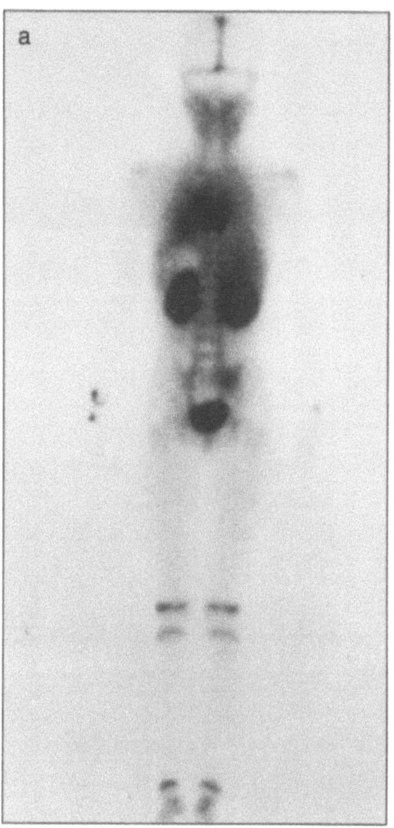

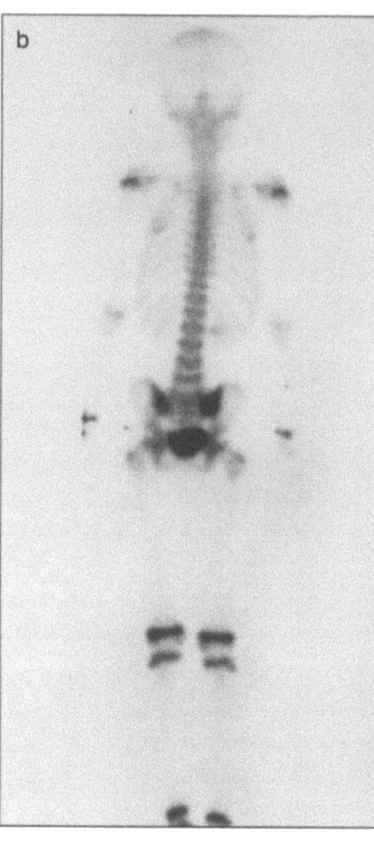

Case 3.3. A 7-year-old boy with back-ache and pyrexia who was generally unwell. Final diagnosis was septic arthritis of the right sacro-iliac joint

Fig. 3.3a. Posterior blood pool whole body scan shows abnormal increased uptake of isotope around the right sacro-iliac joint. Note extravasation of isotope at the injection site in the left hand

Fig. 3.3b. Posterior whole body scan. Asymmetry between the two sacro-iliac joints is noted with marked increased uptake of isotope in the right sacro-iliac joint

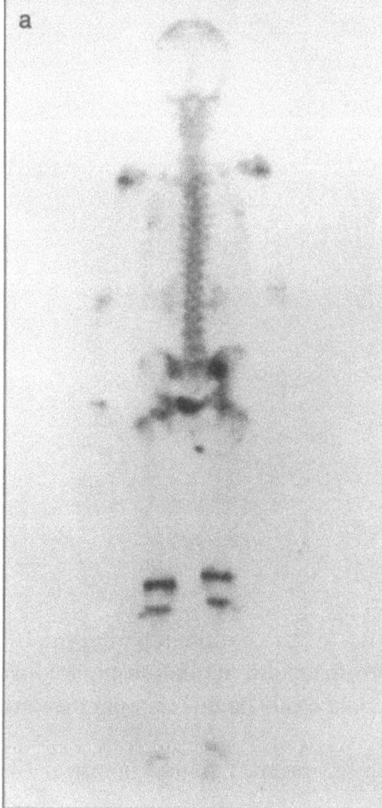

Case 3.4. An 8-year-old girl with backache, pyrexia and signs of sepsis. Final diagnosis was septic arthritis of the right sacro-iliac joint

Fig. 3.4a. Posteroir whole body scan shows increased uptake of isotope in the right sacro-iliac joint

Technical Comment

There is slight rotation of the pelvis; this is presumably the reason for the asymmetry of the hip joints with indistinctness of the epiphyseal plate of the right femoral head. There was no evidence of any sepsis in the right hip.

Teaching Point

Similar appearances may be seen in primary bone tumours (see Case 4.25).

Case 3.5. A 14-year-old boy with recurrent low grade backache and occasional fevers. Final diagnosis was bilateral sacro-ileitis due to clostridium

Fig. 3.5a. Anterior view of the pelvis shows significant abnormal increased uptake of isotope in the left sacro-iliac joint and to a lesser extent in the right sacro-iliac joint

Fig. 3.5b. Posterior view of the pelvis shows, to a better extent, the abnormal uptake in the sacro-iliac joint on the left extending into the iliac wing. The right sacro-iliac joint shows a slight increased uptake of isotope

Fig. 3.5c. Follow-up posterior view of the pelvis 2 years later shows significant improvement in the left sacro-iliac joint and, to some extent, in the right sacro-iliac joint

Fig. 3.5d. Posterior view of the pelvis 3 years following the first scan, when the child still had vague symptoms. This shows asymmetry between the two sacro-iliac joints with improvement on the left, but very little change on the right

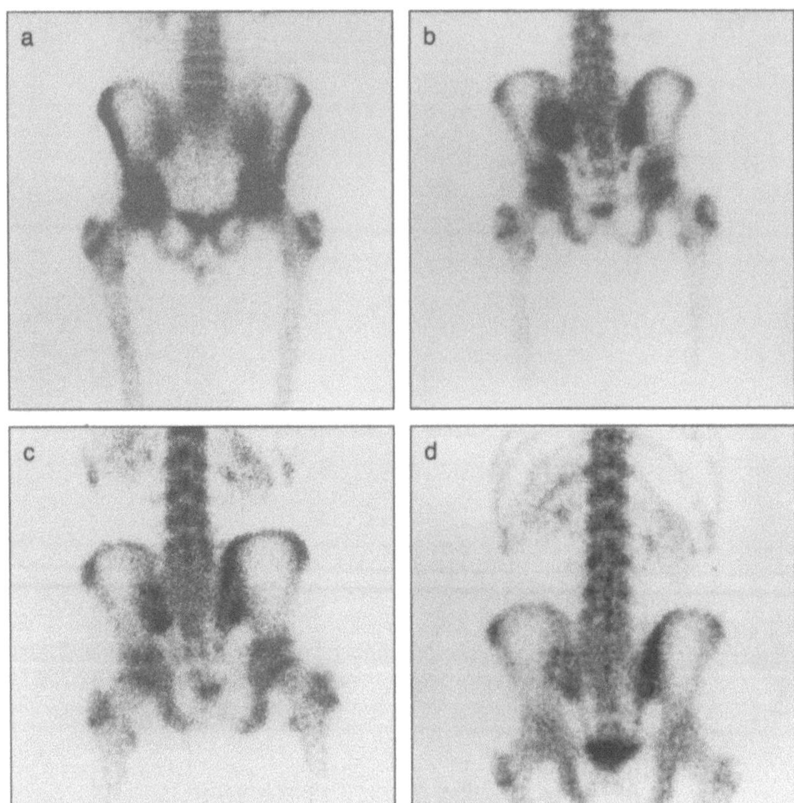

Teaching Point
1. It is difficult to assess the significance of the continuing abnormal increased uptake of isotope in the sacro-iliac joint in relationship to ongoing infection since this appearance could easily be due to reparative new bone formation.
2. Similar appearances may be seen in primary bone tumours (see Case 4.25).

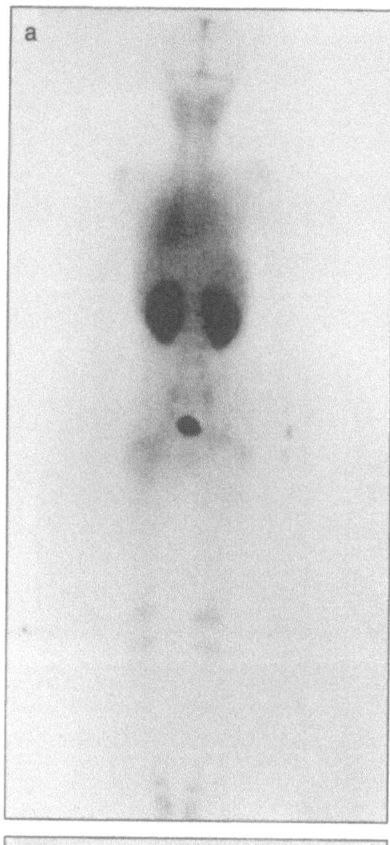

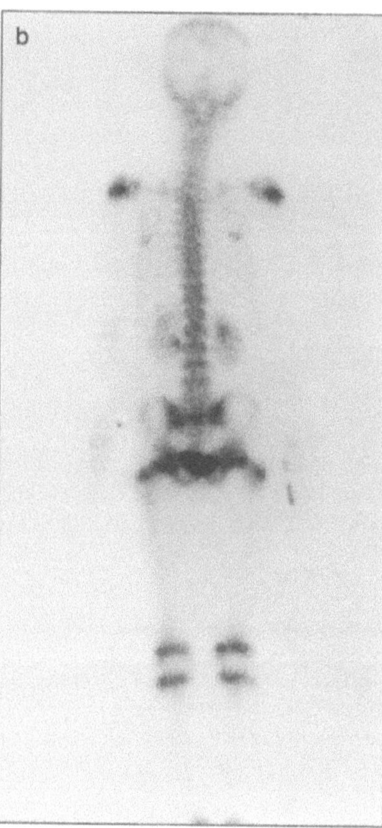

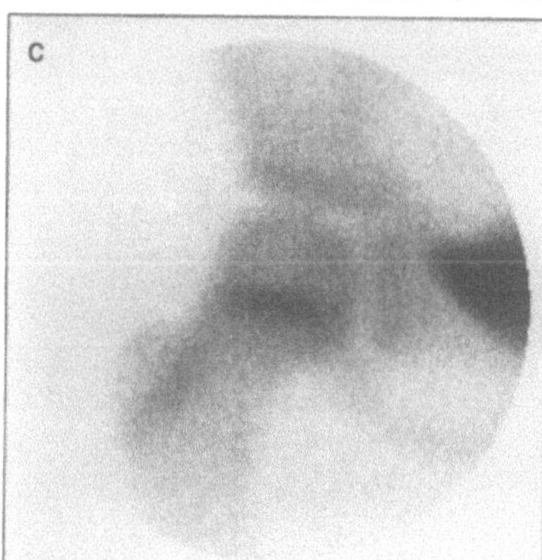

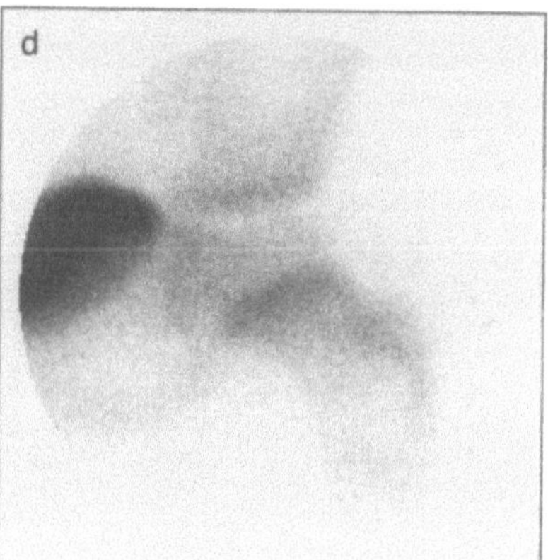

Case 3.6. An 8-year-old boy with acute pain in the left hip. Final diagnosis was septic arthritis of the left hip

Fig. 3.6a. Posterior whole body blood pool image shows slightly increased uptake of isotope in the region of the left hip joint

Fig. 3.6b. Posterior whole body scan is essentially normal

Fig. 3.6c. Pin hole view of the right hip is normal

Fig. 3.6d. Pin hole view of the left hip shows decreased activity in the left femoral head

Teaching Point

Septic arthritis of the hip may have a normal bone scan, this is especially so if only whole body images are obtained and additional posterior and anterior views. Pin hole views are essential but even these may be normal. The decreased activity in Fig. 3.6d presumably is the result of either the infection and/or a joint effusion. The bone scan has failed to show any evidence of osteomyetitis associated with the septic hip.

Case 3.7. A 7-year-old girl with septicaemia and pain in the hip. Final diagnosis was septic arthritis of the right hip

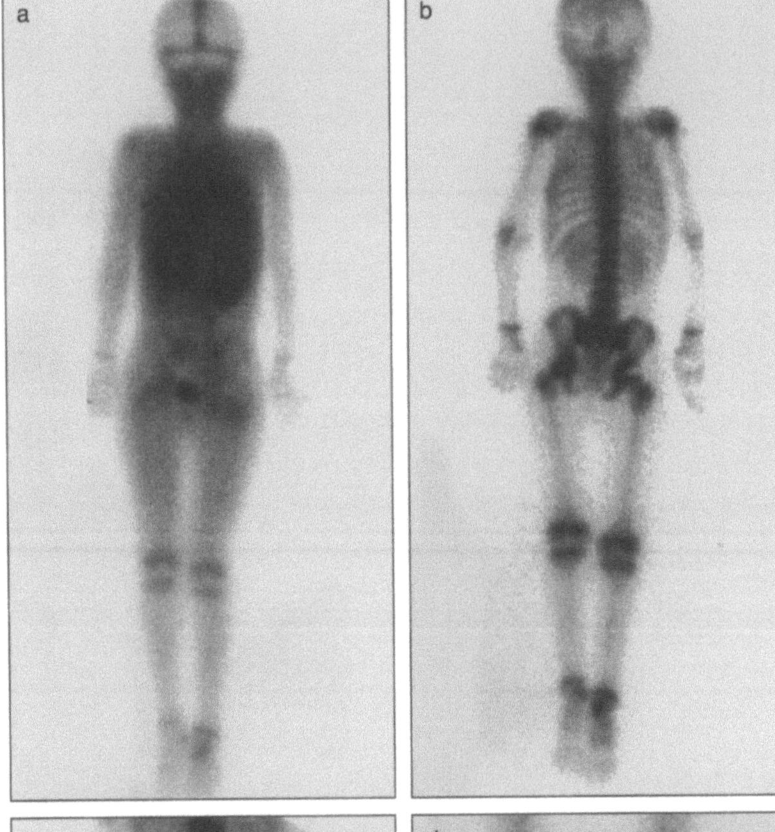

Fig. 3.7a. Posterior whole body blood pool image shows no definite abnormality in the hips, but there is slight increased activity in the right foot and ankle

Fig. 3.7b. Posterior whole body scan shows decreased activity in the region of the right femoral head. Increased activity is noted in the right hind foot

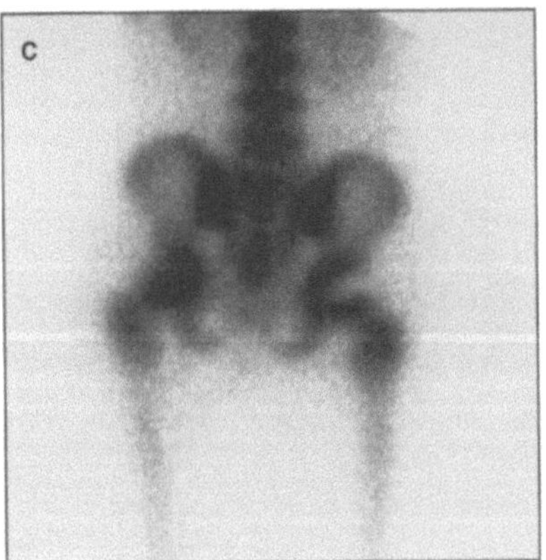

Fig. 3.7c. Posterior view of the pelvis shows absent activity in the right femoral head

Fig. 3.7d. Posterior view of the feet shows generalised increased uptake of isotope throughout the right foot with focal abnormal increased uptake in the posterior bones

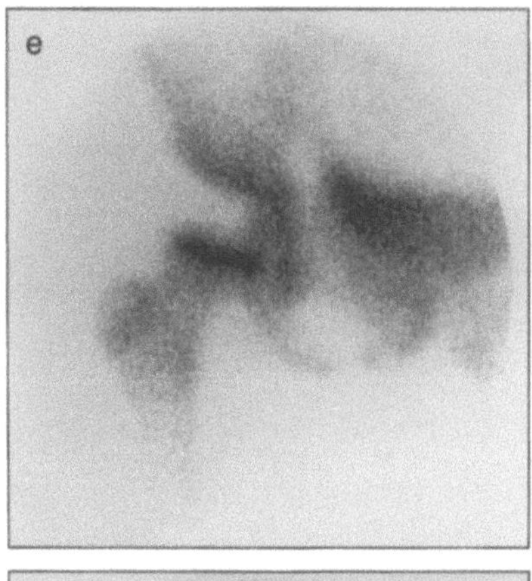

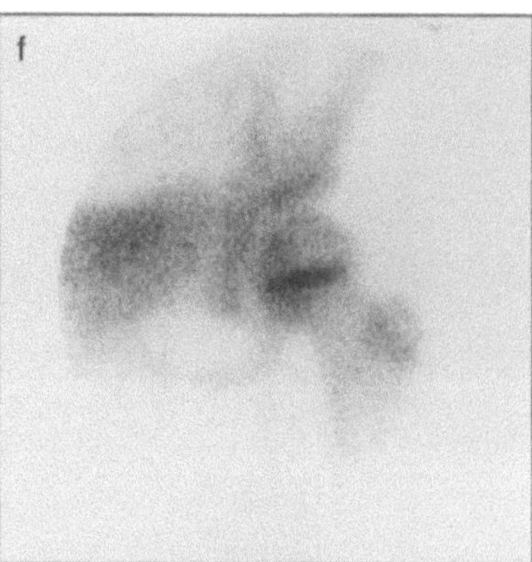

Fig. 3.7e. Pin hole image of the right hip 1 month later shows total absence of activity in the region of the femoral head with, however, preservation of the epiphyseal plate

Fig. 3.7f. Pin hole view of the left hip is normal

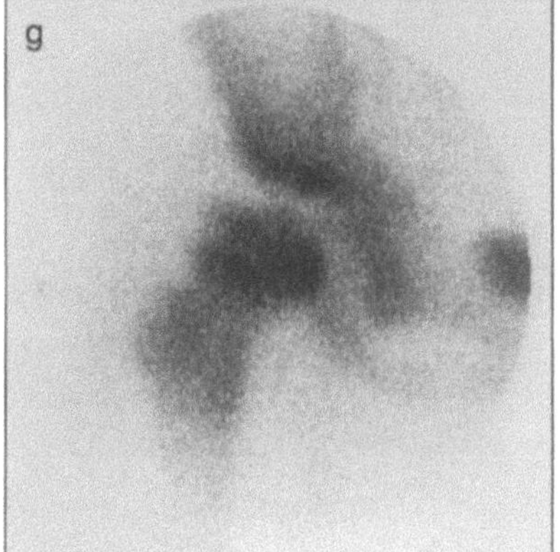

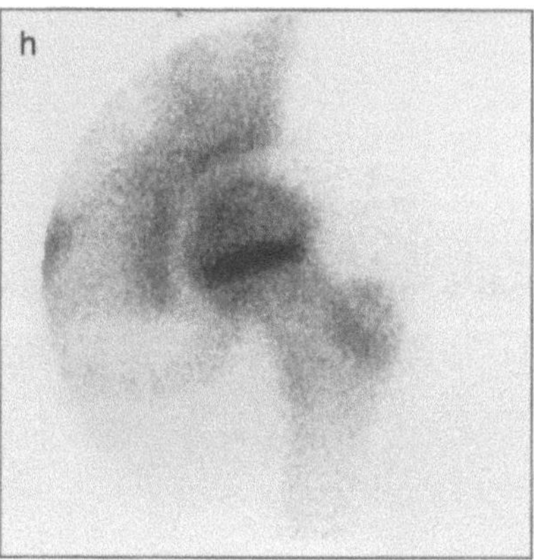

Fig. 3.7g. Follow-up scan 3 months following presentation shows revascularisation of the right femoral head

Fig. 3.7h. Pin hole view of the left hip is normal

Teaching Point

1. In the presence of septic arthritis with no involvement of the adjacent bones, the isotope scan may simply show a cold area which, on this occasion, has caused destruction of the femoral head.
2. Similar appearances of the hip may be seen in Legg-Perthes' disease (see Chap. 6.1).
3. The cause for the increased activity in the right foot was never established. Since the child was treated with antibiotics it remains speculative as to whether there could have been osteomyelitis in the foot.

Case 3.8. A 4-year-old boy with pain in the right hip who was acutely unwell. Final diagnosis was septic arthritis of the right hip

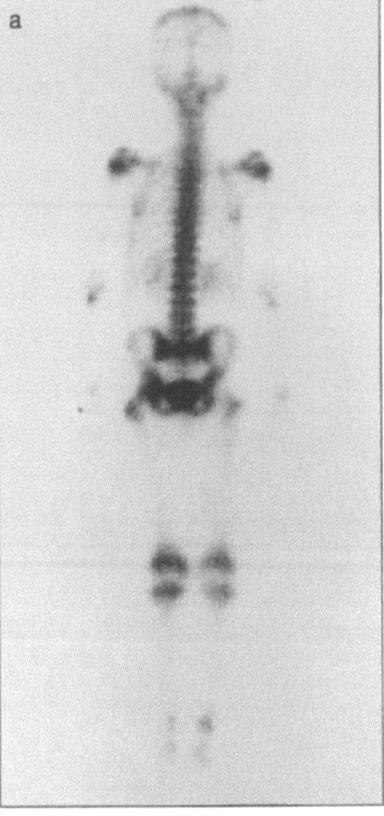

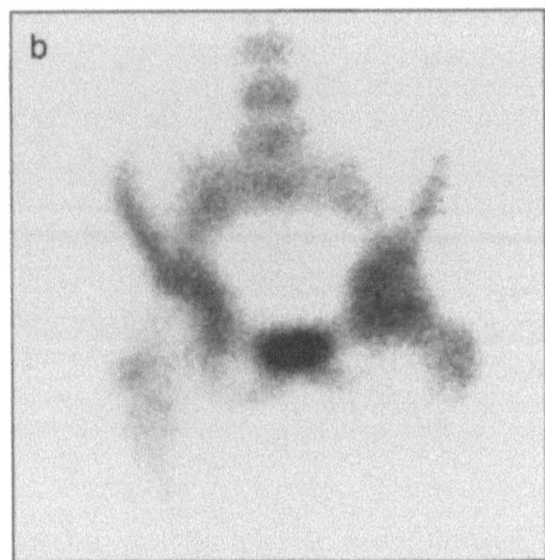

Fig. 3.8a. Posterior whole body scan shows decreased activity in the region of the right femoral capital epiphysis with decreased uptake throughout the growth plates of the right knee

Fig. 3.8b. Anterior view of the pelvis shows total absence of activity in the region of the femoral head and neck with decreased activity in the region of the greater trochanter on the right

Teaching Point

The effect of acute immobilisation on the long bones may be the cause of the decreased uptake of isotope in the growth plates with lack of their normal clarity (also see Case 7.33).

Case 3.9. An 11-month-old boy with septic arthritis of the right knee

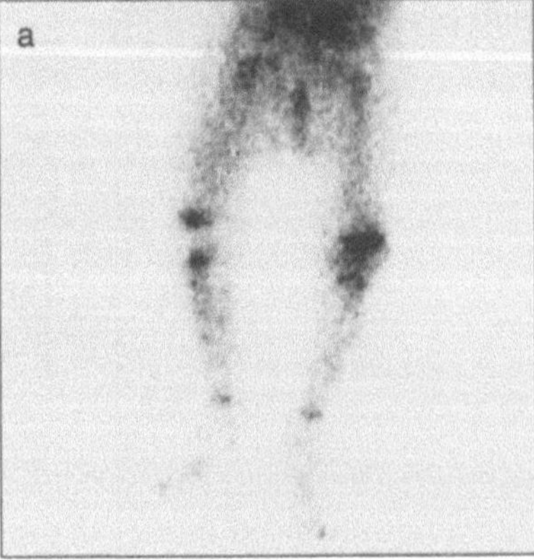

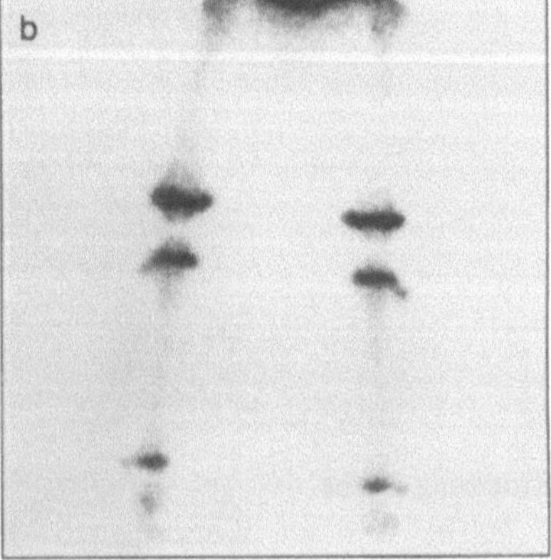

Fig. 3.9a. Posterior blood pool image of the pelvis and lower limbs shows marked increased activity around the right knee. Note the poor positioning of the feet compared to Fig. 3.9b

Fig. 3.9b. Anterior view of the knees shows minimal increased activity in the right distal femoral shaft immediately adjacent to the epiphyseal plate

Teaching Point

If blood pool images are not obtained when infection is suspected, then the diagnosis of septic arthritis becomes more difficult since the 3-h static images may either be normal or show very subtle abnormalities possibly related to the hyperaemia

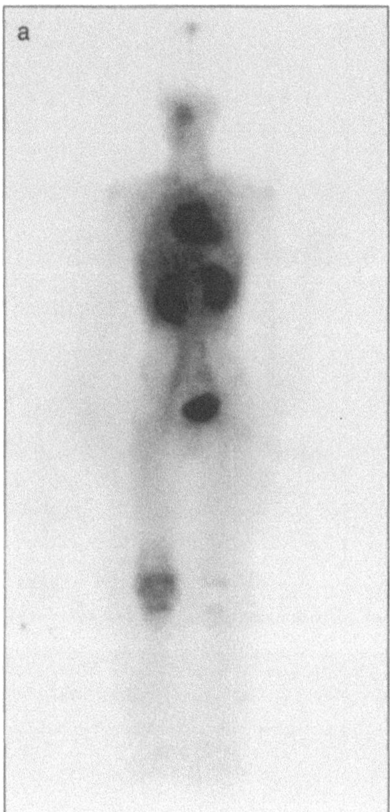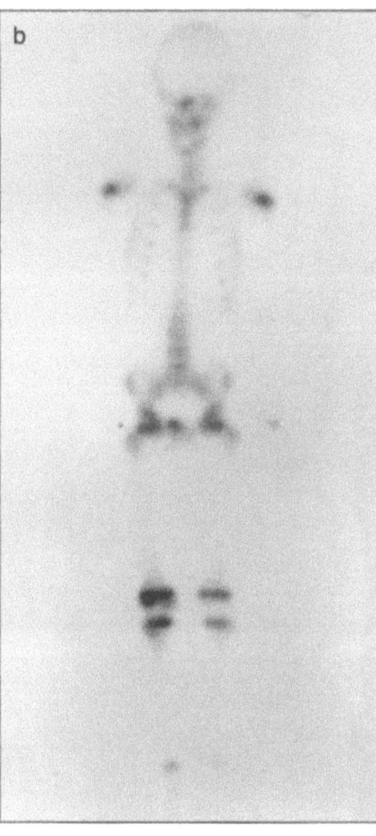

Case 10. A 5-year-old girl with septic arthritis of the right knee and infection of the patella. The child presented with pain and had septicaemia

Fig. 3.10a. Anterior whole body blood pool image shows marked increased activity in the region of the right hip and thigh but most marked around the right knee

Fig. 3.10b. Whole body anterior image shows increased uptake of isotope in the epiphyseal plates around the right knee and ankle

Teaching Point
The increased activity in the growth plates in the presence of acute infection does not indicate osteomyelitis of the adjacent bone but probably reflects the hyperaemia. High-quality spot images of the epiphyseal plates are essential in order to diagnose any underlying osteomyelitis

Case 3.11. An 8-year-old girl with septic arthritis of the left knee

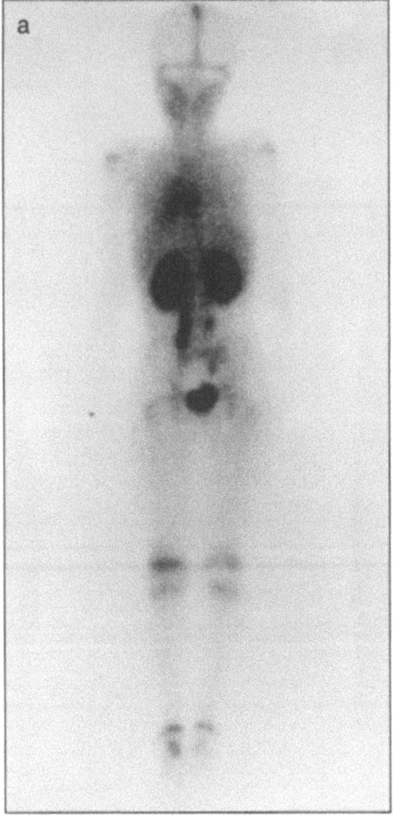

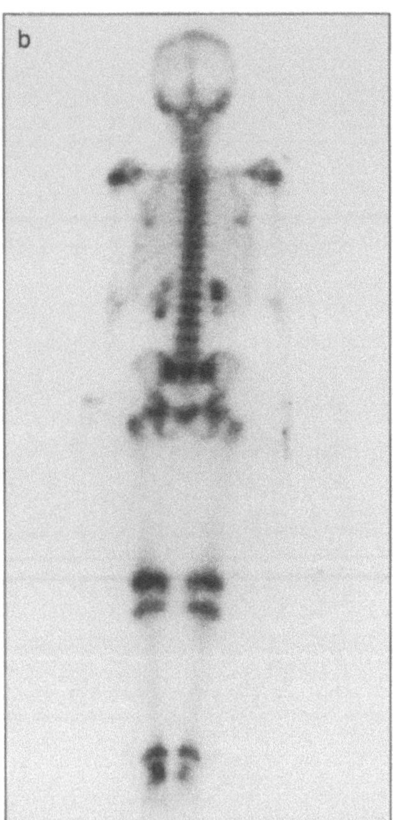

Fig. 3.11a. Posterior whole body blood pool image shows increased uptake of isotope in the epiphyseal plate in the distal left femur and also in the region of the left foot

Fig. 3.11b. Posterior whole body scan shows marked increased uptake of isotope in the distal epiphyseal plate of the left femur as well as increased uptake of isotope around the ankle joint and in the foot on the left

Technical Comment

The appearances of the dilated left ureter on the blood pool whole body image is not borne out on the 3-h whole body image, where the left kidney appears normal.

Teaching Point

Joint aspiration from the knee and blood cultures were both positive and the child was treated with antibiotics. The reason for the increased uptake around the left foot was uncertain. There may have been associated infection in the foot but this was unproven.

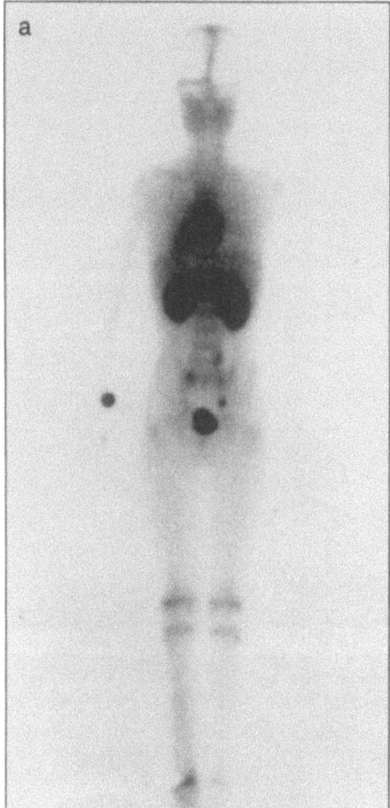

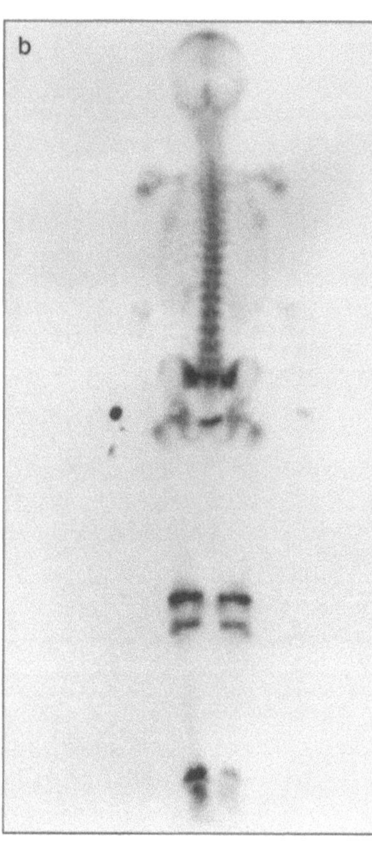

Case 3.12. A 9-year-old girl with septic arthritis of the left ankle

Fig. 3.12a. Posterior whole body blood pool image shows diffuse increased uptake of isotope in the left distal lower limb and left foot

Fig. 3.12b. Posterior whole body image shows focal abnormal increased uptake of isotope in the distal left tibial and fibula epiphyseal plates as well as in the small bones of the foot. Also note the increased activity in the epiphyseal plates around the left knee

Technical Comment

Note extravasation of isotope at the site of the injection in the left hand.

Teaching Point

Aspiration showed septic arthritis of the ankle. The blood pool image suggests that infection was more extensive than simply septic arthritis of the ankle joint and thus hyperaemia is probably the cause of the increased uptake at the growth plates around the left knee. There was no evidence of osteomyelitis in the tibia or fibula.

Case 3.13. A 5-year-old infant with septicaemia due to septic arthritis involving the calcaneus and talus of the left foot

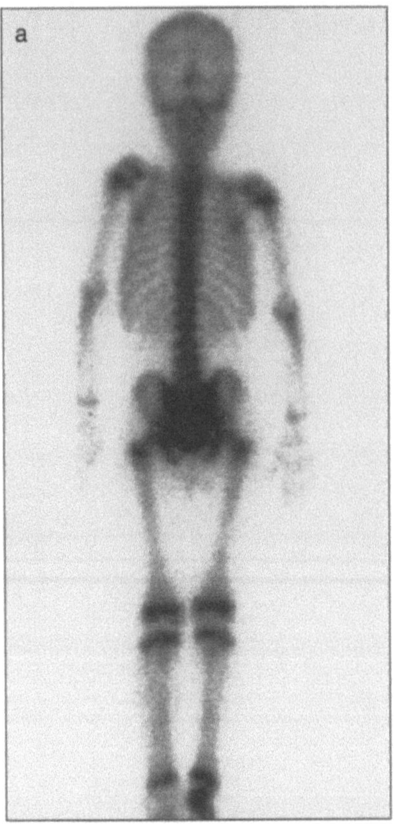

Fig. 3.13a. Posterior whole body image shows decreased uptake of isotope in the left distal tibial epiphysis and also in the foot

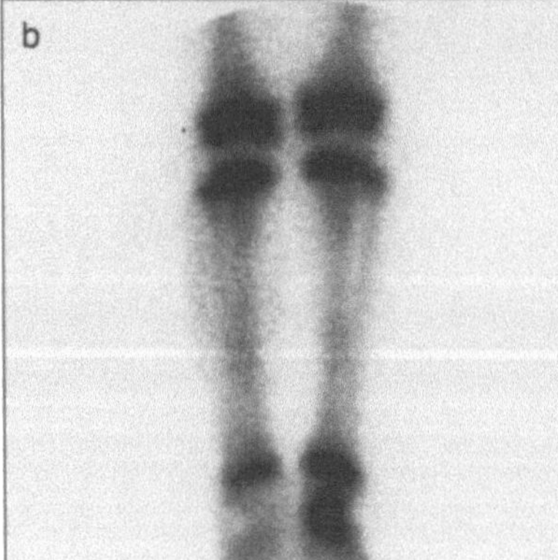

Fig. 3.13b. Posterior view of lower limbs shows generalised decreased activity around the left ankle with further decreased activity in the small bones of the foot

Fig. 3.13c. Lateral view of the feet shows total absence of activity in the left calcaneus and talus

Teaching Point
The reason why some infected joints show increased activity while others show a photopenic area is uncertain and may relate to the amount of fluid/pus in the joint and the associated pressure effect this may have. Note the importance of multiple views, especially in the small bones of the foot to elucidate the extent of the disease.

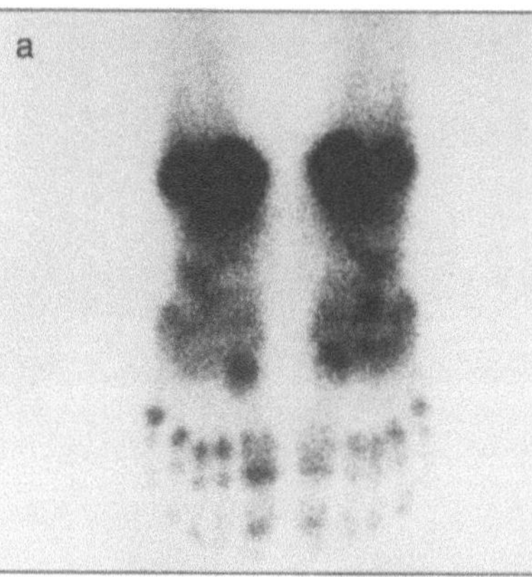

Case 3.14. A 10-year-old boy with pain and evidence of infection in the right lower limb due to septic arthritis of the left first metatarsophalangeal joint

Fig. 3.14a. Posterior view of the feet shows increased activity around the left first metatarsophalangeal joint

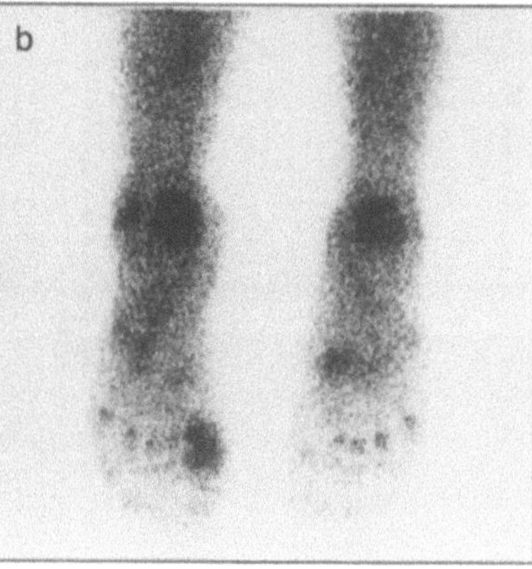

Fig. 3.14b. Posterior blood pool view of the feet at follow-up 3 years later shows marked increased activity around the base of the big toe of the left foot

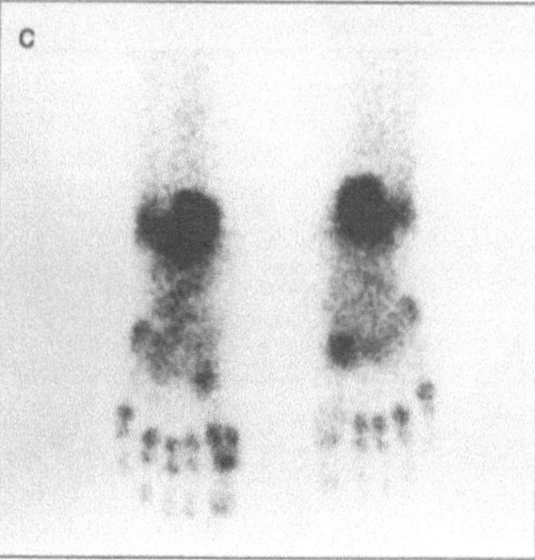

Fig. 3.14c. Posterior view of the feet shows increased uptake of isotope around the first metatarsophalangeal joint. Evidence of chronic osteomyelitis had developed by this stage

3.1.2 Multifocal Arthritis
(2 Cases; Figs. 3.15, 3.16)

Case 3.15. A 6-year-old boy with septicaemia who refused to walk. Final diagnosis was that of multifocal septic arthritis involving the right elbow, left foot and right hip

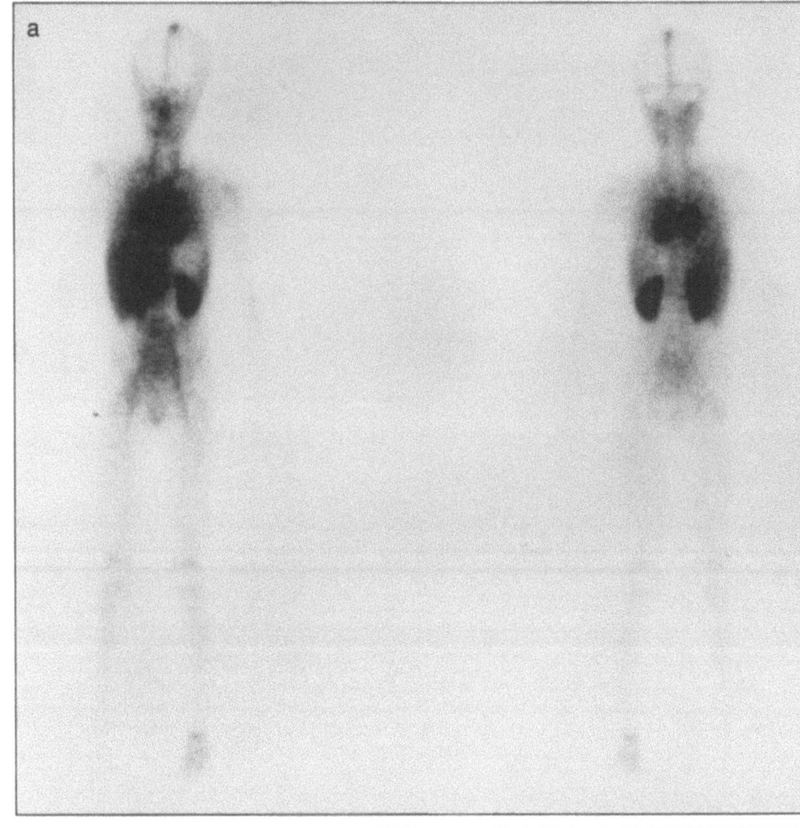

Fig. 3.15a. Blood pool whole body images show increased uptake of isotope in the left foot only

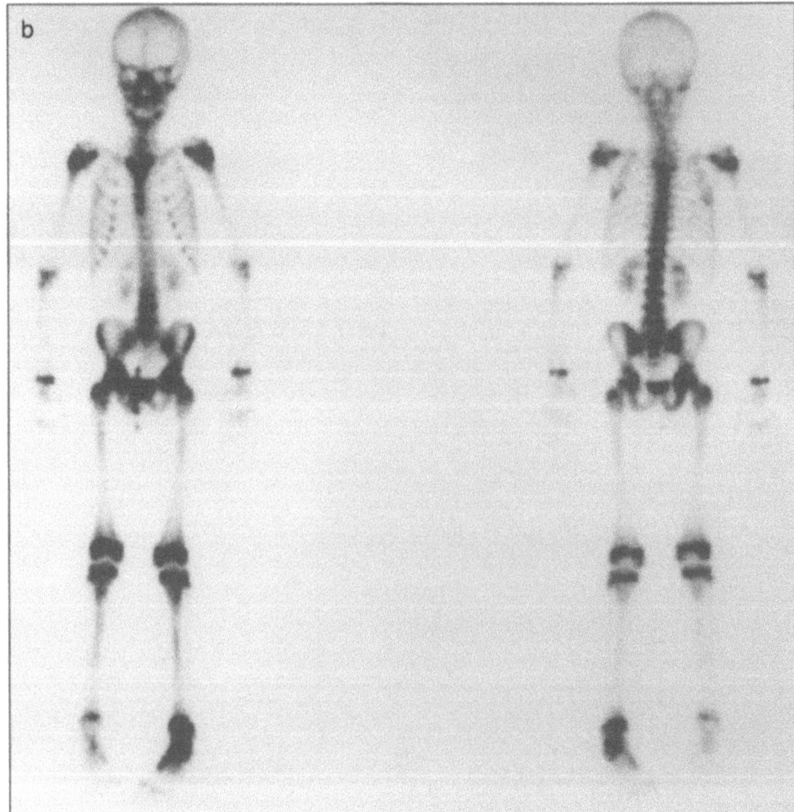

Fig. 3.15b. Whole body scans show abnormal increased uptake of isotope around the left ankle and small bones of the left foot as well as increased uptake of isotope in the right hip (posterior view only) and also around the right elbow

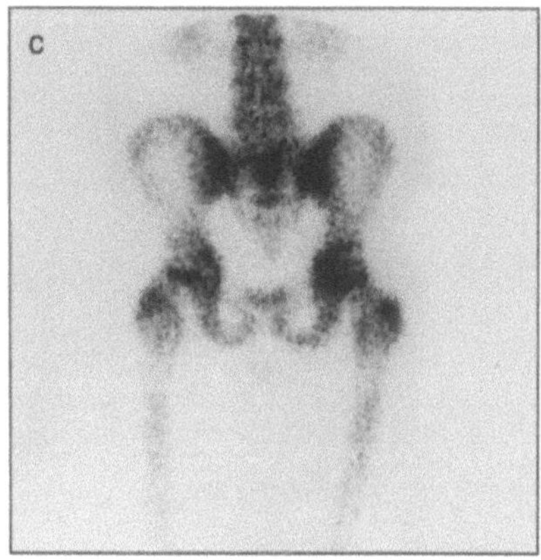 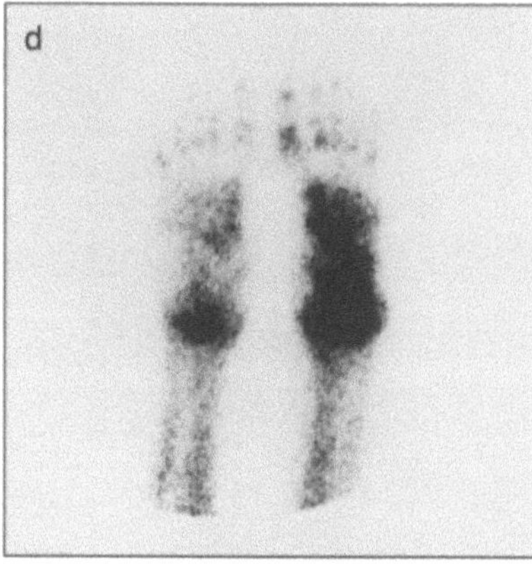

Fig. 3.15c. Posterior view of the pelvis shows asymmetry between the two hip joints with increased uptake on the right compared to the left

Fig. 3.15d. Plantar view of the feet shows increased uptake of isotope in the small bones of the left foot

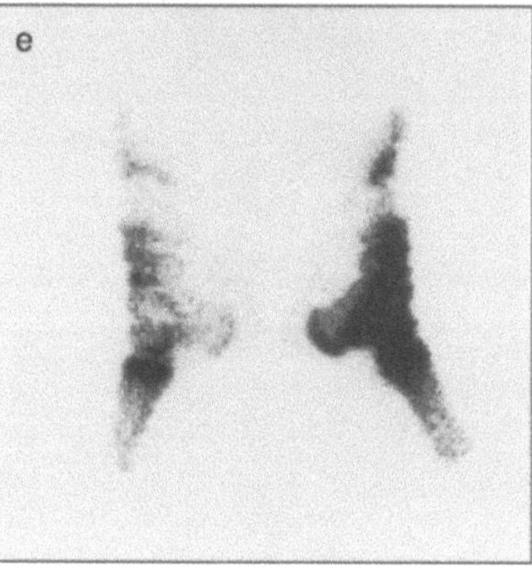

Fig. 3.15e. Lateral view of the feet shows to better advantage that all the small bones of the left foot are involved with slight sparing of the calcaneus

Teaching Point
When infection is suspected, it is important to scan the entire skeleton since multifocal infection may be present.

Case 3.16. An 11-year-old boy with septic arthritis of the right hip and right ankle

Fig. 3.16a. Blood pool whole body image (posterior view) shows marked asymmetry between the hip joints with decreased uptake of isotope in the right hip compared to the left. Asymmetry is also noted around the ankles with increased uptake in the right ankle compared to the left

Fig. 3.16b. Whole body scan (posterior view) shows virtually total absence of activity in the region of the right hip joint whilst the right ankle shows increased activity. Note increased activity throughout both kidneys

Fig. 3.16c. Posterior view of the ankles shows significantly increased activity around the right ankle with loss of clarity of the distal tibial epiphyseal plate

Fig. 3.16d. Lateral view of the feet shows increased activity around the right ankle and slightly increased activity in the calcaneus and talus of the right foot, but no focal increased activity to suggest osteomyelitis in addition to the septic arthritis

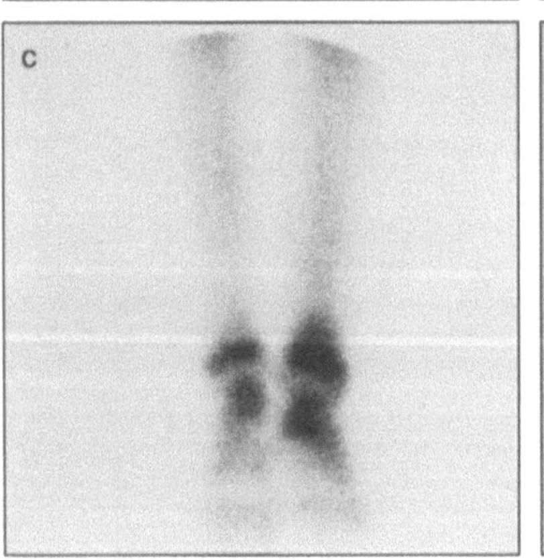

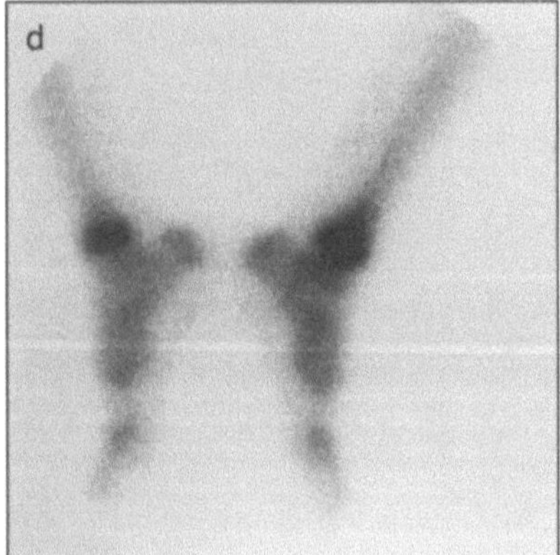

Technical Comment
Note extravasation of isotope in the left hand, the site of the injection.

Teaching Point
Note that the hip shows up as a "cold lesion", while the ankle is "hot". The former is presumably due to the effusion into the hip joint.

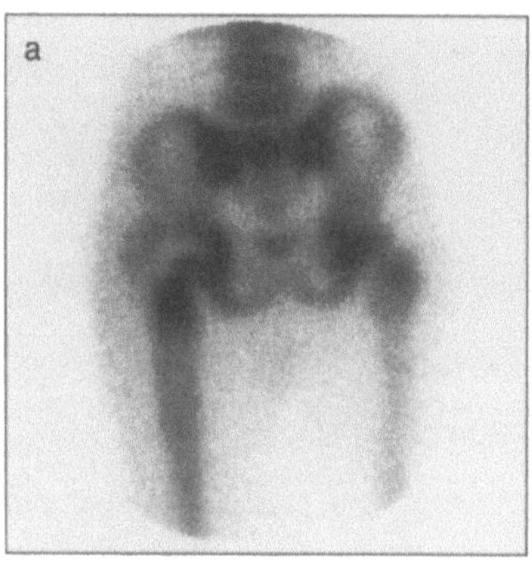 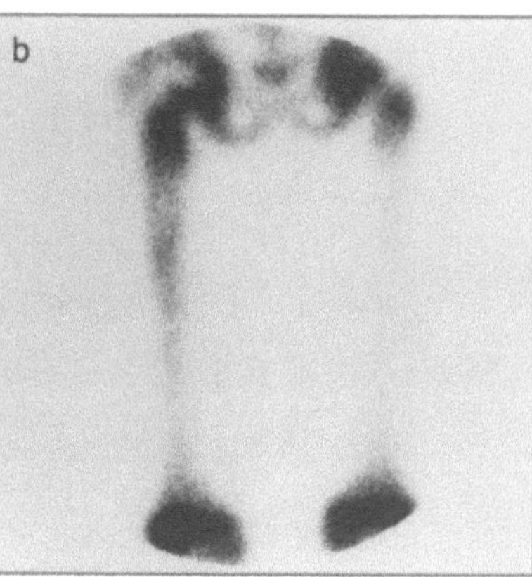

3.1.3 Osteomyelitis as a Complication of Septic Arthritis
(4 Cases; Figs. 3.17–3.20)

Case 3.17. A 4-year-old boy with septic arthritis of the left hip

Fig. 3.17a. Posterior view of the pelvis shows absent activity in the left femoral head with abnormal increase of isotope in the soft tissue lateral to the left hip and in the shaft of the femur

Fig. 3.17b. Posterior view of the femora shows abnormal increased uptake of isotope in the upper third of the shaft of the left femur with a second area in the mid portion of the femur due to osteomyelitis as a complication of the septic arthritis. Absent activity in the left femoral head is again noted

Teaching Point

The accumulation of isotope in the soft tissue adjacent to the septic hip represented an abscess.

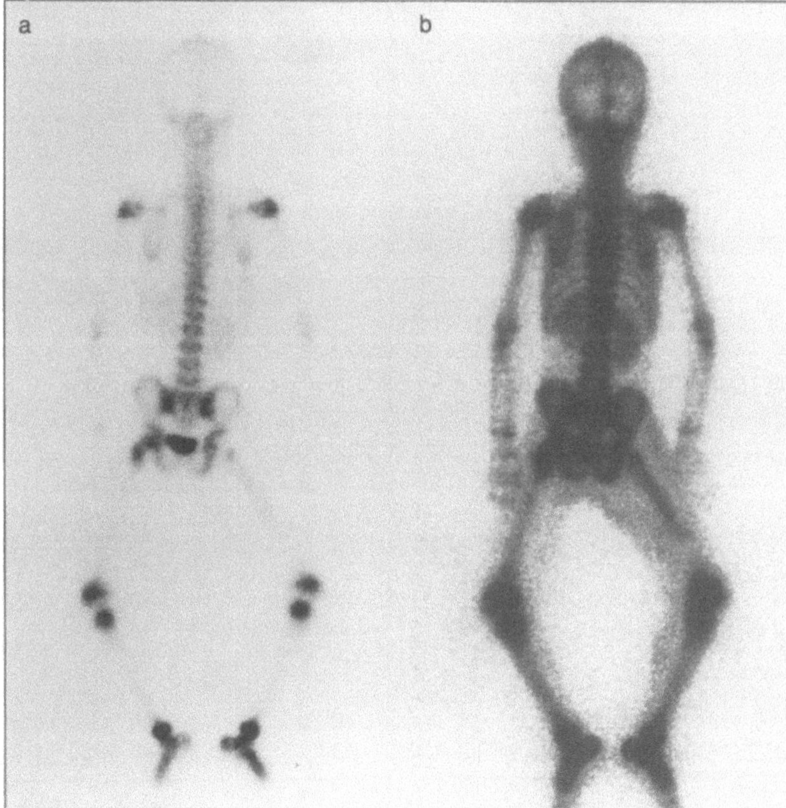

Case 3.18. A 7-year-old boy with pain in the right hip and a limp. Final diagnosis was septic arthritis of the right hip and osteomyelitis of the femur

Fig. 3.18a. Whole body posterior view. The underexposed film shows absence of activity in the region of the right femoral head and neck with decreased activity in the greater trochanter

Fig. 3.18b. Whole body posterior view. The overexposed film reveals a cold area in the distal right femur due to osteomyelitis

Technical Comment

The septic arthritis of the right hip prevents ideal positioning of the lower limbs.

Case 3.19. An 8-year-old boy with septic arthritis of the right hip and osteomyelitis of the femur

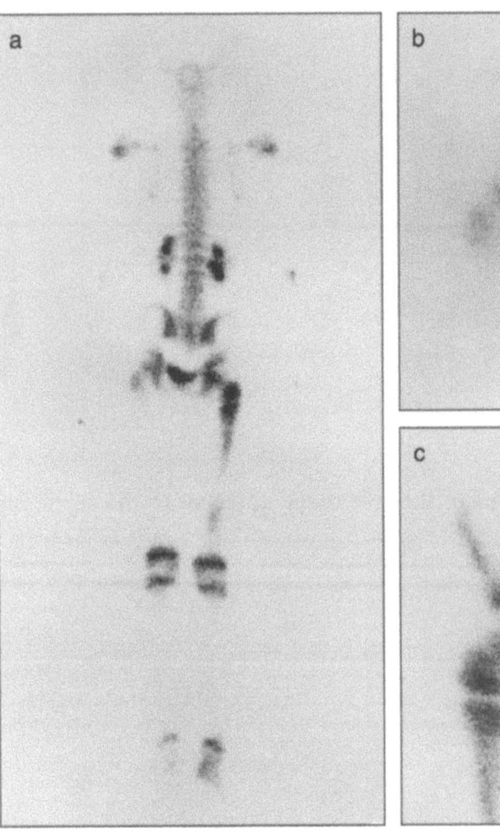

Fig. 3.19a. Whole body scan (posterior view) shows both increased and decreased activity in the right femoral head as well as areas of increased activity of different intensity along the shaft of the right femur and in the right foot

Fig. 3.19b. Posterior view of the pelvis shows an area of total absence of activity and an area of increased activity in the right hip with two areas of abnormal increased activity in the femoral shaft

Fig. 3.19c. Anterior view of the pelvis shows the further extension of the abnormal activity in the right femur into the mid shaft of this bone

Case 3.20. A 4-year-old girl with a long history of being unwell due to osteomyelitis of the right tibia as well as septic arthritis of the right ankle. (This is the same child as in Case 2.15)

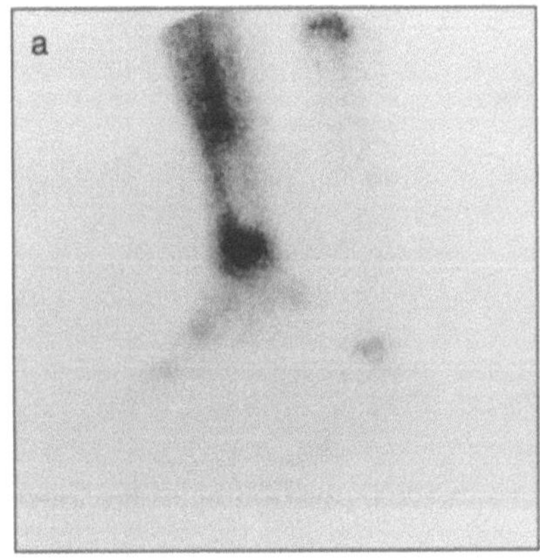
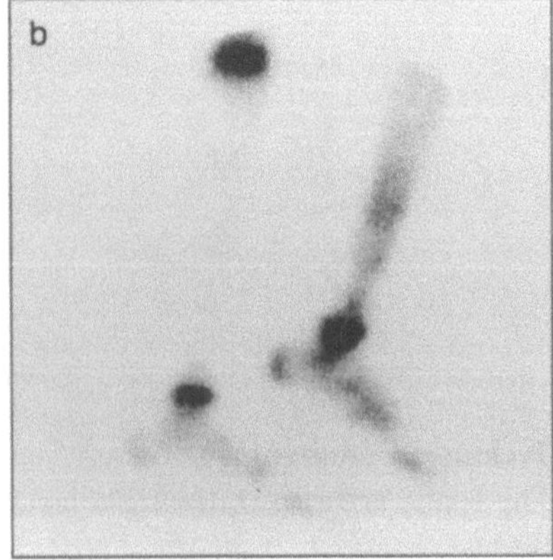

Fig. 3.20a. Lateral blood pool image of the lower limbs shows focal increased uptake in the mid third of the right tibia and the ankle and decreased activity in the lower third of the tibia

Fig. 3.20b. Lateral view of the ankles and feet shows increased activity in the mid third of the right tibia and ankle

3.2 Aseptic Arthritis

3.2.1 Inflammatory Arthritis
(4 Cases; Figs. 3.21–3.24)

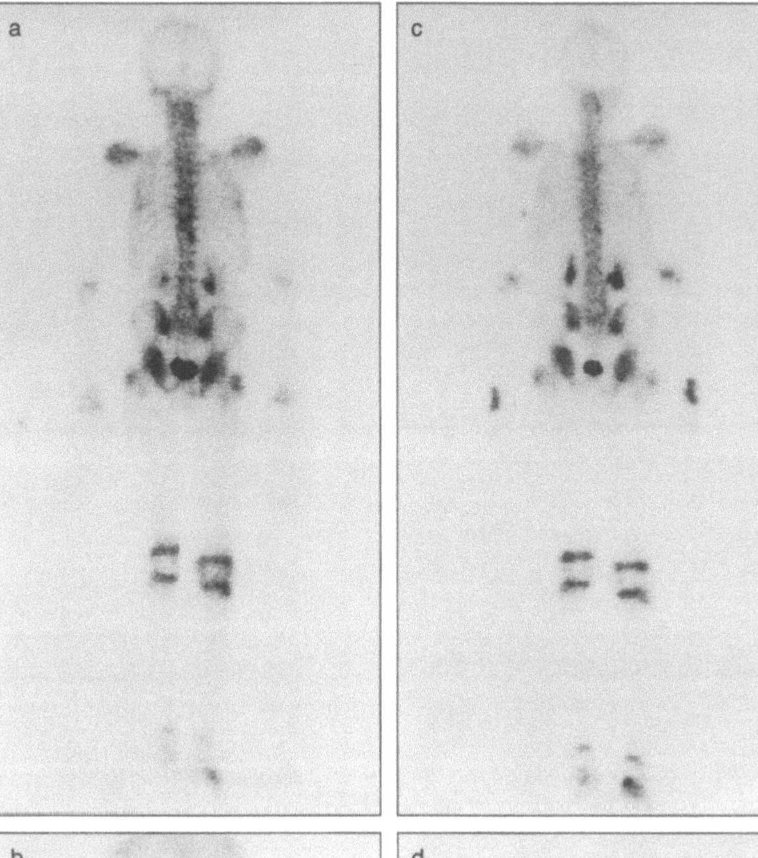

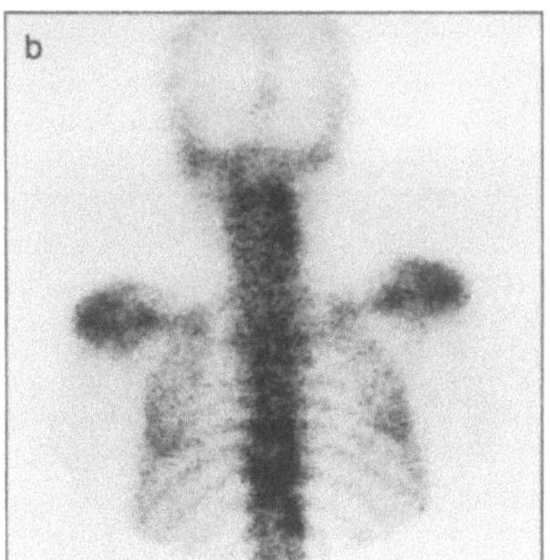

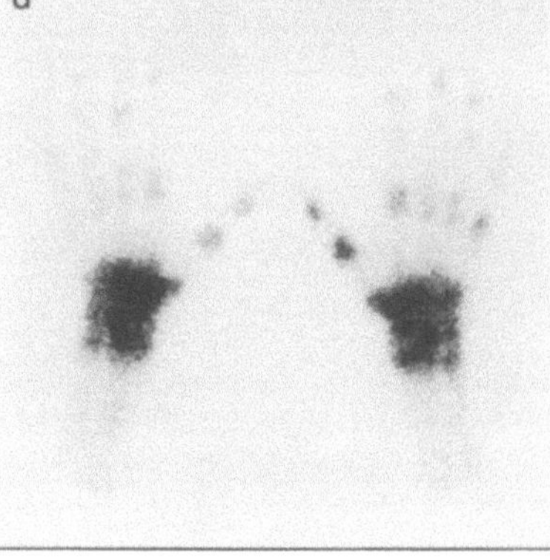

Case 3.21. A 12-year-old girl with severe juvenile rheumatoid arthritis

Fig. 3.21a. Whole body scan (posterior view) shows abnormal uptake in the lower dorsal spine. The epiphyseal plates of the upper limbs and around the ankles are poorly defined. Asymmetry in the feet is noted

Fig. 3.21b. Posterior view of the dorsal and cervical spine shows abnormal increased uptake in the vertebral bodies.
A follow up scan was undertaken 2 years later

Fig. 3.21c. Whole body scan (posterior view) shows abnormal increased uptake of isotope around the wrists. There has been significant improvement in the spine. Asymmetry in the feet is noted

Fig. 3.21d. Palmar view of the hands shows diffuse abnormal increased uptake of isotope in both wrist joints as well as in the interphalangeal joints of the right thumb

Teaching Point
The asymmetry in the feet is of uncertain significance. This could be related to the disease process itself, but the possibility of other pathology cannot be excluded on the bone scan alone.

Case 3.22. A 13-year-old boy with pain in the right knee and ankle, the knee was hot and swollen. Aspiration failed to show any infection and a biopsy was taken which showed juvenile rheumatoid arthritis

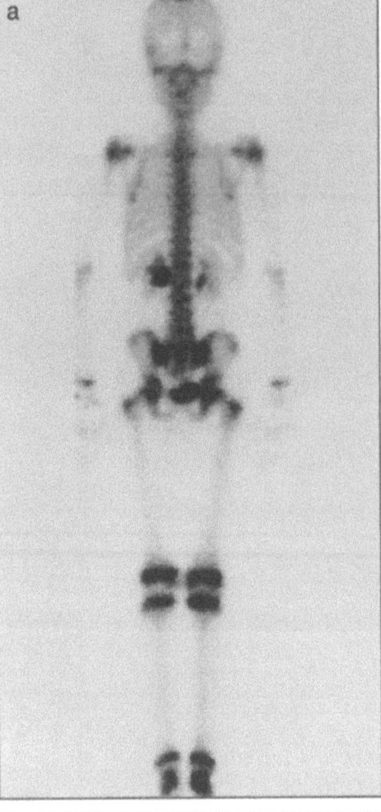

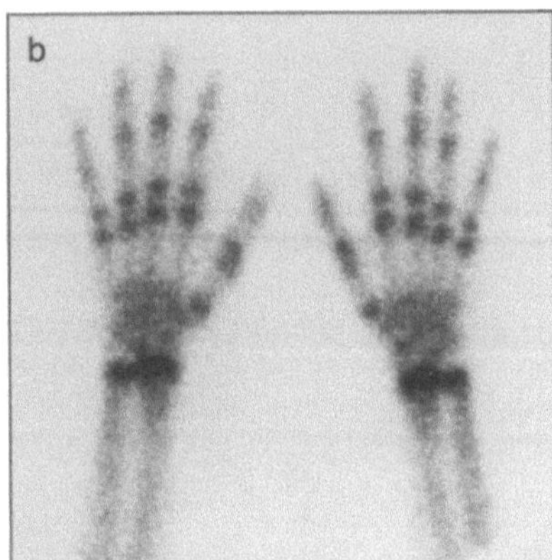

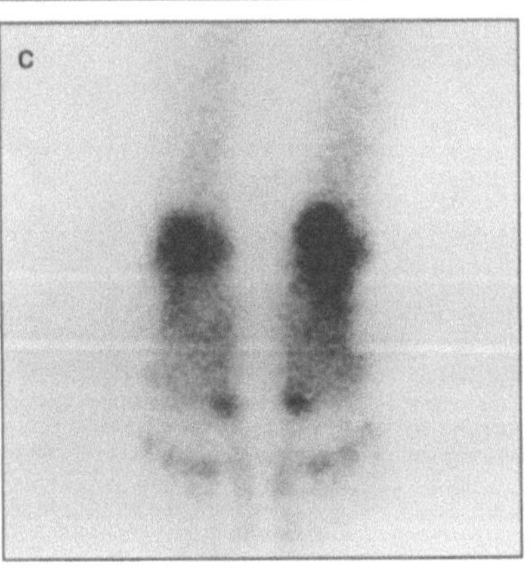

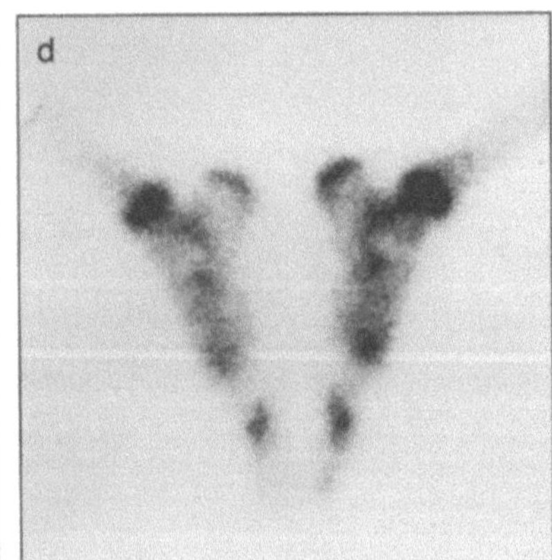

Fig. 3.22a. Whole body scan (posterior view) shows increased uptake in the right knee joint and also around the right ankle. Increased activity is seen in the left renal pelvis

Fig. 3.22b. Palmar view of the hands shows increased activity in the metacarpophalangeal joints

Fig. 3.22c. Posterior view of the feet shows increased activity in the right ankle

Fig. 3.22d. Lateral view of the feet shows the increased activity mainly in the ankle joint and talus of the right foot

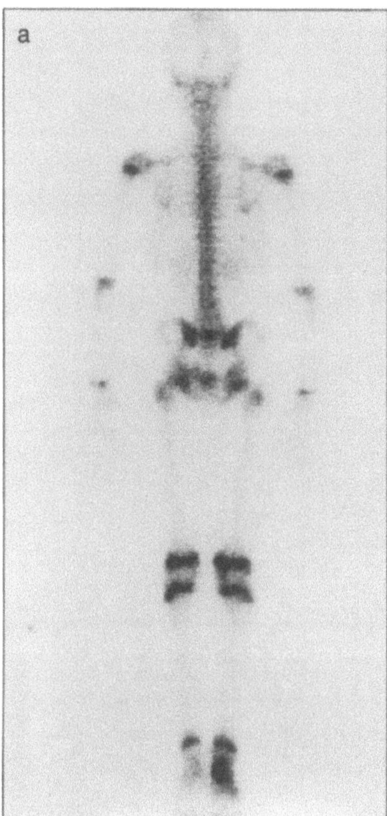

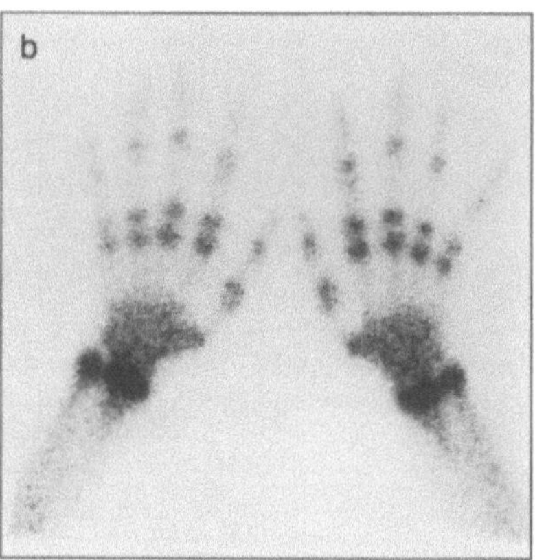

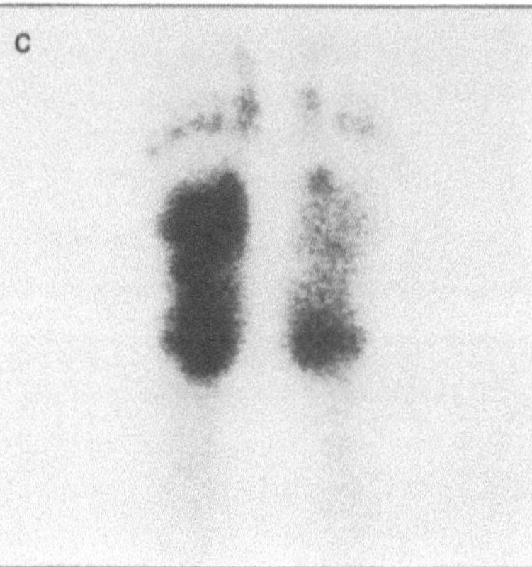

Case 3.23. A 9-year-old girl with a swollen right foot and pain in the left index finger due to juvenile rheumatoid arthritis

Fig. 3.23a. Whole body image shows increased uptake of isotope in the right foot. The hands are poorly seen

Fig. 3.23b. Anterior view of the hands shows abnormal increased uptake of isotope in the proximal interphalangeal joint of the index finger on the left as well as in the metacarpophalangeal joints of the index, middle and ring fingers on the left

Fig. 3.23c. Posterior view of the feet shows generalised increased uptake of isotope throughout the right ankle and foot as well as in the toes

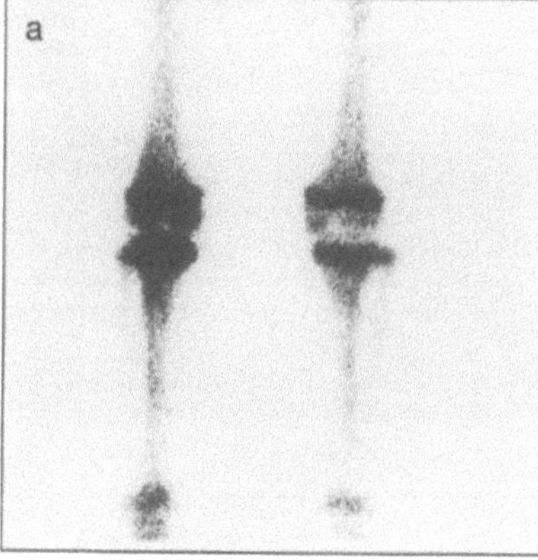

Case 3.24. A 6-year-old girl with rheumatoid arthritis of the left knee and ankle

Fig. 3.24a. Posterior view of the lower limbs shows increased uptake of isotope throughout the left knee with loss of clarity of the epiphyseal plates around the knee and increased uptake of isotope extending into the diaphysis. There is also increased uptake of isotope around the left ankle

Teaching Point

The appearances of the left knee, tibia and ankle are not specific for rheumatoid arthritis and similar appearances could be due to other pathology.

3.2.2 Irritable Hip
(5 Cases; Figs. 3.25–3.29)

Teaching Point

The irritable hip (or transient synovitis) may be either normal on bone scan or show increased activity, as demonstrated below. The main differential diagnosis to be considered is that of Legg-Perthes' disease. The clinical symptoms and signs may be very similar. Differentiation between the irritable hip and Legg-Perthes' disease is then readily made. Less commonly, the hip may show decreased activity and yet return to normal with no changes on X-ray to support the diagnosis of Legg-Perthes' disease. In the early phase with this appearance, differentiation from Legg-Perthes' disease is very difficult. Please compare the images in this section with those in Chap. 6.1, "Legg-Perthes' Disease".

Case 3.25. A 5-year-old girl with pain in the right hip and limping due to transient synovitis

Fig. 3.25a. Posterior view of the pelvis shows asymmetry between the two hip joints with slight increased activity in the right hip compared to the left

Fig. 3.25b. Anterior view of the pelvis fails to show any abnormality

Fig. 3.25c. Posterior magnification view of the pelvis shows the slight increased activity in the right hip involving the roof of the acetabulum as well as the femoral head

Fig. 3.25d. Pin-hole view of the right hip shows generalised increased uptake of isotope in the acetabulum and throughout the femoral head. Note the preservation of the epiphyseal plate

Fig. 3.25e. Pin hole view of the left hip. This is normal

Technical Comment
The settings of the gamma camera for these two pin hole images were the same. Figure 3.25c was acquired with magnification, it is not a post-acquisition computer magnification.

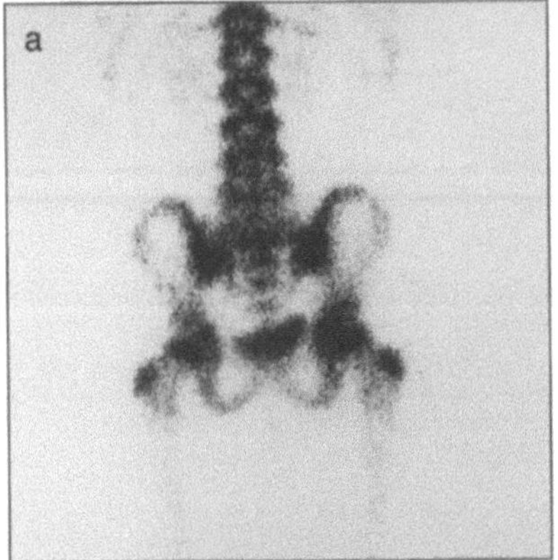
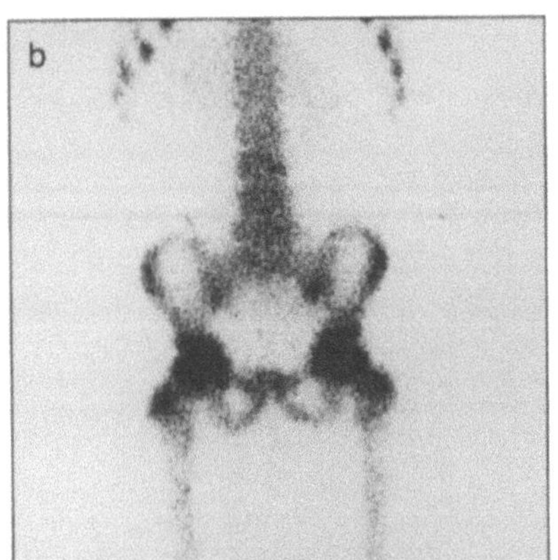
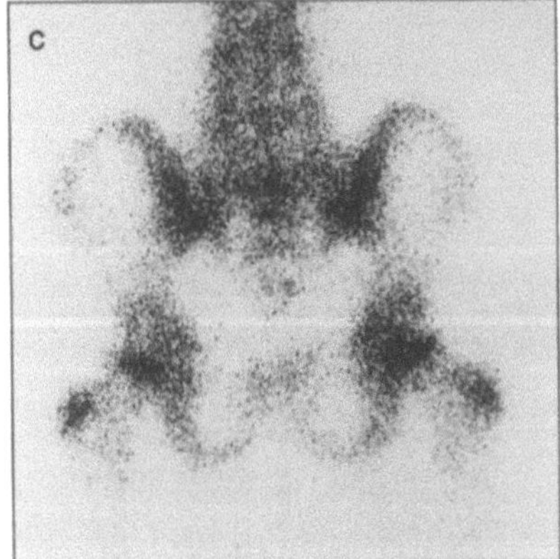
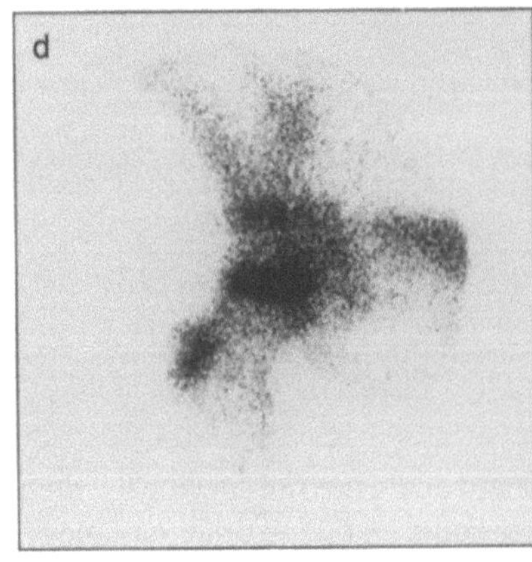
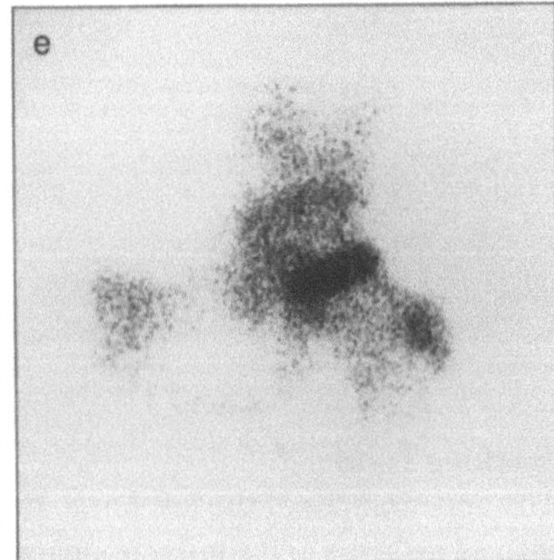

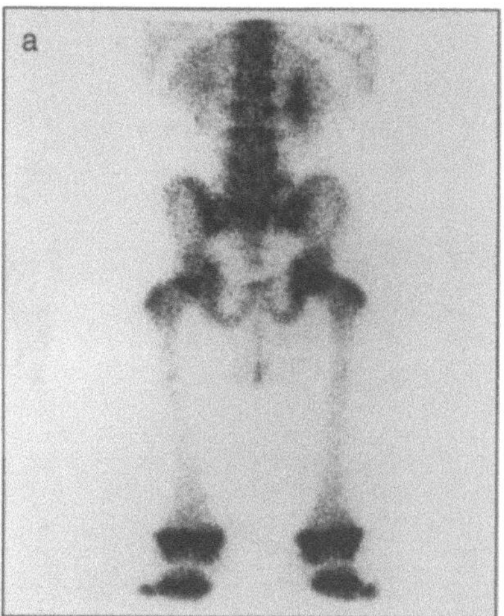

Case 3.26. A 7-year-old boy with pain in the right hip and a limp. Final diagnosis was transient synovitis

Fig. 3.26a. Posterior view of the pelvis shows asymmetry between the two hip joints with increased activity noted on the right compared to the left

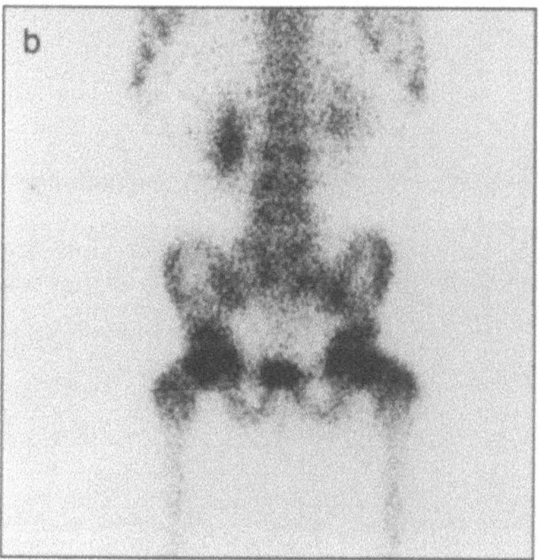

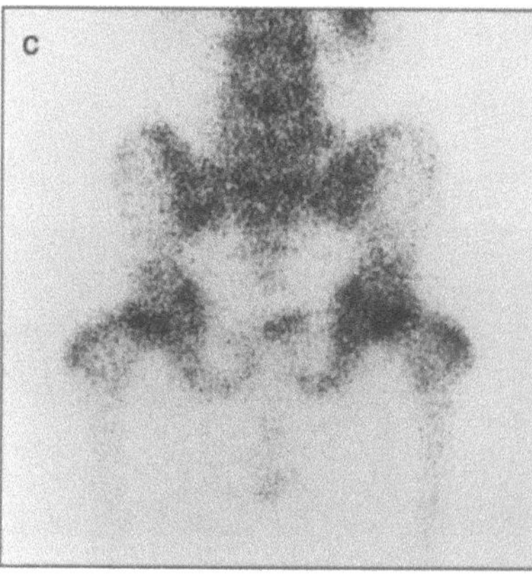

Fig. 3.26b. Anterior view of the pelvis is normal

Fig. 3.26c. Posterior magnification view of the pelvis. There is increased uptake throughout the right hip joint when compared to the left

Case 3.27. A 13-year-old girl with pain in the left hip. This was due to transient synovitis

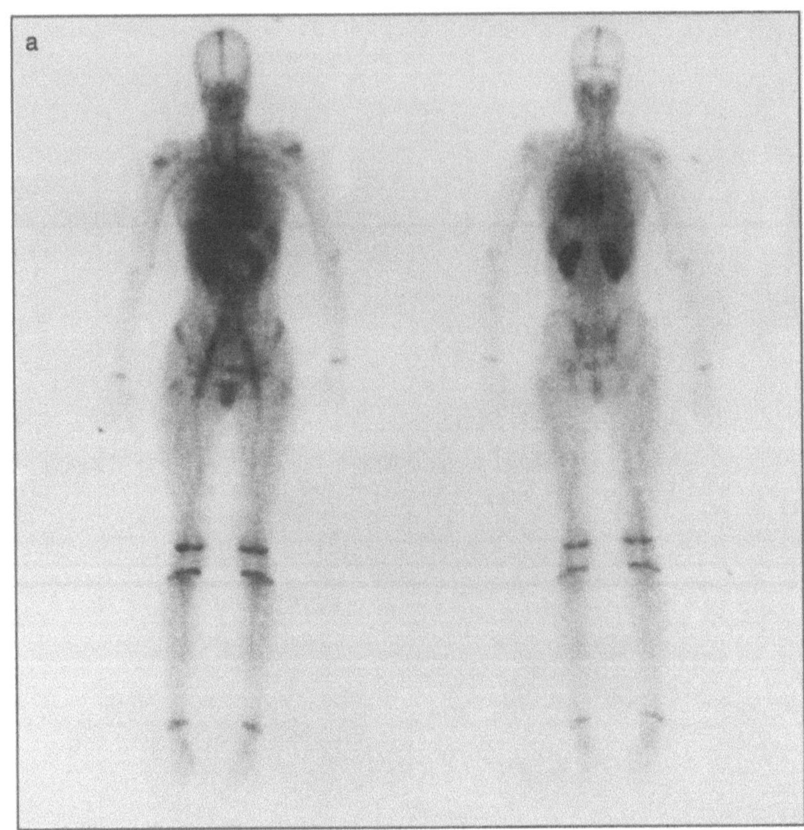

Fig. 3.27a. Whole body blood pool images. There is no asymmetry between the hips

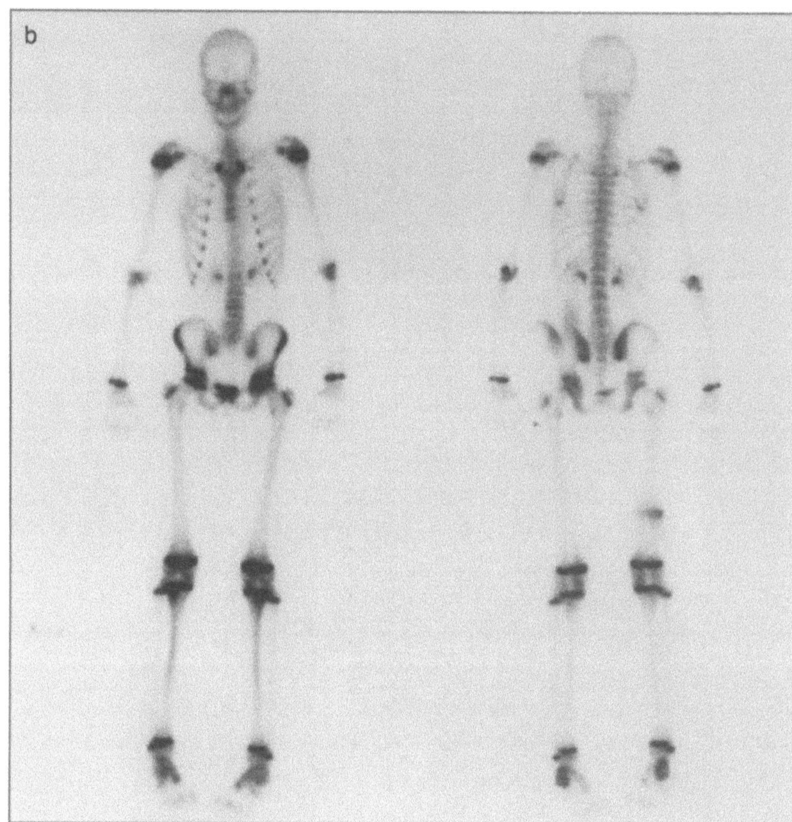

Fig. 3.27b. Whole body scans show increased uptake in the left hip compared to the right with loss of clarity of the epiphyseal plate of the left femoral head. This is best seen on the posterior projection

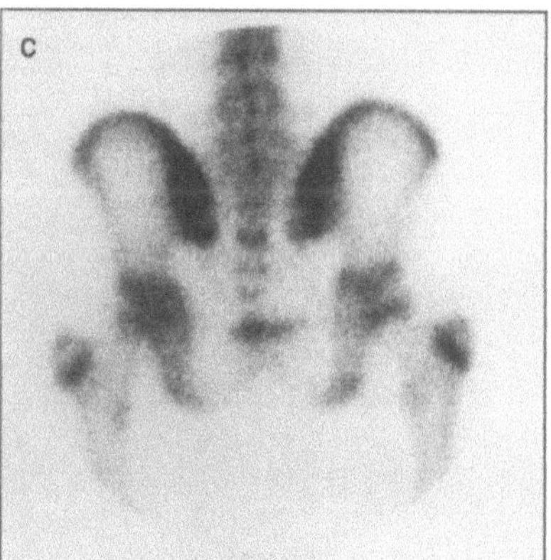

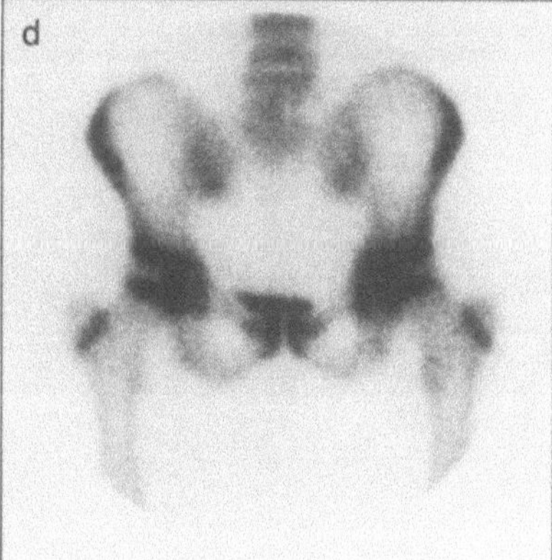

Fig. 3.27c. Posterior view of the pelvis shows loss of clarity of the epiphyseal plate with diffuse increase of isotope throughout the left hip joint

Fig. 3.27d. Anterior view of the pelvis shows only slightly increased activity in the left hip compared to the right

Case 3.28. A 5-year-old boy with transient synovitis of the right hip

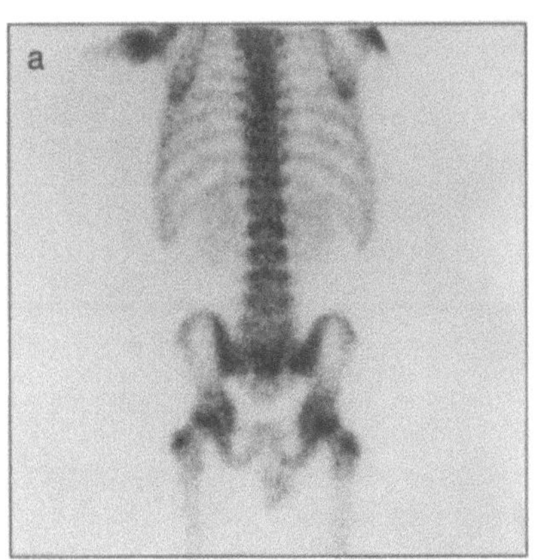

Fig. 3.28a. Posterior view of the spine and pelvis shows increased uptake in the right hip extending throughout the acetabulum

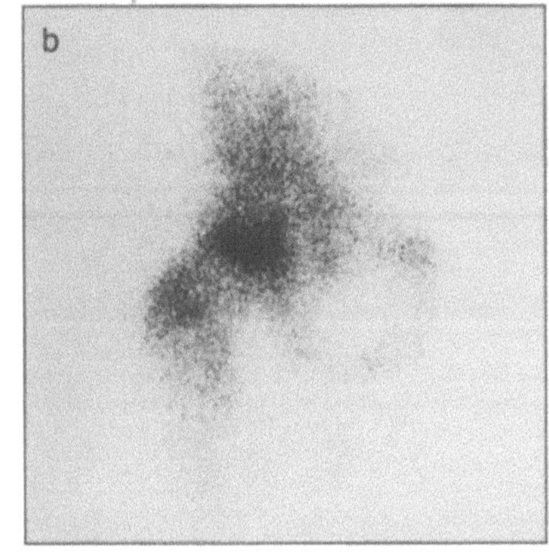

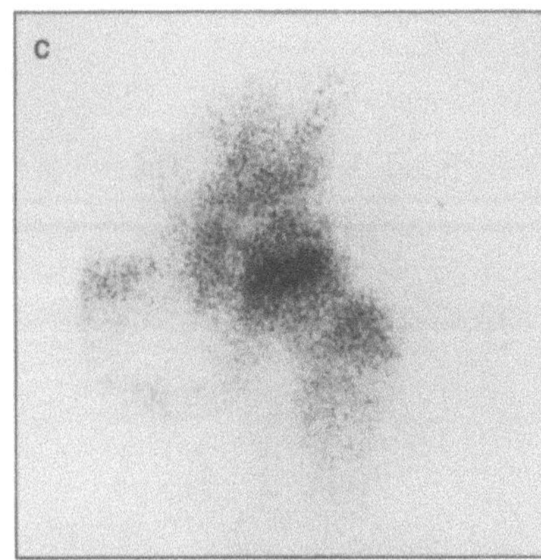

Fig. 3.28b. Pin hole view of the right hip shows diffuse increased uptake of isotope in the right femoral head as well as the acetabulum with loss of clarity of the epiphyseal plate of the femoral head

Fig. 3.28c. Pin hole view of the left hip is normal

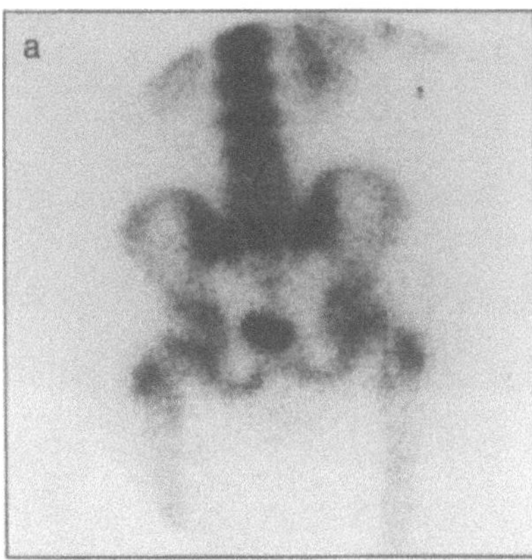

Case 3.29. An 8-year-old boy with pain in the left hip over 8 weeks with a normal radiograph. The child was immobilised and put on traction for a 3-week period and the pain disappeared. Follow-up for 18 months failed to show any abnormality, and the final diagnosis was that of irritable hip

Fig. 3.29a. Posterior image of the pelvis and hips shows decreased activity in the left femoral head

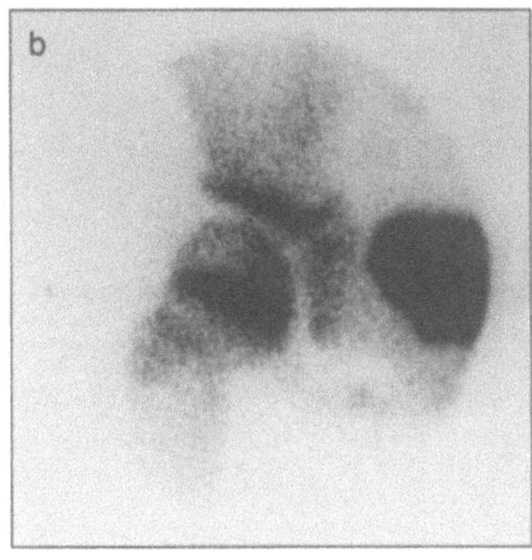

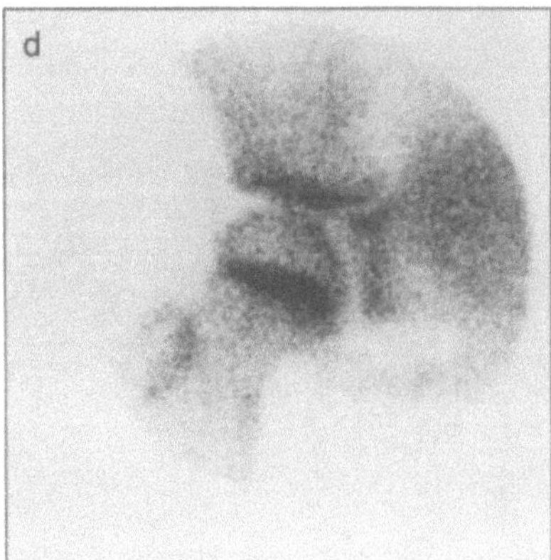

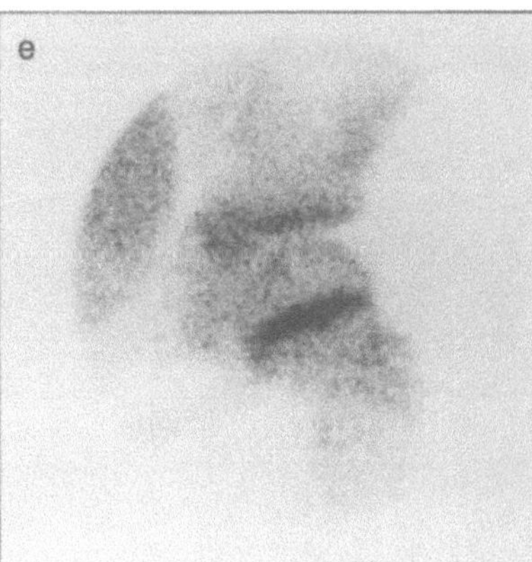

Fig. 3.29b. Pin hole view of the right hip is normal

Fig. 3.29c. Pin hole view of the left hip shows decreased activity throughout the head of the femur, although the outline of the femoral head is preserved

Follow-up bone scan 18 months later.

Fig. 3.29d. Pin hole view of the right hip is normal

Fig. 3.29e. Pin hole of the left hip is normal

Teaching Point

The appearances of the bone scan at presentation are indistinguishable from early Legg-Perthes' disease. Follow-up in this case suggested the diagnosis of irritable hip.

4 Tumours

4.1 Benign Tumours

4.1.1 Osteoid Osteoma
(10 Cases; Figs. 4.1–4.10)

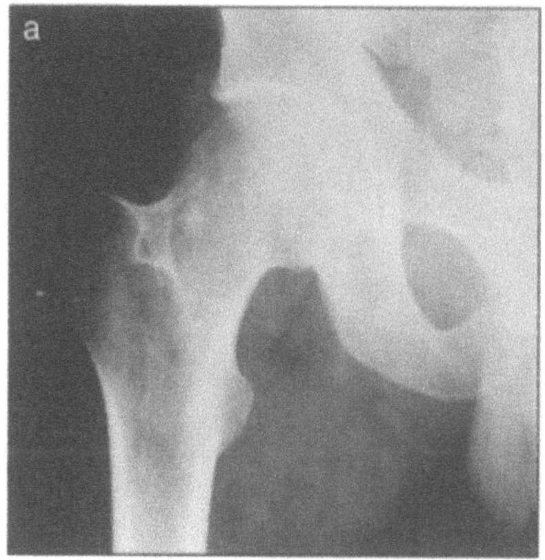

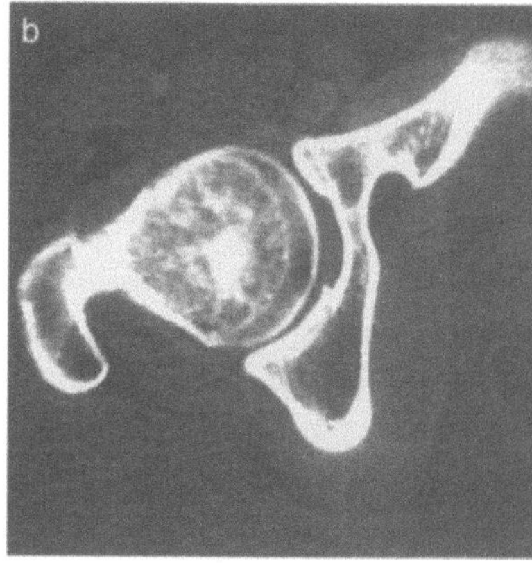

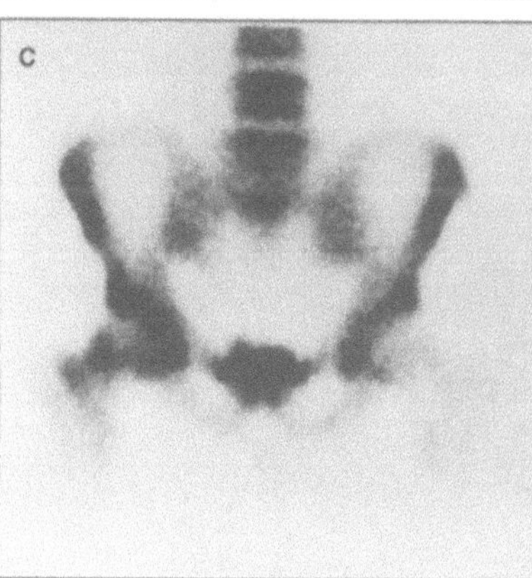

Case 4.1. A 15-year-old boy with pain in the right hip due to an osteoid osteoma

Fig. 4.1a. Radiograph of the right hip. There is a focal area of increased opacity in the neck of the femur, this was considered to be a benign bone island

Fig. 4.1b. Computed tomography (CT) scan shows a focal area of increased attenuation in the neck of the femur but with no surrounding periosteal reaction. This was also considered to be innocent

Fig. 4.1c. Anterior bone scan of the pelvis shows focal abnormal increased uptake of isotope in the neck of the right femur plus generalised increased isotope in the head and shaft

Teaching Point

The bone scan demonstrated that the "bone island" was metabolically active, due to an osteoid osteoma.

Case 4.2. An 18-year-old patient with pain in the right hip; an osteoid osteoma was removed from the neck of the femur

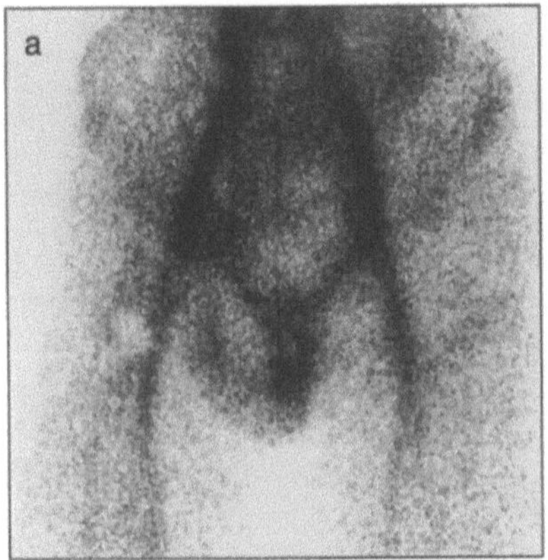

Fig. 4.2a. Anterior blood pool image of the pelvis is unremarkable. The photon-deficient area was caused by a metal object in the right pocket

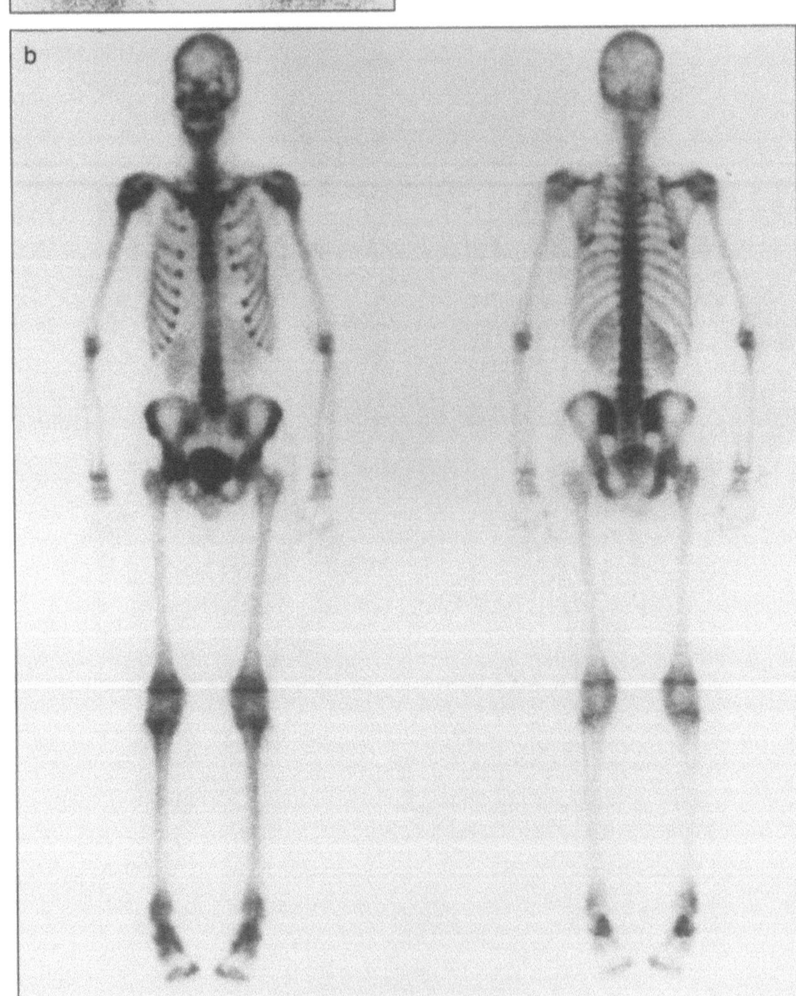

Fig. 4.2b. Whole body scans show slightly increased uptake of isotope in the right hip but the difference compared to the left side is subtle

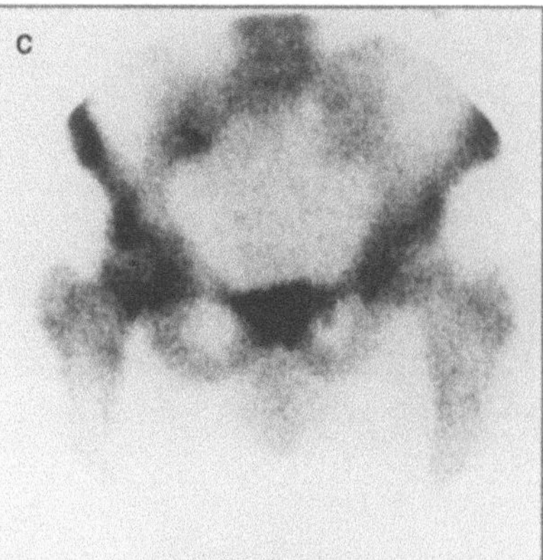

Fig. 4.2c. Anterior image of the pelvis shows focal abnormal increased uptake of isotope in the upper medial aspect of the right femoral neck

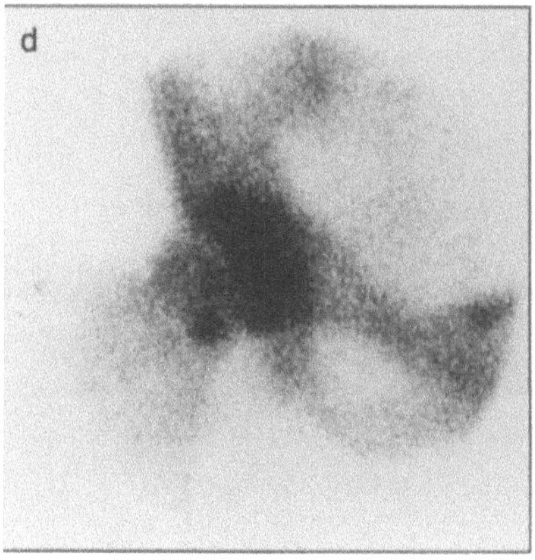
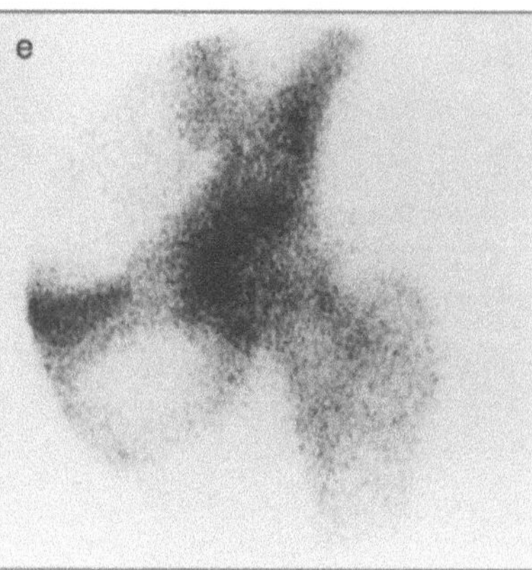

Fig. 4.2d. Pin hole view of the right hip shows the focal abnormal increased uptake of isotope in the osteoid osteoma in the neck of the right femur

Fig. 4.2e. Pin hole view of the left hip is normal

Teaching Point

1. If hip pathology is suspected, pin hole views are essential. This case illustrates the limitations of whole body scanning when looking for osteoid osteoma.
2. An osteoid osteoma is not always "very hot". This child is an example of the atypical appearances on bone scan of an osteoid osteoma.

Case 4.3. A 9-year-old boy with pain in the left hip and a limp due to an osteoid osteoma with atypical isotope features

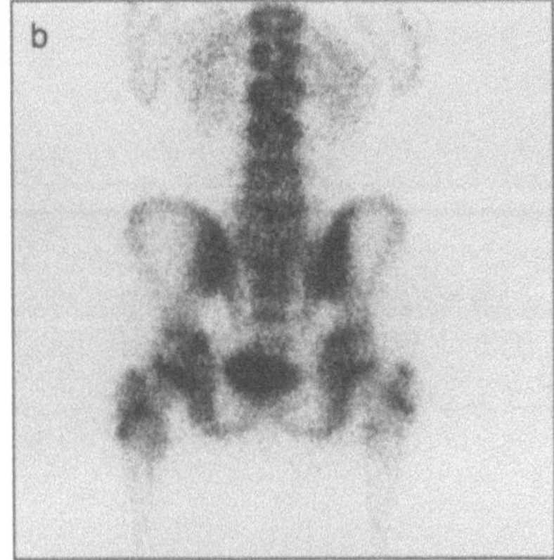

Fig. 4.3a. Blood pool posterior image of the pelvis shows increased activity in the region of the left hip

Fig. 4.3b. Posterior image of the lumbar spine and pelvis shows diffuse increased uptake of isotope in the femoral neck and upper shaft of the left femur

Fig. 4.3c. Anterior image of the pelvis shows diffuse uptake of isotope in the upper left femoral shaft with loss of clarity of the epiphyseal plate of the greater trochanter

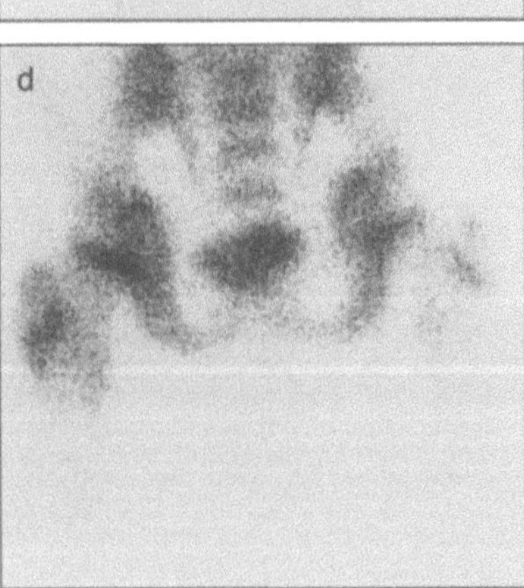

Fig. 4.3d. Posterior magnification scan of the hips fails to reveal a focal abnormality but again demonstrates the diffuse abnormal increased uptake of isotope in the proximal left femoral shaft. Note the increased activity in the epiphyseal plate of both the left femoral head and the left greater trochanter

Teaching Point

These features are not typical of osteoid osteoma but the anatomical site and associated hyperaemia are strongly suggestive of an osteoid osteoma with unusual isotope features. The histology was of a typical osteoid osteoma.

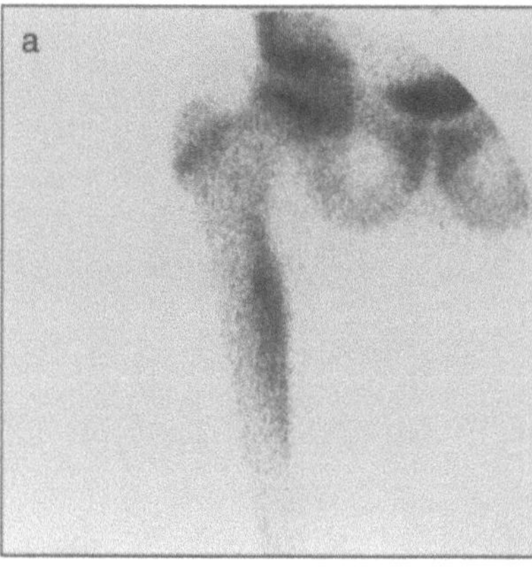

Case 4.4. A 14-year-old girl with pain in the right thigh for 1 year. An osteoid osteoma was removed at surgery

Fig. 4.4a. Anterior image of the right hip and upper femur shows a small focus of intense abnormal increased uptake of isotope surrounded by an area of generalised increased uptake of isotope

Teaching Point

1. Note the difference between the appearances in Cases 4.3 and 4.4. It is easy to overlook the very small focal area of intense increased uptake of isotope in Case 4.3.
2. Similar appearances can be seen with trauma (see Case 5.23).

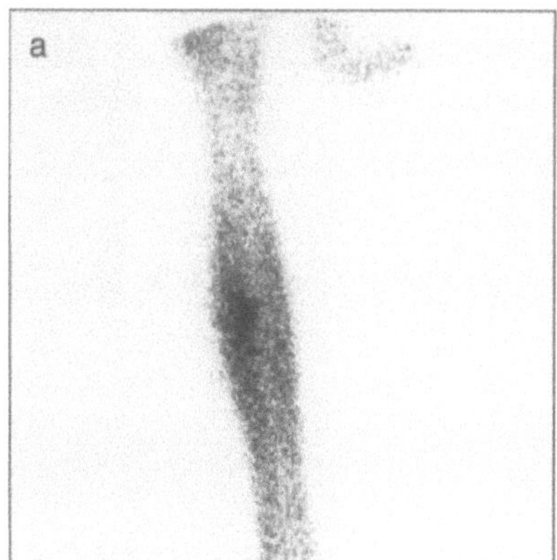
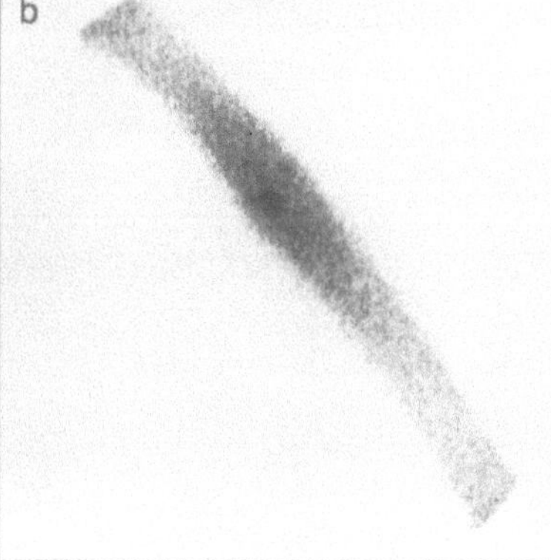

Case 4.5. A 15-year-old boy with pain in the right thigh. An osteoid osteoma was removed at surgery

Fig. 4.5a. Anterior view of the right femur shows focal increased uptake of isotope in the mid shaft surrounded by generalised less intense increased uptake of isotope

Fig. 4.5b. Lateral image of the right femur shows the central nidus with intense increased uptake surrounded by generalised increased uptake of isotope

Teaching Point

These are the typical features of osteoid osteoma.

Case 4.6. A 17-year-old girl with pain in the left hip and thigh. An osteoid osteoma was resected from the upper femoral shaft but the pain persisted following surgery. The first series of scans were undertaken following surgery

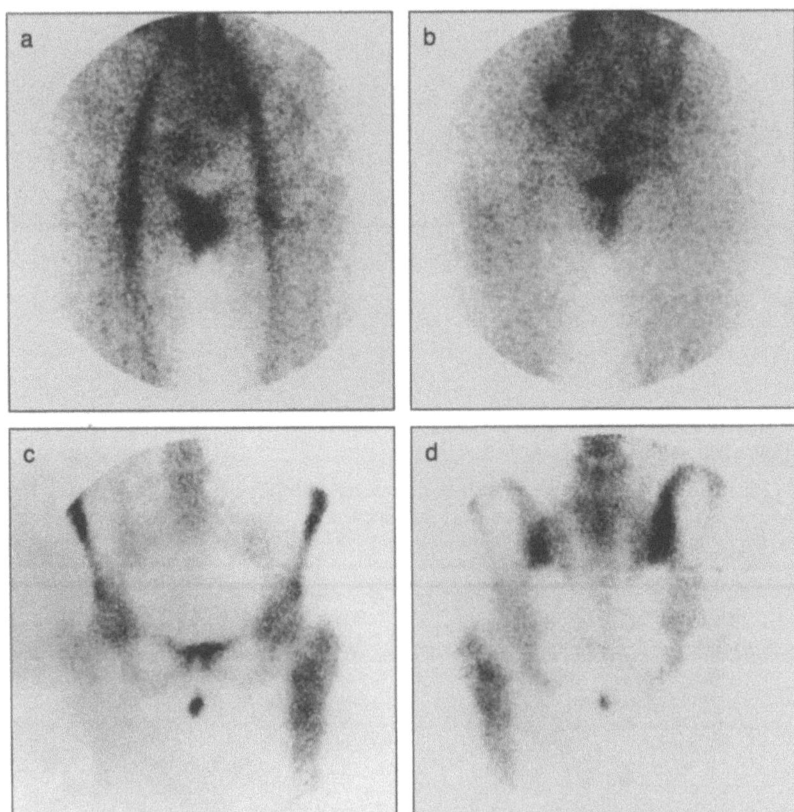

Fig. 4.6a. Anterior blood pool image of the pelvis is unremarkable

Fig. 4.6b. Posterior blood pool image of the pelvis shows slightly diffuse increased uptake of isotope in the upper portion of the left thigh

Fig. 4.6c. Anterior view of the pelvis shows diffuse increased uptake of isotope in the upper third of the shaft of the left femur

Fig. 4.6d. Posterior image of the pelvis and upper femora shows diffuse increased uptake in the shaft of the left femur with a focal area of increased uptake at the level of the lesser trochanter.

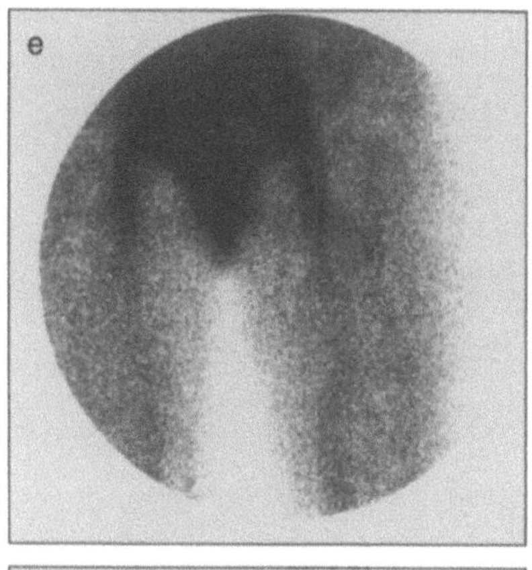

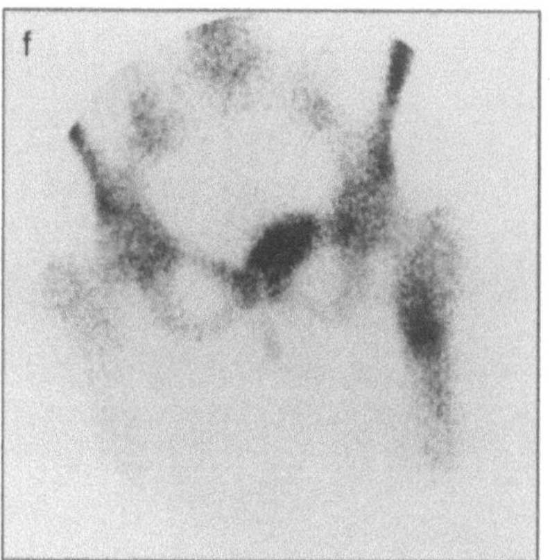

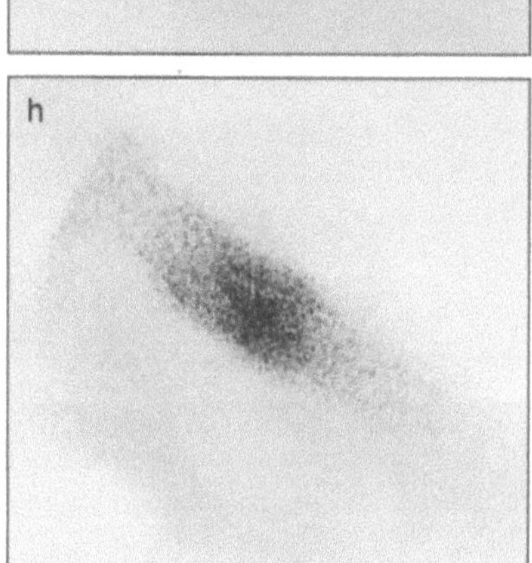

The child remained symptomatic and a repeat bone scan 1 year later was essentially unchanged. She underwent second surgery, the surgeon attempted to remove the osteoid osteoma. However, she returned 2 years following the second surgery, which was 4 years after the first bone scan, with persistent pain in the same region due to incomplete removal of the osteoid osteoma

Fig. 4.6e. Blood pool anterior view of the pelvis is unremarkable

Fig. 4.6f. Anterior view of the pelvis shows focal abnormal increased uptake of isotope in the proximal shaft of the left femur

Fig. 4.6g. Lateral view of the femur shows that the increased uptake of isotope is more marked in the mid and posterior portion of the femur

Fig. 4.6h. Pin hole view of the left upper femur shows a small focus of intense increased uptake of isotope surrounded by an area of generalised increased uptake

Teaching Point

In a patient who has undergone surgery for an osteoid osteoma increased activity at the site of pathology on follow-up bone scan may be difficult to separate the effects of surgery from incomplete removal of the osteoid osteoma or a complication of the surgery.

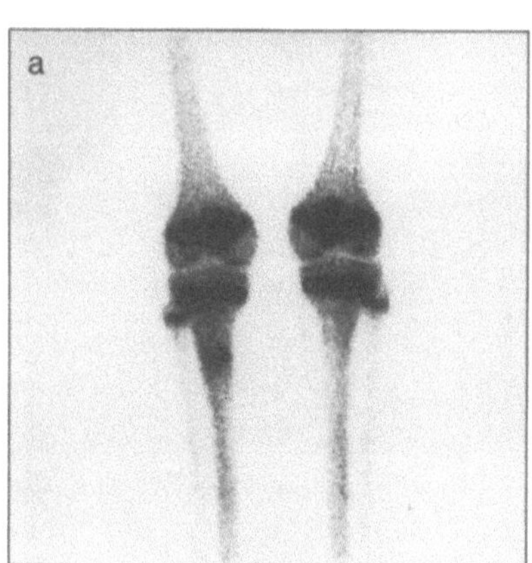

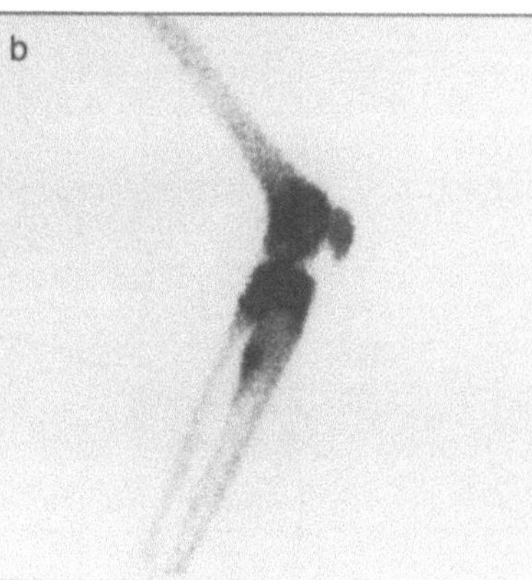

Case 4.7. A 13-year-old boy with pain in the left knee for 1 year. An osteoid osteoma was removed from the left tibia at surgery

Fig. 4.7a. Posterior view of the knees shows focal abnormal increased uptake of isotope in the upper third of the shaft of the left tibia

Fig. 4.7b. Lateral image of the left knee shows the abnormal activity localised to the posterior aspect of the upper shaft of the tibia

Teaching Point

1. These are the typical appearances of an osteoid osteoma on bone scan.
2. A stress fracture can cause a similar appearance but this is an unusual site for a stress fracture (see Cases 5.19 and 5.21).

Case 4.8. An 18-year-old patient with pain in the left tibia. An osteoid osteoma was removed at surgery

Fig. 4.8a. Blood pool image of the lower limbs (posterior view) shows abnormal increased uptake of isotope on the medial aspect of the mid portion of the left calf

Fig. 4.8b. Anterior image of the lower limbs shows focal intense increased uptake of isotope in the mid third of the left tibia with slightly abnormal increased uptake of isotope extending superiorly

Fig. 4.8c. Whole body images show focal intense abnormal increased uptake of isotope on the medial aspect of the mid shaft of the left tibia

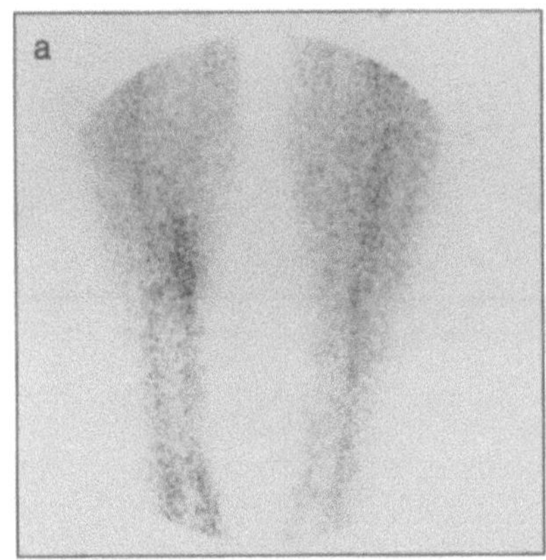
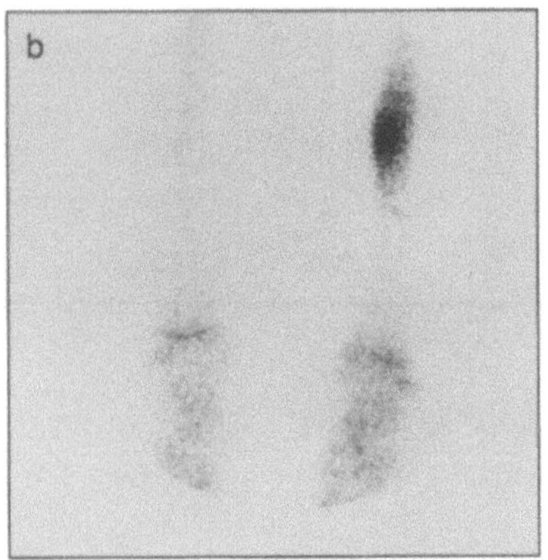
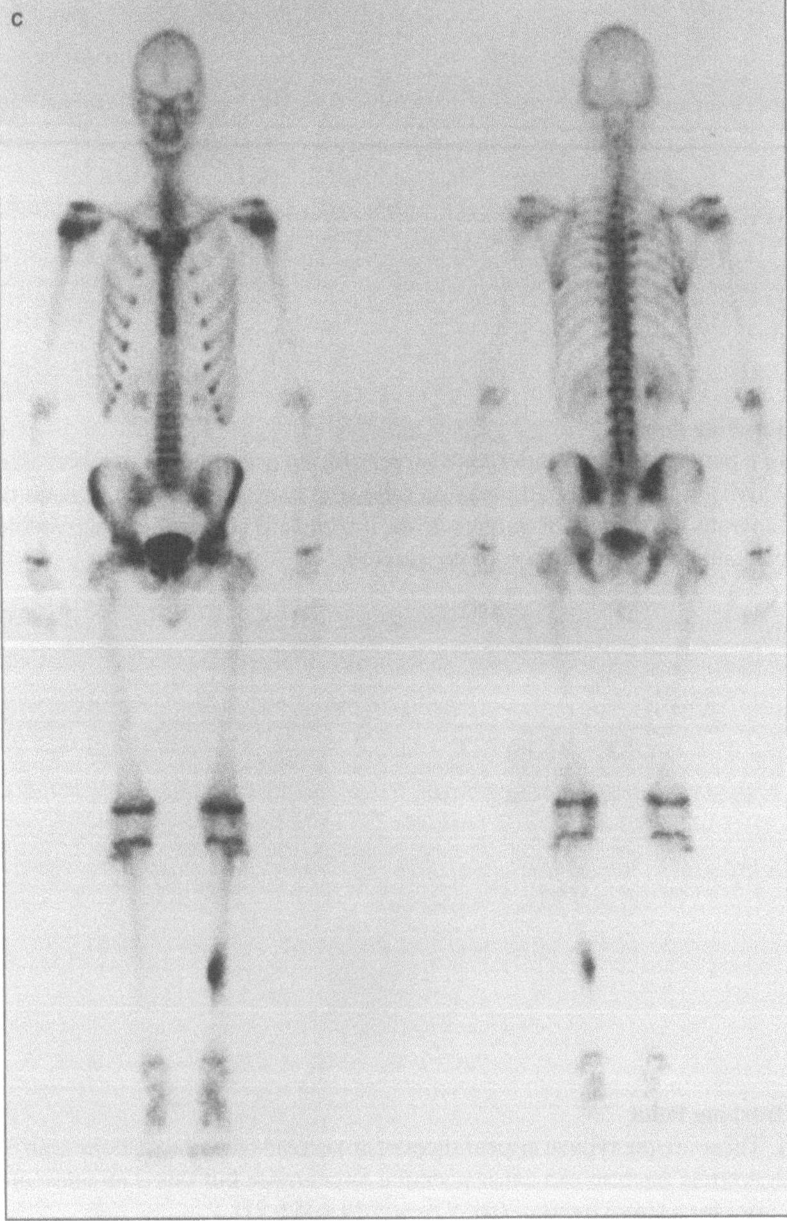

Teaching Point

1. The differential diagnosis includes a stress fracture but the very focal nature of this increased uptake of isotope strongly suggests an osteoid osteoma. Stress fractures are more common in the lower third of the shaft of the tibia rather than at the junction of the mid third and lower third. (see Cases 5.19, 5.21).
2. Similar appearances may be seen in osteoblastoma (see Case 4.14).

Technical Comment

The increased activity seen in the region of the posterior right fourth rib on the whole body image is due to "shine through" from the sterno clavicular joint.

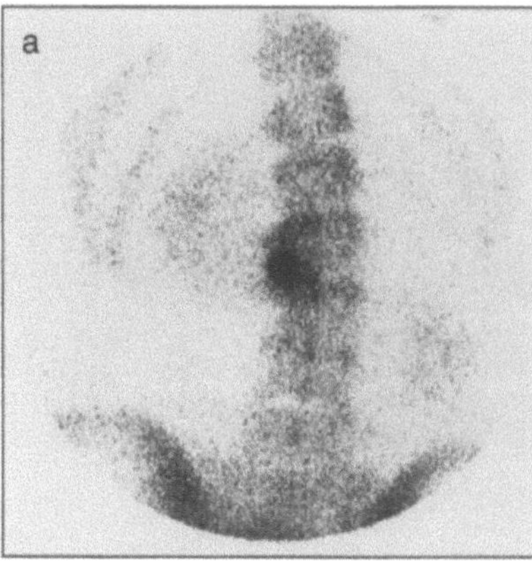

Case 4.9. A 20-year-old patient with pain in the back. An osteoid osteoma at the L2/3 level was removed at surgery

Fig. 4.9a. Posterior view of the lumbar spine shows scoliosis concave to the left. There is focal abnormal intense increased uptake of isotope at the L2/3 level

Teaching Point

1. If single photon emission computed tomography (SPECT) is not undertaken, then a CT scan will be required to localise exactly where the lesion is to assist the surgeon in removing the osteoid osteoma.
2. Similar appearances may be seen with osteoblastoma (see Cases 4.12, 4.13), aneurysmal bone cyst (see Case 4.24), infection (see Case 2.38) or trauma (see Case 5.13).

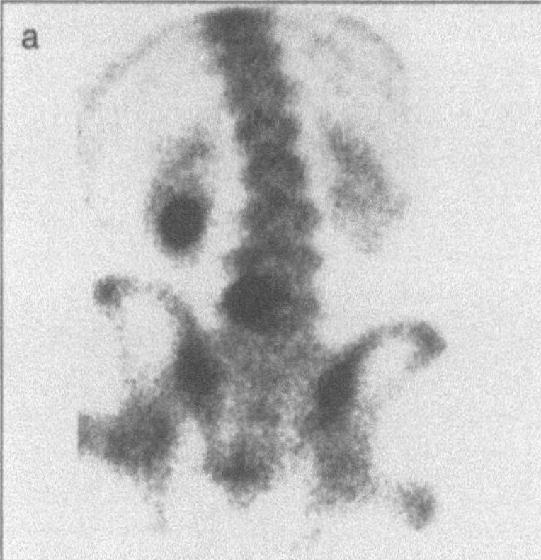

Case 4.10. An 8-year-old boy with backache. An osteoid osteoma at L5 was removed at surgery

Fig. 4.10a. Posterior image of the lumbar spine and pelvis. There is a scoliosis concave to the left. Focal abnormal uptake of isotope is noted at L5. This is shown to lie in the left pars interarticularis at this level

Technical Comment

Note the increased activity in the left renal pelvis due to pelvi-ureteric junction hold-up.

Teaching Point

Similar appearances may be seen with osteoblastoma (see Cases 4.12, 4.13), aneurysmal bone cyst (see Case 4.24), infection (see Case 2.38) or trauma (see Case 5.13).

4.1.2 Osteoblastoma
(4 Cases; Figs. 4.11–4.14)

Case 4.11. A 20-year-old patient with pain in the right elbow due to a recurrence of an osteoblastoma

Fig. 4.11a. Blood pool image of both elbows shows intense focal increased uptake of isotope in the dorsal aspect of the right elbow

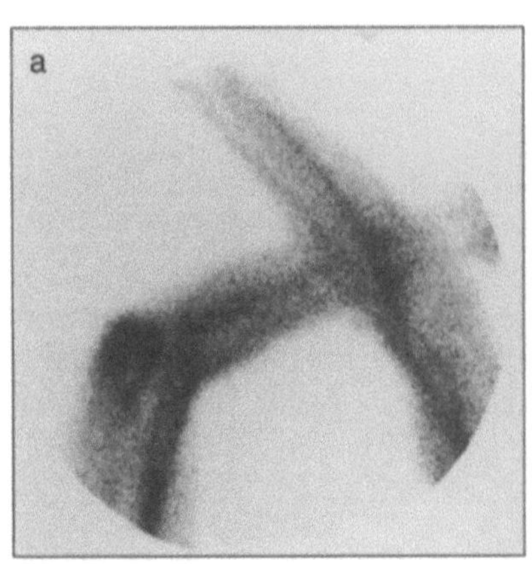

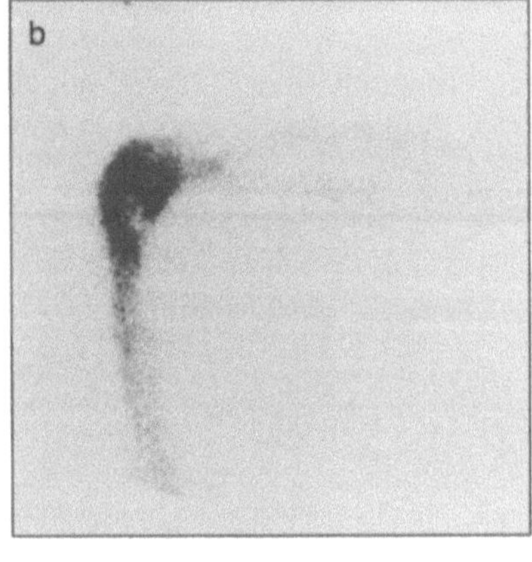

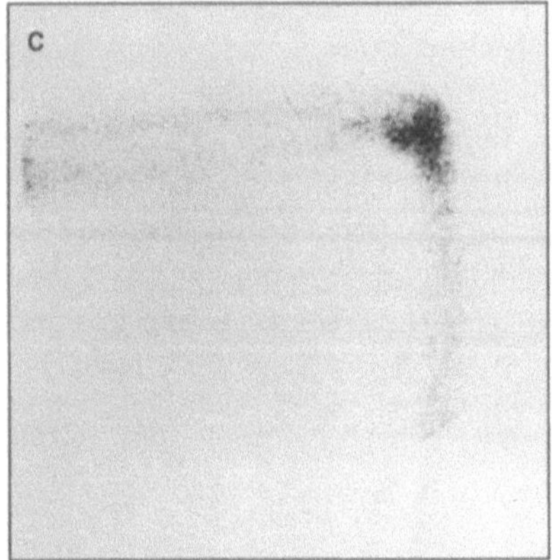

Fig. 4.11b. Lateral view of the right elbow shows intense increased uptake of isotope in the whole elbow

Fig. 4.11c. Lateral view of the left elbow is normal

Technical Comment
Fig. 4.11a, the blood pool image shows the left elbow flexed to 90 degrees, while the right elbow overlies the left and is straight.

Case 4.12. A 13-year-old girl with pain in the back. A benign osteoblastoma in the spine was removed surgically

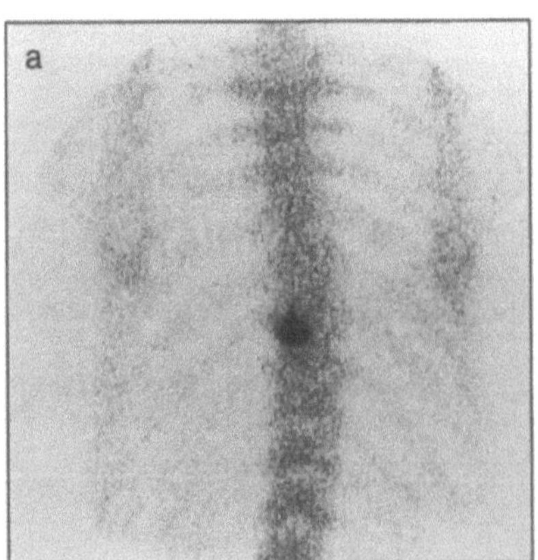

Fig. 4.12a. Posterior image of the thorax and spine. There is focal abnormal increased uptake of isotope in one of the lower dorsal vertebral bodies with a scoliosis concave to the left

Teaching Point
Similar appearances may be seen with osteoid osteoma (see Case 4.9, 4.10) , aneurysmal bone cyst (see Case 4.24), infection (see Case 2.38) and trauma (see Case 5.13).

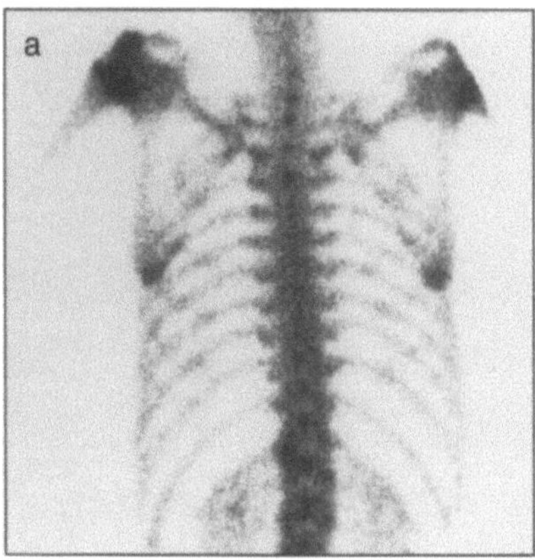

Case 4.13. A 15-year-old boy with pain in the back for over half a year due to an osteoblastoma at the level of D12

Fig. 4.13a. Posterior image of the dorsal spine shows slightly abnormal increased uptake of isotope on the left side of the vertebra at the level of D12

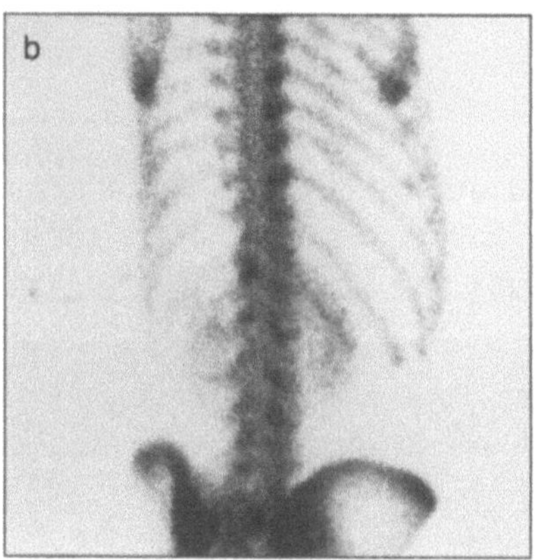

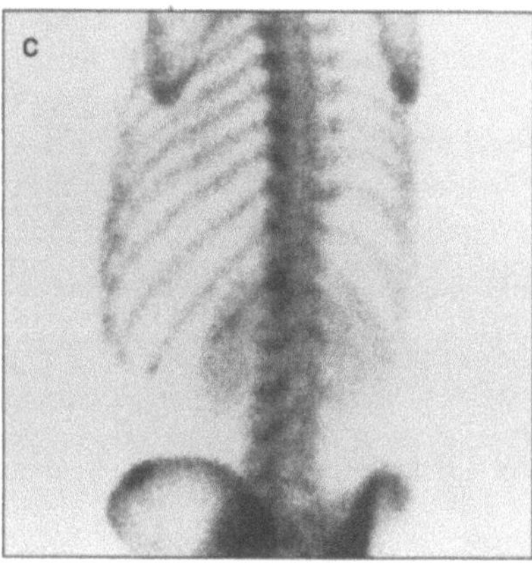

Fig. 4.13b,c. Right posterior oblique and left posterior oblique view of the dorsal spine show the slightly increased uptake of isotope on the left side of the vertebra at the level of D12 to better advantage

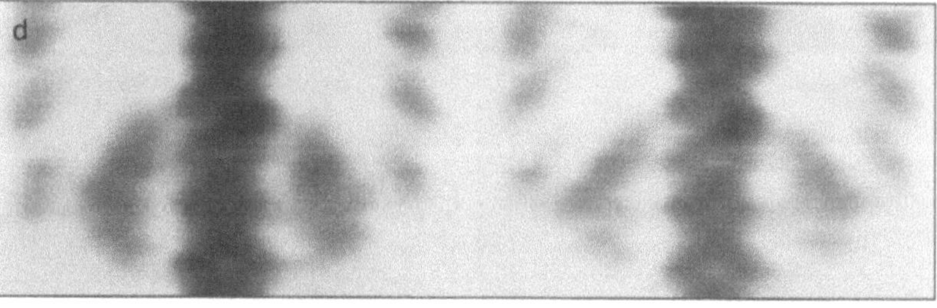

Fig. 4.13d. SPECT coronal slices show the focal abnormal uptake in the body of D12

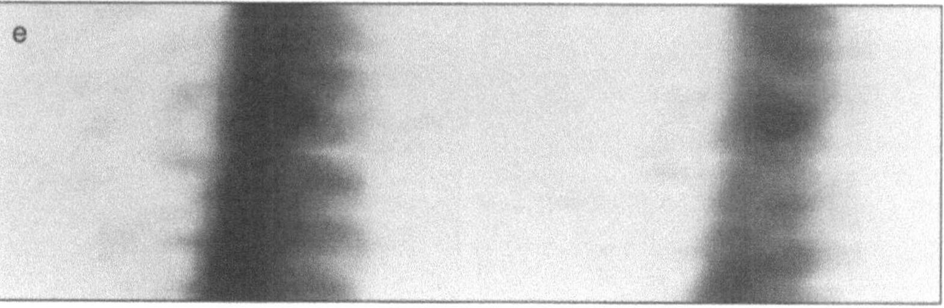

Fig. 4.13e. SPECT sagittal slices show the abnormality to the right of the mid line in the vertebral body

Teaching Point

1. The subtle abnormality on the planar image requires high-quality images to ensure that this abnormality is not missed.
2. To declare a spine normal in the setting of a child with backache, a SPECT should be part of the routine imaging.
3. Similar appearances may be seen with osteoid osteoma (see Cases 4.9, 4.10), aneurysmal bone cyst (see Case 4.24), infection (see Case 2.38) and trauma (see Case 5.13).

Case 4.14. A 10-year-old girl with pain in the right leg. An osteoblastoma was removed surgically from the tibia

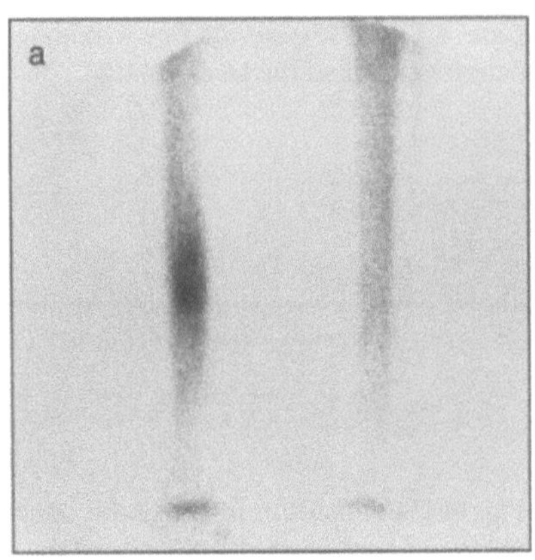

Fig. 4.14a. Anterior view of the lower legs shows focal abnormal increased uptake of isotope in the mid portion of the right tibia; this is slightly more on the medial than on the lateral aspect

Teaching Point

These appearances should be compared to the patient in Case 4.8, who had a diagnosis of an osteoid osteoma. These appearances are non-specific and the differential diagnosis must also include a stress fracture (see Chap. 5.2.1, "Stress Fracture").

4.1.3 Benign Fibrous Cortical Defects

(2 Cases; Figs. 4.15, 4.16)

Case 4.15. A 13-year-old girl with an abnormality on the radiograph of the right knee. The final diagnosis was that of a fibrous cortical defect of the tibia

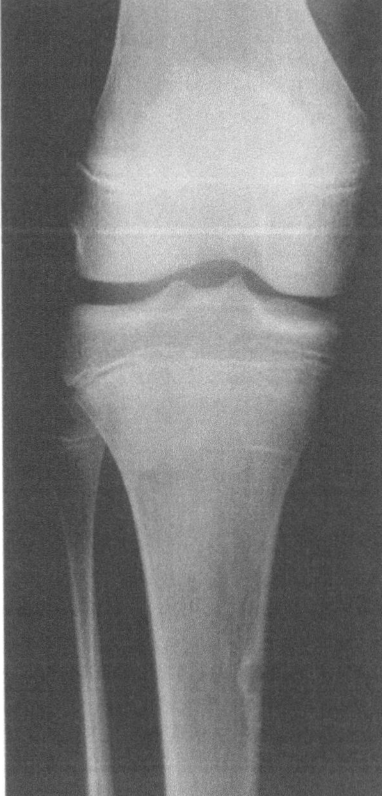

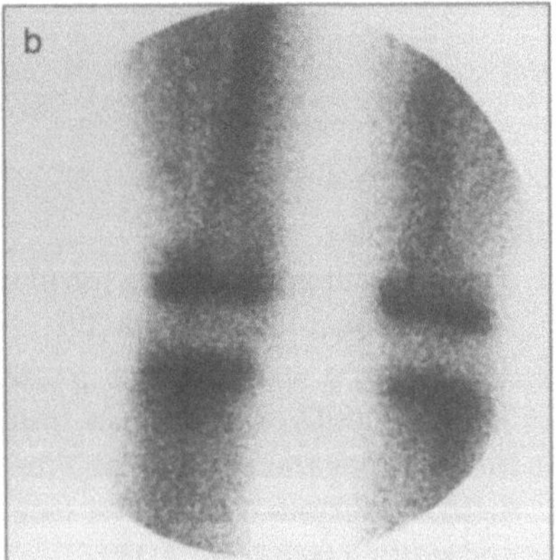

Fig. 4.15a. Radiograph of the right knee. A lytic lesion is seen in the cortex of the upper third of the tibia medially. There is no break in the cortex nor is there a periostal reaction

Fig. 4.15b. Anterior blood pool image of the knees is normal

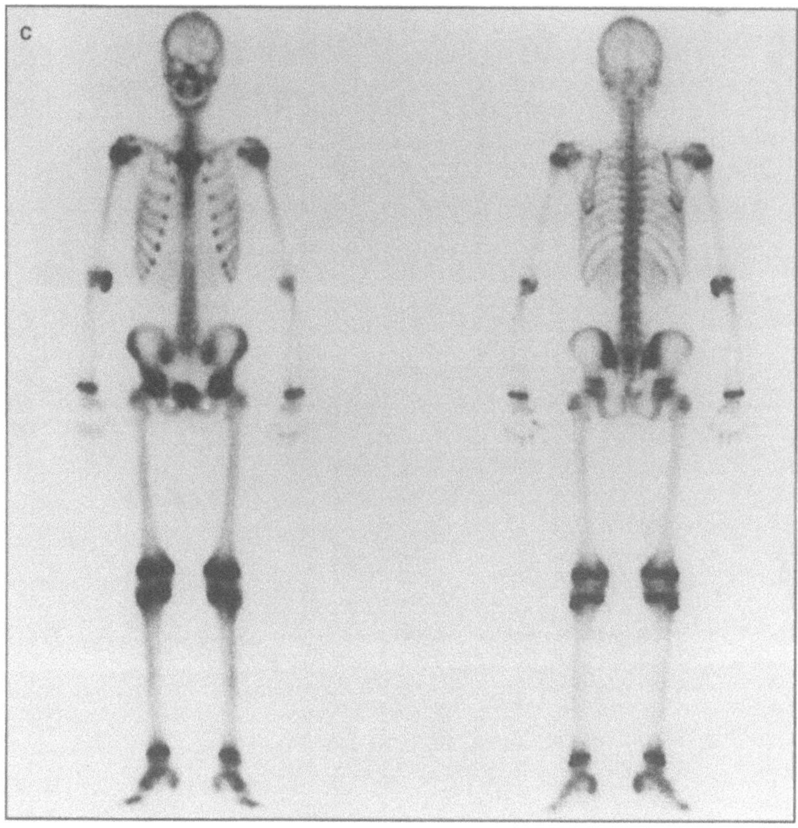

Fig. 4.15c. Whole body scans are normal

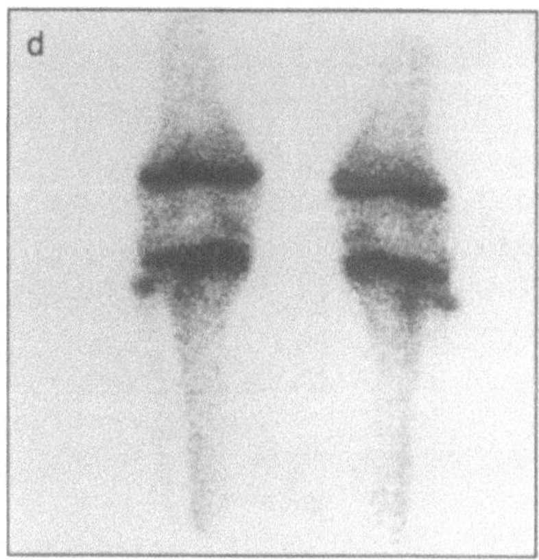

Fig. 4.15d. Anterior image of the knees. Note the normal clarity of the epiphyseal plates. No abnormality is seen

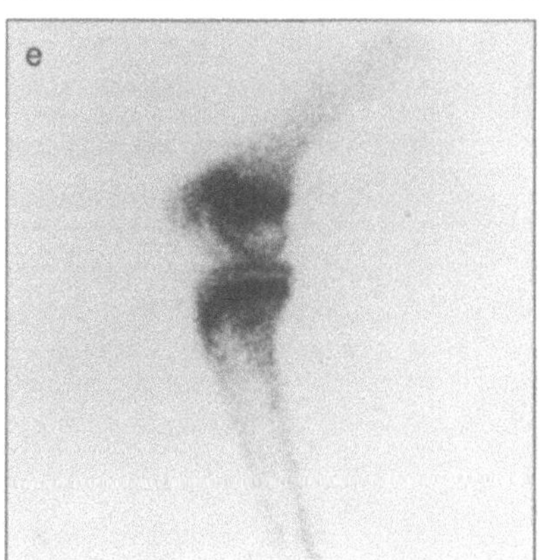

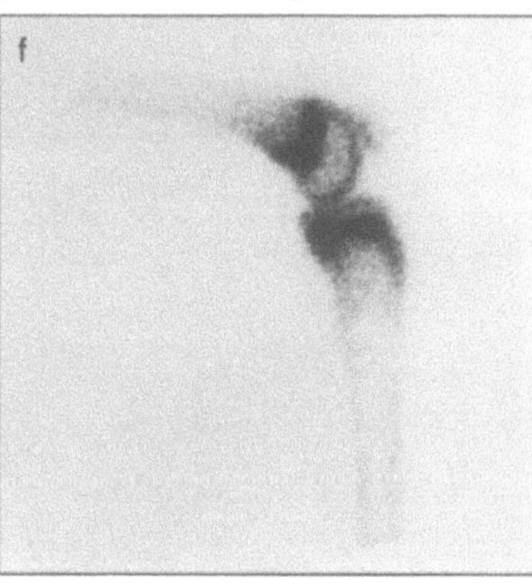

Fig. 4.15e,f. Lateral images of both knees fail to reveal any abnormality

Teaching Point

A benign fibrous cortical defect has no abnormal osteoblastic activity and the bone scan appears normal.

Case 4.16. A 16-year-old girl who was being investigated for a radiological abnormality in the left tibia. The child had no symptoms related to the tibia, the radiographs were reviewed and the final diagnosis was that of a benign fibrous cortical defect

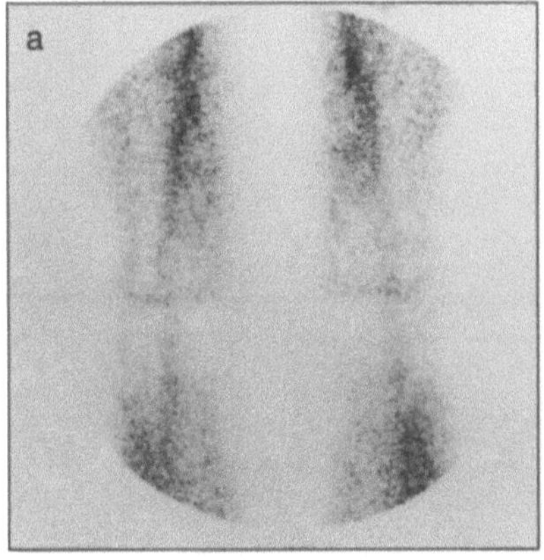 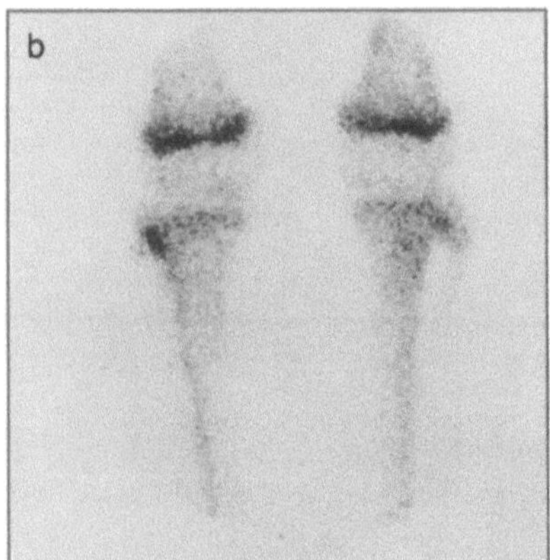

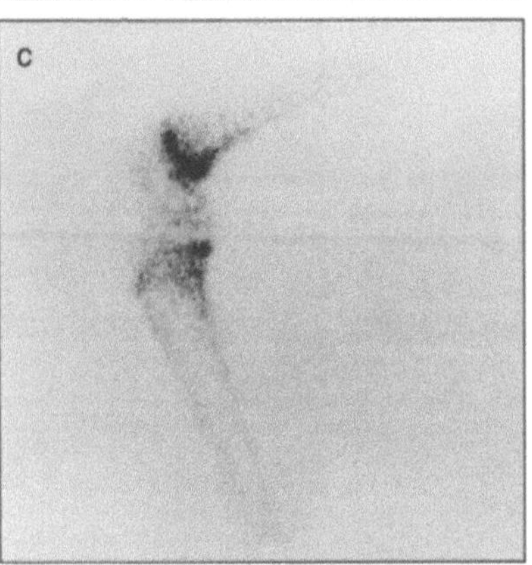 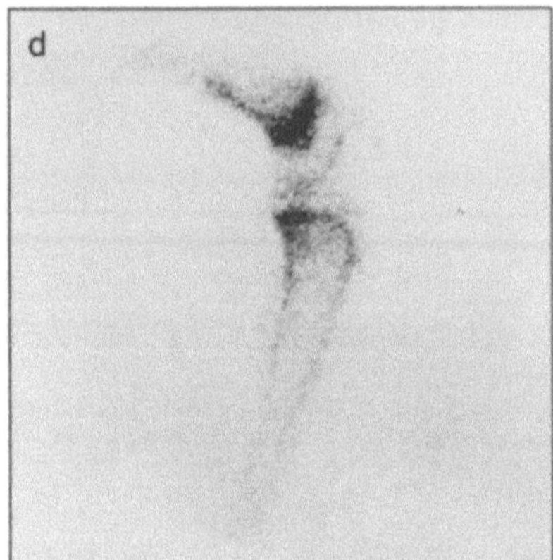

Fig. 4.16a. Anterior blood pool image of the knees is normal

Fig. 4.16b. Anterior image of the knees. Note the normal clarity of the epiphyseal plates. No abnormality is seen in the left tibia. Note the increased uptake of isotope in the head of the right fibula, which was caused by a trauma

Fig. 4.16c,d. Lateral images of the knees fail to reveal any abnormality

4.1.4 Bone Cysts

4.1.4.1 Simple Bone Cysts (2 Cases; Figs. 4.17, 4.18)

Case 4.17. A 4-year-old girl who presented with pain in the left tibia due to a bone cyst

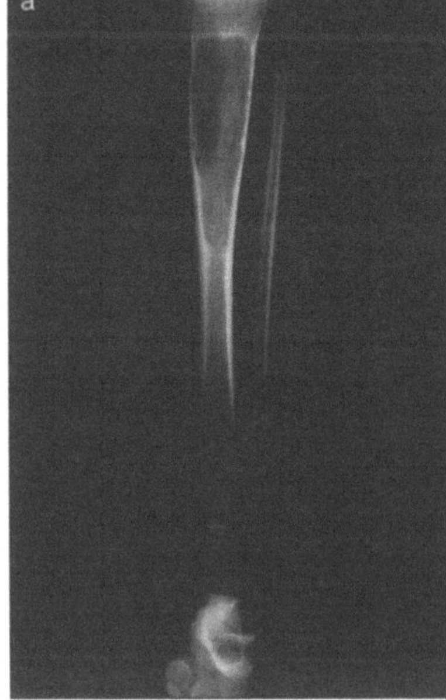 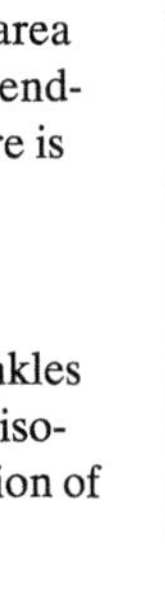 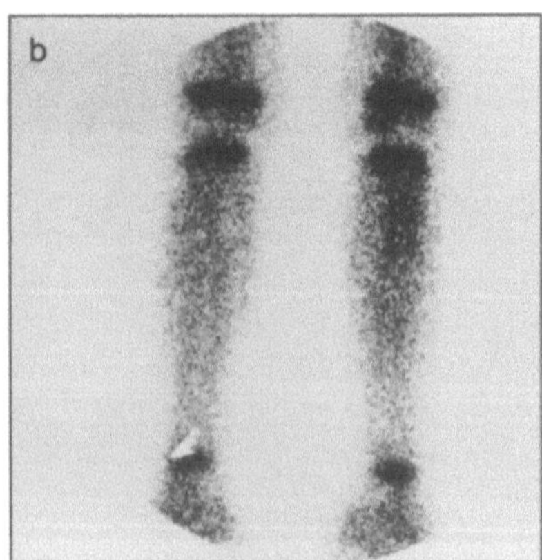

Fig. 4.17a. X-ray of the left tibia and fibula shows a well defined lytic area in the upper third of the tibia extending into the mid shaft. No fracture is seen

Fig. 4.17b. Anterior blood pool image of the knees, tibiae and ankles shows slight increased uptake of isotope in the upper third of the region of the left tibia

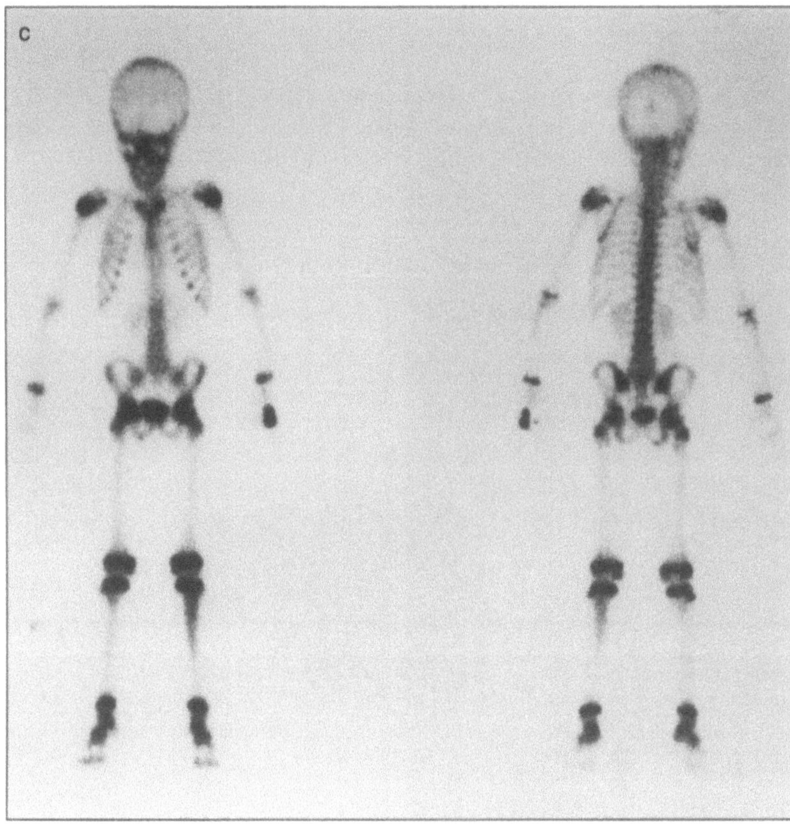

Fig. 4.17c. Whole body images show increased uptake of isotope in the upper half of the left tibia. Note extravasation of isotope in the region of the left hand, the site of the injection

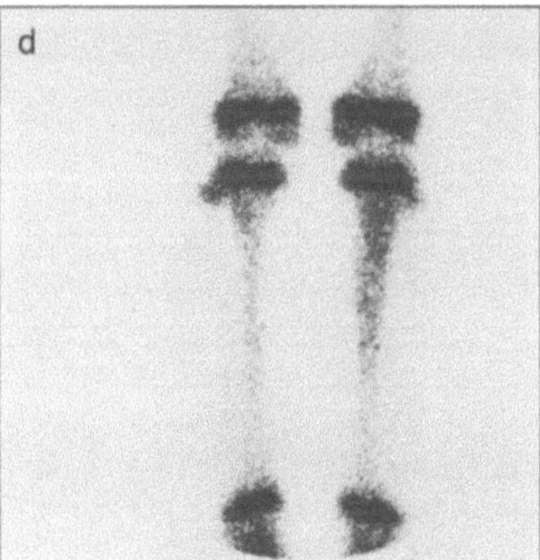

Fig. 4.17d. Anterior image of the knees, tibiae and ankles shows slight increased uptake throughout the upper half of the left tibia

Technical Comment

Note the poor positioning of the feet in Fig. 4.17c compared to Fig. 4.17d.

Teaching Point

A simple bone cyst has usually decreased, normal or slightly increased uptake of isotope. The clinical presentation of pain suggests a complication of the bone cyst. The diffuse nature of the increased uptake of isotope suggests haemorrhage rather than a fracture.

**Case 4.18. A 16-year-old girl with a
bone cyst in the distal right tibia**

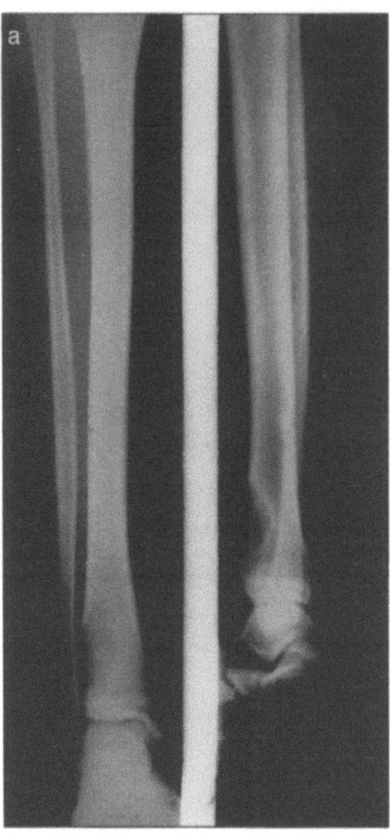

Fig. 4.18a. X-ray images of the right
tibia and fibula (posterior and lateral
views) show a well defined lytic lesion
causing expansion of the tibia

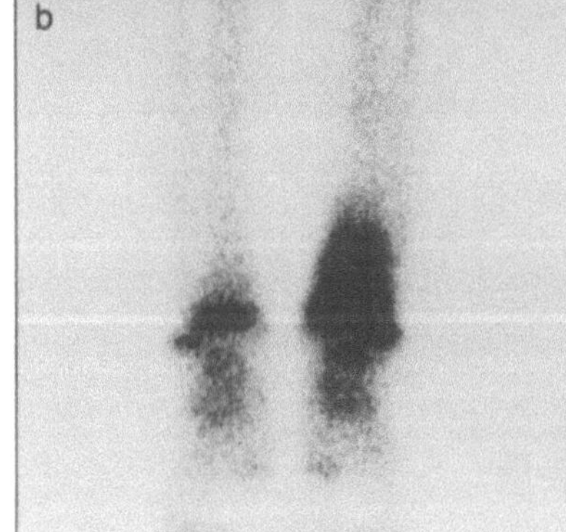

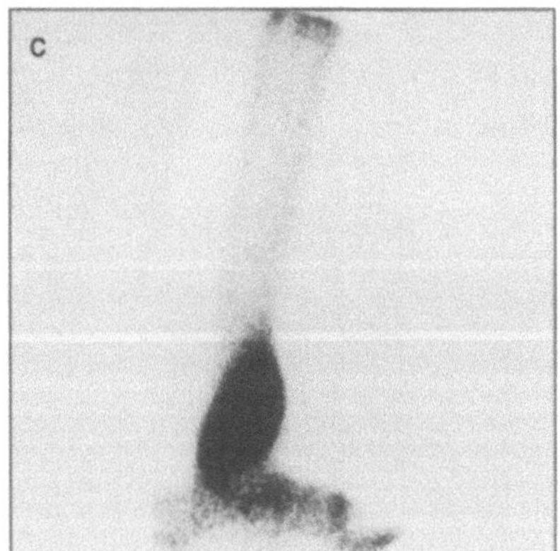

Fig. 4.18b. Posterior image of tibiae,
fibulae, ankles and feet shows marked
increased uptake in the distal end of
the right tibia

Fig. 4.18c. Lateral view of the right
lower limb shows marked increased
uptake of isotope in the distal right
tibia

Teaching Point

1. The diagnosis of a simple bone cyst was confirmed on histology. It is
   unusual for a simple bone cyst to have such an intense osteoblastic activity. No fracture was seen to account for this.
2. Similar appearances may be seen with osteomyelitis (see Case 2.4).

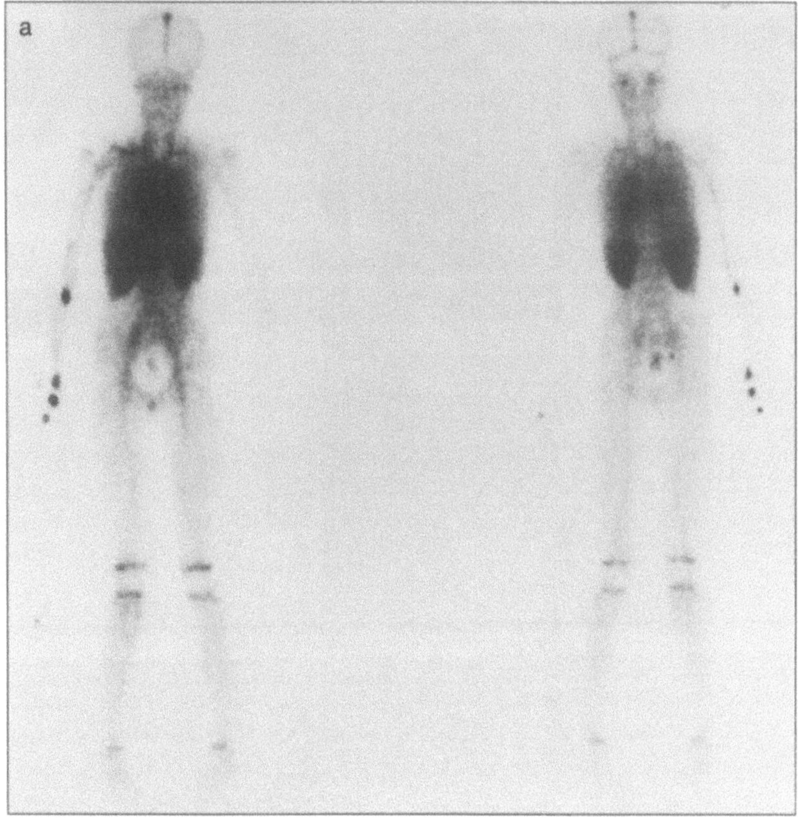

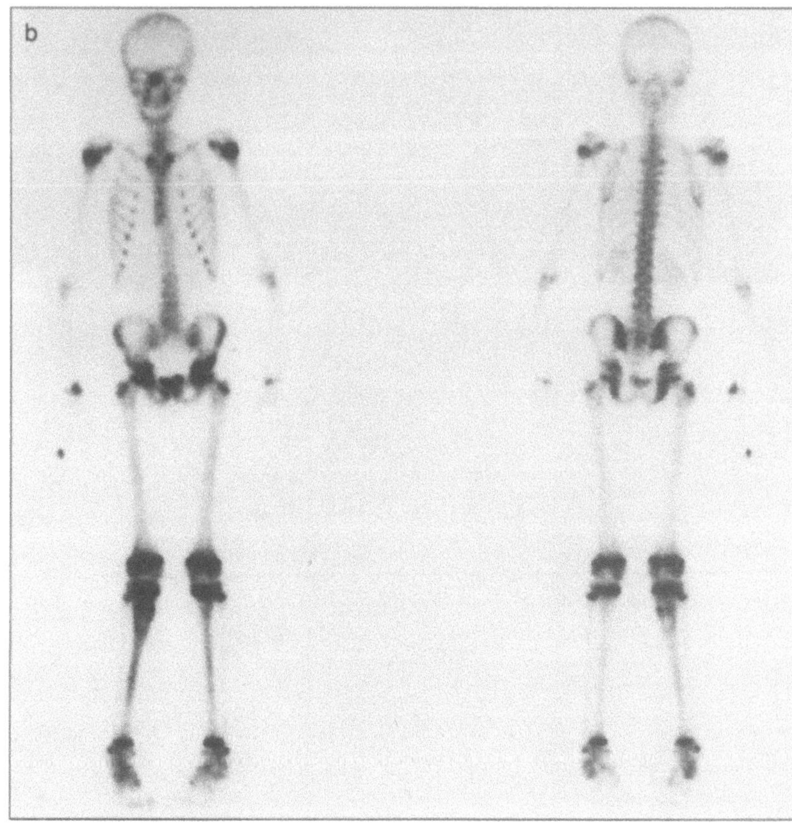

4.1.4.2 Fractures in a Simple Bone Cyst
(5 Cases; Figs. 4.19–4.23)

Case 4.19. An 11-year-old boy who had pain in the right knee following minimal trauma. He had suffered a fracture through a benign bone cyst in the upper right tibia

Fig. 4.19a. Whole body blood pool images show slightly increased uptake of isotope in the upper third of the right tibial diaphysis

Fig. 4.19b. Whole body images show generalised increased uptake of isotope in the upper third of the right tibial shaft with a focal area of intense increased uptake of isotope on the medial aspect, the site of the fracture.

Following surgery and bone graft, a follow-up study was undertaken 1 year after the previous study

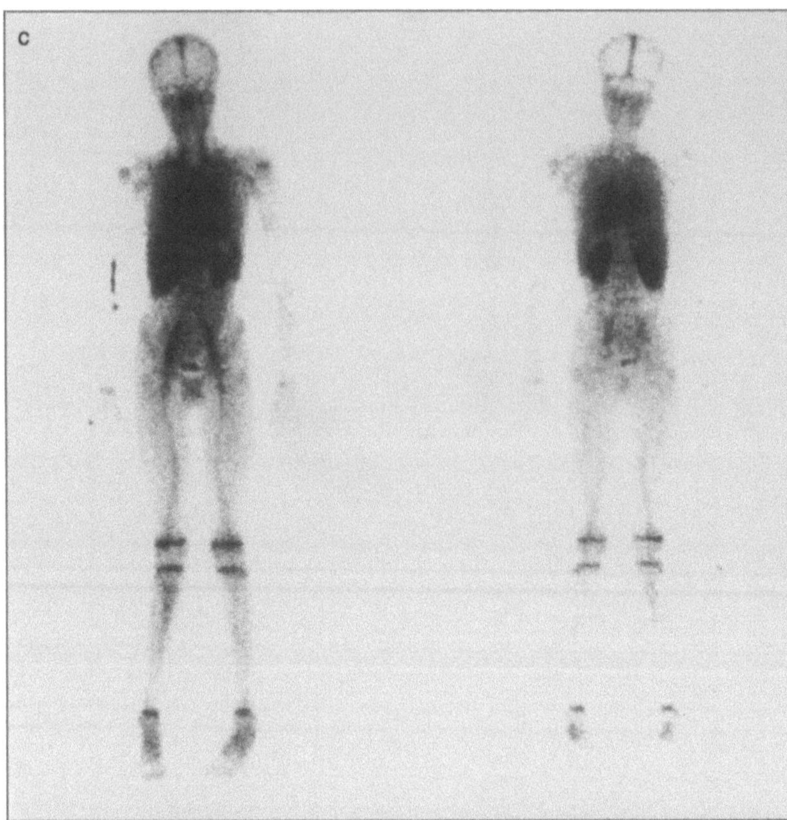

Fig. 4.19c. Blood pool whole body images show diffuse increased uptake of isotope in the upper right tibia; this is more homogeneous than on the previous scan

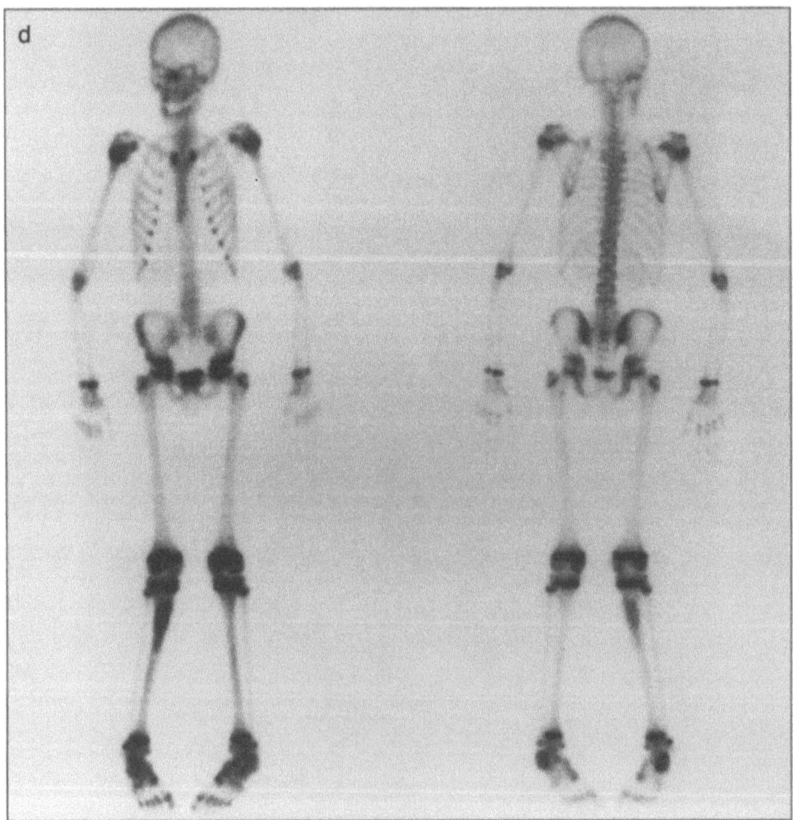

Fig. 4.19d. Whole body scans show diffuse abnormal uptake of isotope in the tupper right tibia

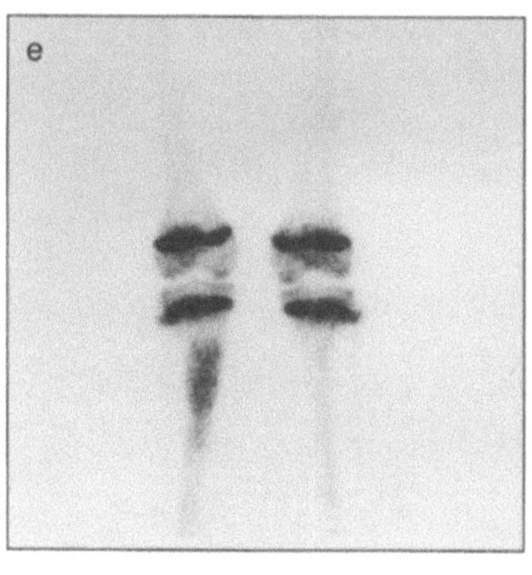

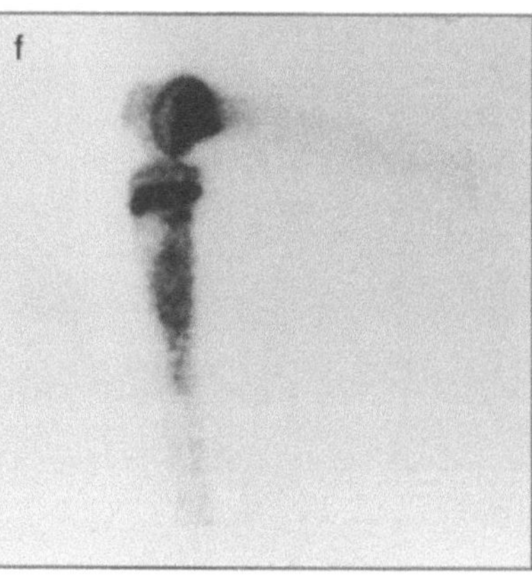

Fig. 4.19e. Anterior image of the knees. A generalised increased uptake of isotope is seen well below the epiphyseal plate of the right tibia, due to a metabolic activity of the implantated bone material

Fig. 4.19f. Lateral image of the right knee shows that the activity is mainly located posteriorly

Technical Comment

1. Note extravasation of isotope in the right hand at the site of the intravenous injection in Fig. 4.19a.
2. Note the isotope has been trapped in the veins of the right shoulder and arm as well as around the elbow in the blood pool phase (Fig. 4.19a), but this has partly cleared by the time the 3-h images have been obtained (Fig. 4.19b).

Teaching Point

The appearances on Fig. 4.19c–f are the result of surgery with bone grafting. The bone may show abnormal increased uptake for many years without complication. See Chap. 5.6 "Post-operative Appearances" and 5.5.1 "Pathological Fracture").

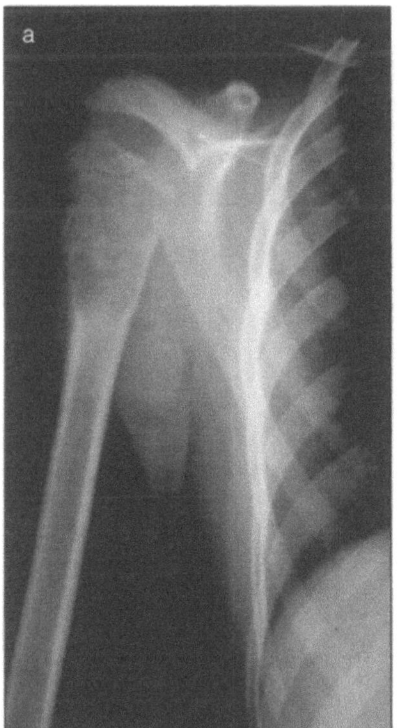

Case 4.20. A 12-year-old girl with pain following minimal trauma due to a fracture through a simple bone cyst in the right upper humerus

Fig. 4.20a. X-ray image of the right hemithorax and right upper humerus shows a well defined lytic lesion in the upper humerus with destruction of the cortex laterally

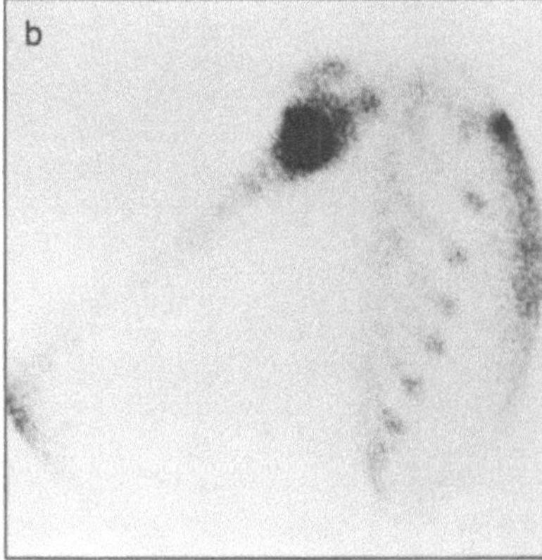

Fig. 4.20b. Anterior image of the right humerus and right hemithorax shows focal increased uptake of isotope in the proximal right humerus

Teaching Point

See Chap. 5.5.1 "Pathological Fracture").

Case 4.21. A 13-year-old girl who fell onto her hands and had pain in the right humerus. The final diagnosis was that of a fracture through a simple bone cyst in the right humerus and a fracture of the right distal radius

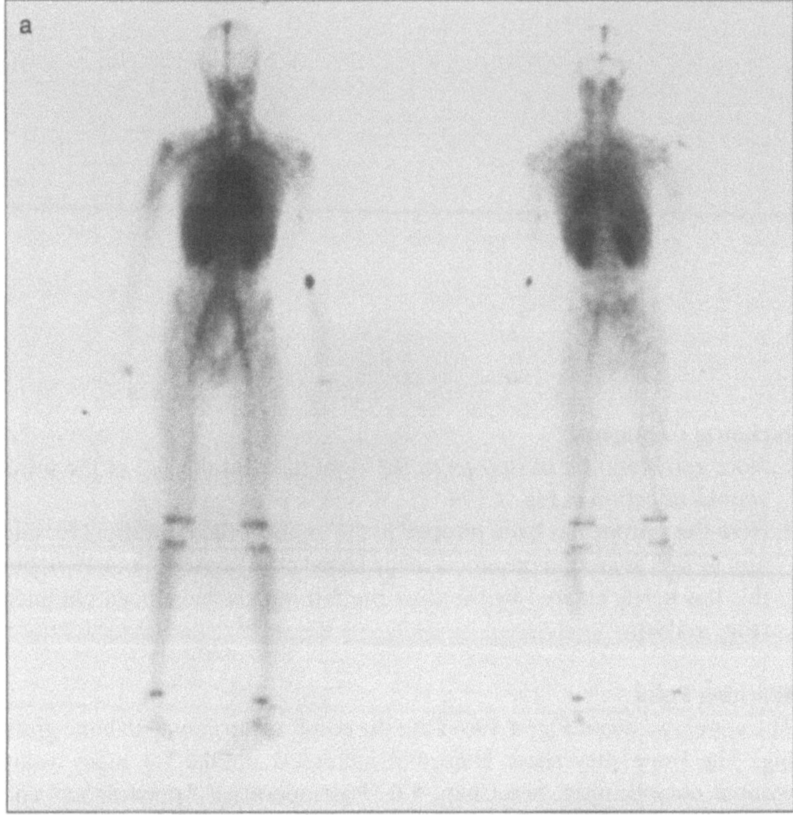

Fig. 4.21a. Whole body blood pool images show abnormal increased distribution of isotope in the upper portion of the right humerus, more obvious on the anterior than on the posterior view. Also note the increased uptake of isotope in the right distal radius

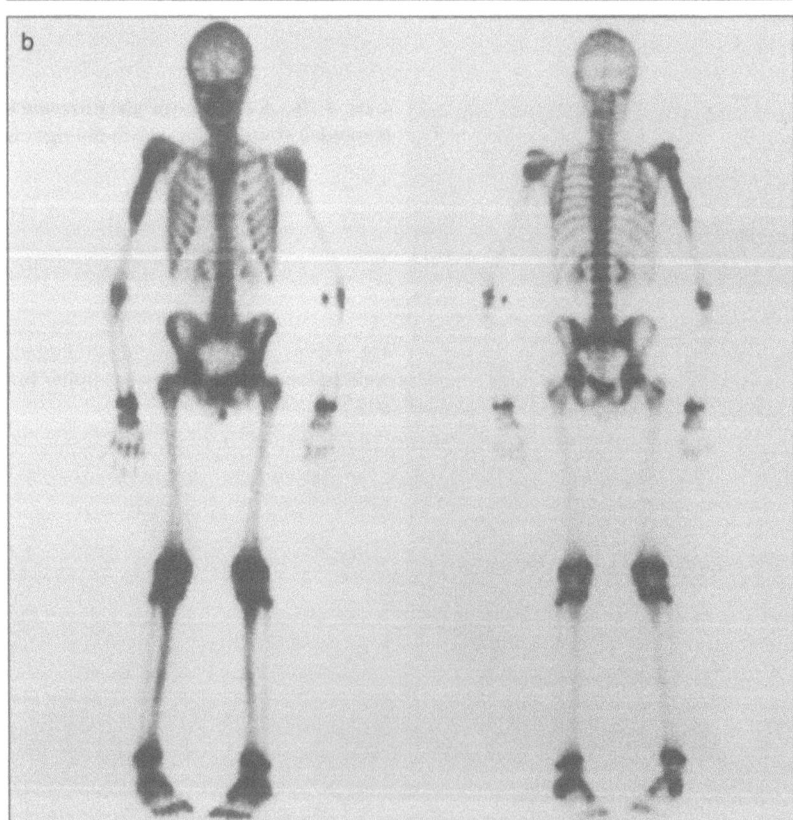

Fig. 4.21b. Whole body images show marked increased uptake of isotope throughout the upper half of the right humerus and the right distal radius

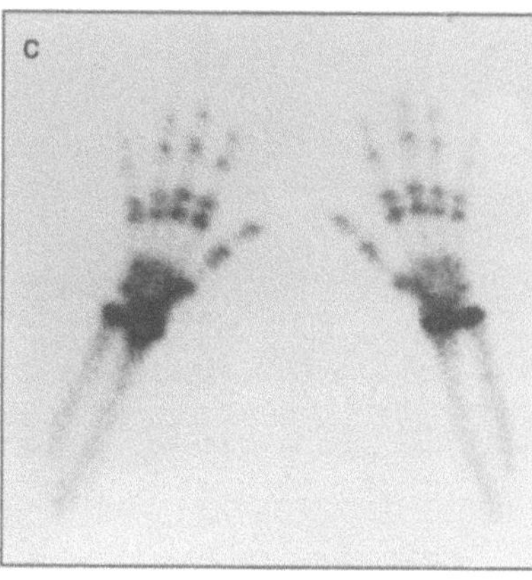

Fig. 4.21c. Palmar view of the hands. There is abnormal increased uptake of isotope most marked in the distal radius on the right. There is slight increased uptake of isotope by the small bones of the wrist on the right. This is presumably due to the associated hyperaemia of the right hand

Technical Comment

Note extravasation of isotope at the site of the injection in the left elbow in Fig. 4.21a,b.

Teaching Point

Similiar appearances could be seen with enchondroma (see Case 7.18).

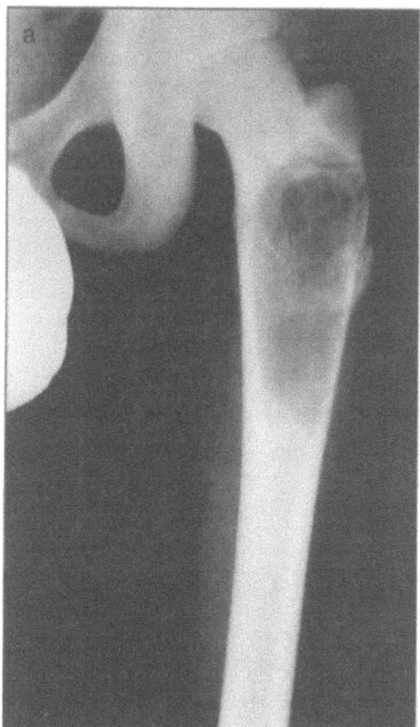

Case 4.22. A 9-year-old boy with a fracture through a bone cyst in the right proximal femur

Fig. 4.22a. X-ray image of the right femur shows a well defined translucent lesion in the upper femoral shaft with a break in the cortex laterally

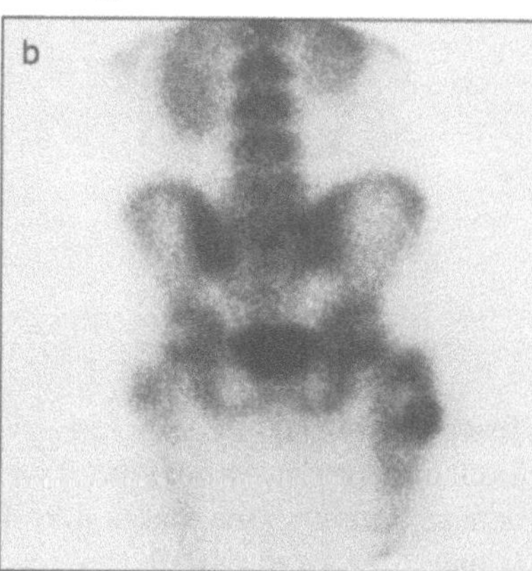

Fig. 4.22b. Posterior view of lumbar spine, pelvis and upper femora shows marked focal increased uptake in the upper right femur, with a "cold" area immediately above

Teaching Point

See Chap. 5.5.1 "Pathological Fracture").

Case 4.23. A 9-year-old boy who had pain in the left arm following minimal trauma due to a fracture through a simple bone cyst in the humerus

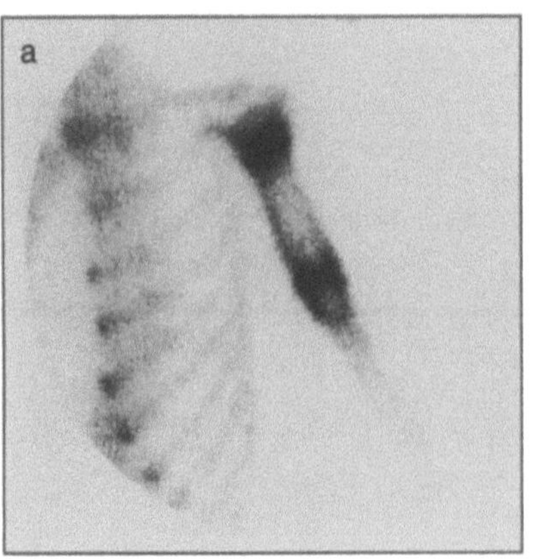

Fig. 4.23a. Anterior image of the left humerus shows decreased activity below the humeral growth plate with an area of marked increased activity at the junction of the upper and middle thirds of the humerus, the site of the fracture

4.1.4.3 Aneurysmal Bone Cysts
(3 Cases; Figs. 4.24–4.26)

Case 4.24. An 8-year-old girl who had progressive weakness of the lower limbs and then was unable to walk. An aneurysmal bone cyst of the lumbar spine at L5 was found to be compressing the spinal canal

Fig. 4.24a. Posterior image of the lumbar spine shows increased uptake of isotope at the L5 level more on the right than on the left

Fig. 4.24b. Magnification image of the spine shows focal abnormal increased uptake of isotope on the right, with additional generalised increased uptake of isotope in the body of L5. The aneurysmal bone cyst was found to lie primarily in the lateral aspect of the bony neural arch

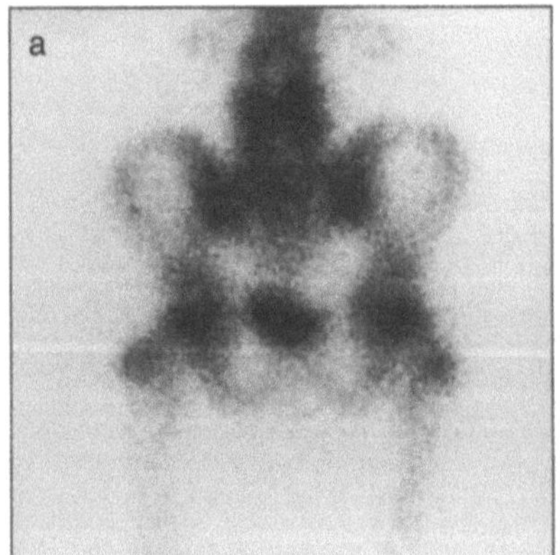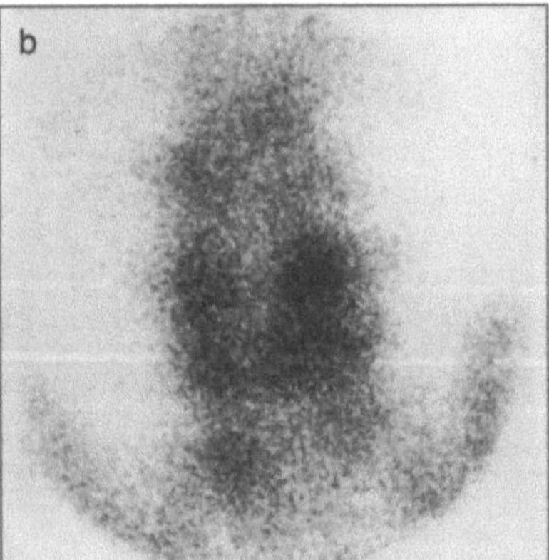

Teaching Point

Similar appearances may be seen in cases of discitis (see Chap. 2.3.3), benign tumours (see Cases 4.9, 4.10, 4.12 and 4.13), spondylolisthesis (Chap. 5.2.3) and trauma (see Case 5.13).

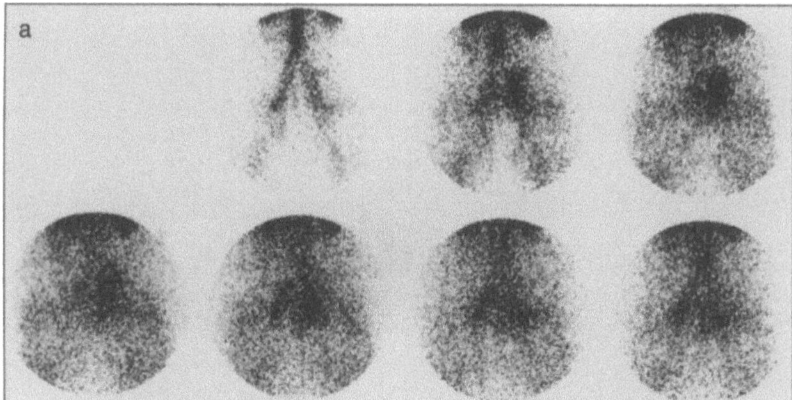

Case 4.25. 14-year-old girl with lower backache due to an aneurysmal bone cyst in the right sacral ala

Fig. 4.25a. Posterior blood flow images show abnormal increase of isotope in the region of the right sacro-iliac joint

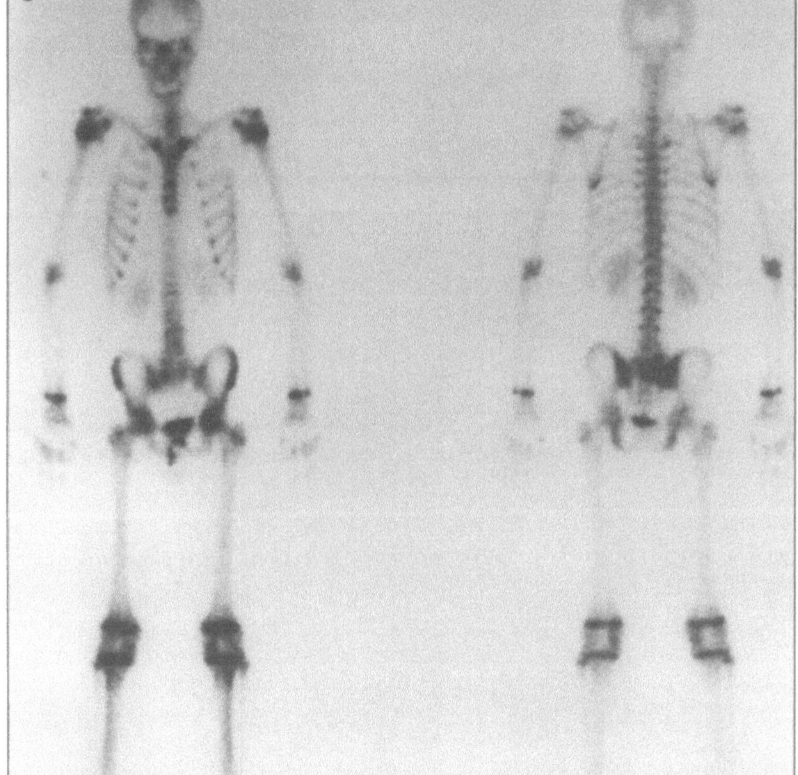

Fig. 4.25b. Whole body scans show abnormal increased uptake of isotope in the right sacro-iliac region, more marked on the sacral side with preservation of the iliac bone

Teaching Point

Similar appearances may be seen with infection (see Cases 3.3–3.5).

Case 4.26. A 10-year-old girl with an aneurysmal bone cyst in the right proximal femur

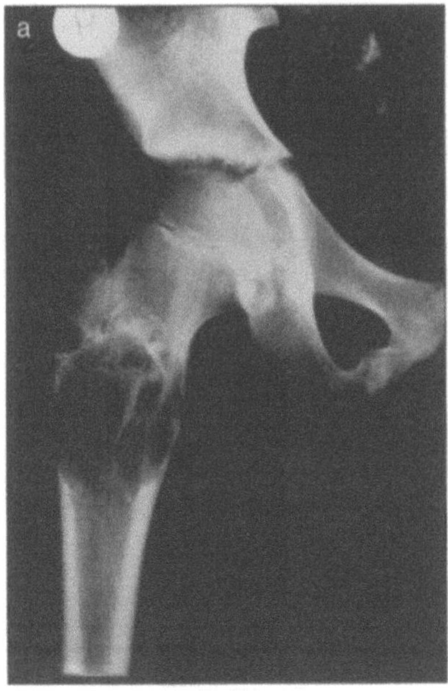

Fig. 4.26a. X-ray of the right upper femur shows a well defined expanded lesion in the upper femoral shaft with translucent and sclerotic areas. The cortical integrity is lost in two places

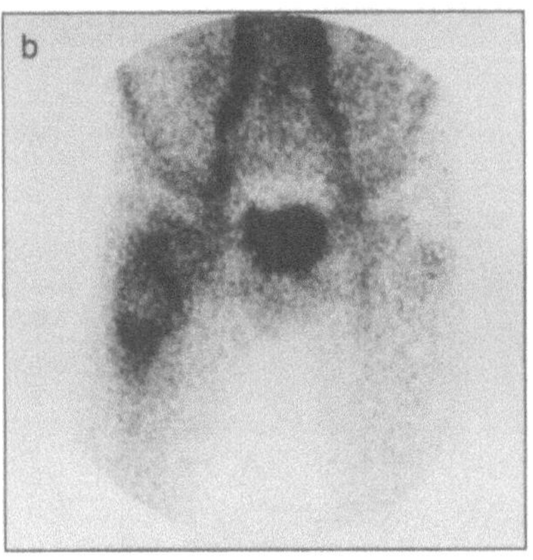

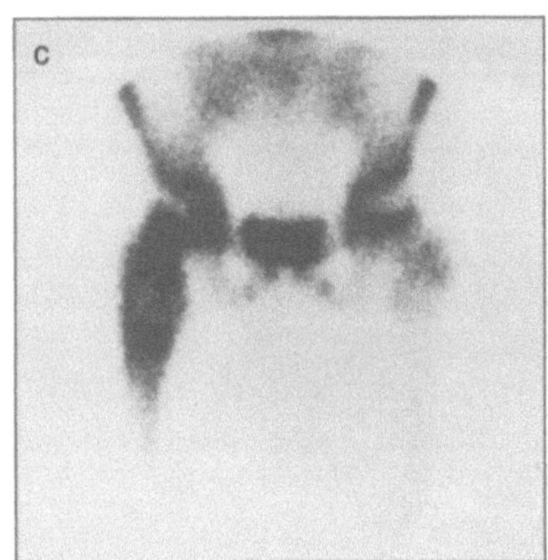

Fig. 4.26b. Anterior blood pool image of the pelvis and upper femora shows increased uptake of isotope in the area of the right proximal femur with an area of decreased uptake in the centre

Fig. 4.26c. Anterior image of the pelvis and upper femora shows marked increased uptake in the right proximal femur with an area of decreased uptake in the centre

4.2 Malignant Tumours

4.2.1 Skeletal Sarcoma

4.2.1.1 Ewing's Sarcoma
(10 Cases; Figs. 4.27–4.36)

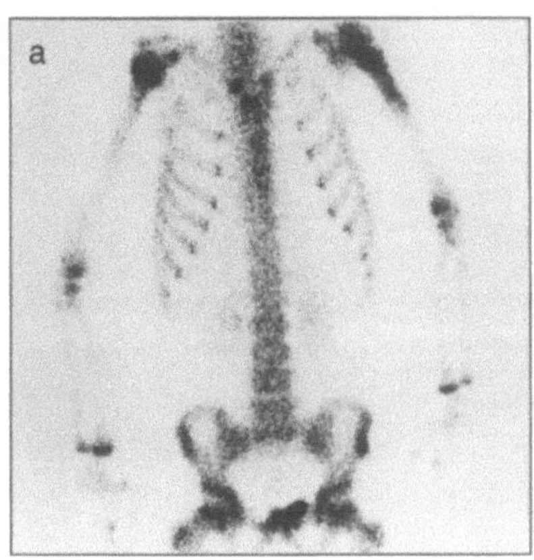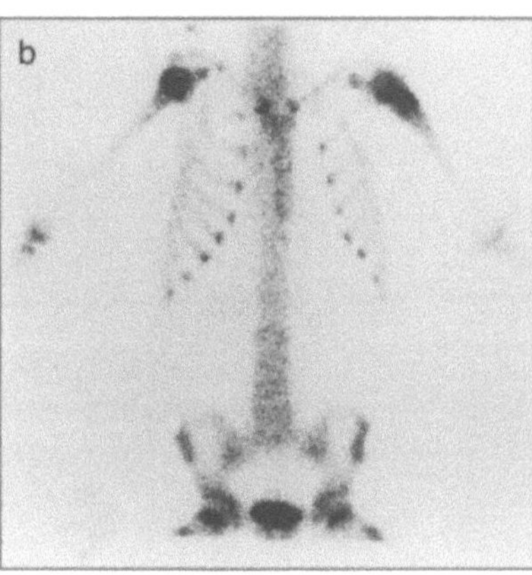

Technical Comment

In Fig. 4.27b, the appearances are due to a combination of therapy of the tumour and a pathological fracture. It is not possible to separate these two out simply on the bone scan.

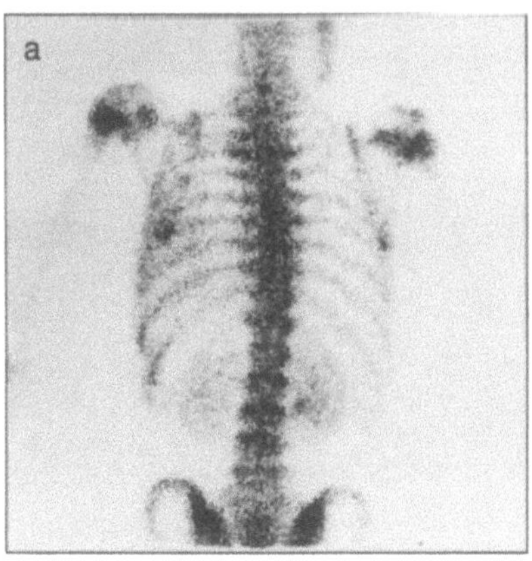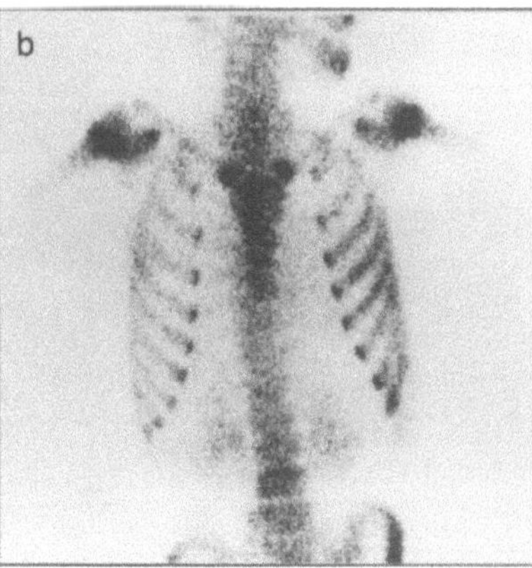

Teaching Point

1. The Ewing's sarcoma was arising from the left fourth rib in its anterior portion but the extensive extra-pleural extent of the mass had a pressure effect on the adjacent ribs causing the increased uptake of isotope (see Cases 5.56, 5.57).
2. Similar appearances may be seen with infection (see Cases 2.22, 2.30, 2.34, 2.35, 6.16–6.18).

Case 4.27. Ewing's sarcoma of the upper left humerus in an 9-year-old boy

Fig. 4.27a. Anterior image of the thorax and upper limbs shows abnormal increased uptake of isotope in the left humerus extending into the mid shaft of the humerus.

Following treatment, the child presented 1 year later with a pathological fracture through the upper humerus

Fig. 4.27b. Follow-up bone scan. Anterior image of the thorax and upper limbs shows increased activity in the upper left humerus which cannot be separated from the adjacent epiphyseal plate

Case 4.28. A 9-year-old girl who presented with pain in her chest due to a Ewing's sarcoma of the left ribs

Fig. 4.28a. Posterior image of the thorax and spine shows diffuse abnormal increased uptake of isotope in the posterior and axillary portions of the lower ribs on the left

Fig. 4.28b. Anterior image of the thorax shows marked abnormal increased uptake of isotope in the anterior portions of the left third, fourth and fifth ribs with diffuse abnormal increased uptake of isotope in the axillary portions of the remaining ribs

Case 4.29. A 9-year-old boy with a
Ewing's sarcoma of the left scapula

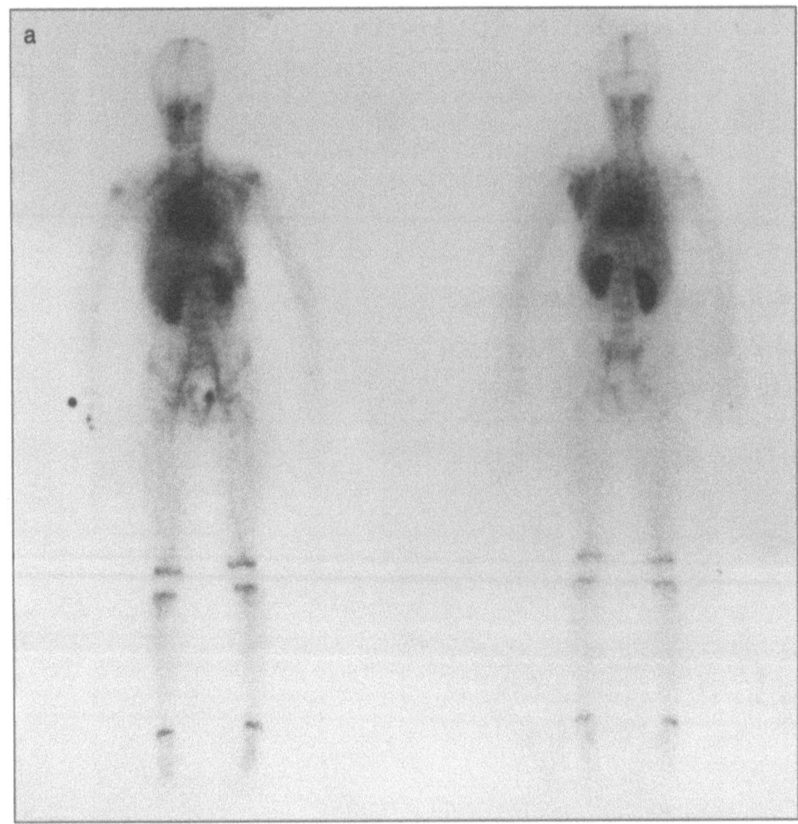

Fig. 4.29a. Blood pool whole body
images show abnormal increased
uptake of isotope in the region of the
left scapula, this is best seen on the
posterior view

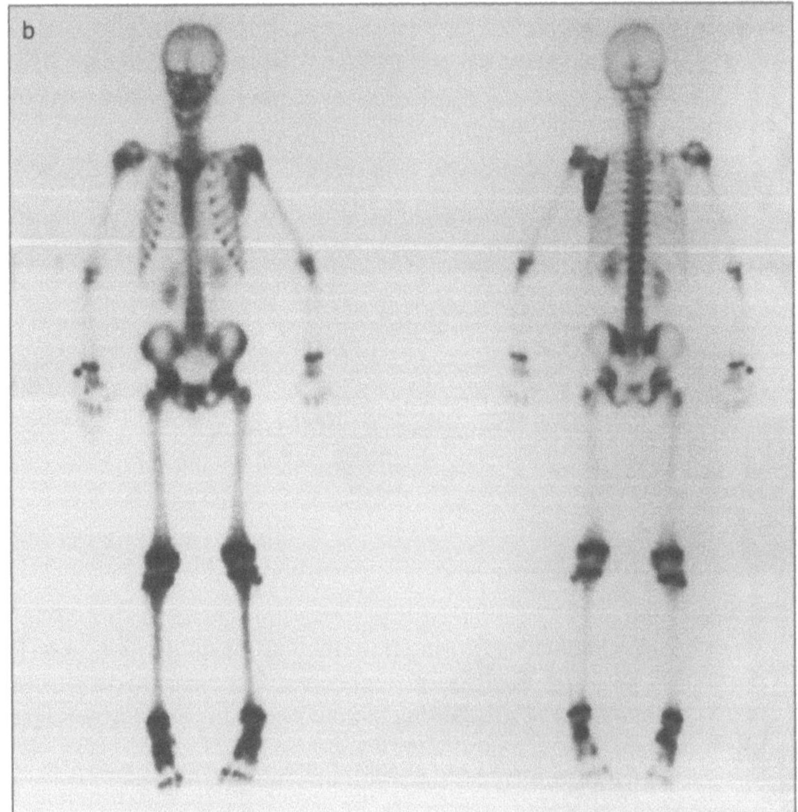

Fig. 4.29b. Whole body scans show
intense abnormal increased uptake of
isotope mainly in the lower and mid
portion of the scapula, again best seen
on the posterior view.

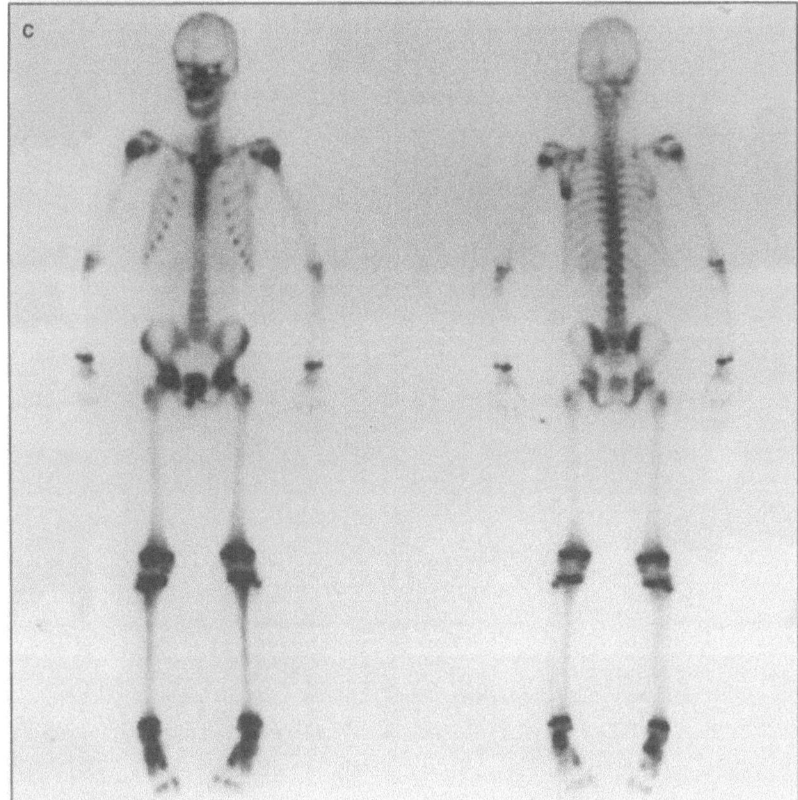

Following full chemotherapy and partial resection of the scapula, a repeat scan was undertaken 4 months later and showed marked improvement

Fig. 4.29c. Whole body images show a small area with abnormal increased uptake at the tip of the left scapula, due to postoperative changes or tumour relapse

Technical Comment
Note extravaxation of isotope at the site of injection at the right hand in Fig. 4.29a,b.

Teaching Point
Compare with soft tissue sarcoma (see Case 4.76). Similar appearances may be seen with infection (see Cases 2.36, 2.37).

Case 4.30. A 12-year-old girl with a Ewing's sarcoma of the right sixth rib

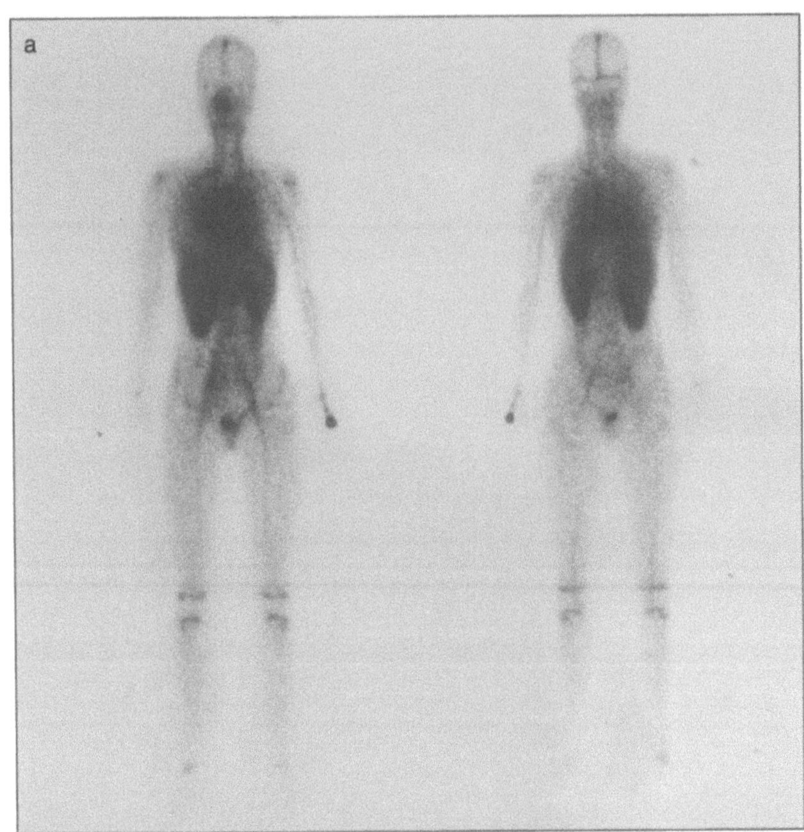

Fig. 4.30a. Blood pool whole body images are unhelpful. Note the isotope in the veins of the left upper limb following the injection of isotope

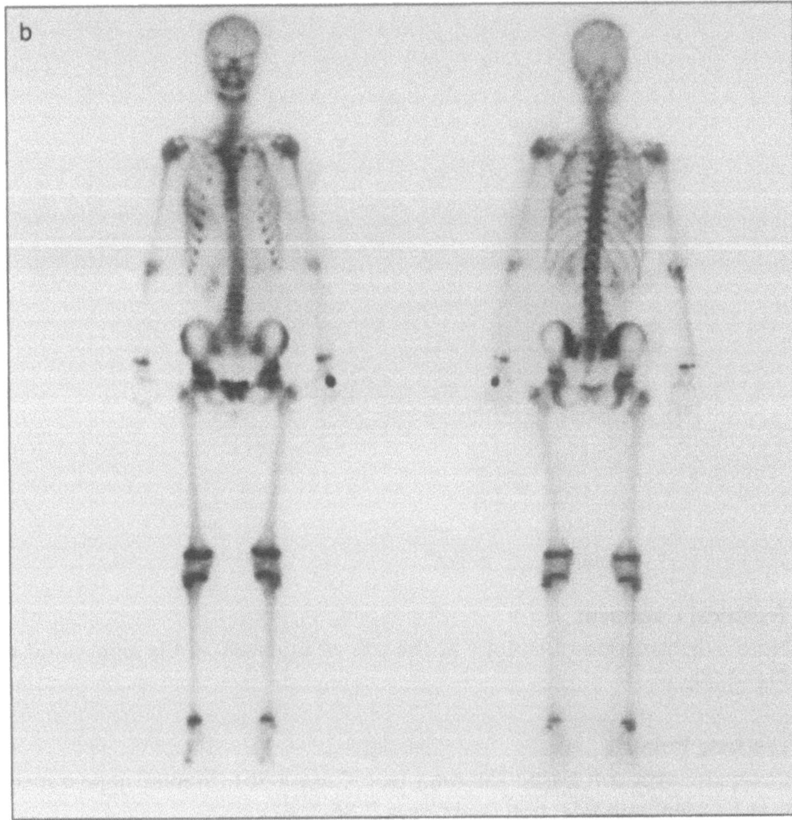

Fig. 4.30b. Whole body images show focal abnormal increased uptake of isotope in the anterior portion of the right sixth rib with increased uptake in the adjacent fifth rib

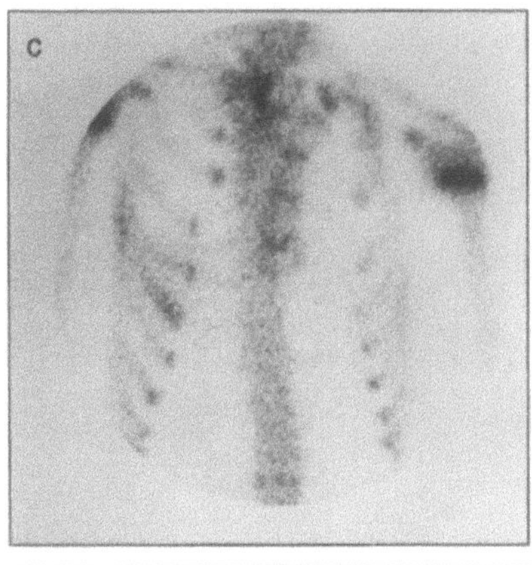

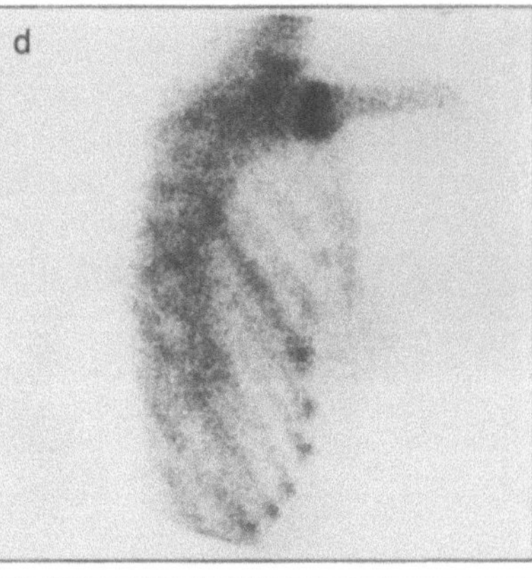

Fig. 4.30c. Anterior image of the thorax shows the abnormal ribs

Fig. 4.30d. Right lateral image of the chest shows that the sixth rib is involved almost in its entirety and there is, in addition, slight increased uptake of isotope in the rib above this. There is also evidence of uptake in soft tissues adjacent to the rib.

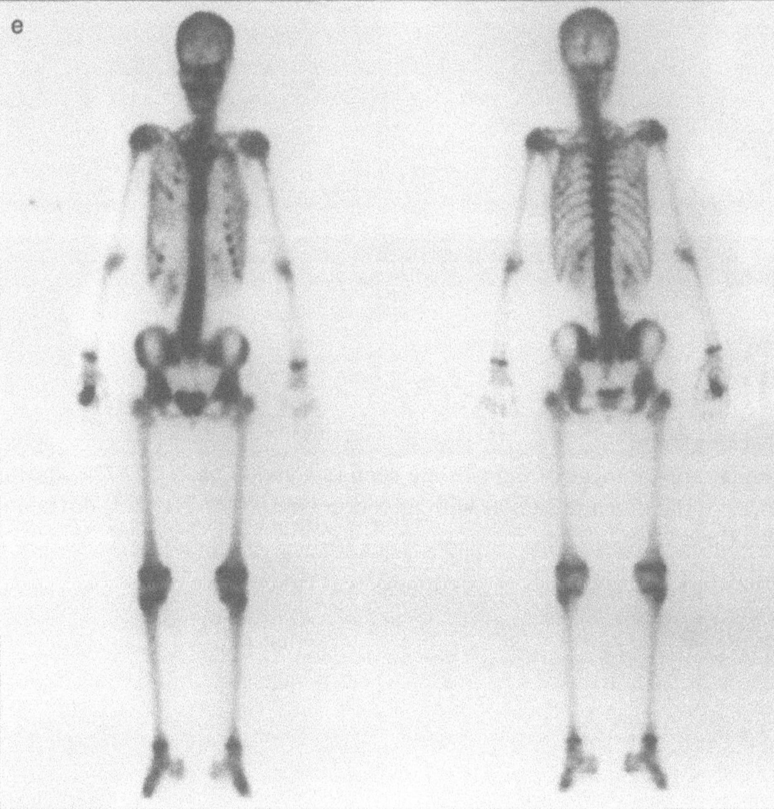

Following chemotherapy and surgery, the child underwent a follow-up bone scan 1 year later

Fig. 4.30e. Whole body bone scans show absence of activity in the region of the anterior portions of the right ribs, the area of rib resection

Fig. 4.30f. Right posterior oblique image of the ribs shows absent activity in the mid ribs following rib resection but there is still focal abnormal increased uptake of isotope in a short posterior segment of one of the right mid ribs, due to either tumour recurrence or effect of surgery

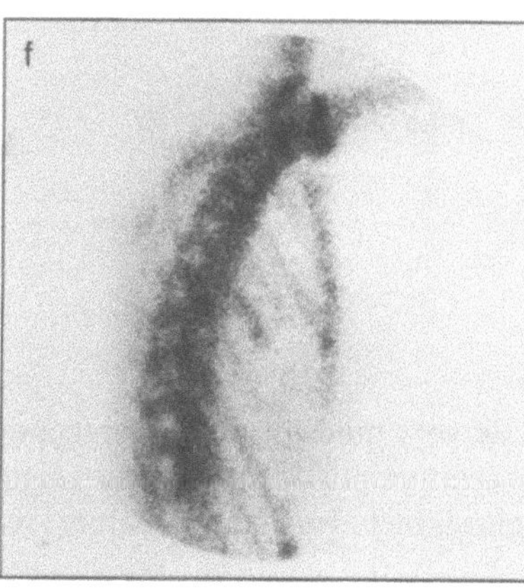

Technical Comment

Note extravasation of isotope at the injection site in the left wrist in Fig. 4.30a,b and in the right wrist in Fig. 4.30e.

Teaching Point

Similar appearances may be seen with infection (see Cases 2.22, 2.30, 2.34, 2.35, 6.16–6.18) or trauma (see Cases 5.56 and 5.57).

Case 4.31. A 2-year-old girl presented with a swelling on the back due to a Ewing's sarcoma of the rib. The child was treated with chemotherapy and represented with distant metastases 2 years later

Fig. 4.31a. At diagnosis. Posterior image of the thorax shows abnormal increased uptake of isotope in the left tenth and 11th ribs. The primary tumour was arising in the tenth rib with a mass effect causing displacement of the 11th rib

Fig. 4.31b. Posterior image of the lower limbs is normal.

Two years later the child represented with distant metastases

Fig. 4.31c. Posterior image of the thorax is normal

Fig. 4.31d. Posterior image of the lower limbs shows diffuse abnormal increased uptake of isotope throughout the left tibia due to Ewing's sarcoma. It was considered that this was a metastasis from the primary rather than a new secondary Ewing's sarcoma

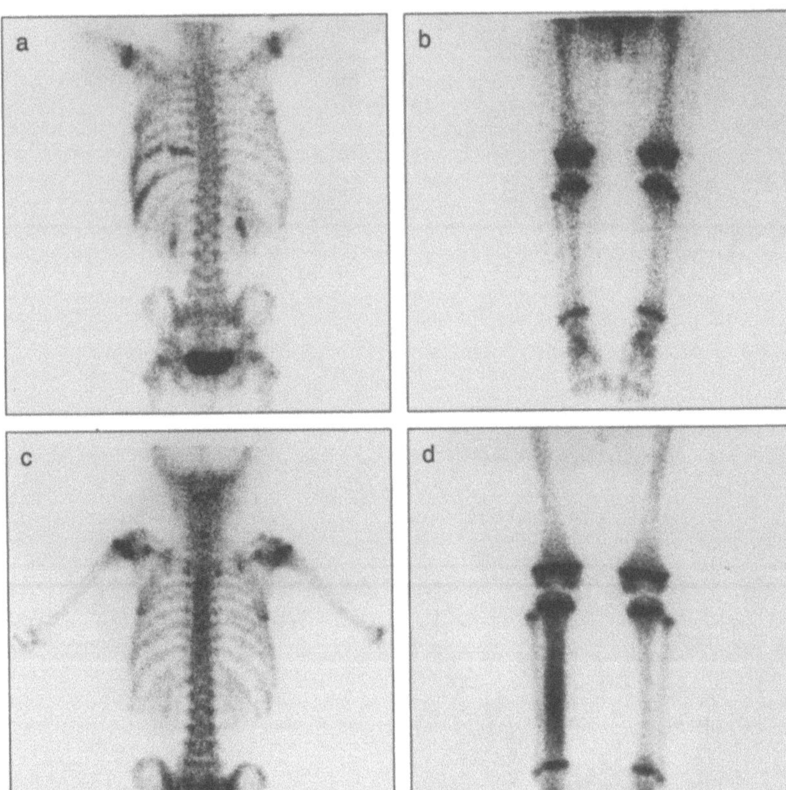

Teaching Point

Similar appearances of the ribs are seen in Cases 5.56, 5.57. The appearances of the tibia are similar with infection (see Cases 2.1, 2.2) or trauma (see Case 5.40).

Case 4.32. A 16-year-old girl with pain in the right leg. This was due to Ewing's sarcoma of the mid portion of the right fibula

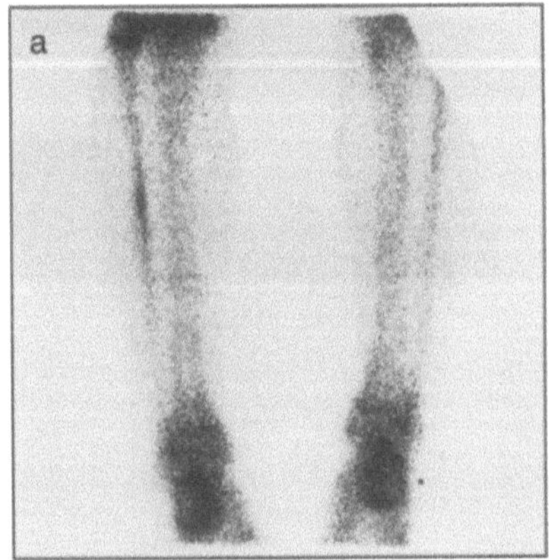

Fig. 4.32a. Anterior image of the lower legs shows abnormal increased uptake of isotope in the mid shaft of the right fibula

Teaching Point

Note that Ewing's sarcoma may stimulate very mild osteoblastic reaction and thus produces subtle signs on bone scintigraphy. The bone scan signs are non-specific and the differential diagnosis includes a stress fracture (see Cases 5.15, 5.22).

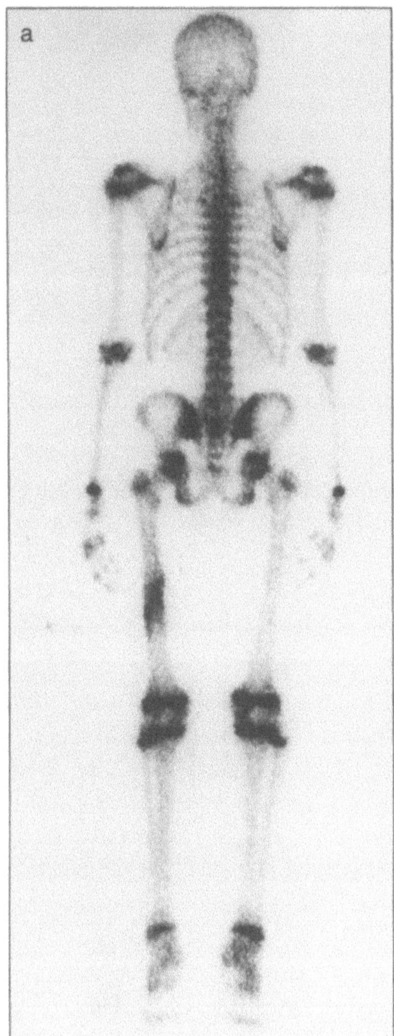
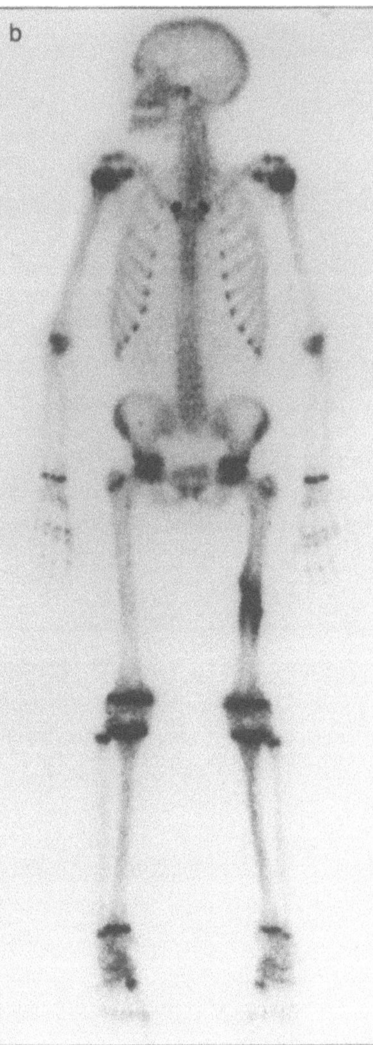

Case 4.33. A 10-year-old boy with a Ewing's sarcoma of the left femur

Fig. 4.33a. Posterior whole body scan shows abnormal increased uptake of isotope in the mid portion of the left femur. Asymmetry between the feet is noted

Fig. 4.33b. Anterior whole body scan confirms the abnormal increased uptake of isotope in the mid portion of the femur. Again the difference between the feet is noted

Teaching Point

No pathology was found in the feet and the suggestion that the authors make as to the difference in the appearances in the feet may be related to the fact that the child was limping for a short period due to the pain from the Ewing's sarcoma. Note, however, that the sacro-iliac joints appear symmetrical and there is no difference between the epiphyseal plates around the knees. These factors are against there having been a significant abnormal gait for any length of time.

Case 4.34. A 1-year-old boy with a Ewing's sarcoma in the left femur

Fig. 4.34a. Anterior blood pool image of the pelvis and lower limbs shows abnormal increased uptake of isotope in the region of the mid portion of the left thigh with decreased isotope in the left hemipelvis

Fig. 4.34b. Anterior image of the pelvis and lower limbs shows abnormal increased uptake of isotope in the mid portion of the left femur. There is again decreased uptake of isotope in the left hemipelvis

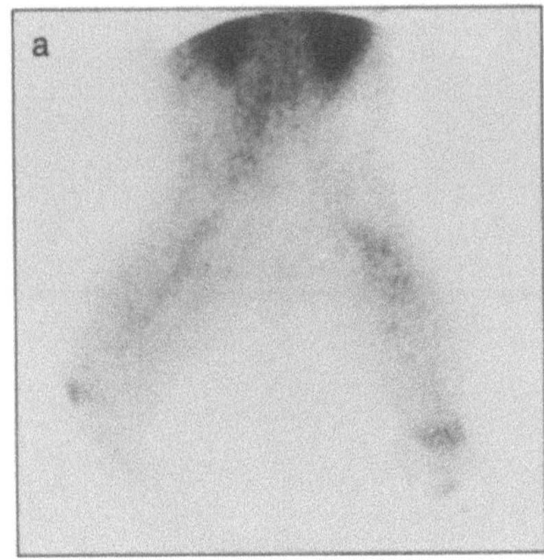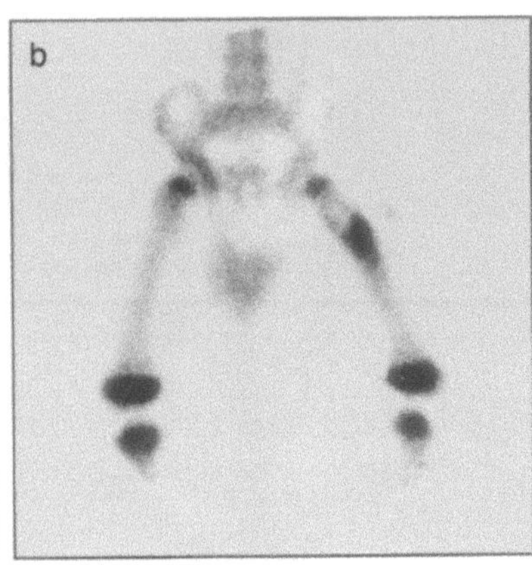

Technical Comment
Note the poor positioning of the lower limbs with the left leg being lateral and the knees are not together.

Case 4.35. A 14-year-old girl with Ewing's sarcoma of the distal left femur

Fig. 4.35a. Blood pool anterior view of the knees. There is increased uptake of isotope in the distal left femur

Fig. 4.35b. Anterior image of the knees shows abnormal increased uptake of isotope in the distal left femoral diaphysis extending to the epiphyseal plate. In the central portion of this increased activity is an area of decreased activity

Fig. 4.35c. Lateral image of the left knee shows the abnormal increased activity extending ventrally and this may well be the cause for the non-homogeneous distribution as noted in Fig. 4.35b

Fig. 4.35d. Lateral image of the right knee is normal.

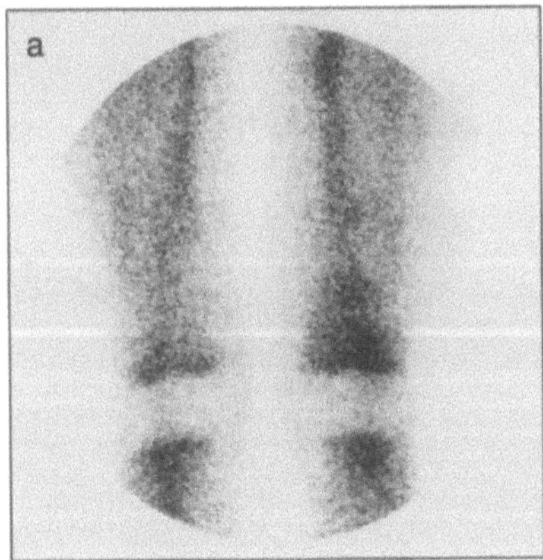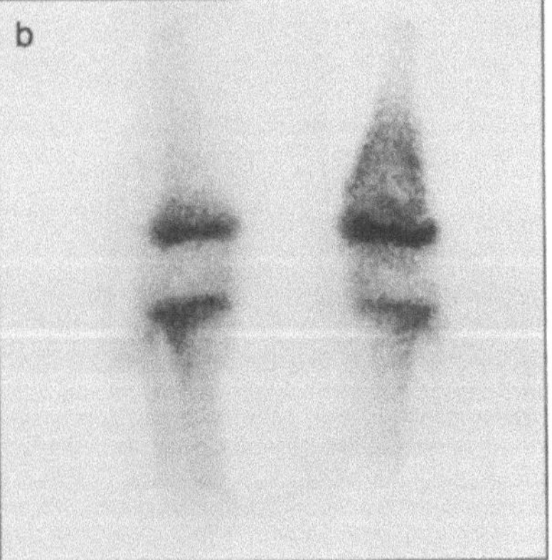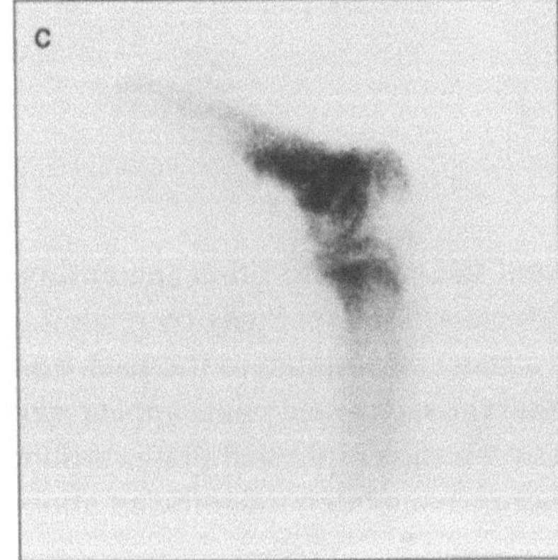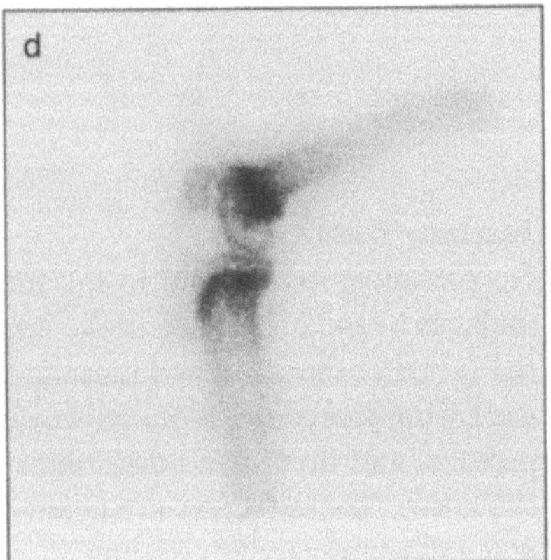

124

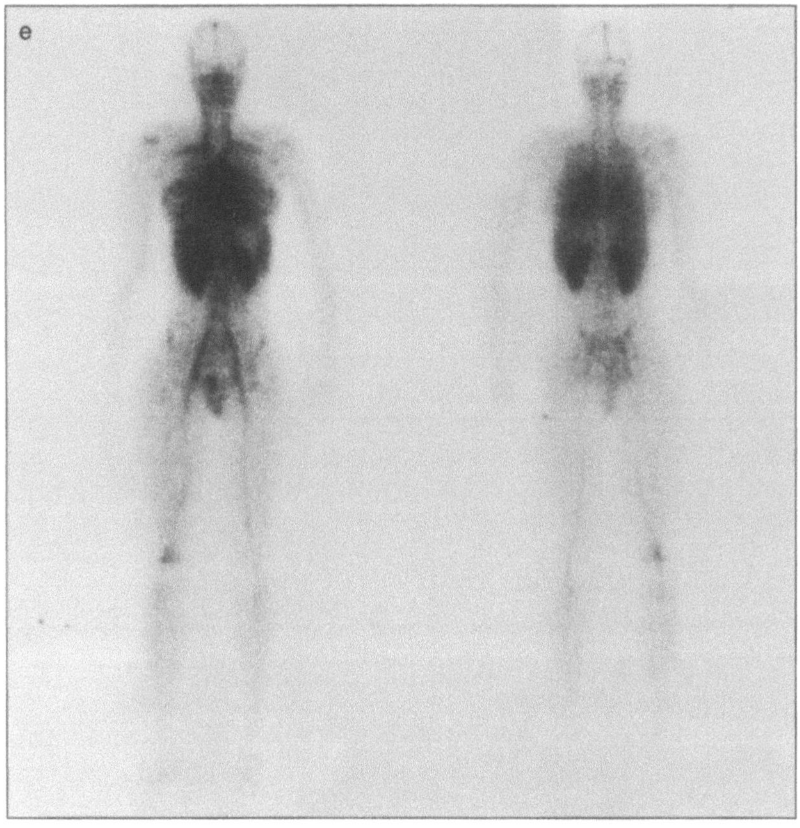

The child underwent chemotherapy and did well for a period of time but returned some 4 years later with pain in the opposite knee

Fig. 4.35e. Blood pool whole body scans 4 years later show abnormal increased uptake of isotope in the distal right femur and the right shoulder

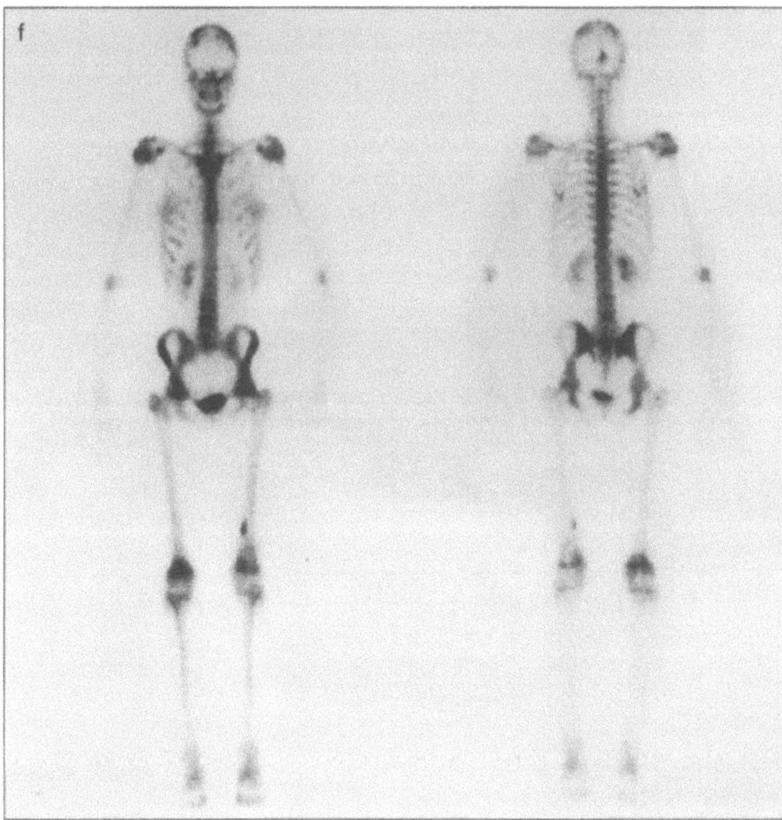

Fig. 4.35f. Whole body scans show abnormal increased uptake of isotope in the skull vault, the right shoulder and in the original primary tumour in the distal left femur but with a new skip lesion above this. There is, in addition, increased activity in the distal right femur. These were all due to deposits

Technical Comment
Fig. 4.35f, note the increased uptake in the region of the breasts on the anterior view; the patient was 18 years of age.

Case 4.36. A 13-year-old girl with primary multifocal Ewing's sarcoma

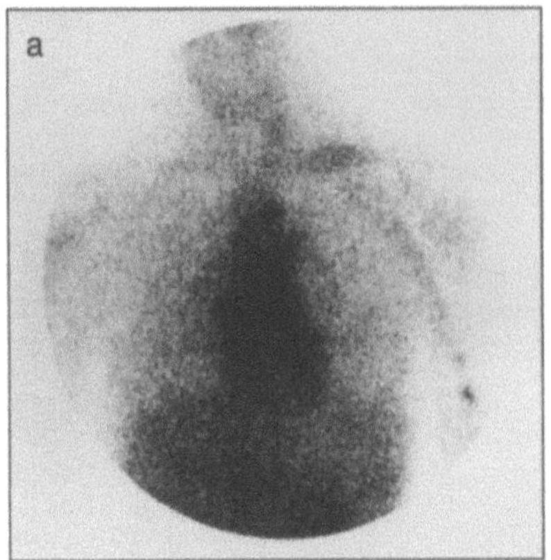

Fig. 4.36a. Blood pool anterior image of the chest shows abnormal increased uptake of isotope in the region of the left clavicle

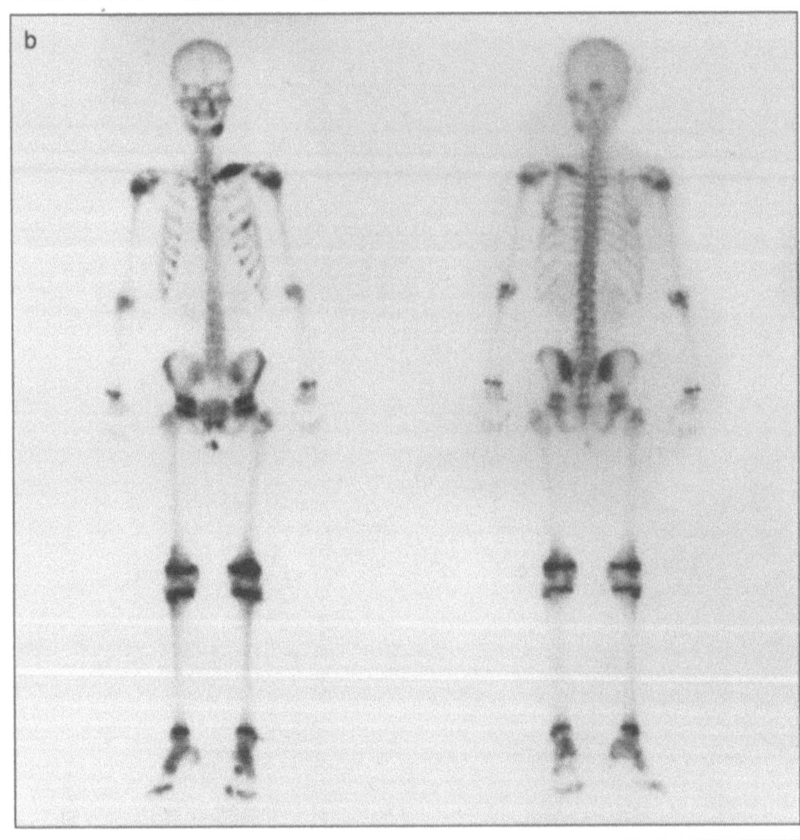

Fig. 4.36b. Whole body scans show abnormal increased uptake of isotope in the left clavicle, on the left side of the mandible, in the anterior left fifth rib and in the occipital bone of the skull

Fig. 4.36c. Left lateral image of the skull shows abnormal increased uptake in the mandible, occiput and left clavicle

Fig. 4.36d. Right lateral image of the skull fails to show the occipital lesion as clearly, as on Fig. 4.36c. The mandibular and clavicular lesions are again noted

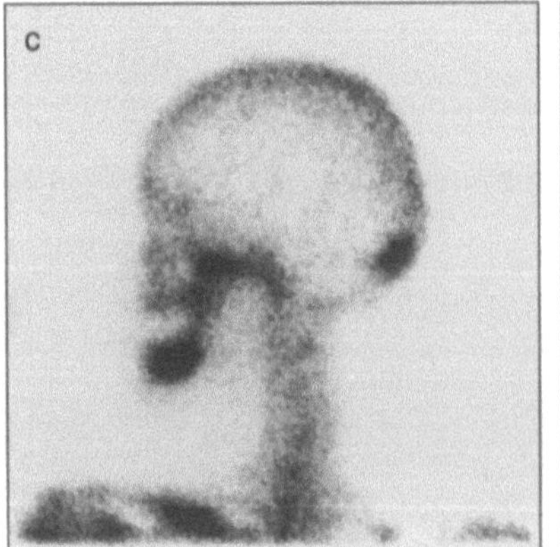

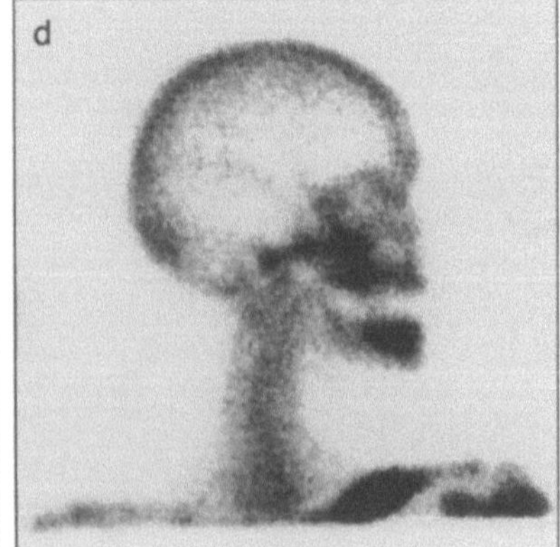

Teaching Point
Similar appearances may be seen with infection (see Cases 2.21, 2.28) or trauma (see Case 5.3).

4.2.1.2 Osteogenic Sarcoma
(14 Cases; Figs. 4.37–4.50)

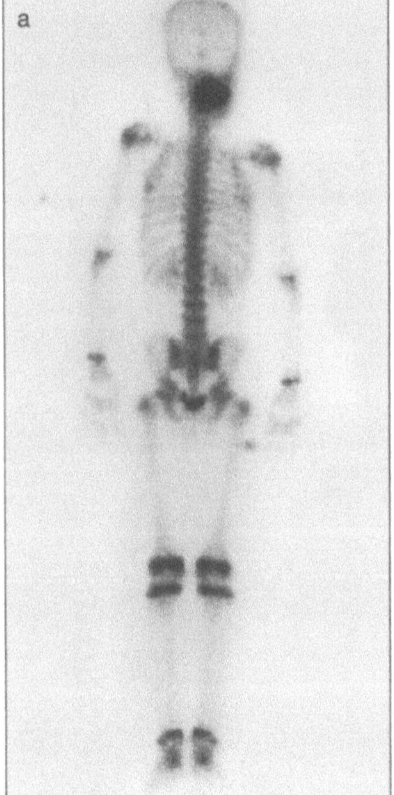

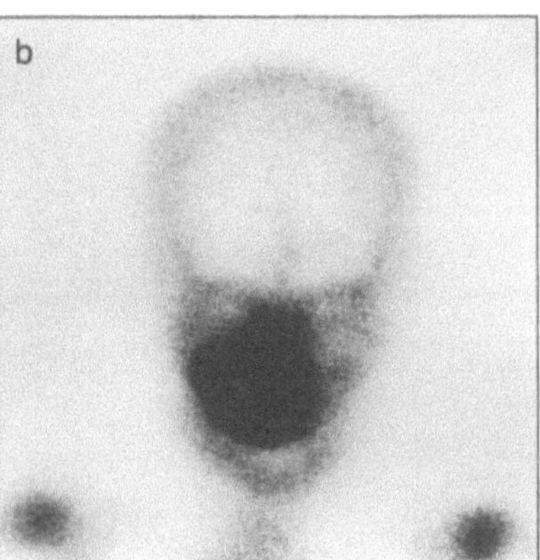

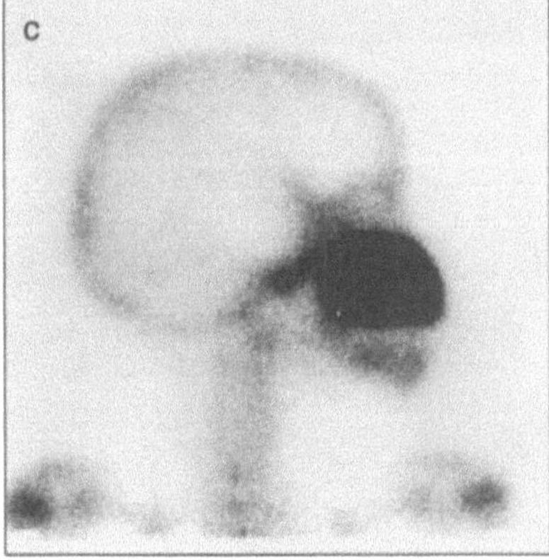

Case 4.37. A 10-year-old girl with a swelling of the face. An osteogenic sarcoma was arising from the maxilla

Fig. 4.37a. Whole body posterior scan shows focal abnormal uptake of isotope in the mid face

Fig. 4.37b,c. Anterior and right lateral images of the skull show that the abnormal increased uptake of isotope involves the entire mid face

Technical Comment

Note activity in the regions of the soft tissues of the upper aspect of the right thigh; this was due to contamination and was not seen on the spot views (not shown).

Teaching Point

1. With this intense increased uptake of isotope, it is impossible to be certain the origin of the tumour and CT scans were helpful.
2. Similar appearances can be seen with a primitive neuroectodermal tumour (PNET; see Case 4.54).

Case 4.38. A 20-year-old patient with pain on the right side of the face due to an osteogenic sarcoma of the right maxilla

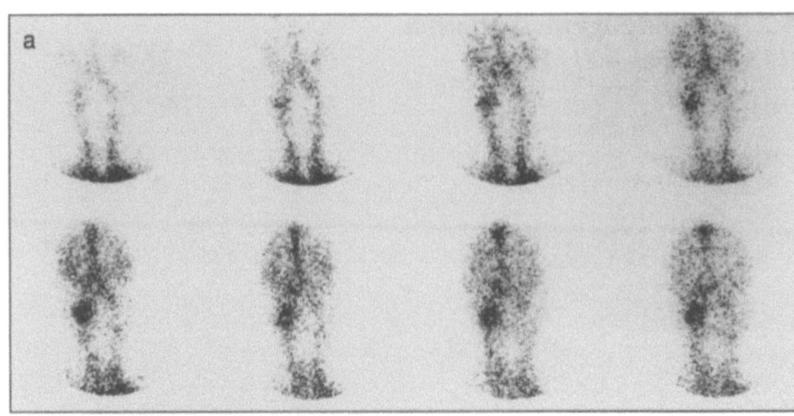

Fig. 4.38a. Blood flow images of the face and head show focal abnormal increased uptake of isotope on the right side

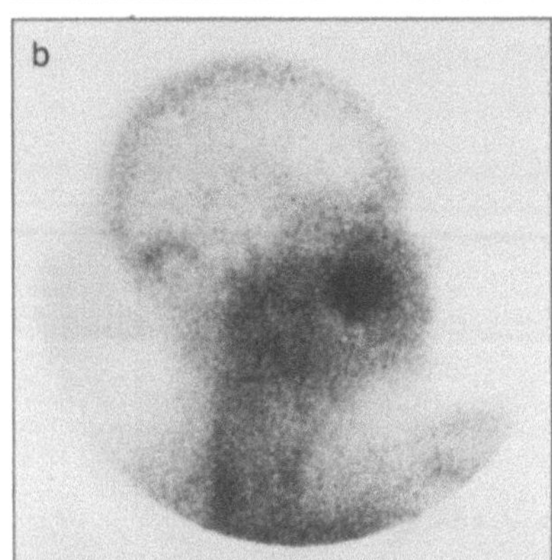

Fig. 4.38b. Blood pool right lateral image of the skull shows increased uptake in the region of the maxilla

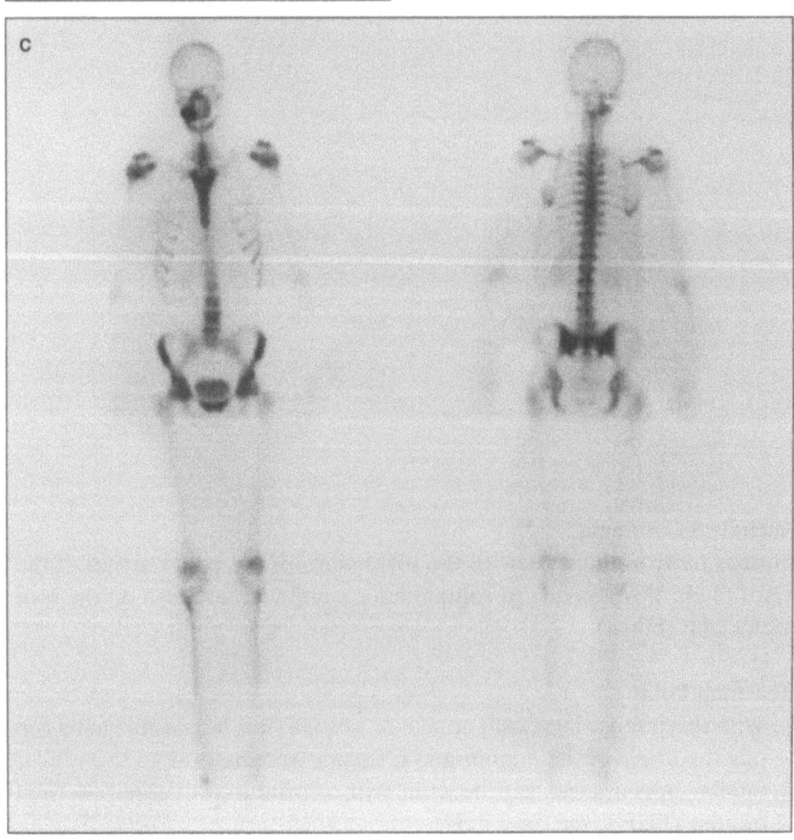

Fig. 4.38c. Whole body scans show intense abnormal increased uptake of isotope, better seen on the anterior than on the posterior view

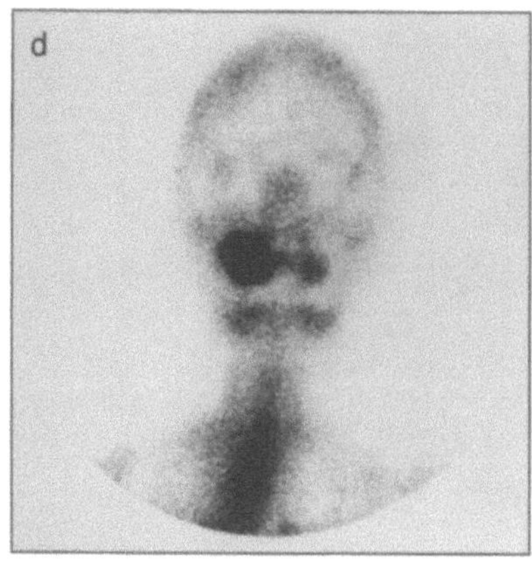 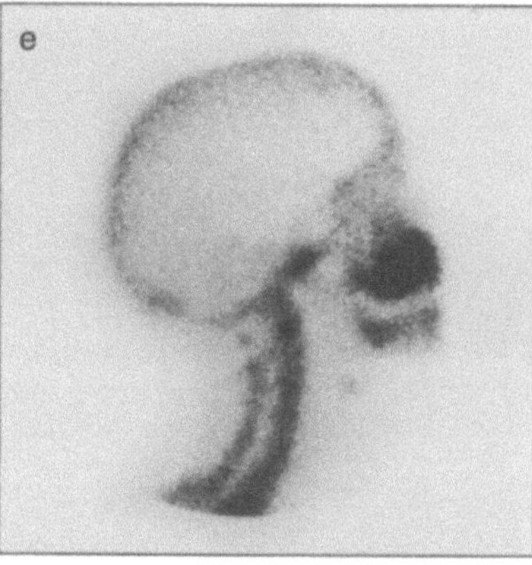

Fig. 4.38d. Anterior image of the skull shows marked increased uptake of isotope in the region of the right maxilla

Fig. 4.38e. Right lateral image of the skull shows the increased activity is confined to the inferior portion of the maxilla.

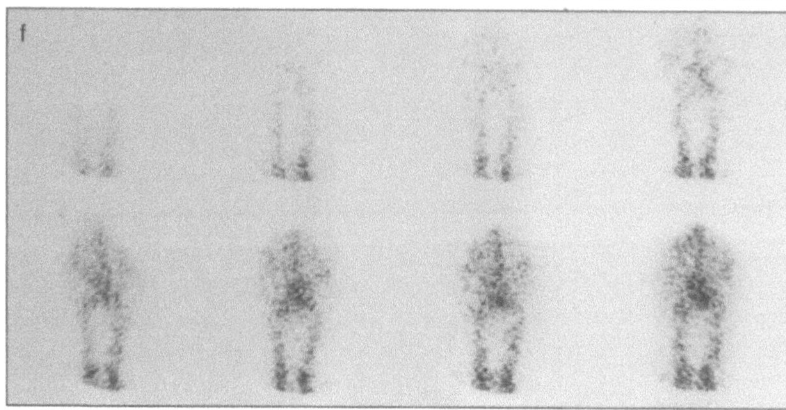

The patient was treated with chemotherapy and had routine follow-up. The scan done 2 years following the diagnosis was essentially normal

Fig. 4.38f. Blood flow. No abnormality is seen

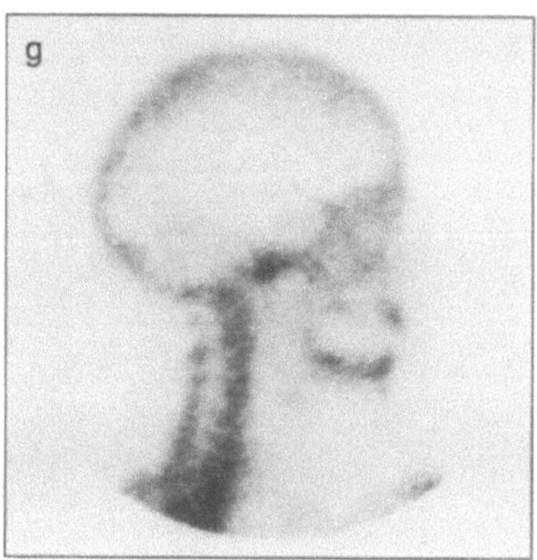

Fig. 4.38g. Right lateral image of the skull. There is a photon-deficient area in the inferior aspect of the mandible in the region of the hard palate

Teaching Point

Similar appearances could be seen with a PNET tumour (see Case 4.54).

Case 4.39. A 2-year-old boy with limited movement and pain in the right arm due to an osteogenic sarcoma of the upper end of the humerus. (Follow-up scan shown in Case 4.77)

Fig. 4.39a. Posterior blood pool image of the thorax and shoulders is normal

Fig. 4.39b. Right lateral image of the skull, anterior thorax and right arm shows the abnormal increased uptake of isotope in the proximal right diaphysis extending to the growth plate

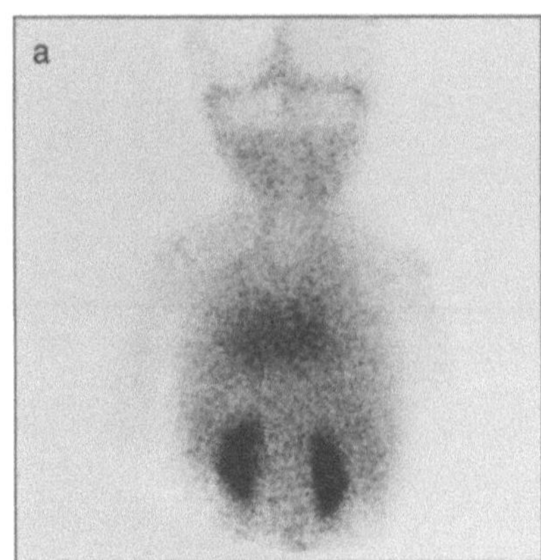
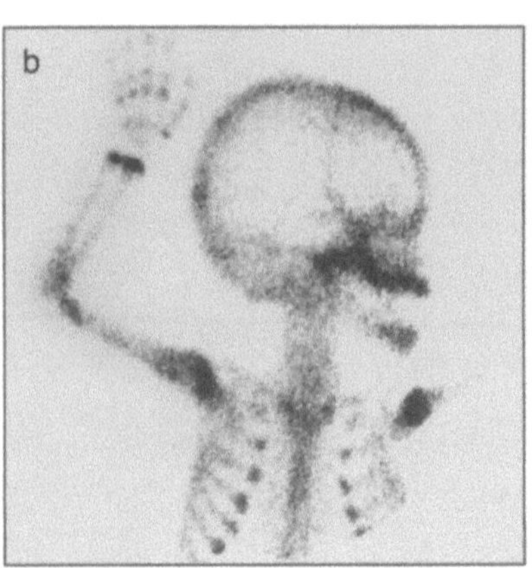

Case 4.40. An 11-year-old girl with swelling and pain of the left forearm due to an osteogenic sarcoma

Fig. 4.40a. Palmar image of the forearms shows abnormal uptake of isotope in the distal two thirds on the left. There are areas of intense increased uptake of isotope with other areas of only slight increased uptake. The lesion extends into the proximal radius. The increased uptake of isotope in the ulna was simply due to the pressure effect of the mass

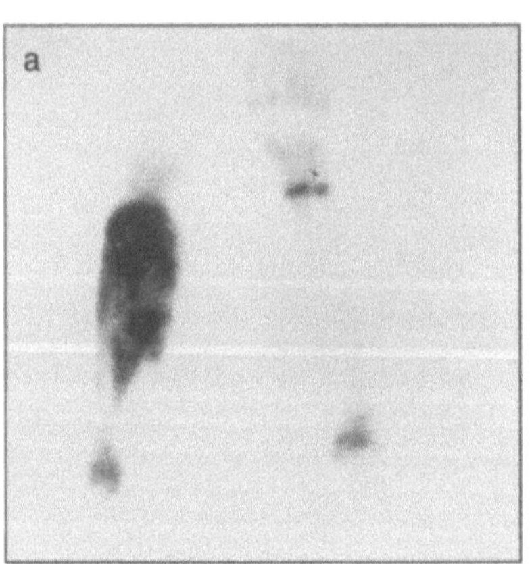

Teaching Point
1. The irregular uptake does suggest the possibility of a chondrosarcoma rather than an osteogenic sarcoma, but biopsy is the final arbiter.
2. Similar appearances with pressure effect are seen in Cases 5.56 and 5.57.

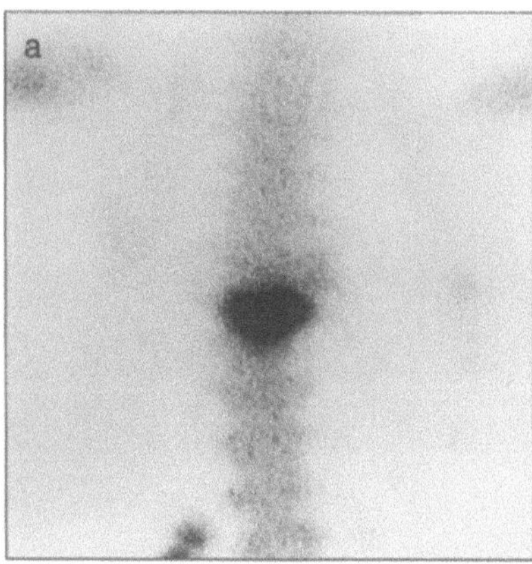

Case 4.41. A 6-year-old boy who had bladder symptoms and also weakness of the lower legs; this was due to a primary osteogenic sarcoma of one of the mid thoracic vertebral bodies

Fig. 4.41a. Posteror image of the thorax and spine shows focal intense increased uptake of isotope in a solitary mid dorsal vertebra.

Follow-up post-operative bone scan 3 months later

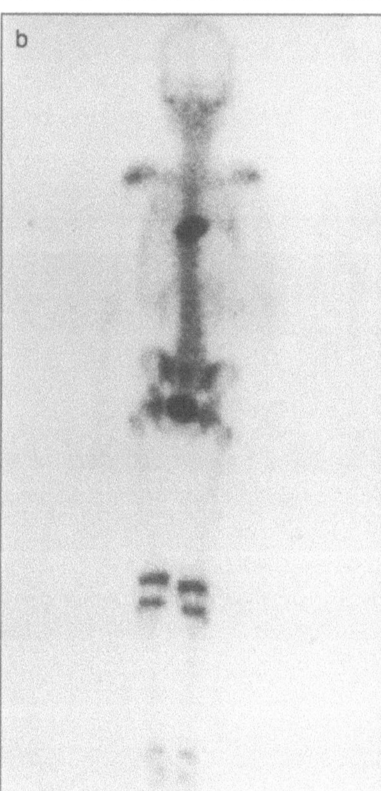

Fig. 4.41b. Whole body scan following surgery (posterior view) shows intense abnormal increased uptake of isotope in the mid dorsal spine which is seen to extend into the soft tissues. Absent activity in the posterior ribs on the right is noted

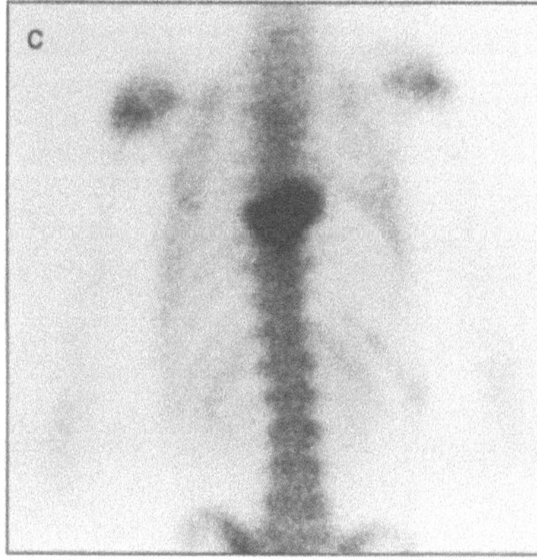

Fig. 4.41c. Posterior image of the spine and thorax shows the abnormal increased uptake of isotope in the spine as well as the photon-deficient areas in the ribs on the right

Technical Comment

1. The settings on the whole body scan are low because of the intense uptake by the tumour and therefore the absent ribs cannot be seen.
2. Scans in Fig. 4.41b,c were obtained following surgical rib resections.

Case 4.42. A 6-year-old girl with pain in the left thigh due to a primary osteogenic sarcoma in the proximal femur

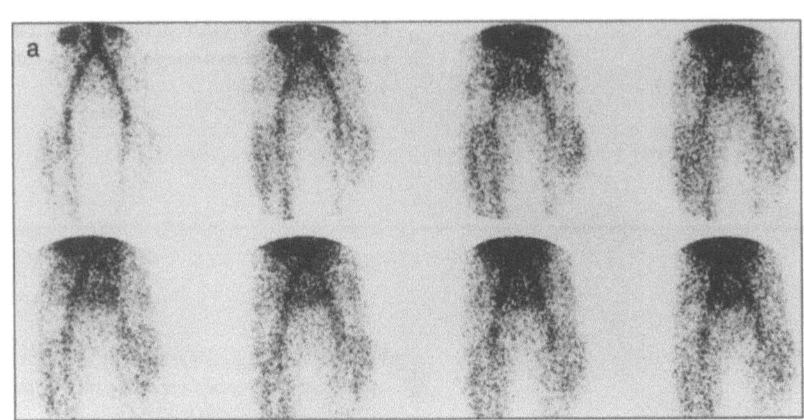

Fig. 4.42a. Anterior blood flow images show only minimal increased activity in the left thigh

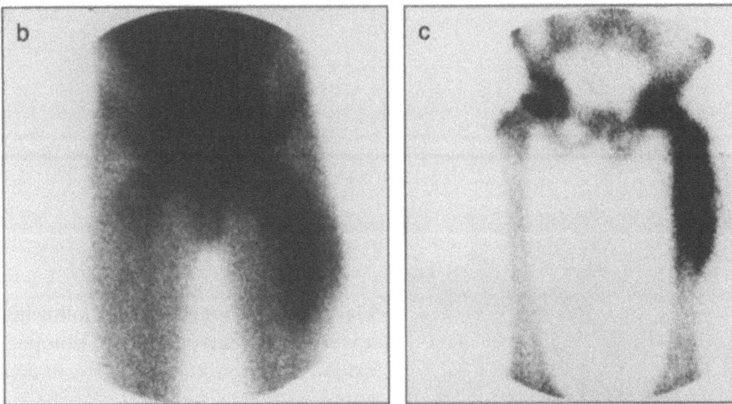

Fig. 4.42b. Anterior blood pool image of pelvis and upper femora shows quite marked increase of isotope in the proximal left thigh

Fig. 4.42c. Anterior image of the pelvis and upper femora shows that the lesion probably does not involve the neck of the femur on the left

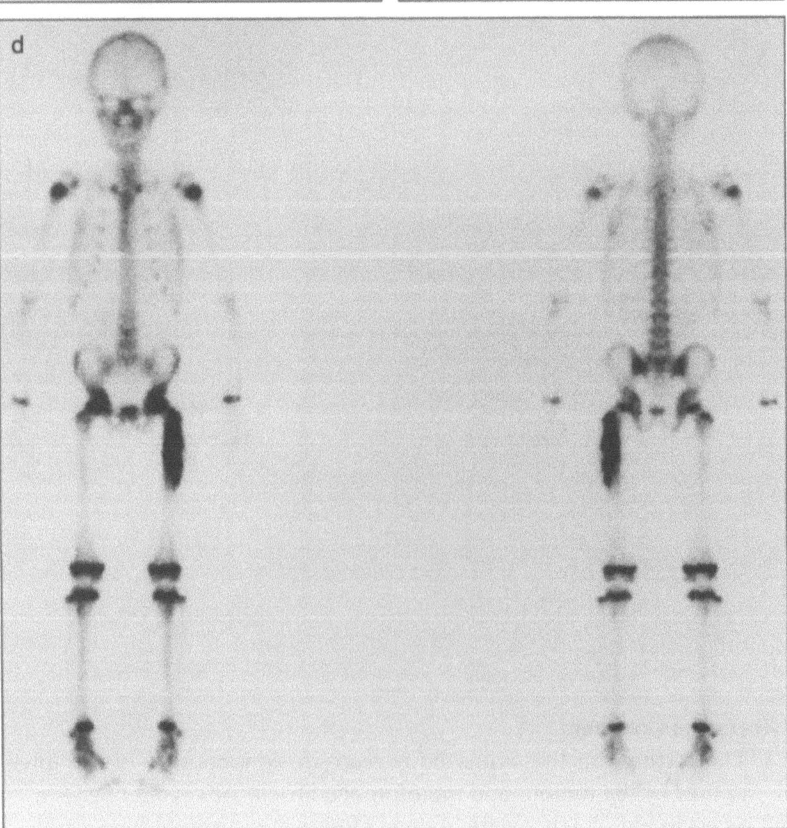

Fig. 4.42d. Whole body scans show abnormal increased uptake of isotope extending from the proximal left femur down the shaft to the mid portion of the femur. No metastases are seen

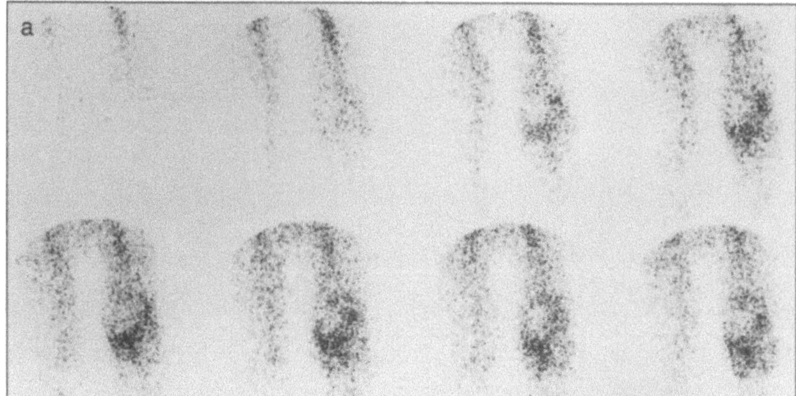

Case 4.43. An 8-year-old boy with pain in the leg due to a primary osteogenic sarcoma of the distal left femur

Fig. 4.43a. Anterior blood flow images show increased uptake of isotope in the region of the distal left femur

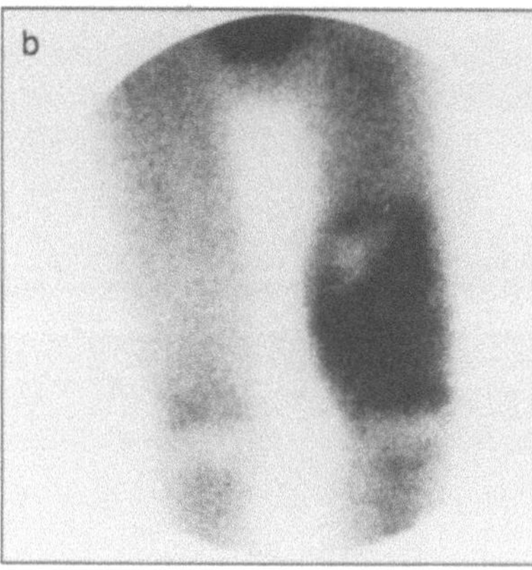

Fig. 4.43b. Blood pool anterior image of the knees shows marked abnormal increased uptake of isotope in the distal half of the left femur with increased uptake of isotope in the upper tibia as well

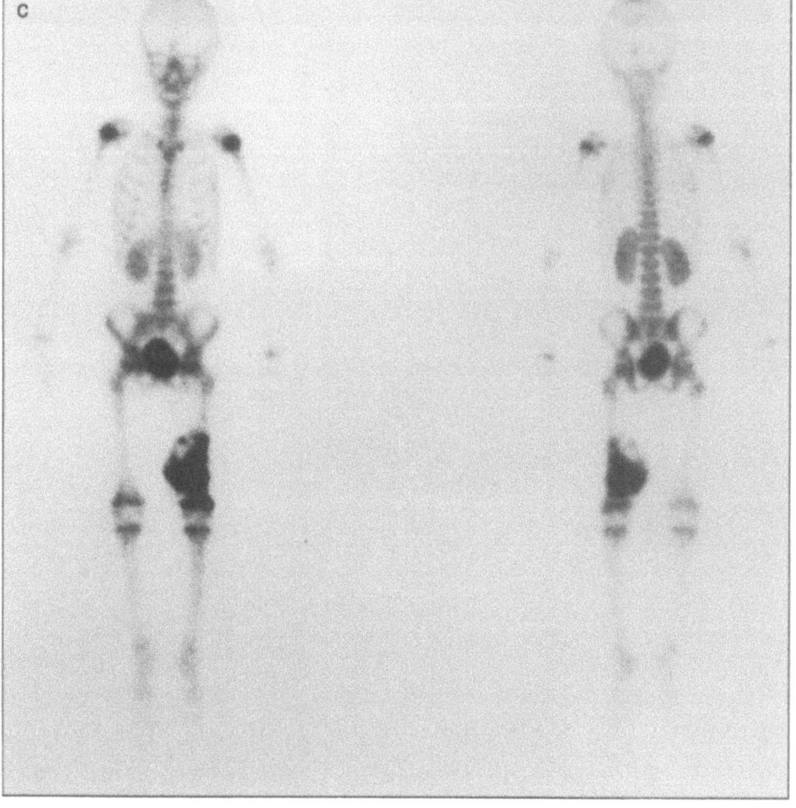

Fig. 4.43c. Whole body scans show marked abnormal increased uptake of isotope in the lower half of the left femur. The epiphyseal plate is still seen quite clearly, suggesting that the origin of the lesion is in the diaphysis of the distal femur

Teaching Point
1. Note the marked retention of radiotracer by both kidneys. This scan was undertaken before chemotherapy was started and the reason for the uptake by the kidneys is uncertain.
2. The increased uptake in the proximal tibial epiphyseal plates is presumably related to the general hyperaemia of the left knee.

Case 4.44. **A 9-year-old boy with pain and a limp due to osteogenic sarcoma of the distal right femur with distant metastases at presentation**

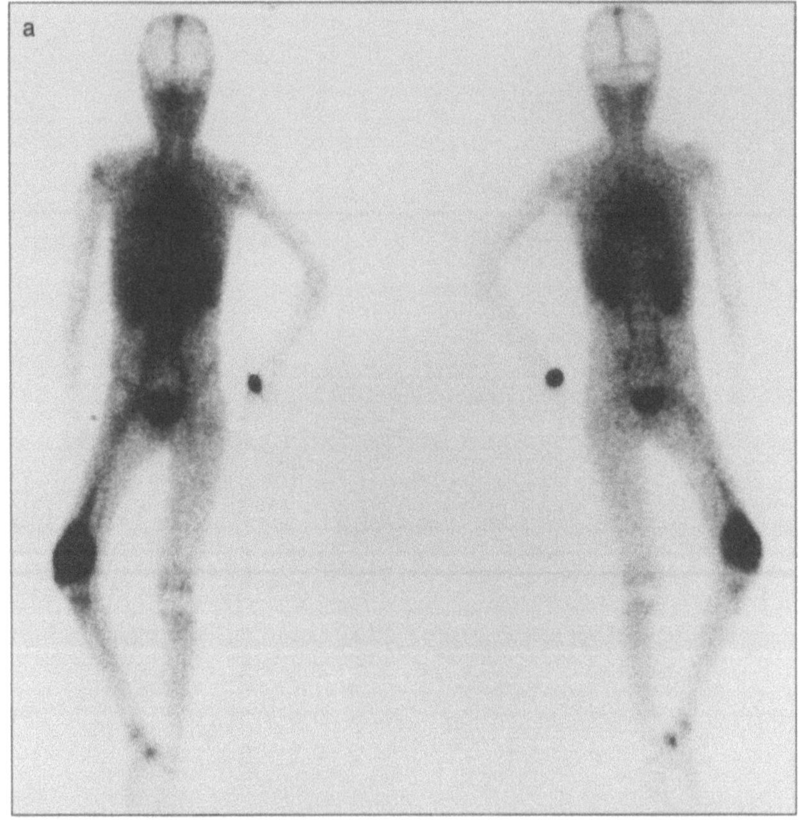

Fig. 4.44a. Whole body blood pool images show intense abnormal increased uptake of isotope in the distal right femur with extension into the mid shaft of the femur. There is also increased uptake of isotope in the right ankle

Fig. 4.44b. Whole body scans show abnormal uptake extending from the distal right femoral condyles proximally into the mid shaft of the femur with a small skip lesion. Abnormal activity is also noted in the right foot, the right proximal humerus and the right hip

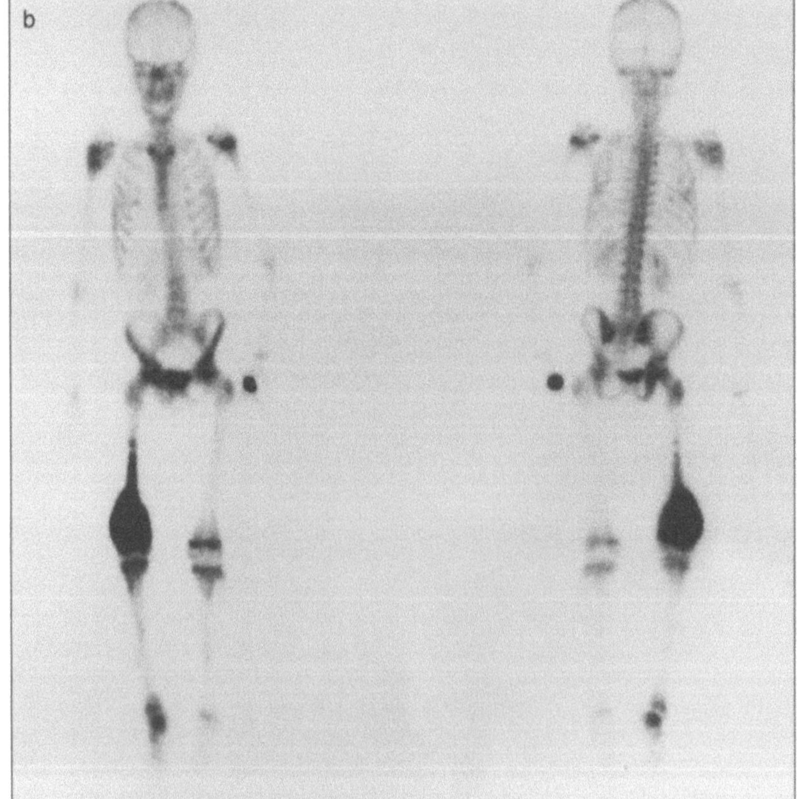

Technical Comment

Note extravasation at the site of injection in the left hand.

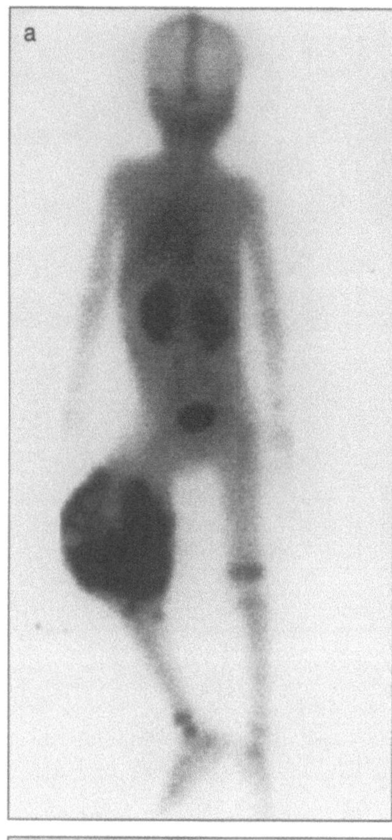
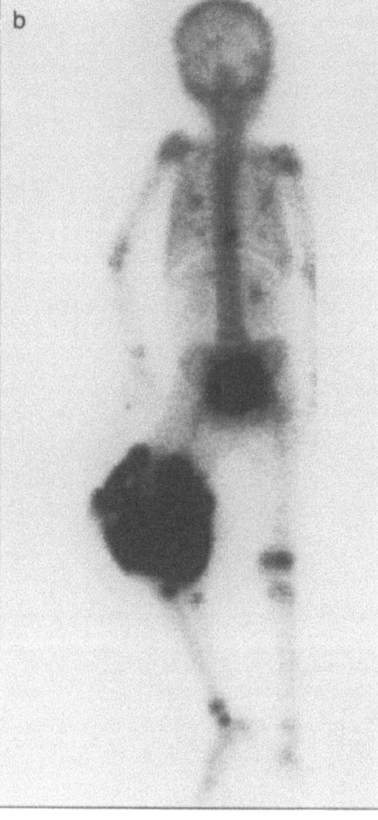

Case 4.45. A 4-year-old boy who presented with a large swelling of the left thigh. The history was of many months duration and the child was suffering from a primary osteogenic sarcoma of the left femur with distant metastases in ribs, spine and lungs

Fig. 4.45a. Posterior blood pool whole body image shows the mass in the distal left femur with intense uptake of isotope. This is not homogeneous with areas of slightly decreased uptake of isotope noted. The normal anatomy of the knee joint has been lost. Abnormal uptake around the left ankle is noted

Fig. 4.45b. Posterior whole body scan shows abnormal uptake of isotope in the mass on the left. The femur cannot be separated from the mass. Abnormal uptake is also noted in the lower thoracic vertebrae, in the thorax and around the left ankle

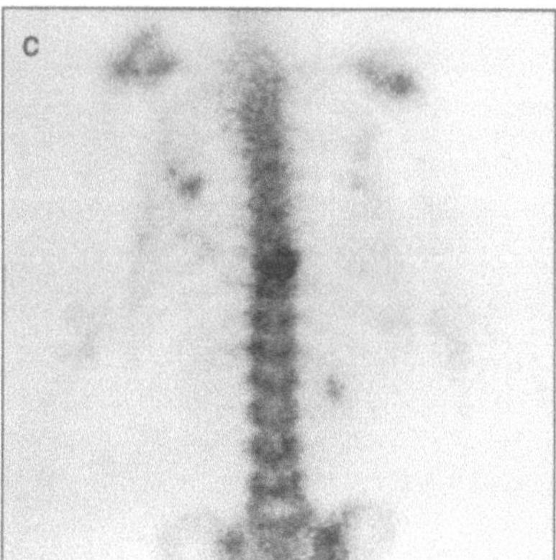
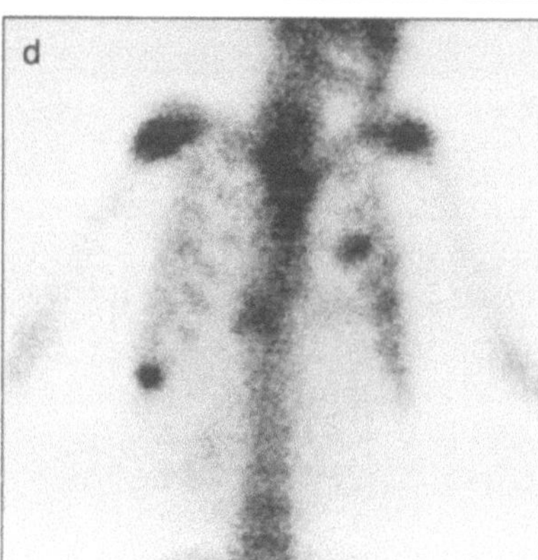

Fig. 4.45c. Posterior image of the spine shows the abnormal vertebral body to better advantage. Abnormal uptake is noted overlying the ribs

Fig. 4.45d. Anterior image of the thorax shows the pulmonary and rib metastases

Technical Comment

The quality of these scans is not ideal in that the bladder is not empty and the positioning of the child is not perfect. There is also slight movement on Fig. 4.45d. This reflects how unwell the child was and that these scans are not technically ideal but remain diagnostically adequate.

Teaching Point

It may be difficult to distinguish between pulmonary metastases from rib metastases and in these cases SPECT of the thorax may be useful, if the CT scan of the lungs is normal.

135

Case 4.46. A 6-year-old boy with pain in the left leg due to primary osteogenic sarcoma with distant metastases

Fig. 4.46a,b. Whole body scans show abnormal increased uptake of isotope in the expanded lower left femur. There are areas within this which show decreased uptake of isotope. In the mid shaft of the left femur there is also increased uptake of isotope as is in the proximal femur. Abnormal increased uptake of isotope is also noted in the proximal ends of both tibiae and the proximal ends of both humeri as well as in the anterior superior iliac bone on the left and the thoracic and lumbar spine. Pulmonary metastases are also noted

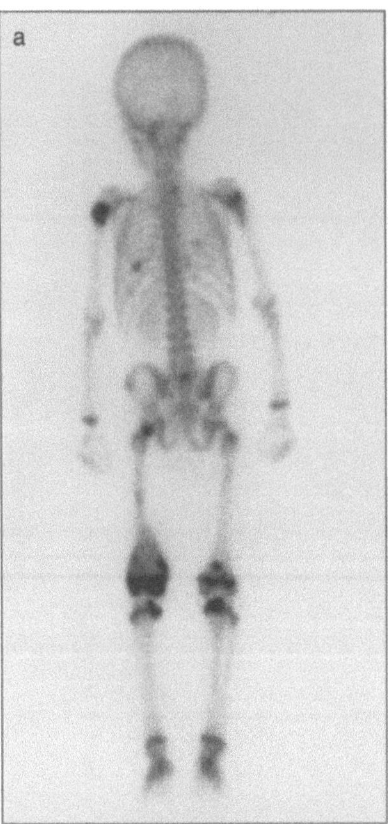
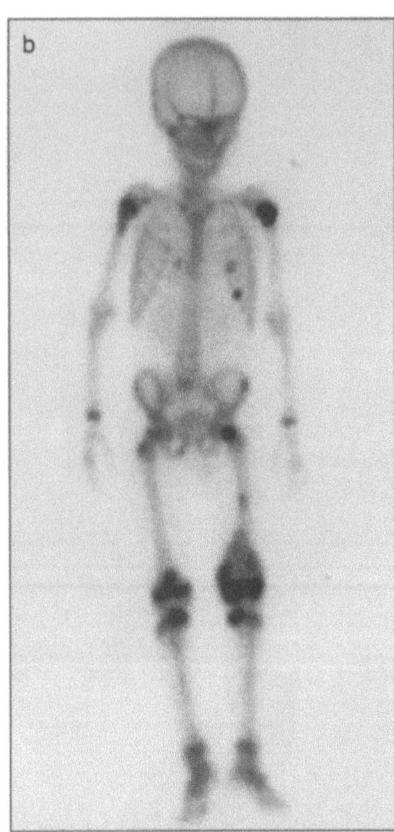

Case 4.47. A 12-year-old boy who presented with multifocal osteogenic sarcoma

Fig. 4.47a. Whole body posterior scan shows multiple areas of abnormal increased uptake of isotope. These include the skull vault, humeri, vertebrae, pelvis, femora and tibiae

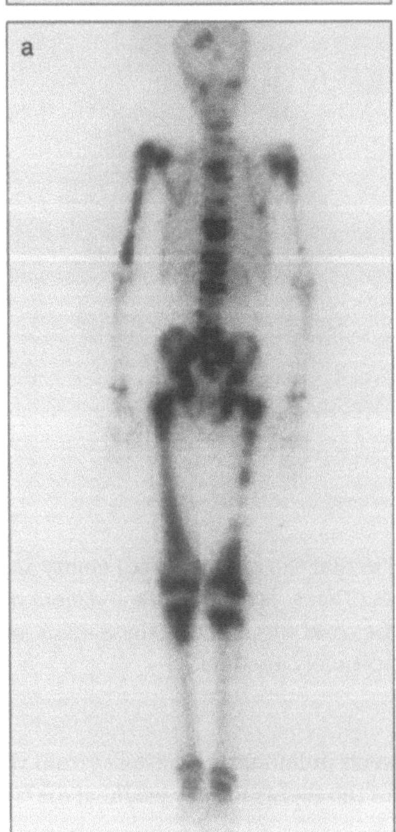

Teaching Point
The difference between primary osteogenic sarcoma with metastases at diagnosis from multifocal osteogenic sarcoma is a combination of the extent of the other lesions and the fact that no one lesion predominates in the multifocal form.

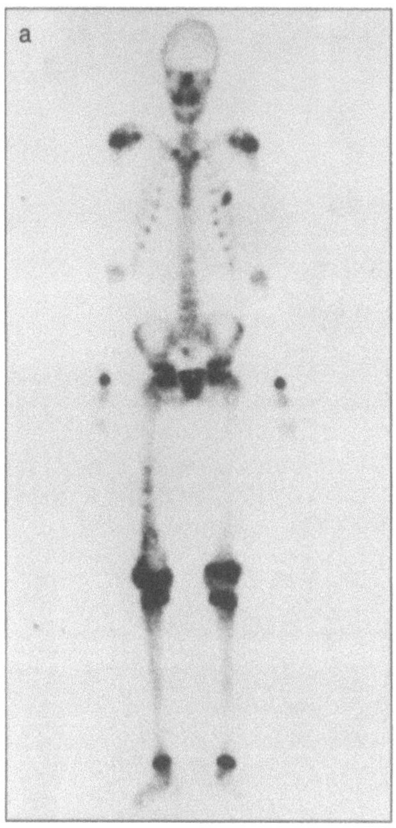
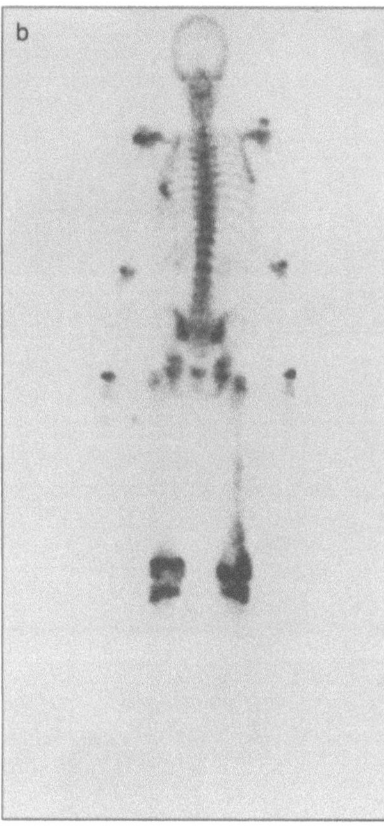

Case 4.48. A 10-year-old boy with pain in the right thigh due to primary osteogenic sarcoma who, at presentation, had distant metastases

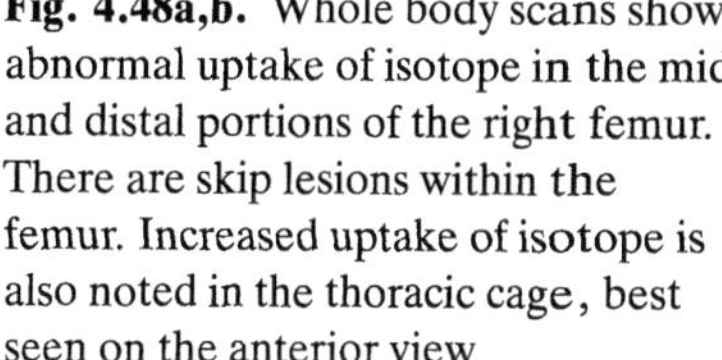

Fig. 4.48a,b. Whole body scans show abnormal uptake of isotope in the mid and distal portions of the right femur. There are skip lesions within the femur. Increased uptake of isotope is also noted in the thoracic cage, best seen on the anterior view

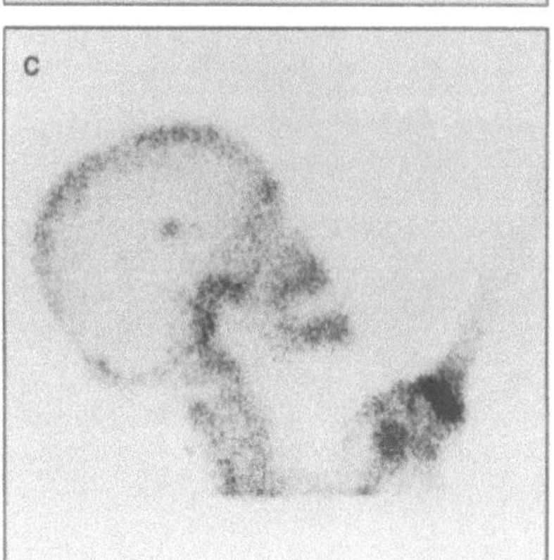

Fig. 4.48c. Right lateral image of the skull shows focal abnormal increased uptake of isotope in the right temporo-parietal region

Case 4.49.　A 16-year-old boy with primary osteogenic sarcoma of the upper right tibia

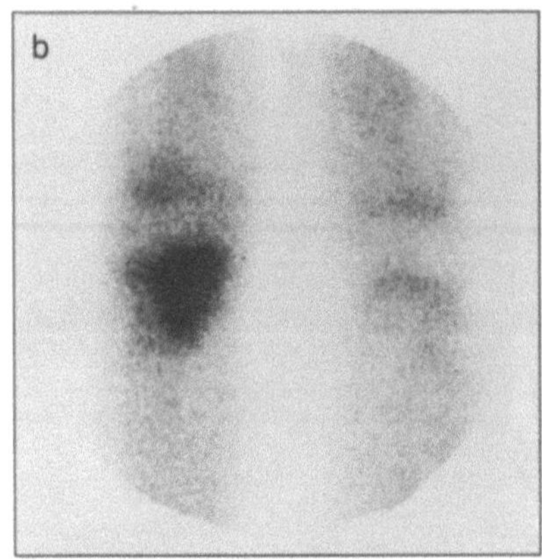

Fig. 4.49a. Anterior blood flow images of the knees show abnormal uptake in the proximal right tibia

Fig. 4.49b. Anterior blood pool image of the knees shows marked increased uptake of isotope in the medial aspect of the right proximal tibia

Fig. 4.49c. Whole body scans show abnormal uptake in the metaphysis and diaphysis of the proximal right tibia, better seen on the posterior than on the anterior view. Increased uptake of isotope is noted in the right foot and distal femur on the right

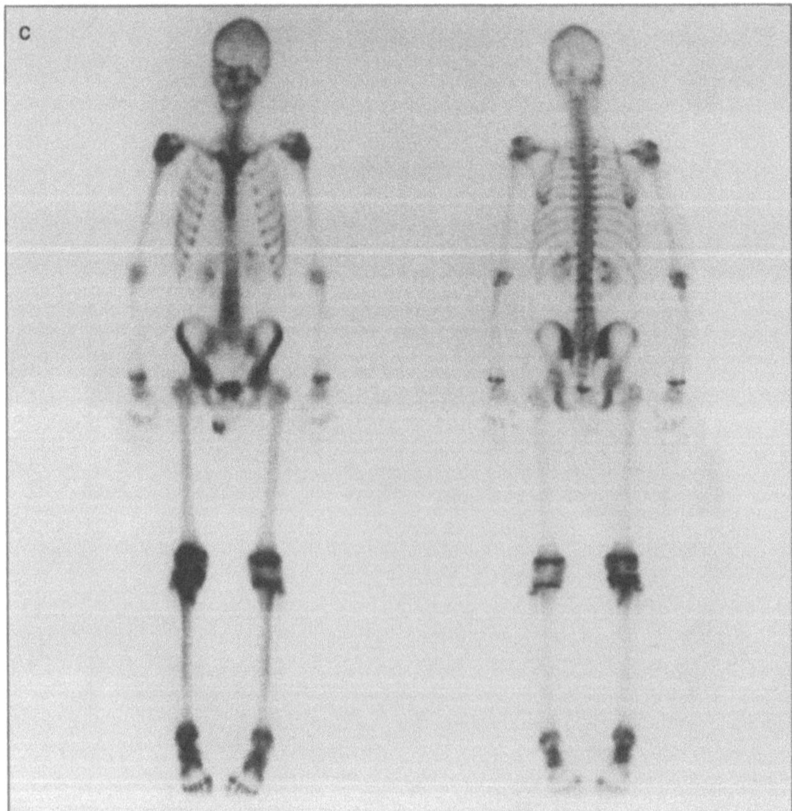

Technical Comment

It would have been advantageous to have done spot magnification images of the knees to assess the proximal tibia to better advantage.

Teaching Point

Similar appearances are seen with infection (see Case 2.5) and Langerhans' histiocytosis (see Case 4.85).

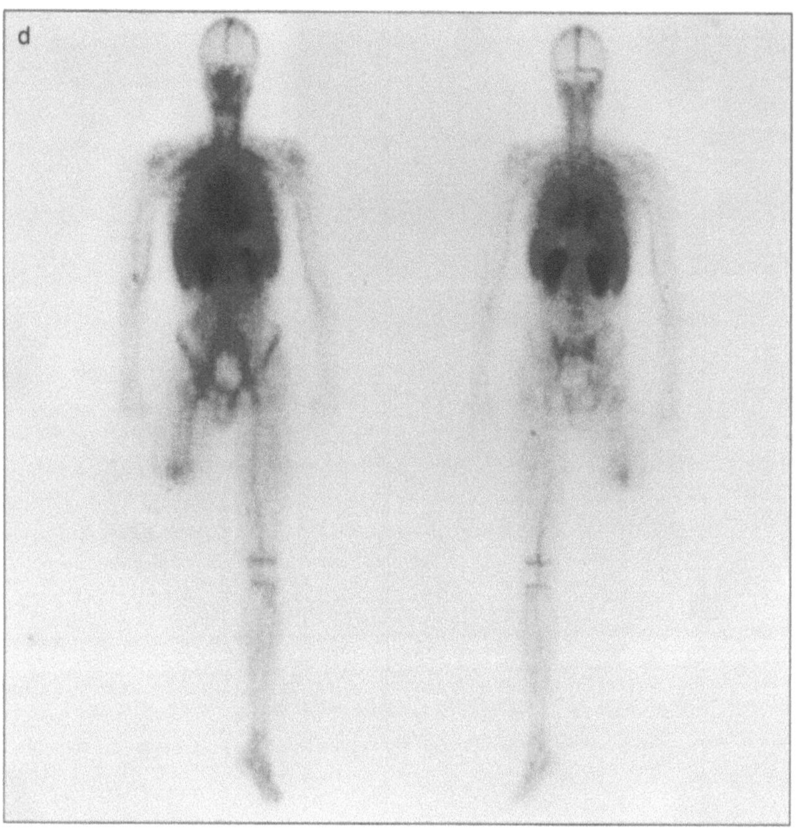

Following chemotherapy and amputation, follow-up scans were obtained 2 months later.

Fig. 4.49d. Whole body blood pool images show increased uptake of isotope around the distal end of the amputation site in the right femur

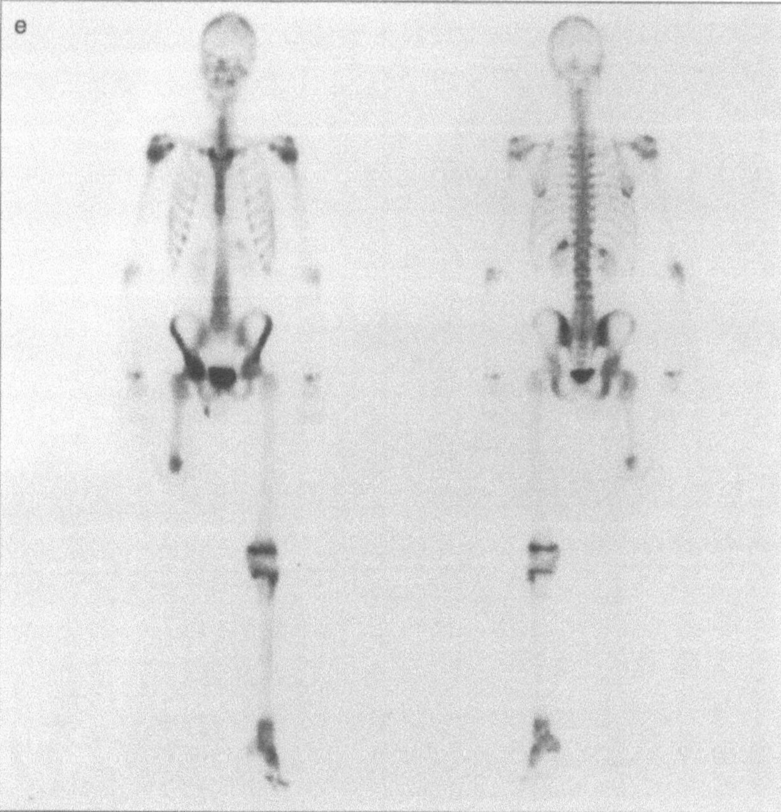

Fig. 4.49e. Whole body images show increased uptake in the distal right femur. These appearances were noted on subsequent follow-up scans over a period of a further 2 years, but no metastases were noted at this site. Generalised increased uptake of isotope is seen in the right hip extending to the ischeum tuberosity. (For follow-up images, see Case 5.73)

Teaching Point
The cause for this increased uptake at the amputation site and the right hip was related to an artificial limb.

Case 4.50. A 20-year-old patient with an osteogenic sarcoma in the left femur and multiple metastases

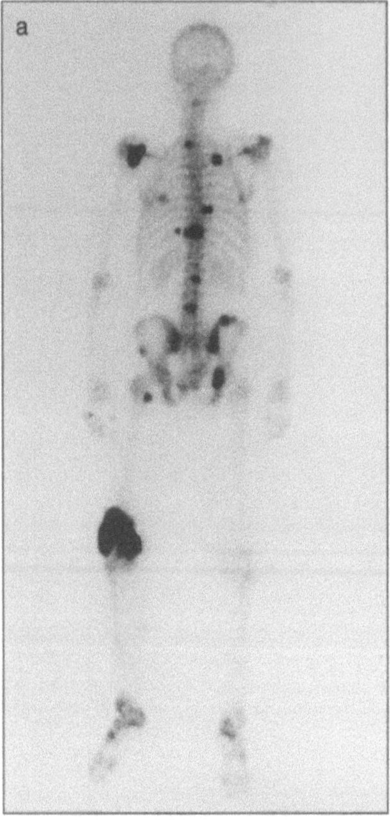
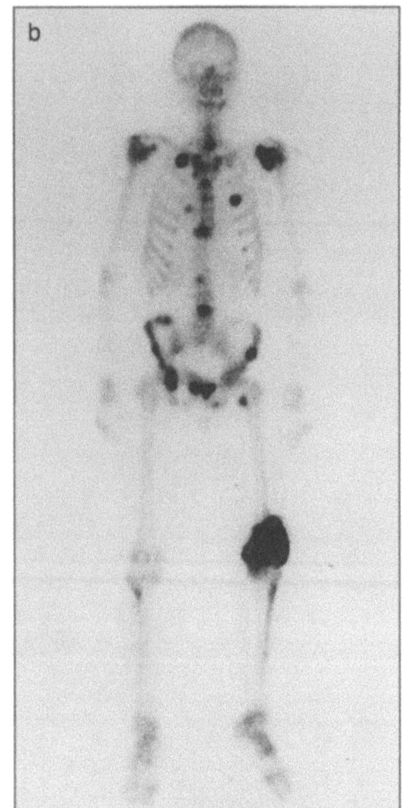

Fig. 4.50a,b. Whole body scans show intense abnormal increased uptake of isotope in the distal left femur. Multiple abnormal areas of increased uptake of isotope throughout the spine, pelvis, left shoulder and upper left femur are seen. The extent of involvement of the bony pelvis is more marked on the anterior scan

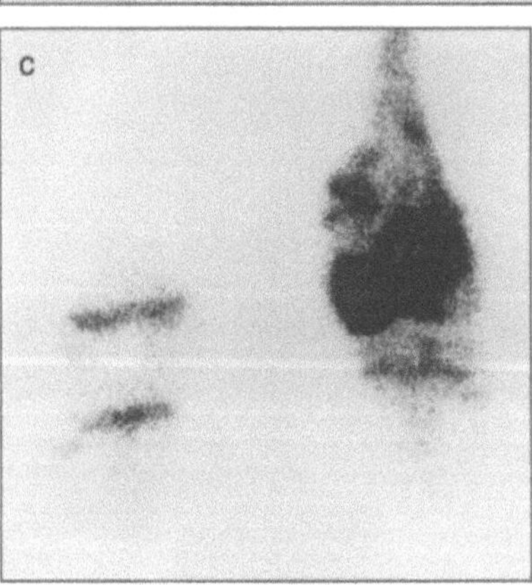

Fig. 4.50c. Anterior image of the tumour shows the extent to better advantage

4.2.1.3 Chrondrosarcoma
(2 Cases; Figs. 4.51, 4.52)

Teaching Point
Chondrosarcoma may be suggested from the bone scan appearances where there is not homogeneous intense increased uptake of isotope but rather areas with absent activity surrounded by areas of increased activity.

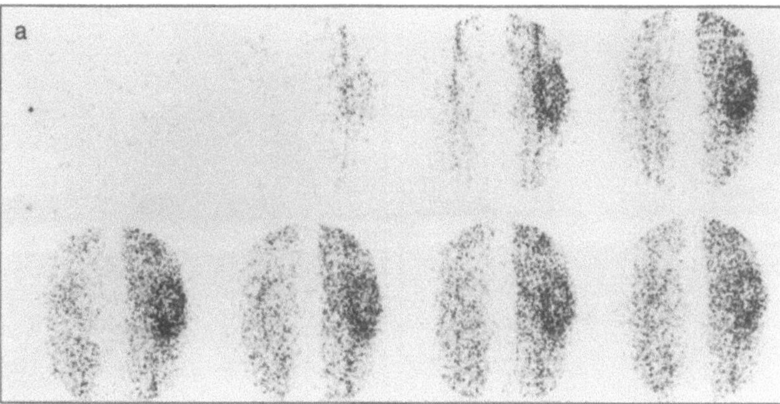

Case 4.51. An 11-year-old boy with a primary chondrosarcoma of the proximal left tibia

Fig. 4.51a. Anterior blood flow images show abnormal increased uptake of isotope in the region of the left knee laterally

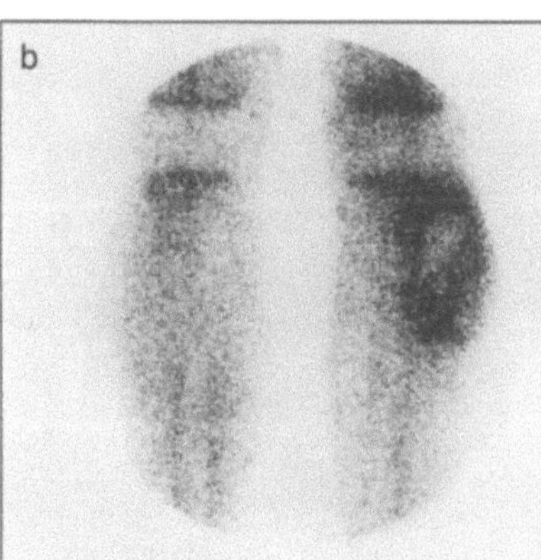

Fig. 4.51b. Anterior blood pool image of the knees shows abnormal increased activity on the lateral aspect of the left knee

Fig. 4.51c. Anterior image of the knees shows loss of clarity of the left tibial epiphyseal plate. The fibula cannot be clearly seen. There are multiple areas of focal abnormal increased uptake of isotope and it is not possible on this image to separate the fibula from the tibia

Fig. 4.51d. Lateral lateral image of the left knee shows that most of the tumour lies posteriorly. Note the focal areas of intense increased uptake of activity with adjacent areas of decreased activity

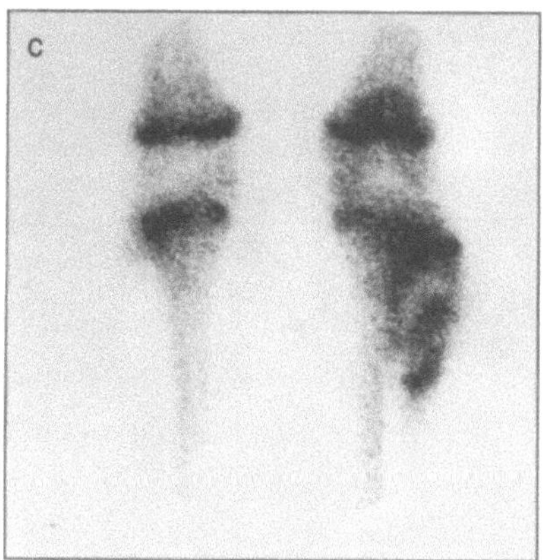

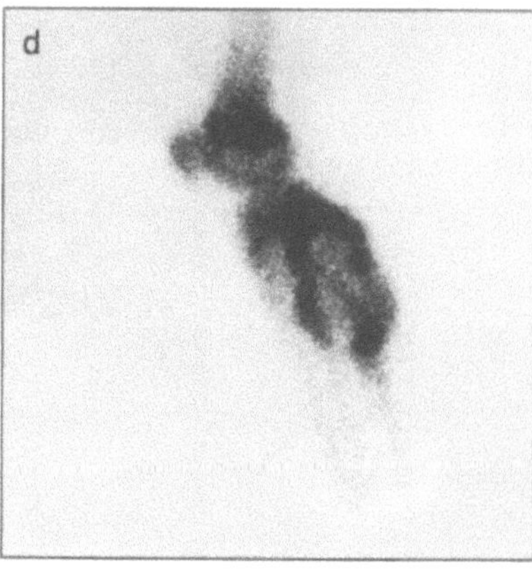

Teaching Point
It is impossible from these images to know whether the tumour arose from the tibia or fibula.

Case 4.52. A 15-year-old boy with pain around the knee due to a chondrosarcoma of the distal right femur

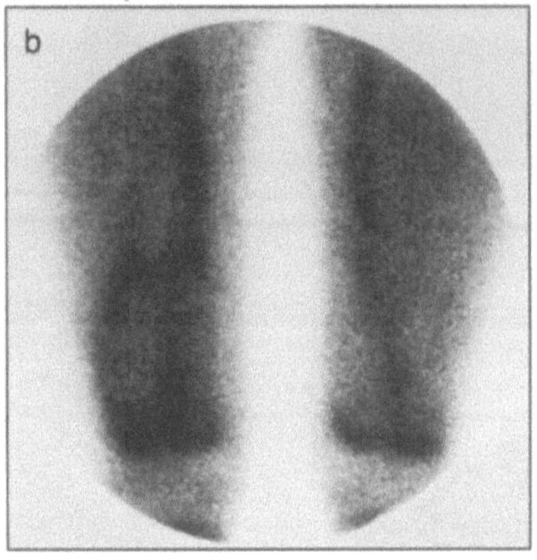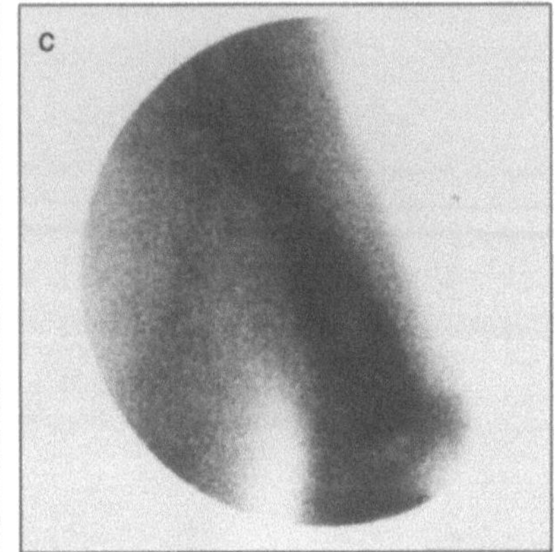

Fig. 4.52a. Blood flow images fail to reveal any asymmetry around the knees

Fig. 4.52b. Anterior blood pool image of the distal femora shows abnormal increased uptake of isotope in the distal femur on the right

Fig. 4.52c. Lateral blood pool image of the right femur shows increased uptake of isotope in the distal third of the femur

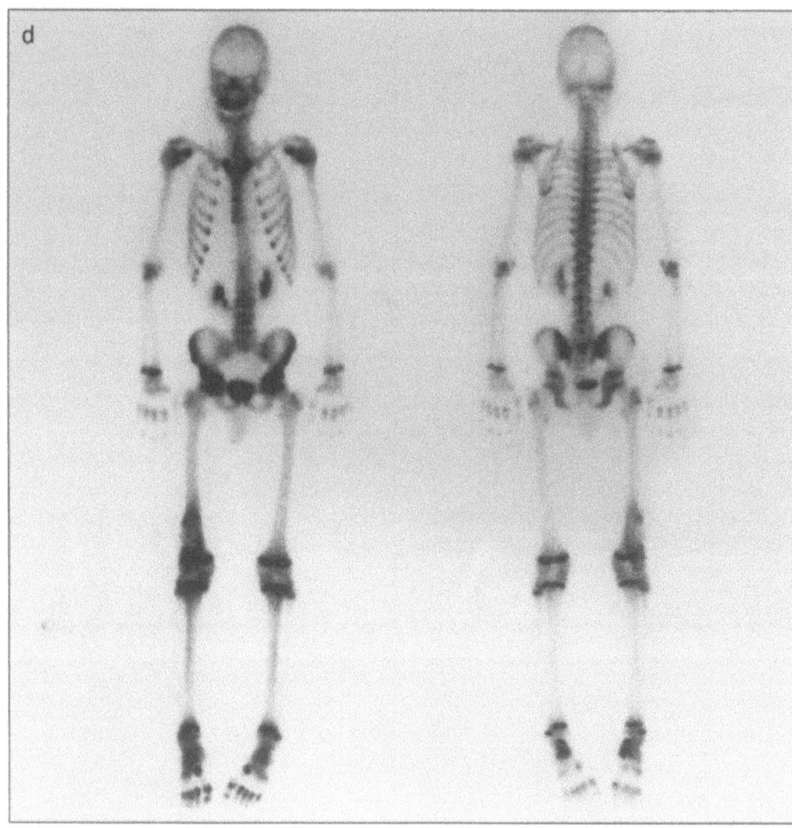

Fig. 4.52d. Whole body images show abnormal uptake of isotope in a non-homogeneous fashion in the lower right femur. The position of the right kidney is rather low and the axes of the collecting systems of both kidneys are abnormal, suggesting a horseshoe kidney

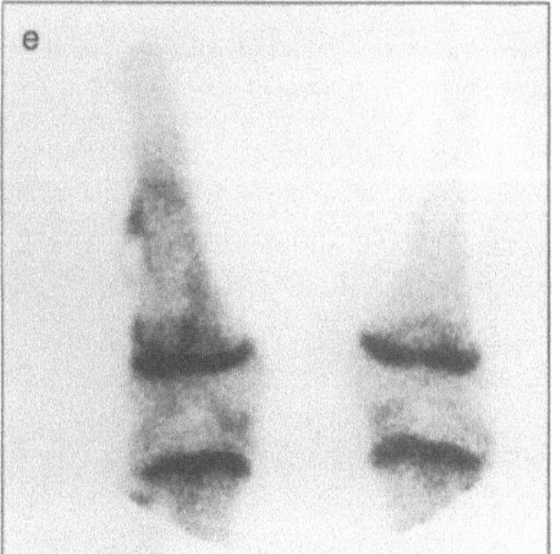 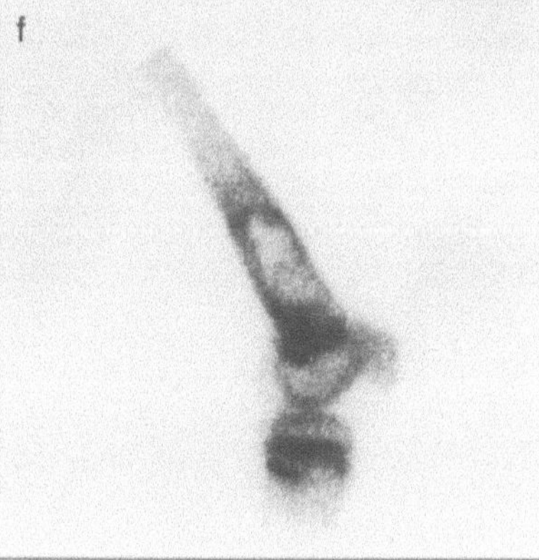

Fig. 4.52e,f. Anterior and lateral images of the knees show to better advantage the focal areas of increased and decreased uptake of isotope in the distal right femur

Technical Comment

The kidneys were not investigated but the appearances on the whole body images strongly suggest a horseshoe kidney.

4.2.2 Neuroectodermal Tumours

4.2.2.1 Primitive Neuroectodermal Tumours
(3 Cases; Figs. 4.53–4.55)

Case 4.53. A 13-year-old girl, unwell for some time, who presented with anaemia and an abdominal swelling. A retrohepatic mass was discovered on ultrasound and CT, the biopsy of this mass and also an adjacent rib revealed a primitive neuroectodermal tumour (PNET)

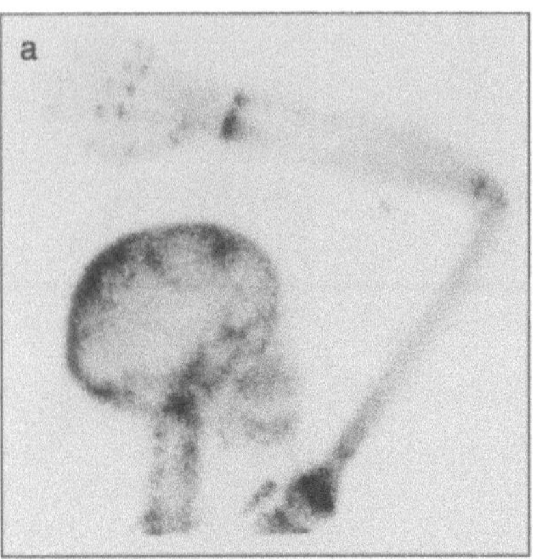

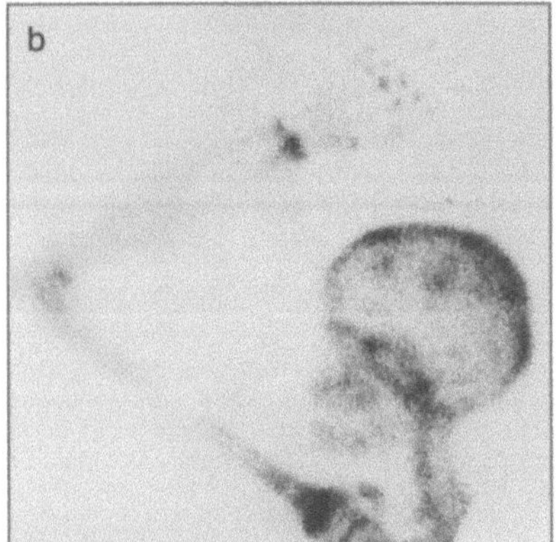

Fig. 4.53a. Right lateral image of the skull and right arm shows abnormal increased uptake of isotope in the skull vault. Abnormal increased uptake of isotope is also noted in the proximal right humerus. The epiphyseal plates of the distal radius and ulna are indistinct

Fig. 4.53b. Left lateral image of the skull and left arm shows abnormal uptake of isotope in the skull vault and the proximal left humerus. The distal radial and ulna epiphyses are indistinct

Fig. 4.53c. Posterior image of the thorax and lumbar spine. Multiple ribs show abnormal increased uptake of isotope, the abnormal upper humeri are again seen. Patchy abnormal increased uptake of isotope is noted in some vertebral bodies (D12, L2 and L4) whilst other vertebral bodies show decreased activity (L1 and left lateral aspect of L2). Note the abnormal distribution of isotope in the kidneys

Fig. 4.53d. Posterior image of the lumbar spine and pelvis. Virtually total absence of activity is noted at L5 with decreased activity again noted at L1 and, to a lesser extent, L2. The epiphyseal plates around the femoral necks are lost and there is increased uptake of isotope in the femoral necks

Fig. 4.53e. Left posterior oblique image of the thorax shows similar features on the left side as are noted on the right

Fig. 4.53f. Right posterior oblique image of the ribs shows to better advantage patchy areas of increased and decreased uptake in the ribs and also in the dorsal spine

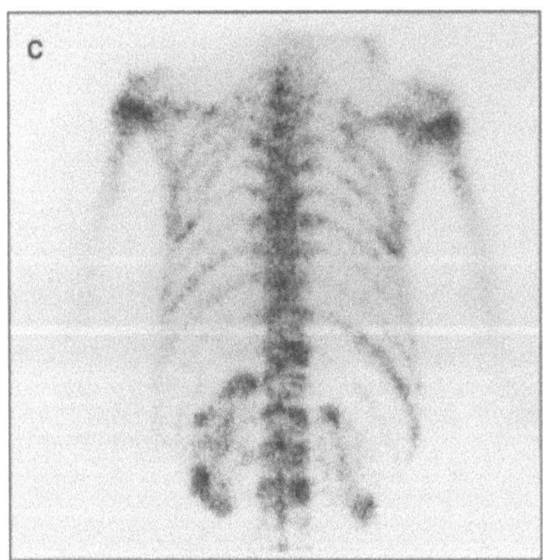

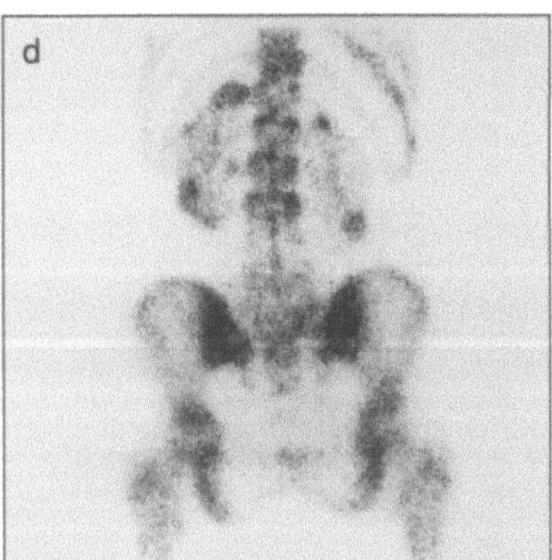

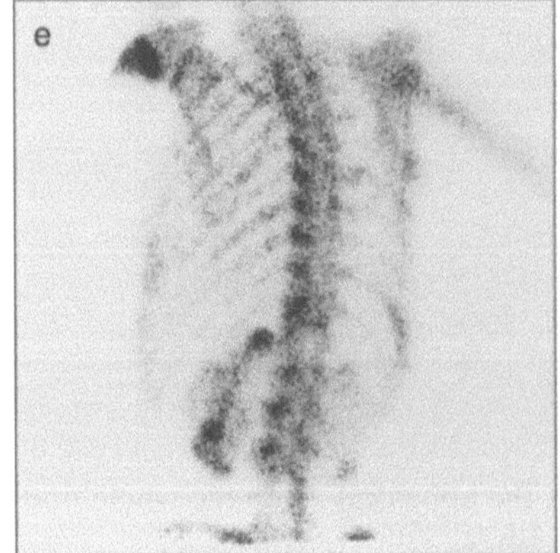

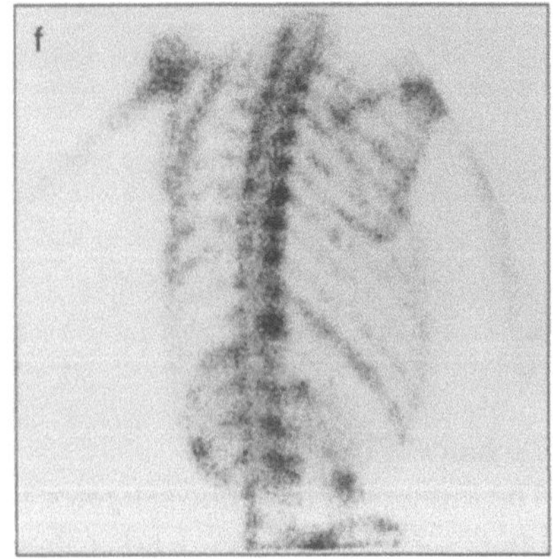

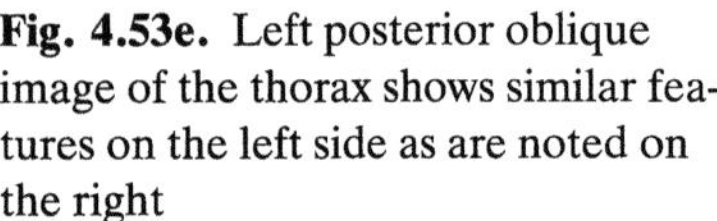

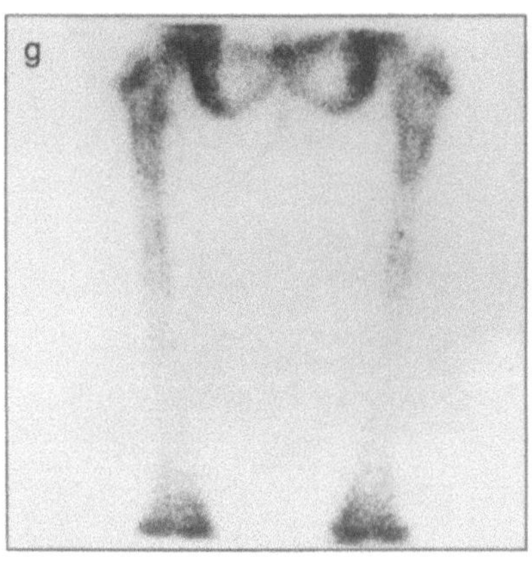
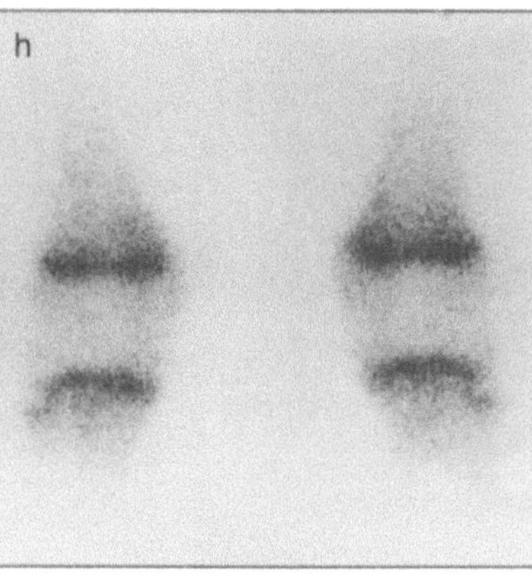

Fig. 4.53g. Posterior image of the femora shows patchy abnormal distribution of isotope with areas of both increased and decreased activity. The epiphyses around the knees are indistinct with abnormal uptake of isotope in the metaphyses

Fig. 4.53h. Posterior magnification image of the knees. The previous described abnormalities are seen to better advantage

Teaching Point

Similar appearances as noted in Fig. 4.53c may be seen in children with sickle cell disease (see Chap. 6.3, "Sickle Cell Disease").

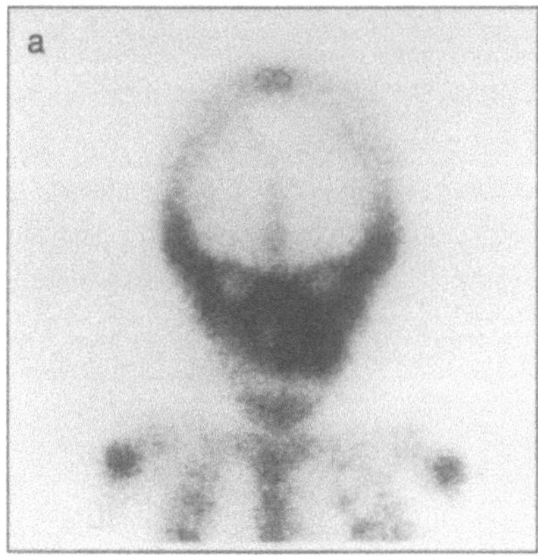
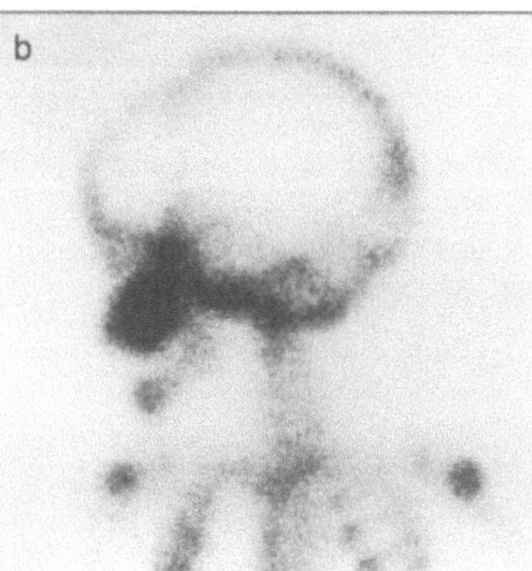

Case 4.54. A 6-month-old baby boy with swelling of the cheek for 10 days, which on biopsy proved to be a PNET tumour

Fig. 4.54a. Anterior image of the skull and facial bones shows focal abnormal increased uptake of isotope in the midface on the left

Fig.4.54b. Left lateral image of the skull shows focal abnormal increased uptake of isotope in the region of the maxilla

Teaching Point

Note the similarity between the isotope appearances of this child and that of the children with primary osteogenic sarcoma of the maxilla (Cases 4.37, 4.38). Whilst bone scanning remains a very sensitive technique for the detection of increased osteoblastic activity, it is non-specific and further specific investigations are required.

Case 4.55. A 15-year-old girl with pain in the pelvis due to a PNET tumour of the ileum

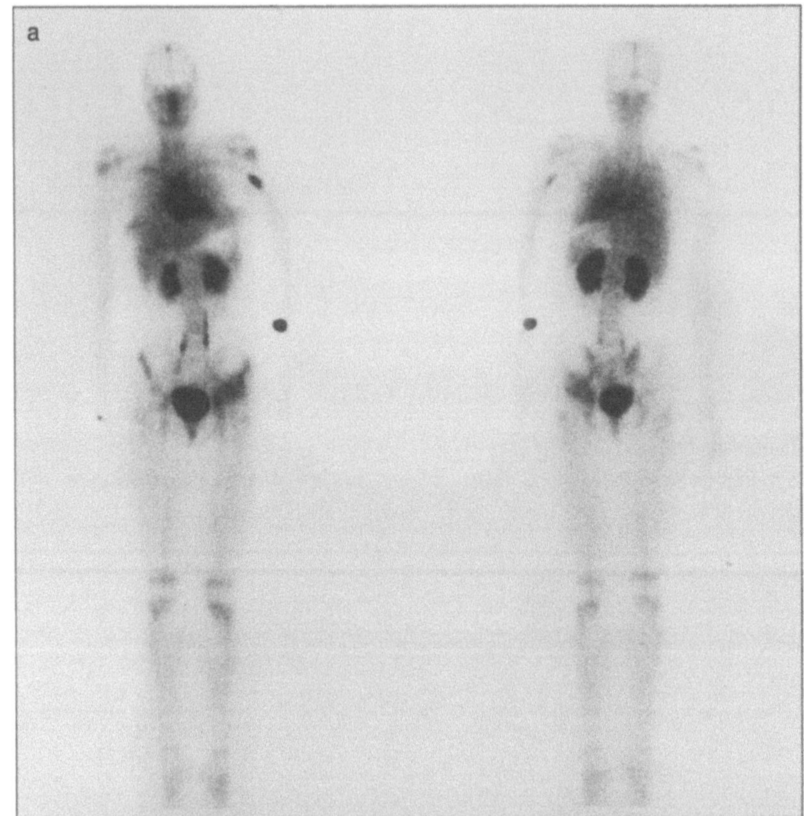

Fig. 4.55a. Whole body blood pool images show increased uptake of isotope in the left hemipelvis. Note extravasation of isotope in the left hand. This is the site of the injection

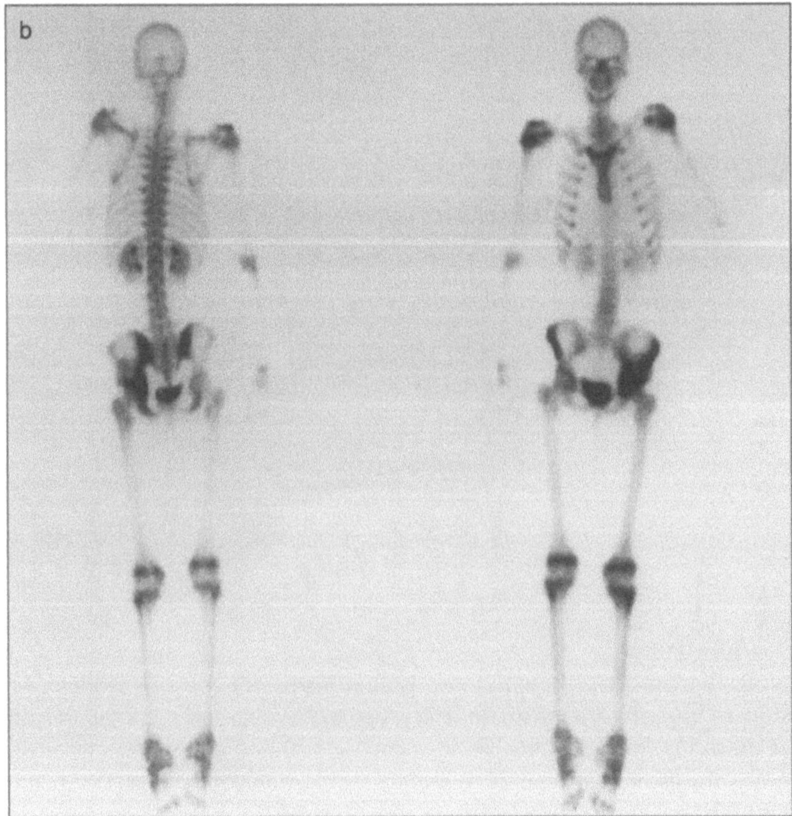

Fig. 4.55b. Whole body scans show increased uptake in the region of the left hemipelvis due to the PNET tumour.

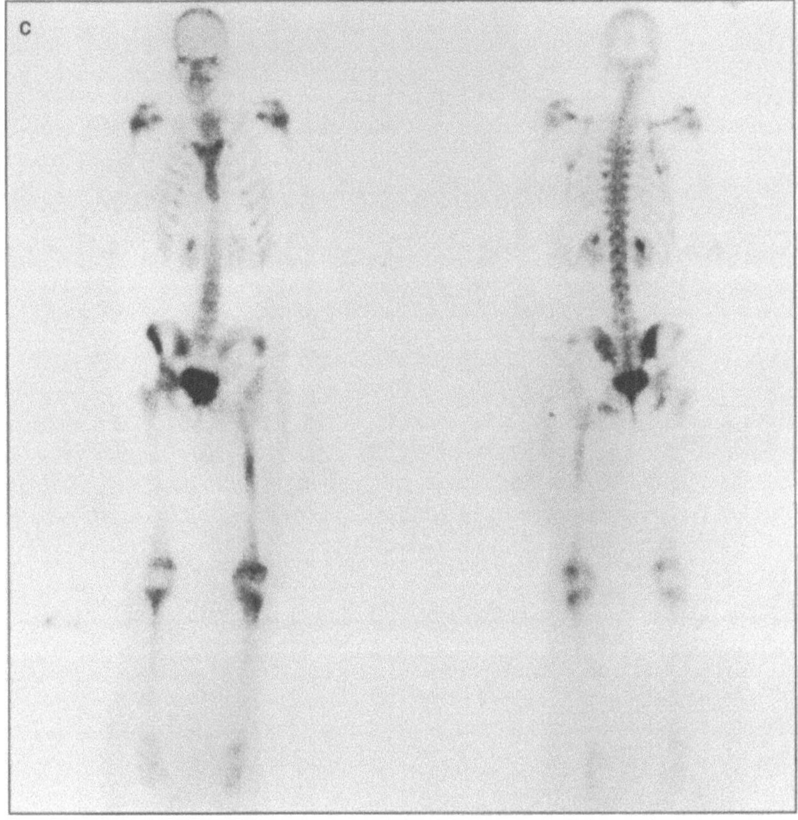

A follow-up bone scan was undertaken after hemipelvectomy with an artificial hemipelvis and total prosthetic replacement of the left hip

Fig. 4.55c. Whole body images show a photon-deficient area in the region of the left hemipelvis and the left upper femur. There is increased uptake of isotope in the mid shaft of the left femur due to surgery

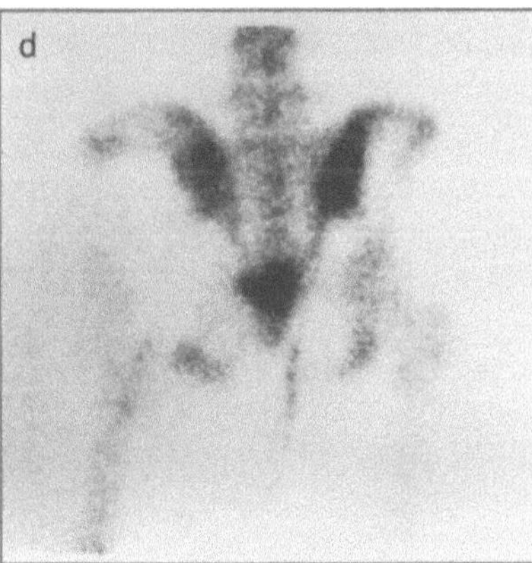

Fig. 4.55d. Posterior image of the pelvis again shows the photon-deficient area throughout the left hemipelvis

4.2.2.2 Neuroblastoma
(7 Cases; Figs. 4.56–4.62)

Case 4.56. A 15-month-old girl who was noted to have a lump above the left clavicle. The mass was a neuroblastoma with distal involvement of the skeleton (stage IV neuroblastoma)

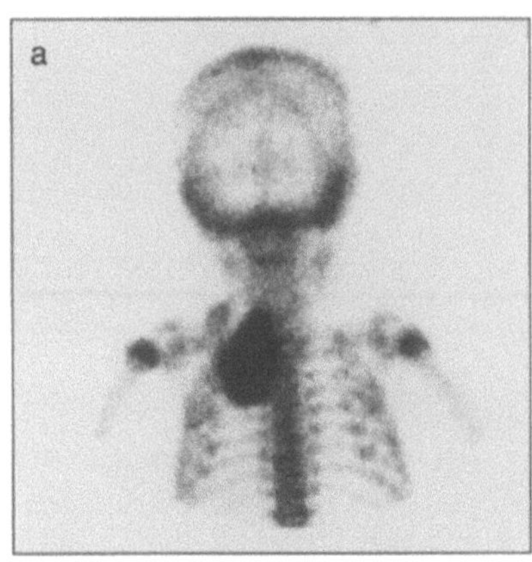

Fig. 4.56a,b. Posterior images of the skull thorax, spine and pelvis reveal intense abnormal increased uptake of isotope in the left upper thorax extending up into the neck which is not confined to the bones. This corresponds closely to the extent of the mass seen on chest X-ray. Multiple focal areas of increased uptake of isotope are seen in the ribs; some of these are due to the anterior normal costochondral junctions. The lateral abnormalitis are due to skeletal involvement by neuroblastoma

Fig. 4.56c. Right anterior oblique image of the chest and pelvis shows the mass in close proximity to the spine. Note the normal hot costochondral junctions

Fig. 4.56d. Anterior image of the pelvis and lower limbs. There is abnormal increased uptake of isotope in the distal left femoral shaft

Fig. 4.56e. Posterior image of the pelvis and lateral lower limbs shows the abnormal increased uptake of isotope in the distal left femoral metaphysis extending into the diaphysis.

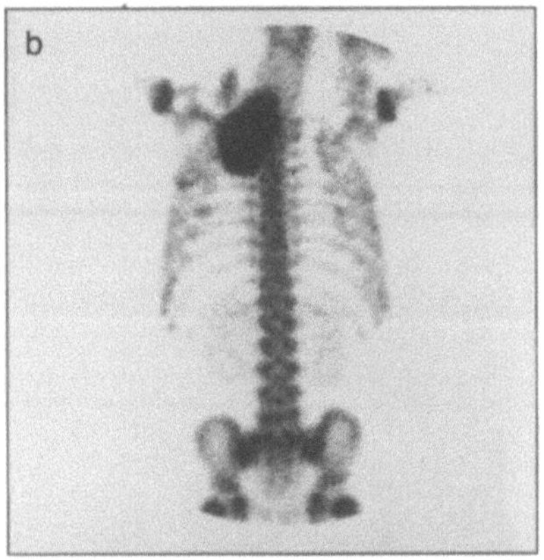

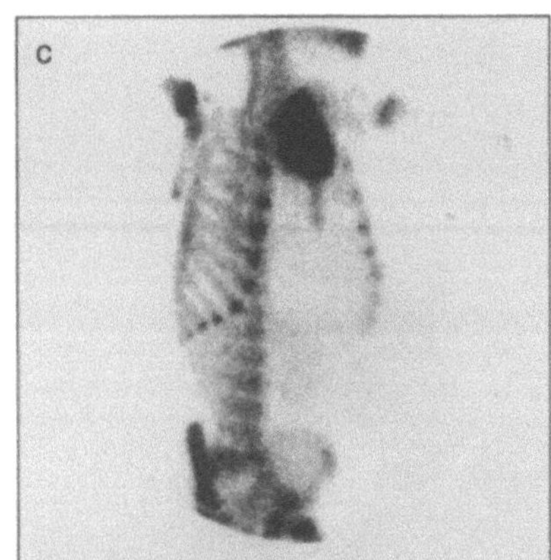

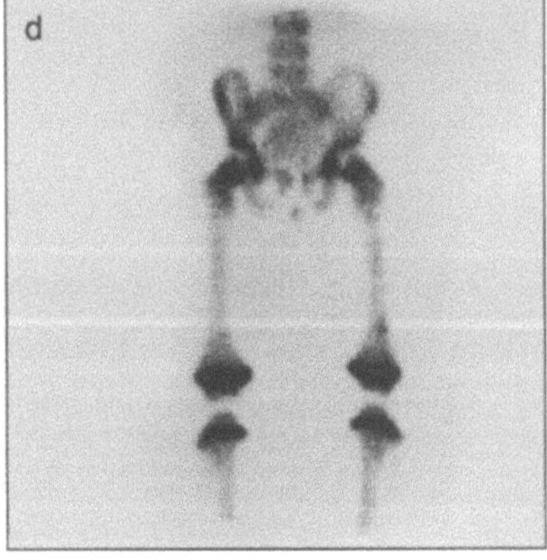

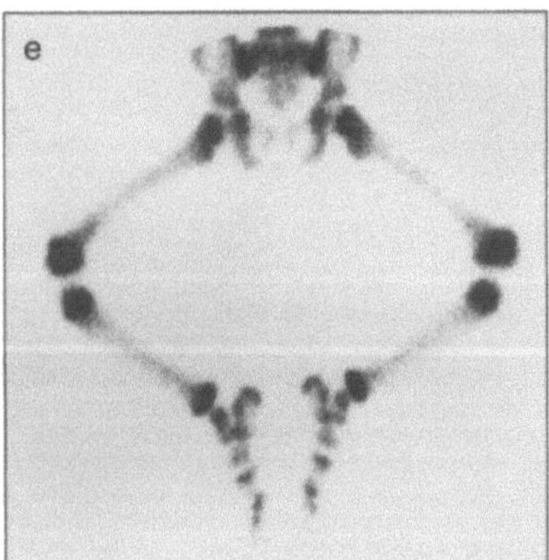

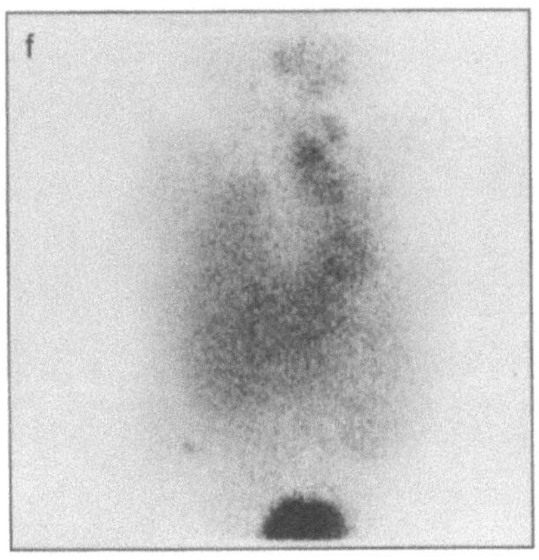

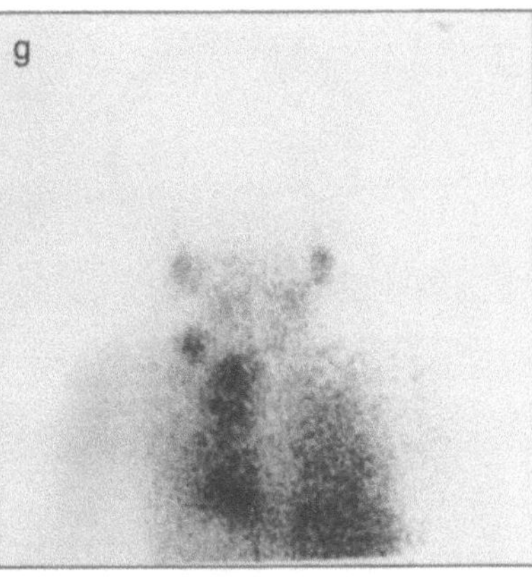

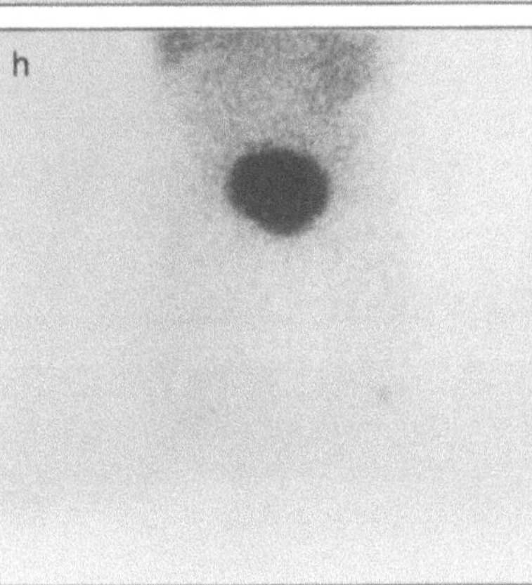

An iodine-123 metaiodobenzylguani-
dine (MIBG) scan was undertaken

Fig. 4.56f. Anterior 24-h I 123 MIBG
image of the chest and pelvis shows
uptake of isotope in the tumour.
Uptake of isotope is also noted in the
heart and liver as well as in the bladder. The distribution in these latter
three organs is normal

Fig. 4.56g. Posterior 24-h
I 123 MIBG image of the thorax.
Abnormal uptake of isotope is noted in
the mass and also in the supraclavicu-
lar area which is independent of the
mass. Activity in the heart is again
noted

Fig. 4.56h. Anterior 24-h I 123 MIBG
image of the lower limbs. Abnormal
focal increased uptake of isotope is
noted in the femoral shaft on the left.
This is rather faint but corresponds to
the abnormal area seen on the bone
scan

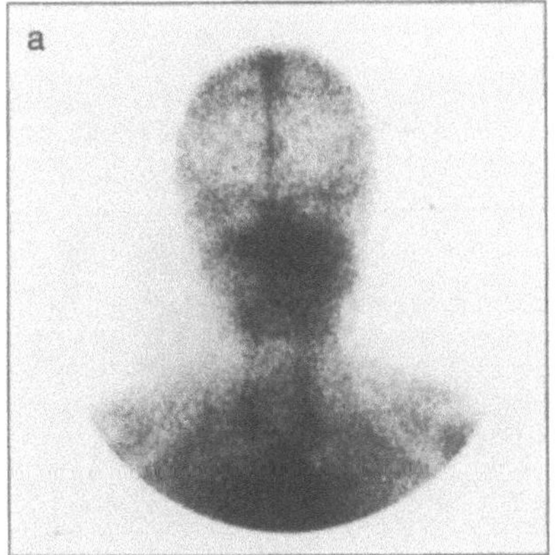

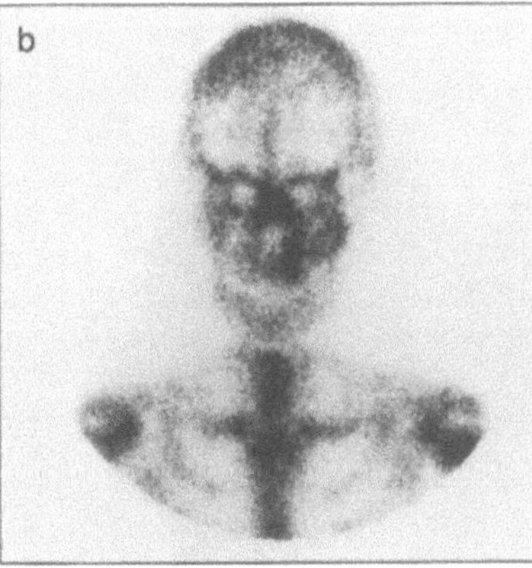

**Case 4.57. A 10-year-old girl who pre-
sented with stage IV neuroblastoma**

Fig. 4.57a. Anterior blood pool image
of the skull shows abnormal increased
uptake of isotope on the left side of the
face

Fig. 4.57b. Anterior image of the
skull shows abnormal increased uptake
of isotope in the skull vault and also on
the left side of the face laterally
(Continued on p. 148)

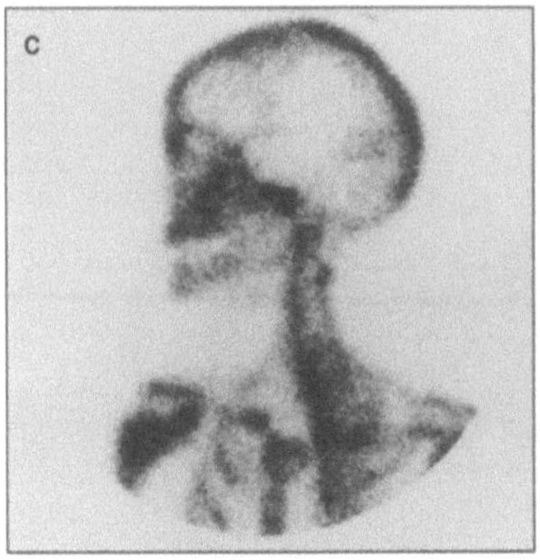

Fig. 4.57c. Left lateral image of the skull shows abnormal increased uptake of isotope in the skull vault and also in the region of the maxilla (compare with Fig. 4.57d)

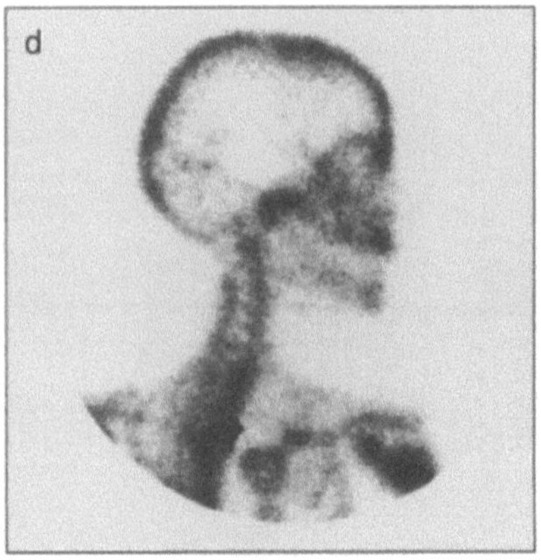

Fig. 4.57d. Right lateral image of the skull shows the abnormal skull vault but the facial bones are virtually normal

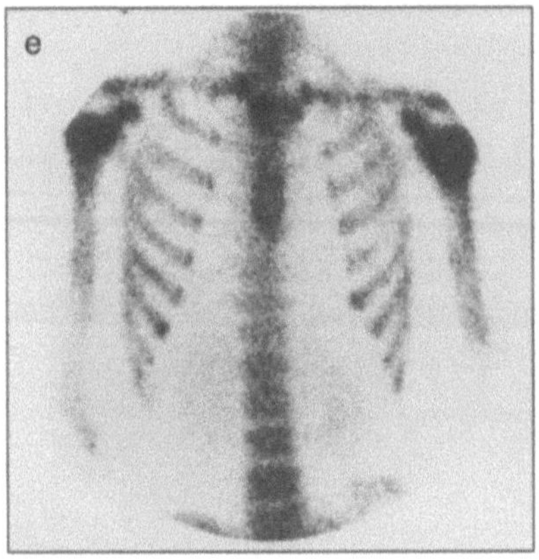

Fig. 4.57e. Anterior image of the thorax shows abnormal increased uptake of isotope in the anterior ends of the ribs bilaterally as well as abnormal uptake in the clavicles and humeri

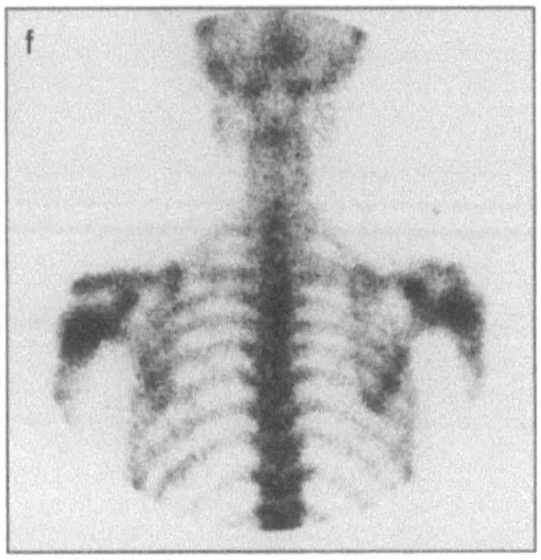

Fig. 4.57f. Posterior image of the thorax shows abnormal uptake in the upper humeri and the posterior ribs especially on the left

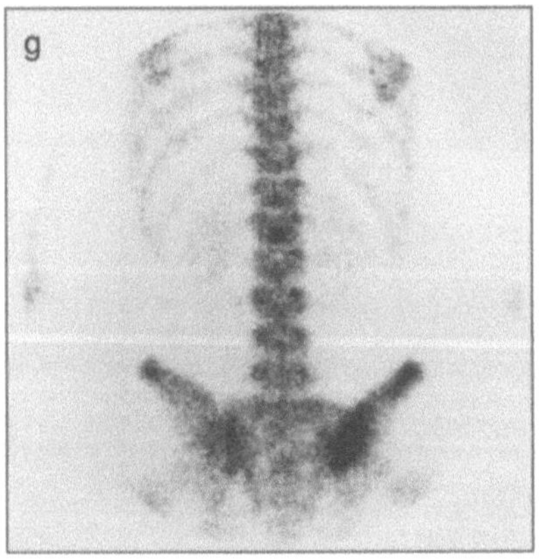

Fig. 4.57g. Posterior image of the spine and pelvis in a sitting position shows abnormal uptake of isotope in the upper lumbar spine and in the right hemipelvis

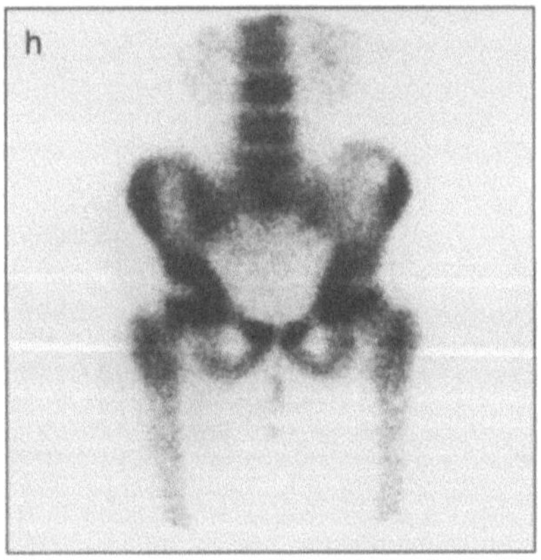

Fig. 4.57h. Anterior image of the pelvis shows abnormal uptake of isotope in both iliac crests and in the upper femora

Fig. 4.57i. Posterior image of the pelvis shows abnormal increased uptake in the right hemipelvis and upper femora

Fig. 4.57j. Posterior image of the knees shows loss of clarity of the epiphyseal plates with abnormal activity extending from the epiphyseal plates into the diaphyses of the femora and tibiae.

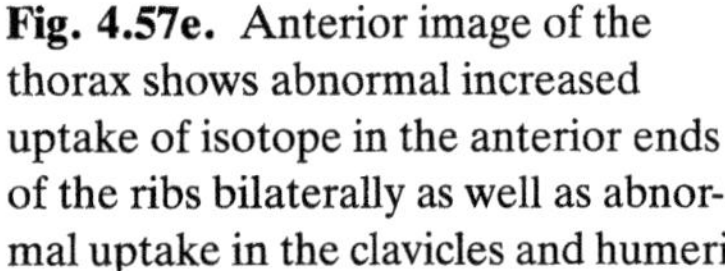

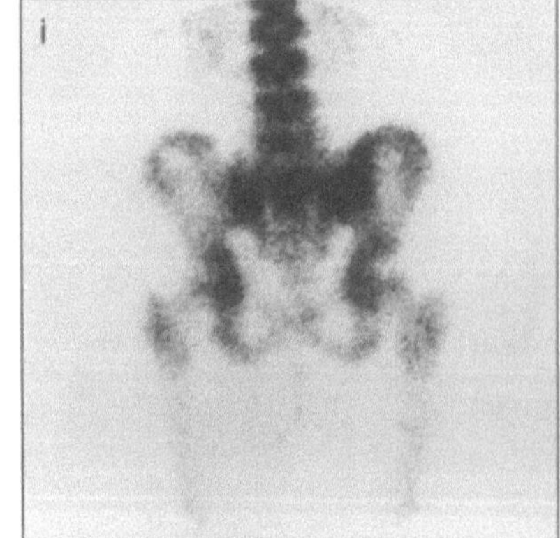

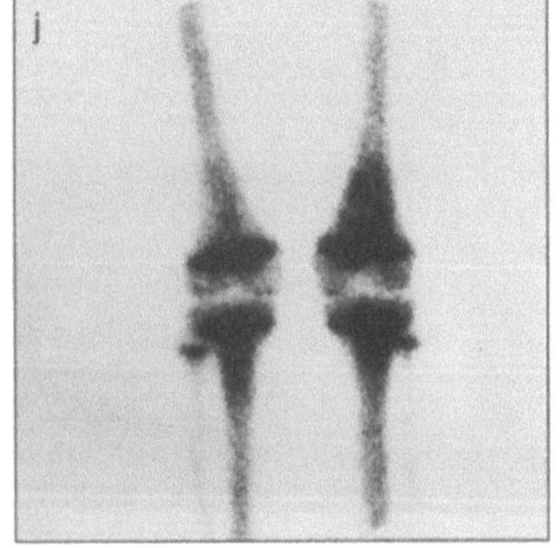

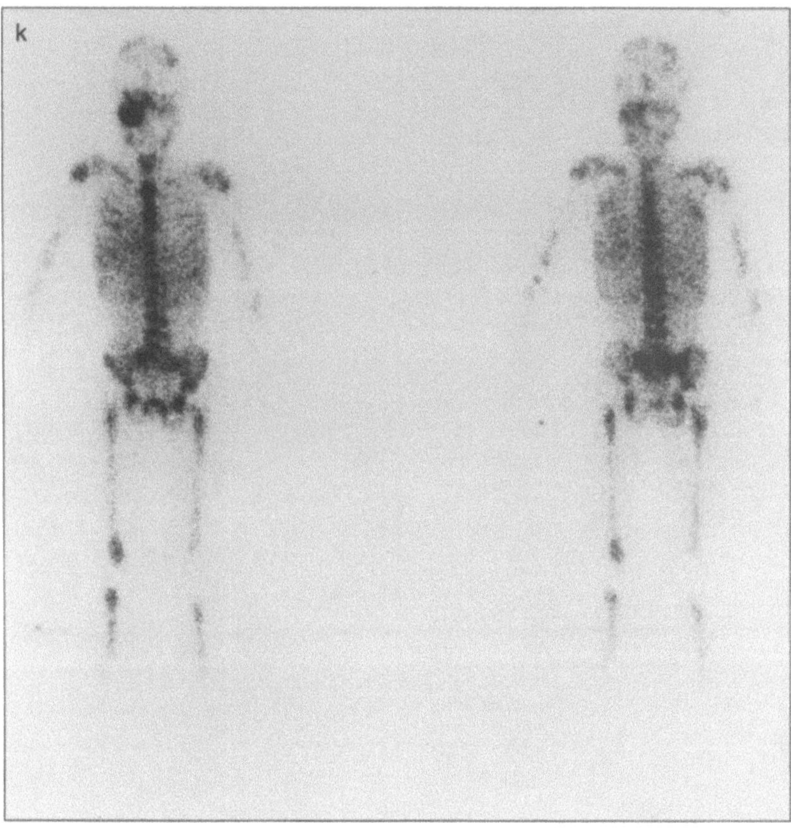

An iodine-123 MIGB scan was undertaken

Fig. 4.57k. I 123 MIBG whole body scans at 24 h show diffuse uptake by the skeleton. The soft tissue mass in the face shows intense abnormal increased uptake of isotope

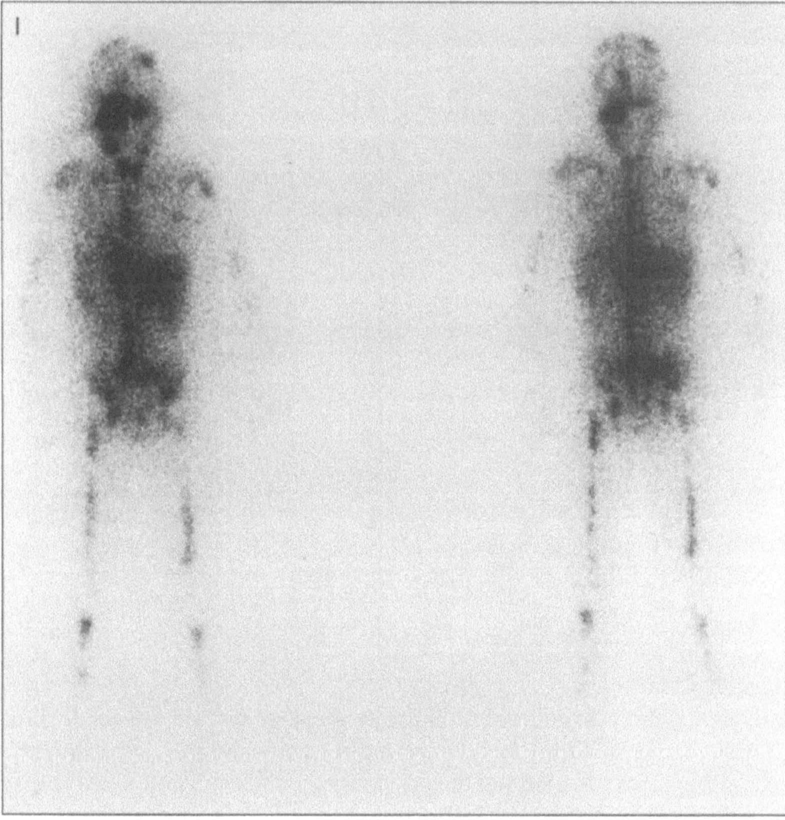

Fig. 4.57l. The child was treated with MIBG therapy and images were obtained 1 week after the injection of the I 131 MIBG. Abnormal uptake is noted in the skeleton and the tumour

Case 4.58. A 4-year-old boy presenting with a limp was found to have stage IV neuroblastoma

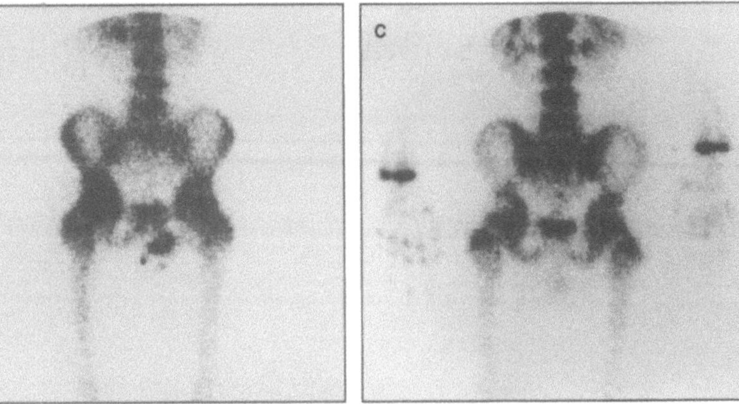

Fig. 4.58a. Posterior image of the thorax and lumbar spine shows abnormal increased uptake of isotope in a soft tissue mass in the lower chest on the right

Fig. 4.58b. Anterior image of the pelvis shows abnormal increased uptake of isotope in the right hip

Fig. 4.58c. Posterior image of the pelvis shows the abnormal right hip again.

An iodine-123 MIBG scan was taken

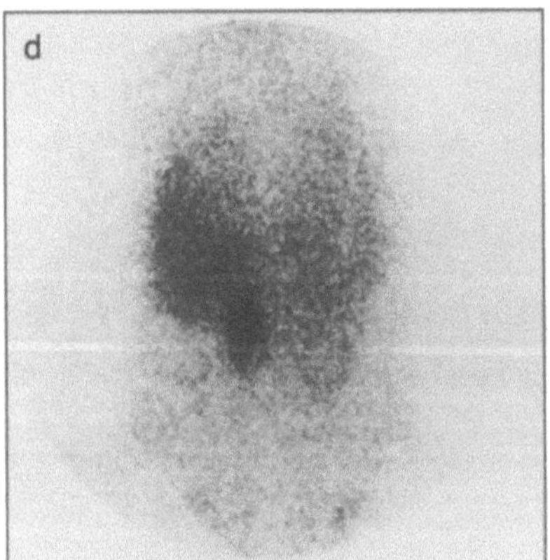

Fig. 4.58d. Posterior 24-h I 123 MIBG image of the thorax shows the mass taking up the MIBG. Isotope is also noted in the liver and to a lesser extent the heart is seen on this view which is normal

Teaching Point
Frequently thoracic neuroblastoma may be stage I disease, especially in the young. These children frequently have normal urinary catecholamine excretion but as this case and the previous case show it is important to stage all patients with neuroblastoma.

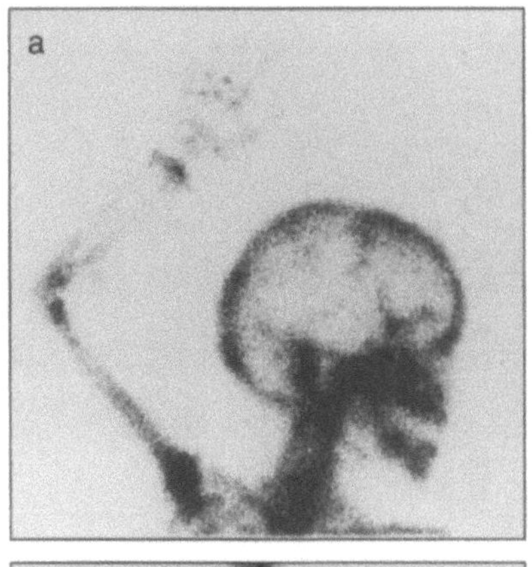

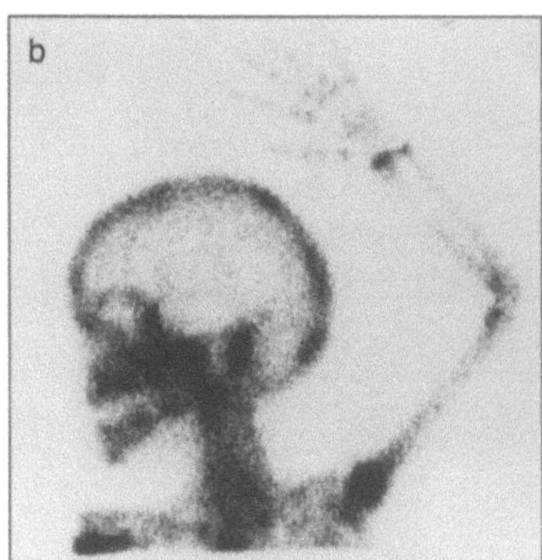

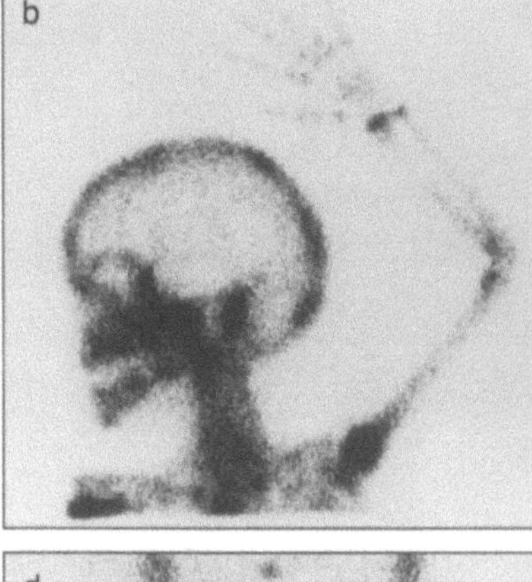

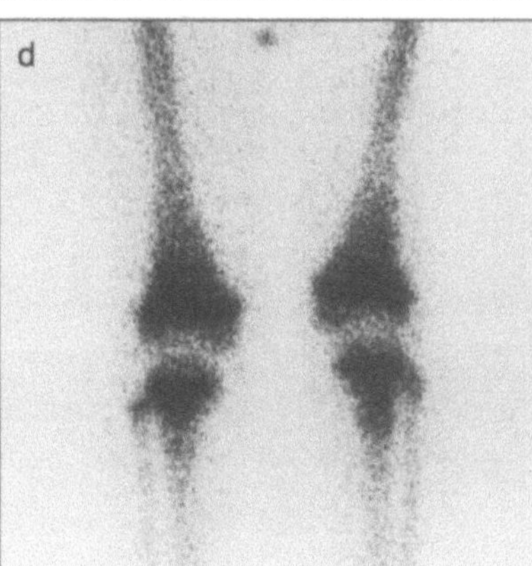

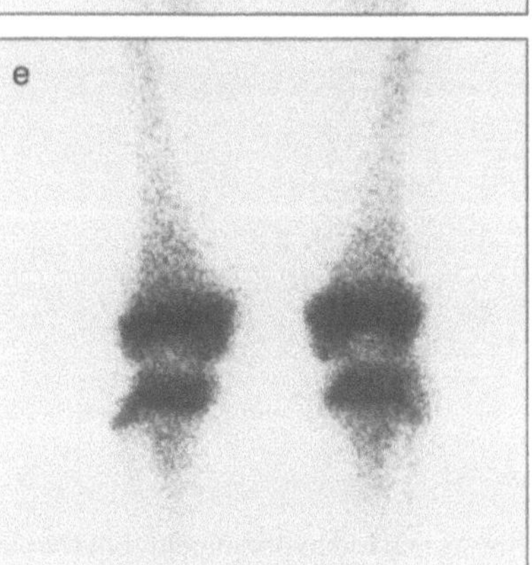

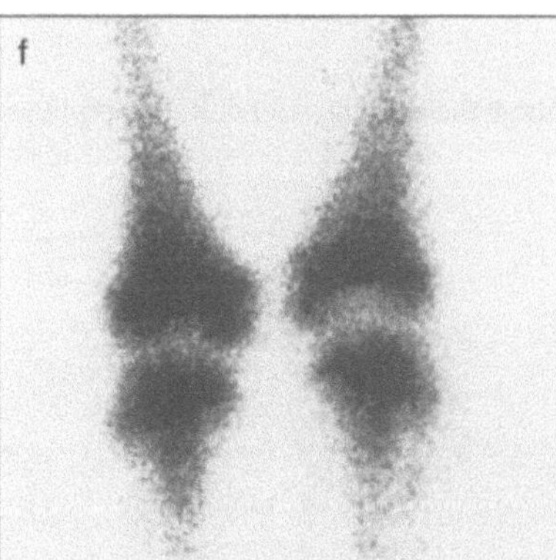

Case 4.59. A 3-year-old girl who was ill and anaemic was found to have stage IV neuroblastoma

Fig. 4.59a. Right lateral image of the skull and right arm shows abnormal uptake of isotope in the vault, right upper humerus and radius

Fig. 4.59b. Left lateral image of the skull and left arm shows abnormal uptake of isotope in the vault. The humerus is normal on this side

Fig. 4.59c. Anterior image of the thorax and pelvis shows uptake in the tumour on the left side of the abdomen as well as in both femoral necks

Fig. 4.59d. Posterior image of the knees shows loss of clarity of the epiphyseal plates around the knees due to infiltration by the neuroblastoma.

The girl went into complete remission following chemotherapy. A follow-up bone scan 5 months later was normal

Fig. 4.59e. Posterior image of the knees shows the normal, well defined epiphyseal plates.

Three months later the child relapsed and a further bone scan was undertaken which showed diffuse skeletal involvement

Fig. 4.59f. Posterior image of the knees shows loss of clarity of the epiphyseal plates around the knees due to infiltration by the neuroblastoma

Teaching Point
High-quality images of the epiphyseal plates are required to adequately assess the skeleton.

Case 4.60. A 7-year-old boy who was anaemic with an abdominal mass. He was found to have stage IV neuroblastoma

Fig. 4.60a. Right lateral image of the skull and right arm shows abnormal uptake of isotope in the vault and right upper humerus. The epiphyseal plates around the wrist are indistinct due to neuroblastoma infiltration

Fig. 4.60b. Left lateral image of the skull and left arm shows abnormal uptake of isotope in the vault. The humerus is less involved on this side. The proximal radius and ulna show abnormal increased uptake of isotope

Fig. 4.60c. Posterior image of the thorax and pelvis fails to show uptake by the tumour but the left kidney is displaced laterally and downwards. There are areas of both decreased uptake of isotope in the vertebral bodies as well as one area of increased uptake at L2. The ribs also show patchy increased uptake of isotope

Fig. 4.60d. Posterior image of the knees shows loss of clarity of all the epiphyseal plates around the knees due to infiltration by the neuroblastoma and an area of increased uptake in the distal right femur.

The boy went into complete remission following chemotherapy. Follow-up bone scans 4 and 13 months later were normal

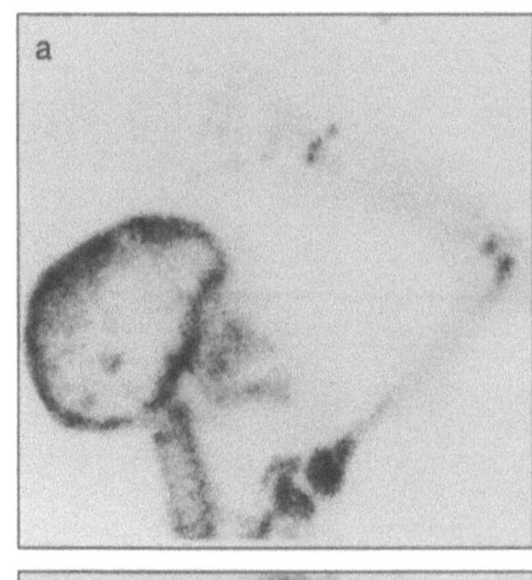
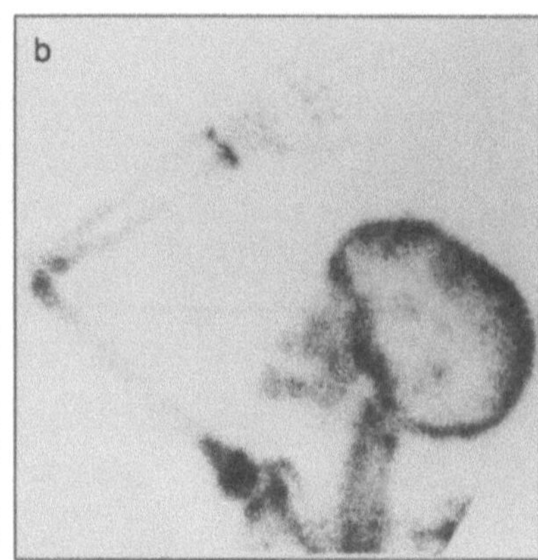
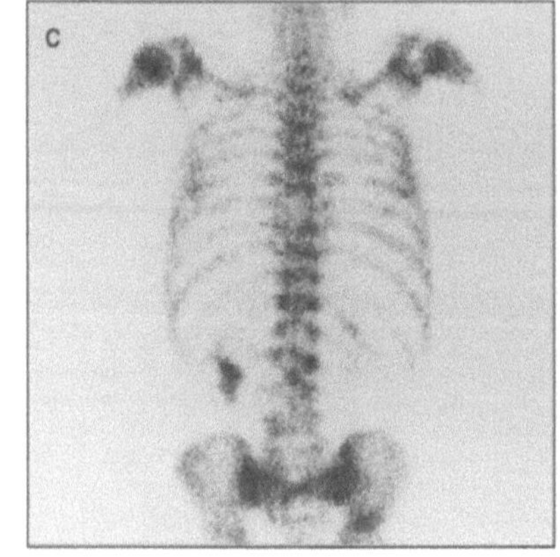
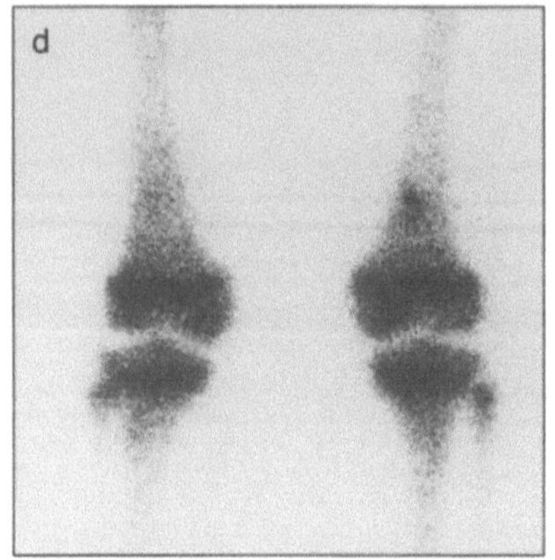
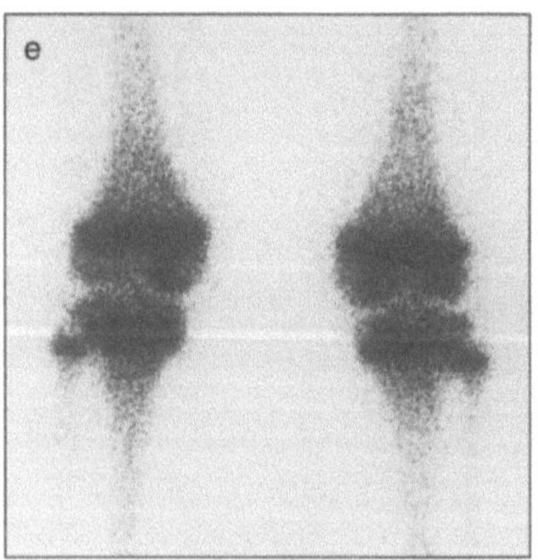
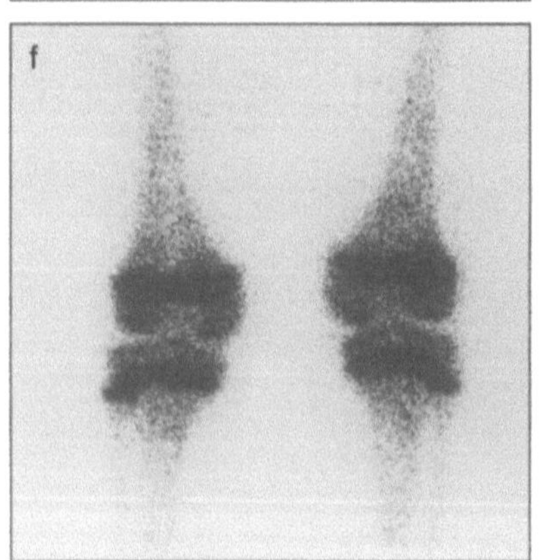

Fig. 4.60e. Posterior image of the knees shows marked improvement, but the clarity of the epiphysical plates of the left femur and left tibia medially are still indistinct.

Fig. 4.60f. Posterior image of the knees show the normal, well defined epiphyseal plates 13 months later

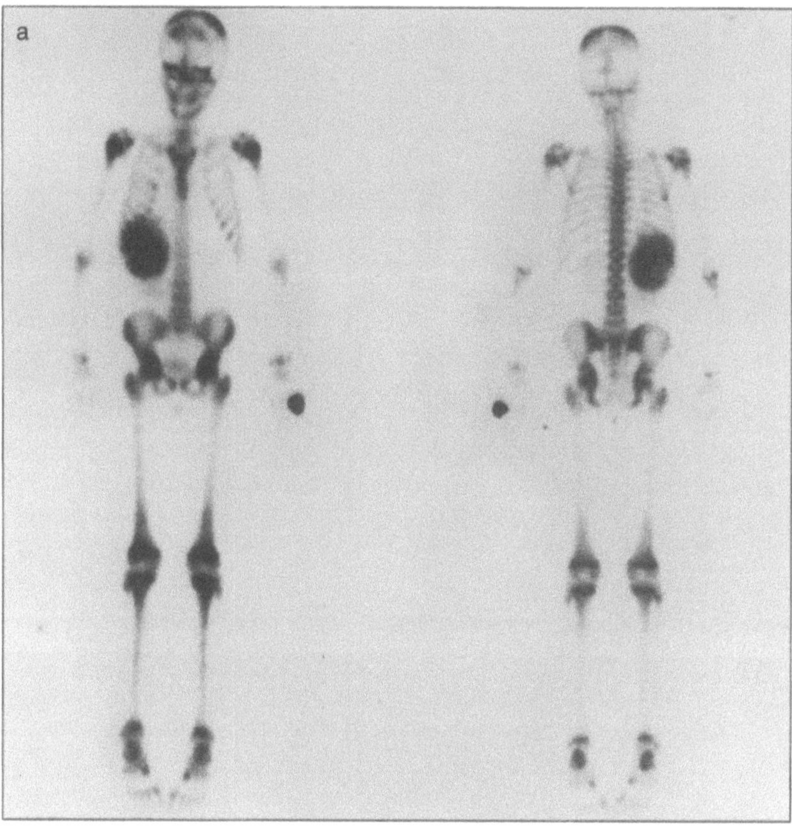

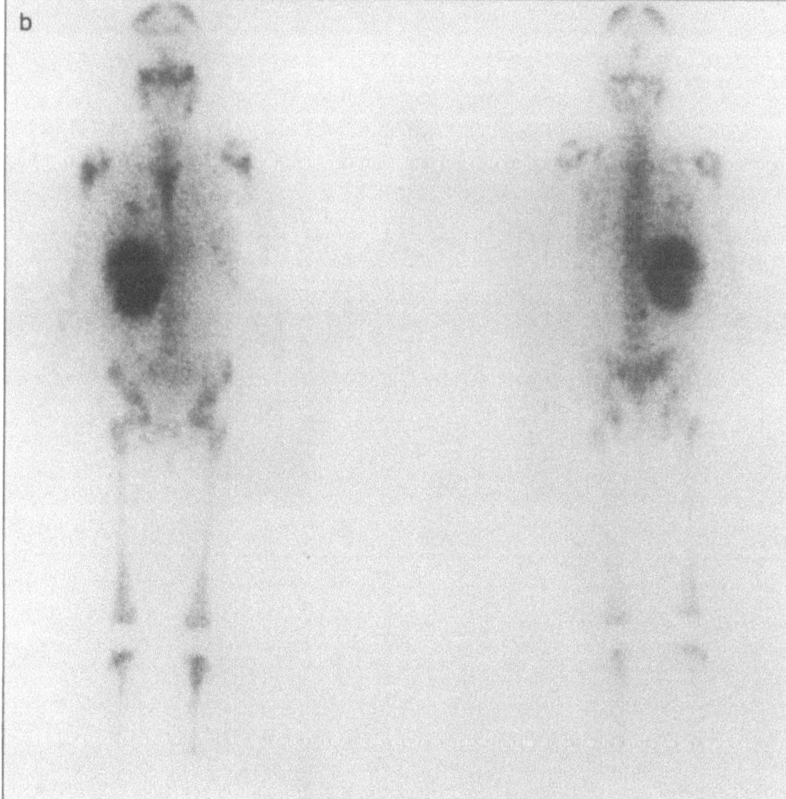

Case 4.61. A 10-year-old girl with stage IV neuroblastoma

Fig. 4.61a. Whole body scans show abnormal uptake by the abdominal mass on the right side of the abdomen. The skeleton has abnormal uptake in the skull, the facial bones, the humeri, the spine, femora and tibiae.

An I 123 MIGB scan was undertaken

Fig. 4.61b. Whole body I 123 MIBG scan at 20 h shows uptake of isotope by the tumour as well as diffuse uptake throughout the skeleton

Teaching Point

1. Neuroblastoma is more commonly seen in the younger children but may be found in patients in the third or fourth decade of life.
2. The loss of clarity of the epiphyseal plates which have remained "hot" around the knees is evidence of involvement by neuroblastoma on bone scan.

Case 4.62. A 4-year-old girl with stage IV neuroblastoma

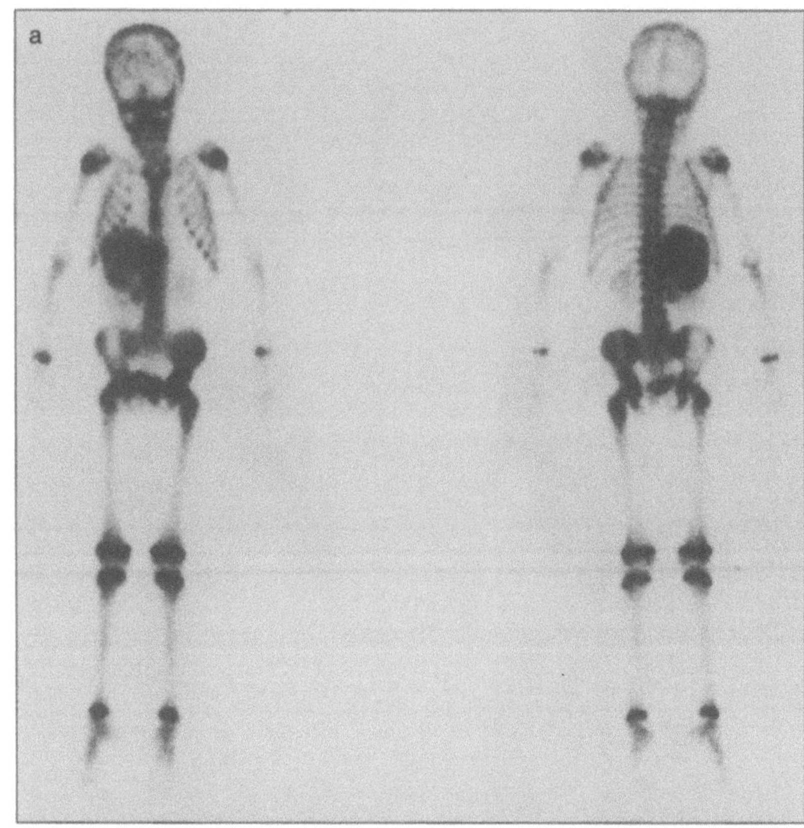

Fig. 4.62a. Whole body scans show intense abnormal increased uptake of isotope in the tumour. Abnormal uptake of isotope is also noted in the spine, the left hemipelvis, femora, knees and skull

Fig. 4.62b. Posterior image of the thorax and lumbar spine shows uptake of isotope in the tumour as well as abnormal increased uptake in both the dorsal and lumbar spine

Fig. 4.62c. Posterior image of the lumbar spine and pelvis shows abnormal increased uptake of isotope in the left hemipelvis and also in the proximal femora more marked on the left than on the right.

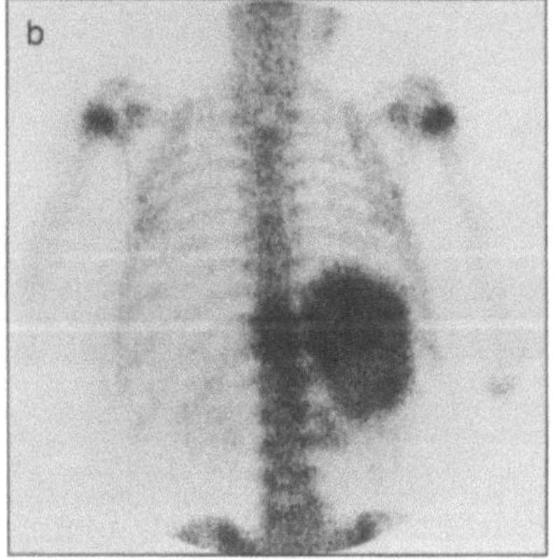

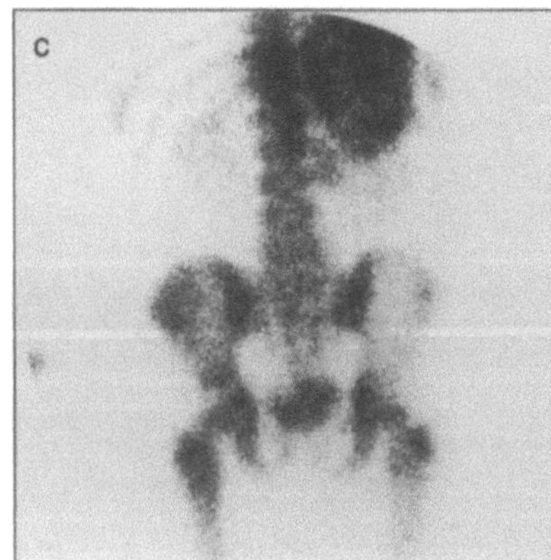

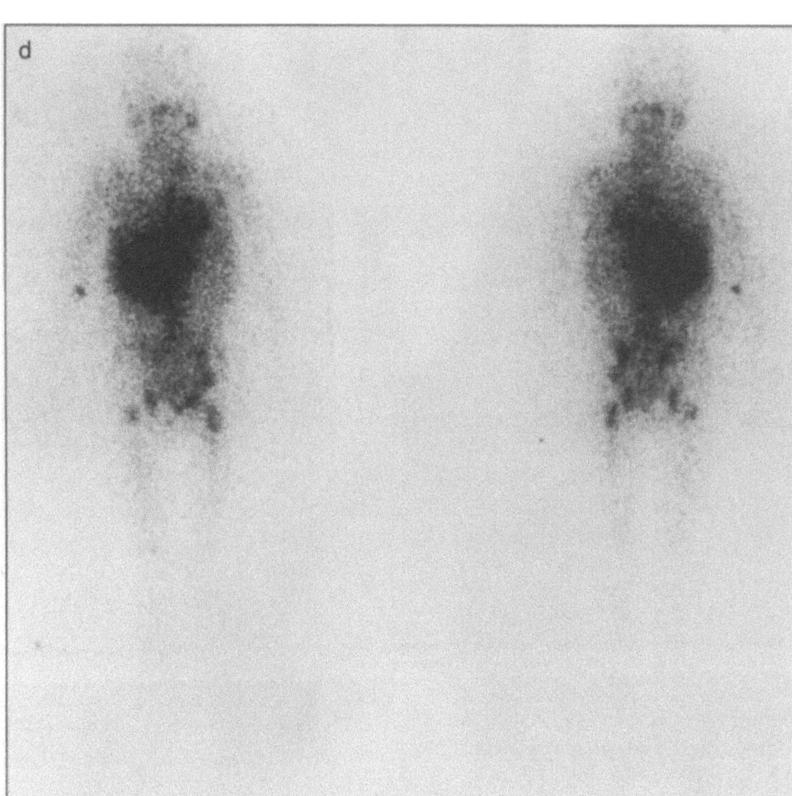

An I 123 MIBG scan was undertaken

Fig. 4.62d. Whole body I 123 MIBG scan at 25 h shows abnormal uptake by the tumour mass in the upper abdomen. Uptake is also noted in the pelvis and upper femora

Technical Comment
The high uptake by the tumour in Fig. 4.62d prevents visualisation of the spine.

4.2.2.3 Phaeochromo-cytoma
(1 Case; Fig. 4.63)

Case 4.63. A 12-year-old girl who presented with diffuse pain throughout the skeleton and was also noted to be hypertensive. The child was found to be suffering from a phaeochromocytoma with bony deposits

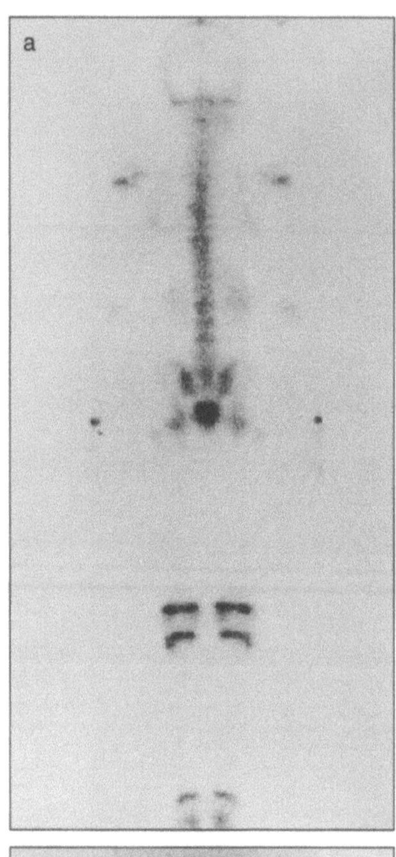

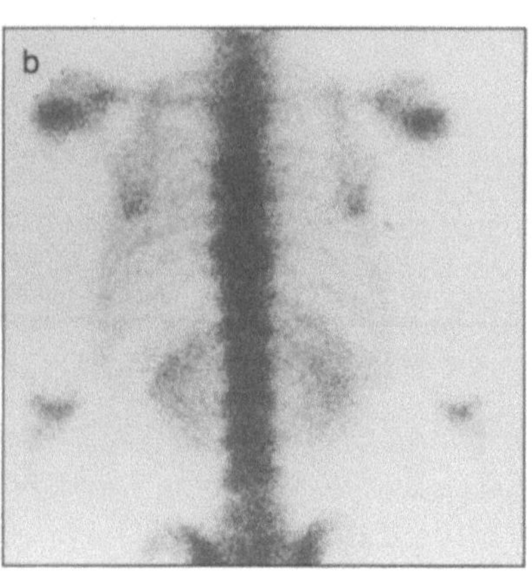

Fig. 4.63a. Posterior whole body image shows abnormal uptake of isotope in the spine

Fig. 4.63b. Posterior image of the thorax shows an abnormal uptake in both the dorsal and lumbar spine.

An I 123 MIBG scan was undertaken

Fig. 4.63c. Posterior whole body I 123 MIBG scan at 20 h shows multiple areas of increased uptake of isotope in the spine and also in the left shoulder

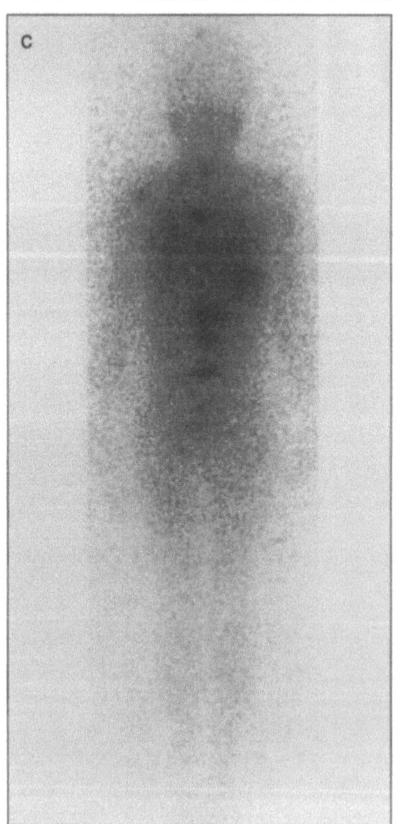

Teaching Point
The primary tumour is not taking up the I 123 MIBG even though the deposits are positive.

4.2.3 Reticular Endothelial System Malignancy

4.2.3.1 Hodgkin's Lymphoma
(3 Cases; Figs. 4.64–4.66)

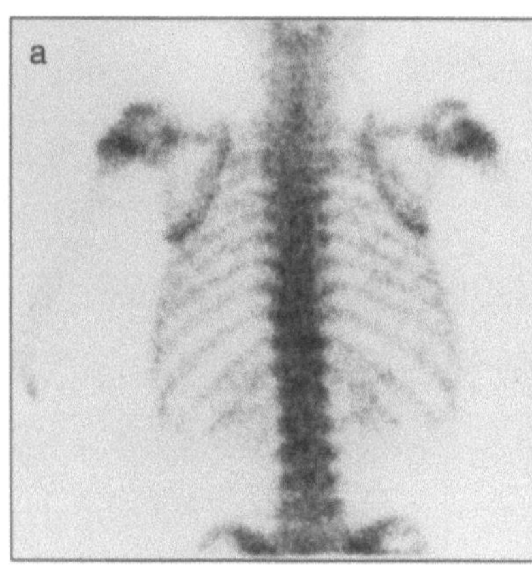

Case 4.64. An 8-year-old boy with Hodgkin's disease. He had stage IV disease with recurrence of the disease 6 months after the onset

Fig. 4.64a. Posterior view of the cervical, dorsal and lumbar spine as well as the shoulder girdle shows focal abnormal increased uptake of isotope in the right side of D11

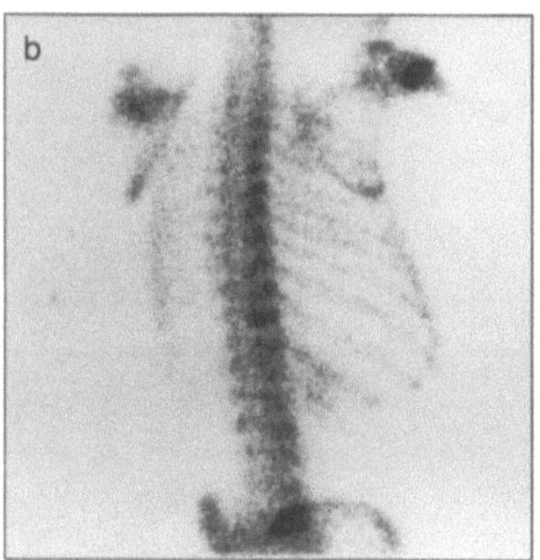

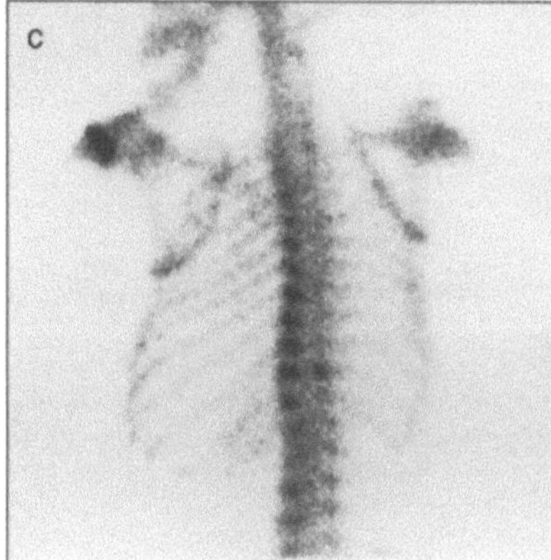

Fig. 4.64b. Right posterior oblique view of the thoracic cage and lumbar spine shows focal abnormal increased uptake of isotope in the body of D11 on the right side

Fig. 4.64c. Left posterior oblique view of the dorsal and upper lumbar spine shows only a small spot with increased activity in D11.

Five months later, a repeat bone scan was undertaken

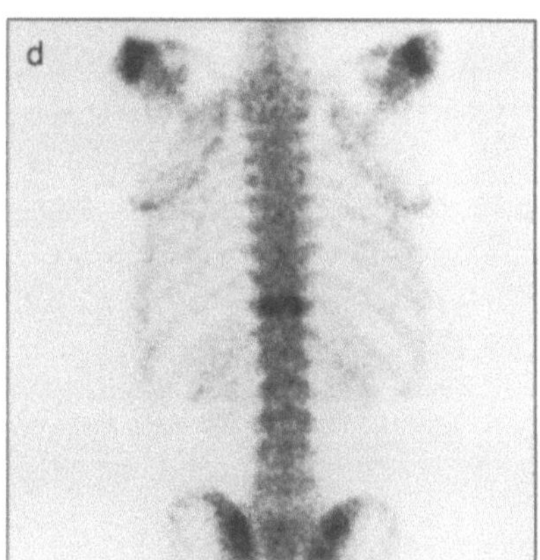

Fig. 4.64d. Posterior view of the dorsal and lumbar spine shows diffuse increased uptake of isotope in the body of D11

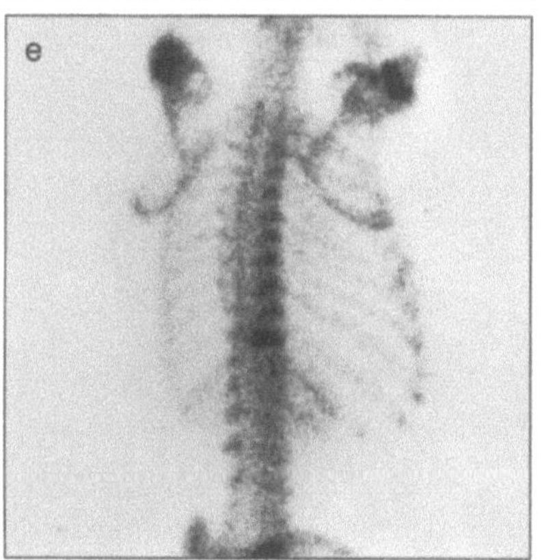

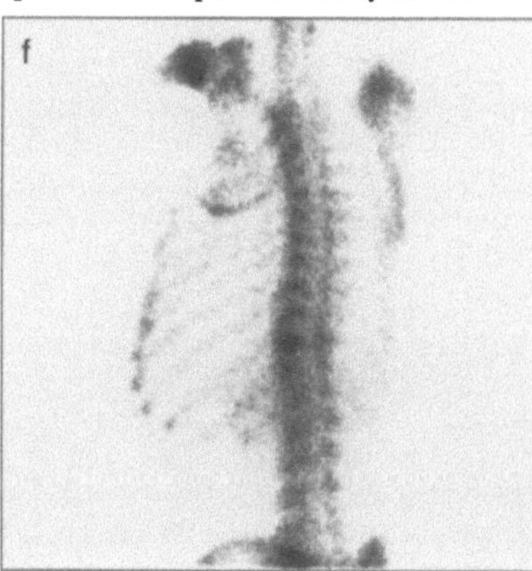

Fig. 4.64e. Right posterior oblique view of the dorsal and lumbar spine shows abnormal increased uptake in the body of D11

Fig. 4.64f. Left posterior oblique view of the thoracic cage, dorsal and lumbar spine shows abnormal increased uptake of isotope in the body of D11.
(continued on p. 160)

The next bone scan was undertaken 3 months later.

Fig. 4.64g. Posterior view of the dorsal and lumbar spine shows slightly abnormal increased uptake of isotope in the body of D11

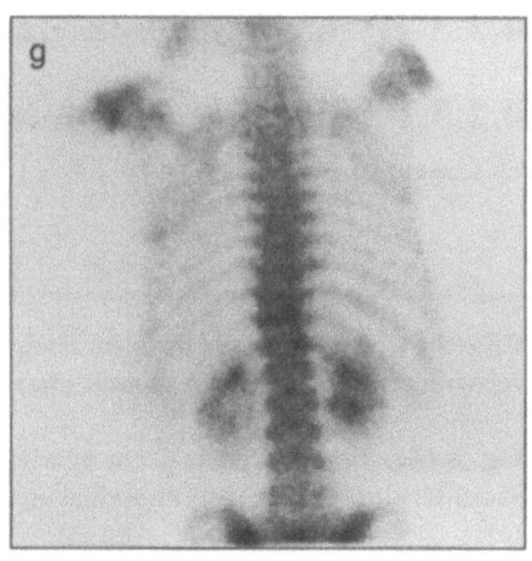

Fig. 4.64h. Right posterior oblique view shows a very slightly abnormal increased uptake of isotope in the body of D11

Fig. 4.64i. Left posterior oblique view of the dorsal and lumbar spine shows abnormal increased uptake of isotope in the body of D11.

One week later a gallium-67 scan was undertaken

Fig. 4.64j. Gallium 67 scan posterior view at 48 h shows no evidence of any focal abnormal uptake in the spine. Activity is seen in the liver wich is normal

Fig. 4.64k. Gallium 67 scan anterior view of the thorax and the upper abdomen shows abnormal increased uptake of isotope in the mediastinum confirming stage IV disease but showing that the uptake in the spine on the last bone scan was reparative new bone formation rather than Hodgkin's disease

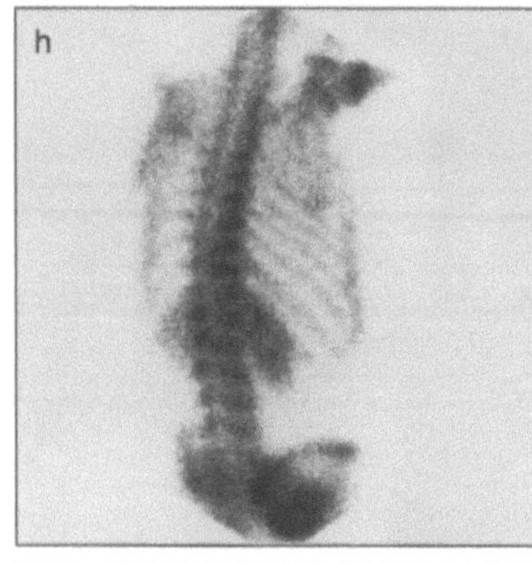
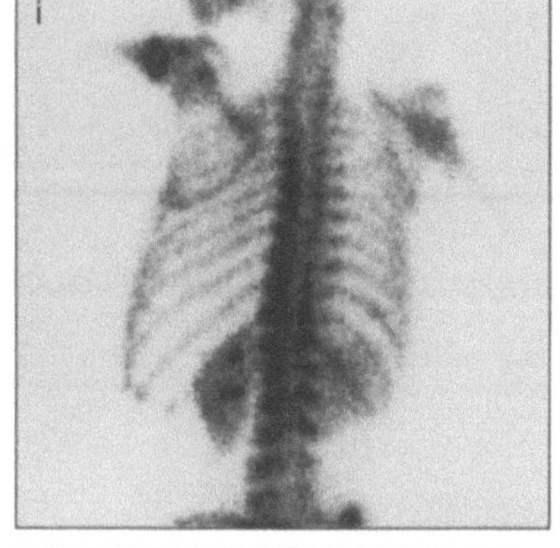
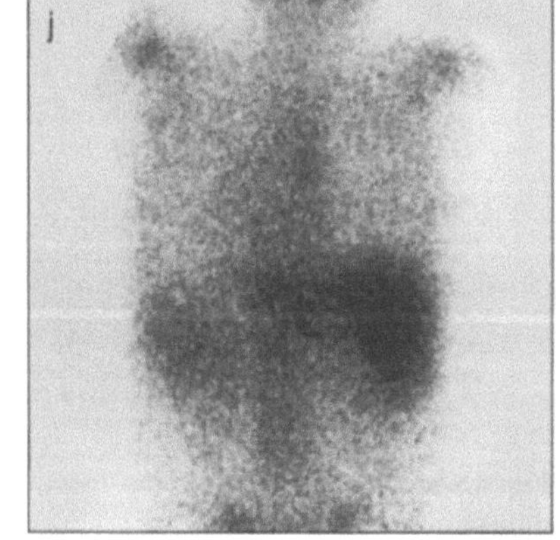
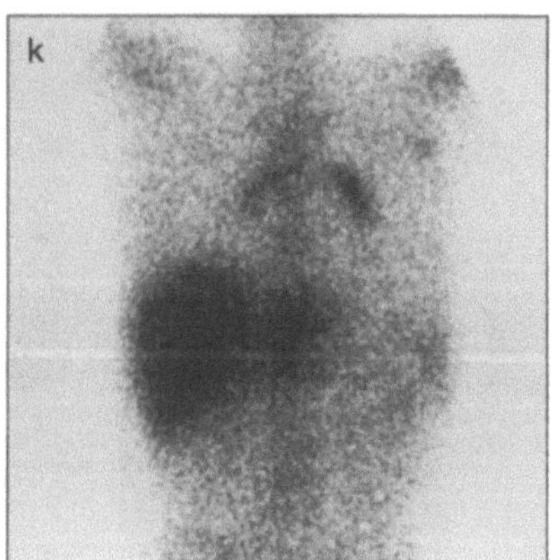

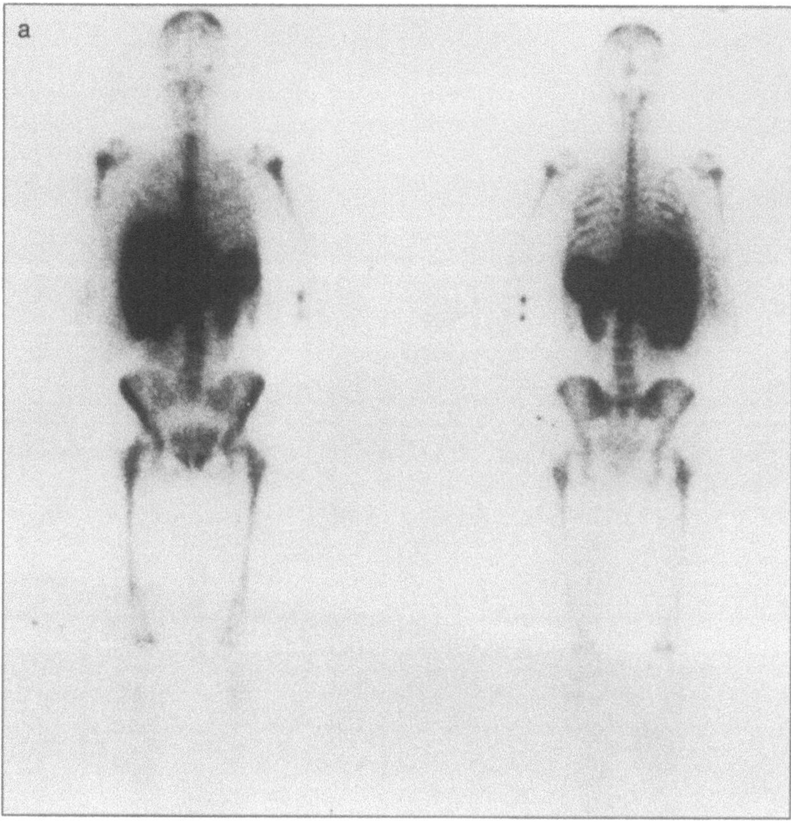

Case 4.65. An 18-year-old girl with a 1-month history of being unwell and anaemic. She was found to have disseminated Hodgkin's disease

Fig. 4.65a. Bone marrow whole body scans with Tc 99m nanocolloid show intense abnormal increased uptake of isotope in the enlarged liver and spleen. There is abnormal uptake of isotope in the proximal humeri as well as in both femora. The decreased activity in the upper thorax is caused by radiotherapy

Fig. 4.65b. Whole body bone scans show abnormal increased uptake of isotope in the skull vault. Increased uptake of isotope is also noted in the shafts of the femora as well as the proximal diaphyses of the tibiae. Well defined linear absent activity is seen in the posterior aspects of the rips bilaterally. This corresponds to the radiotherapy field

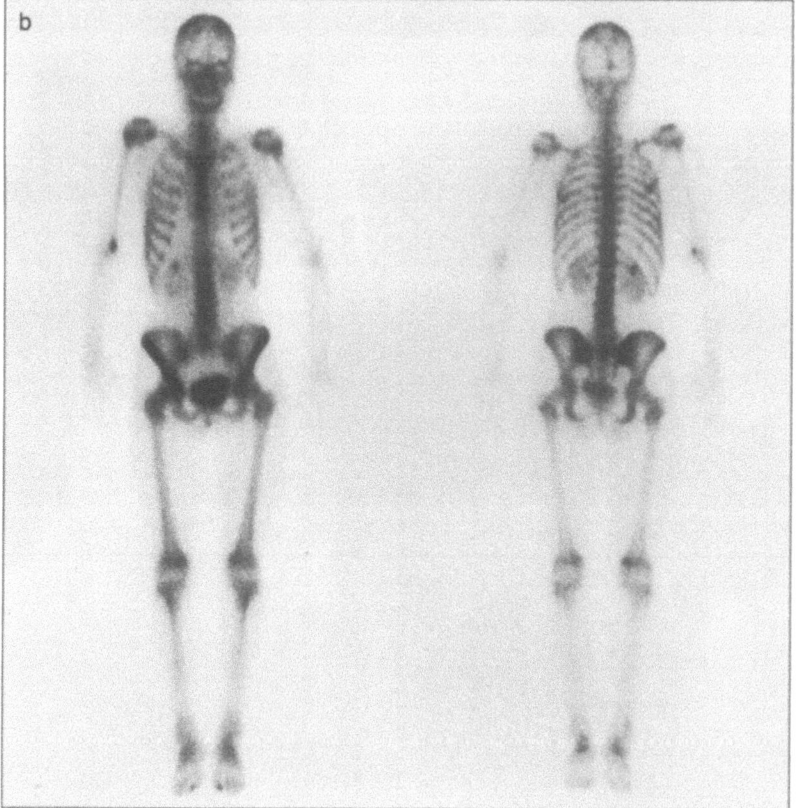

Technical Comment

1. Focal increased uptake of isotope is noted in the upper calyx of the right kidney; this is presumably due to a dilated calyx.
2. Note extravasastion of isotope in the left elbow (Fig. 4.65a) and the right elbow (Fig. 4.65b), the sites of injection.

Teaching Point

1. The epiphyseal plates are difficult to evaluate at this age since skeletal maturation varies and some children have already closed their growth plates around the knees at this age.
2. For effect of radiotherapy also see Case 5.77.

Case 4.66. A 14-year-old girl with Hodgkin's disease stage IV

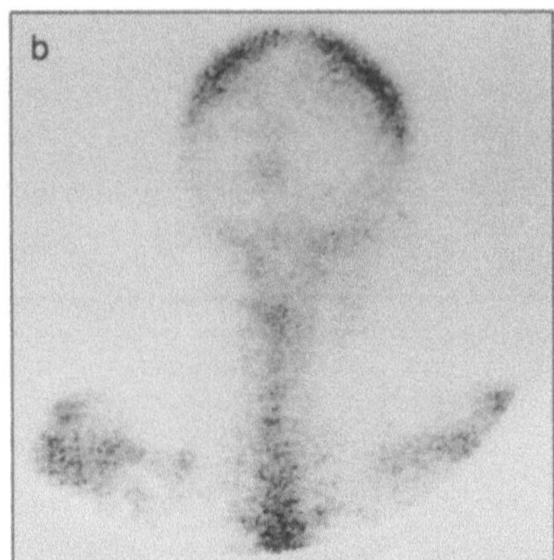

Fig. 4.66a,b. Anterior and posterior views of the skull show abnormal accumulation in the vault bilaterally

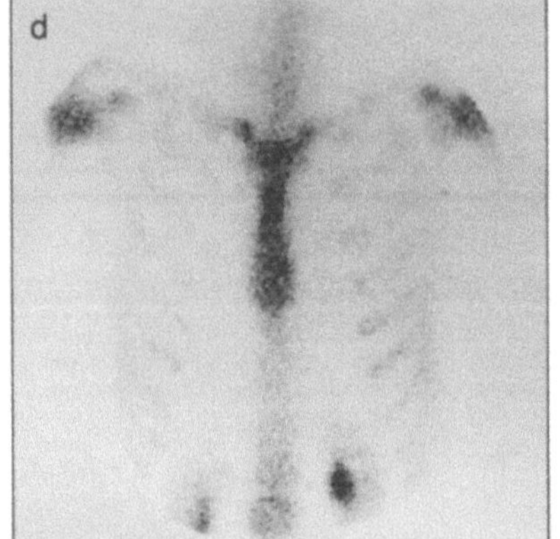

Fig. 4.66c. Posterior view of the thorax and upper lumbar spine shows only slightly increased uptake of isotope in the posterior left lower ribs. There is also abnormal increased retention of the tracer by the left kidney

Fig. 4.66d. Anterior view of the thorax and upper abdomen is normal. The retention of the tracer in the left kidney is again noted

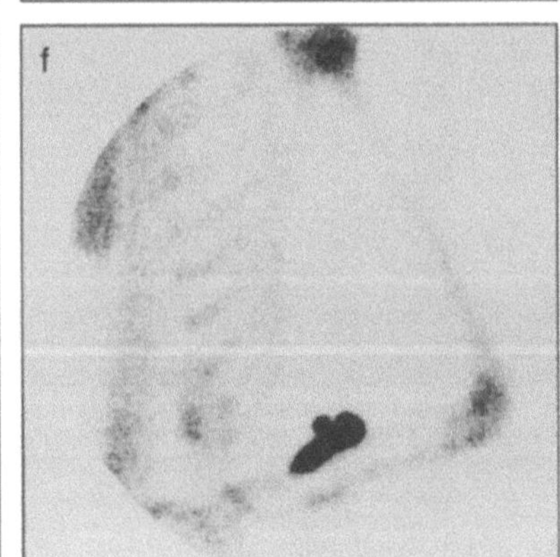

Fig. 4.66e, f. Anterior views of the upper limbs show abnormal increased uptake of tracer in the distal humeri and forearm bones. Note extravasation at the injection site in the left forearm

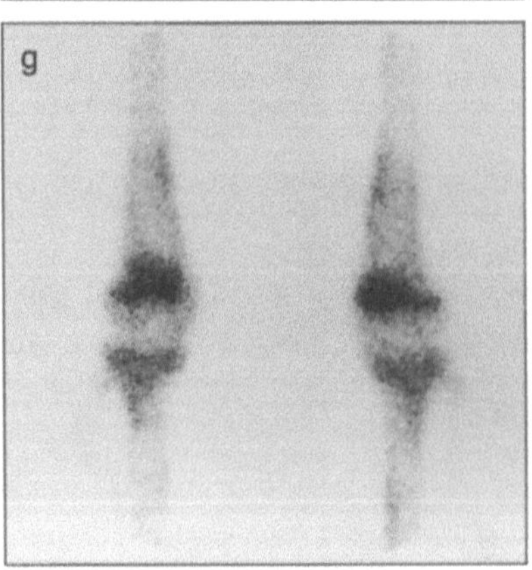

Fig. 4.66g. Posterior view of the knees shows abnormal increased uptake of isotope in the distal femora and proximal tibiae

162

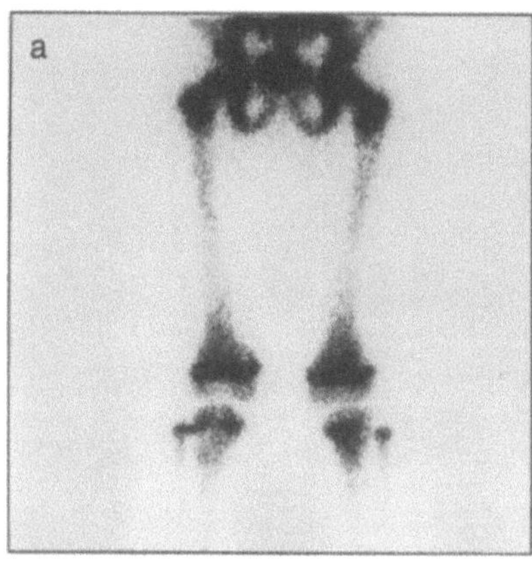

4.2.3.2 Non-Hodgkin's Lymphoma
(1 Case; Fig. 4.67)

Case 4.67. A 5-year-old boy who was found to have a non-Hodgkin's lymphoma (B cell)

Fig. 4.67a. Posterior image of the lower limbs shows abnormal increased uptake of isotope around the diaphyses and metaphyses of the knees. There is also a photon-deficient area in the upper lateral aspect of the left tibia

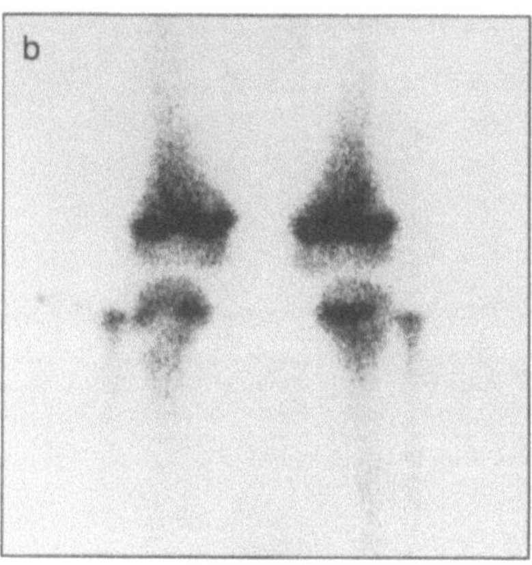

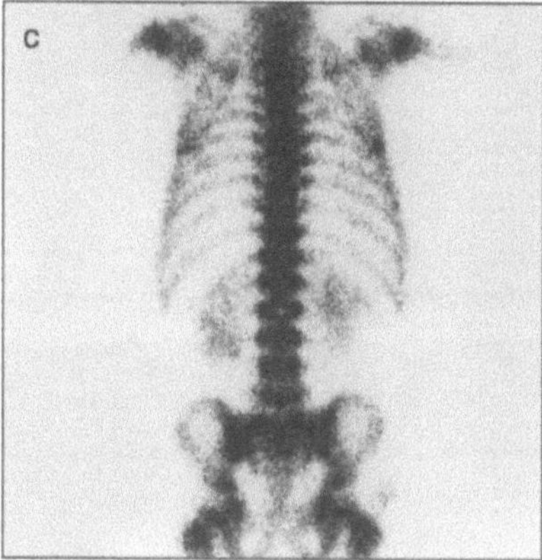

Fig. 4.67b. Posterior magnified image of the knees. The loss of clarity of the epiphyseal plates is seen to better advantage. Note the fibulae are involved as well. The photon-deficient area in the upper left tibia is again noted

Fig. 4.67c. Posterior image of the spine and pelvis shows abnormal increased uptake of isotope in the femoral necks. Note the unusual appearances of the kidneys.

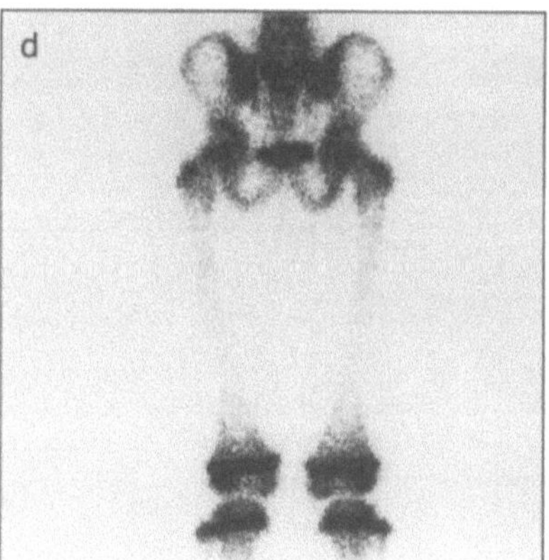

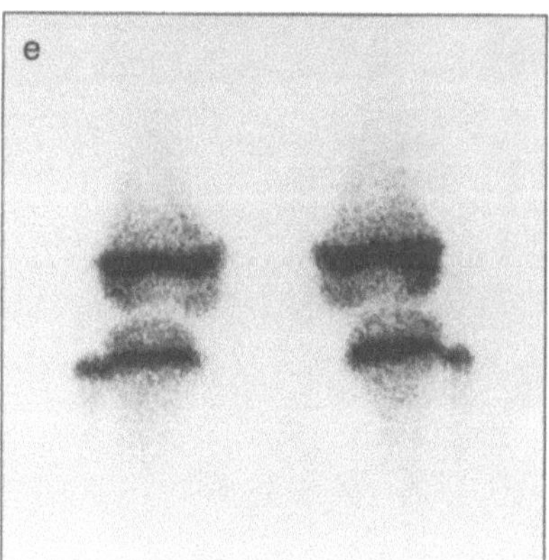

Following chemotherapy, the child went into complete remission. A follow-up bone scan was obtained 7 months after the original bone scan

Fig. 4.67d. Posterior image of the pelvis and knees. This is now normal

Fig. 4.67e. Magnification posterior image of the knees. The epiphyseal plates are now clearly seen and the knees appear normal

Technical Comment

Note the importance of obtaining the knees in the centre of the gamma camera with magnification and with the feet internally rotated into the "radiographic neutral position" so that the fibula may be separated from the tibia.

4.2.3.3 Leukaemia
(3 Cases; Figs. 4.68–4.70)

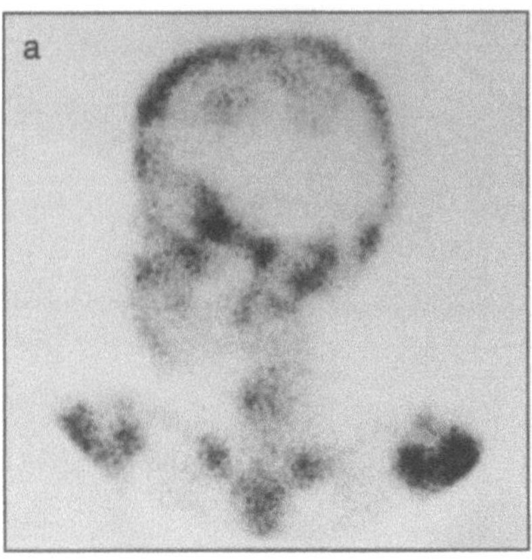

Teaching Point
Routine bone scans are not undertaken in children with leukaemia. Children may present with focal signs or symptoms without an established diagnosis, and a bone scan may then be indicated which suggests a diffuse process such as leukaemia. Children known to be suffering from leukaemia may present with focal pain in which a complication (e.g. fracture or infection) is suspected, then a bone scan is indicated.

Case 4.68. An 8-year-old boy with acute lymphoblastic leukaemia and diffuse involvement of the bone marrow

Fig. 4.68a. Left lateral image of the skull shows abnormal uptake of isotope in the skull vault

Fig. 4.68b. Posterior image of the thorax shows focal abnormal increased uptake of isotope in multiple ribs

Fig. 4.68c. Anterior image of the thorax. The abnormal ribs are again noted. There is also abnormal increased uptake of isotope in the humeri more marked on the left than on the right. Note activity in the enlarged spleen

Fig. 4.68d. Posterior image of the dorsal and lumbar spine shows decreased uptake of isotope at L5 and increased uptake in the ribs

Fig. 4.68e. Posterior image of the lower limbs shows abnormal increased uptake of isotope around the knees and also throughout the tibiae

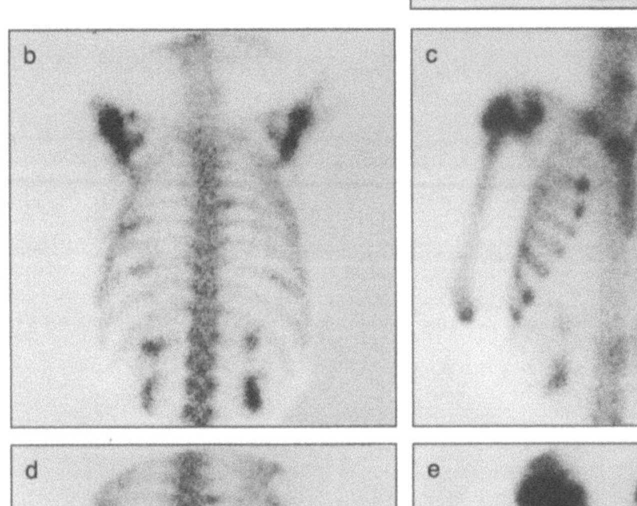

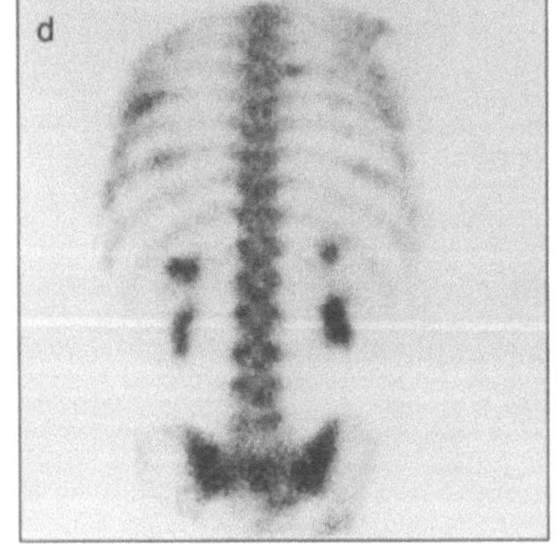

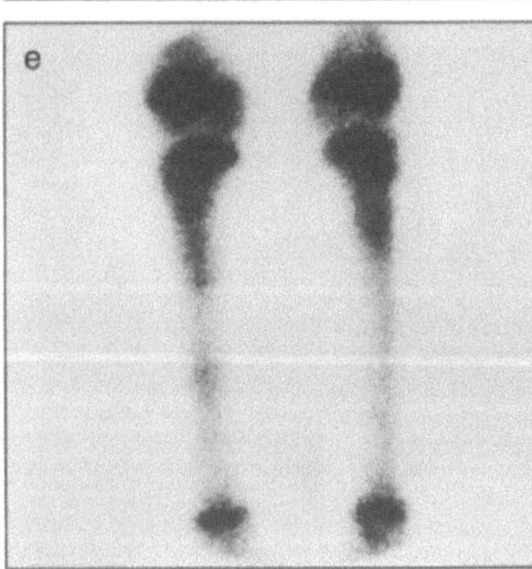

Technical Comment
Retention of isotope in the pelvis of both kidneys; these might possibly be renal duplications.

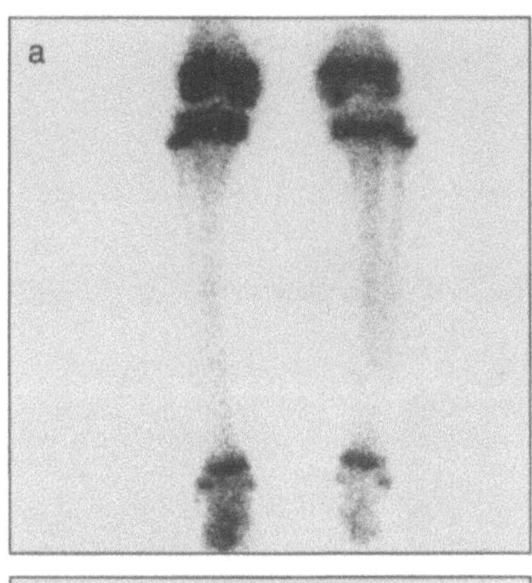
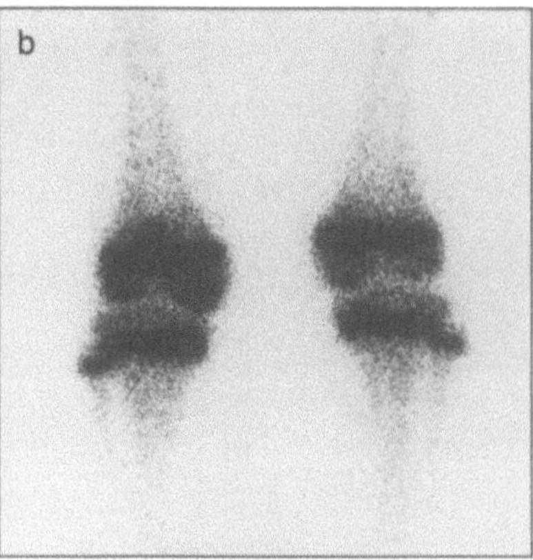
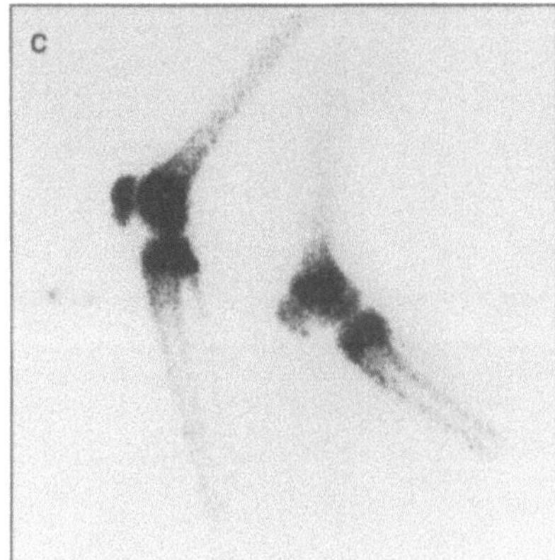
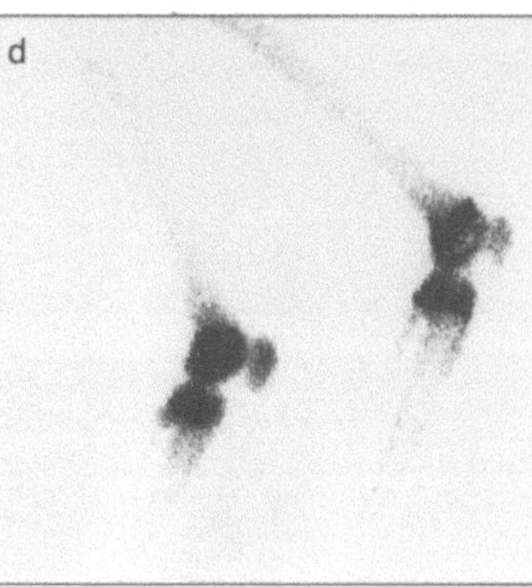

Case 4.69. 9-year-old boy with acute pain and an effusion in the left knee. This was due to acute lymphoblastic leukaemia

Fig. 4.69a. Posterior image of the knees and lower limbs shows increased uptake of isotope around the left knee, left ankle and foot

Fig. 4.69b. Posterior magnification image of the knees shows abnormal increased uptake of isotope immediately above the medial aspect of the left femoral epiphyseal plate

Fig. 4.69c. Lateral image of the knees (the right knee is in the medial lateral position whilst the left knee is in the lateral lateral position). There is marked increased uptake of isotope in the left patella

Fig. 4.69d. Opposite lateral image of the knees (medial lateral view of the left knee and the lateral lateral view of the right knee). The increased uptake in the left patella is again noted

Teaching Point
1. It is an unusual but well recognised presentation of acute leukaemia for there to be a solitary bony lesion which later develops into the full blown acute lymphoblastic leukaemia picture.
2. The cause for the increased uptake of isotope in the left ankle remains conjectural.

Case 4.70. A 9-year-old girl with a two months history of pain in the back; this was due to acute lympho-blastic leukaemia

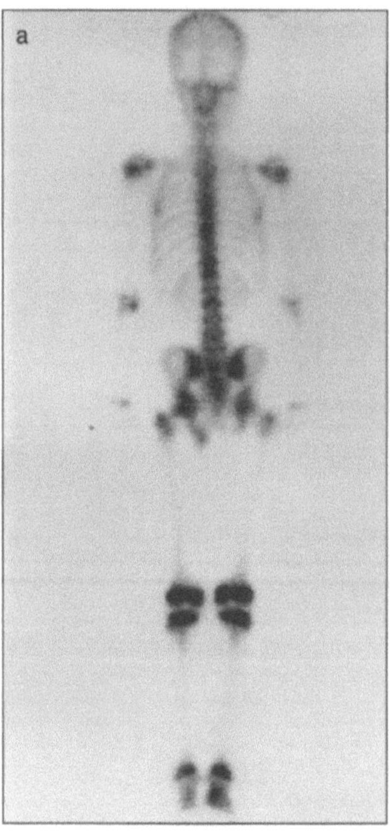

Fig. 4.70a. Posterior whole body scan shows patchy abnormal increased uptake of isotope in the dorsal and lumbar spine and the right sacro-iliac joint. The knees appear normal. There is increased activity in the right foot. The cause for this was presumed to be the leukaemia

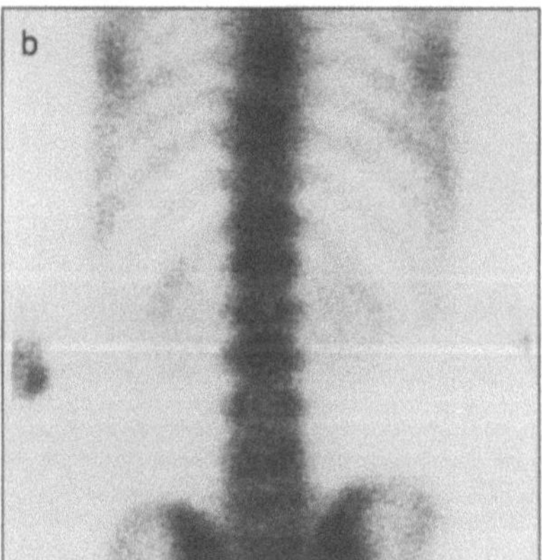

Fig. 4.70b. Posterior image of the spine shows focal abnormal increased uptake of isotope in some of the dorsal and lumbar spine vertebrae whilst other vertebrae remain normal

Teaching Point.
As in Case 4.69, the skeleton may be involved early on when the acute lymphoblastic leukaemia has not yet manifested itself in a generalised form.

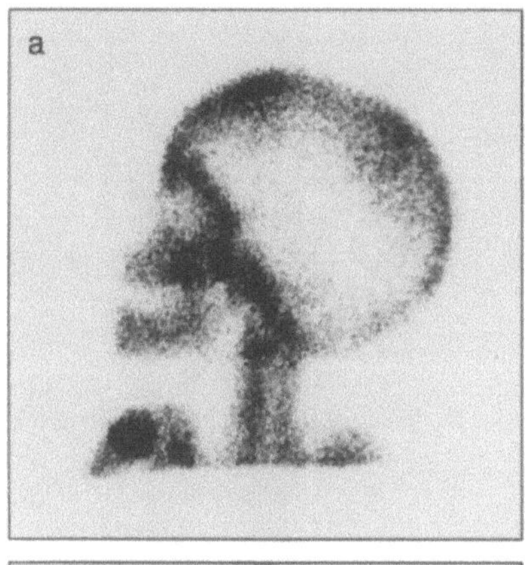
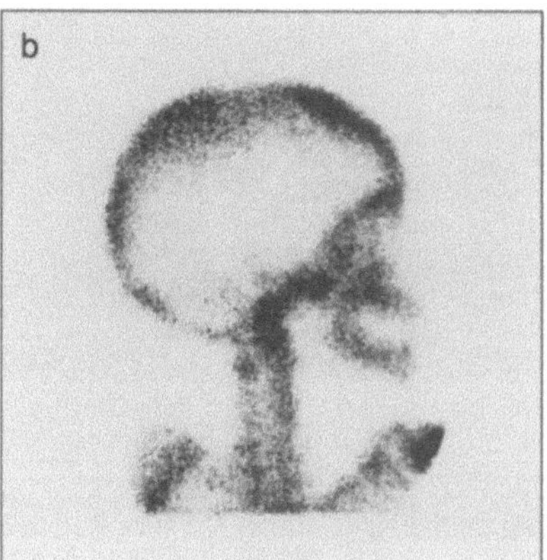
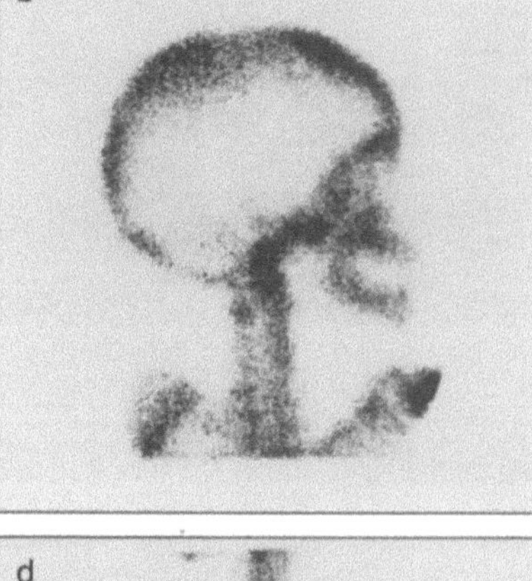
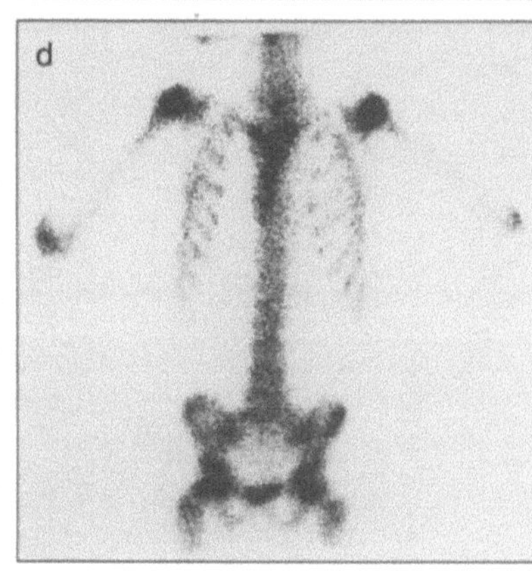
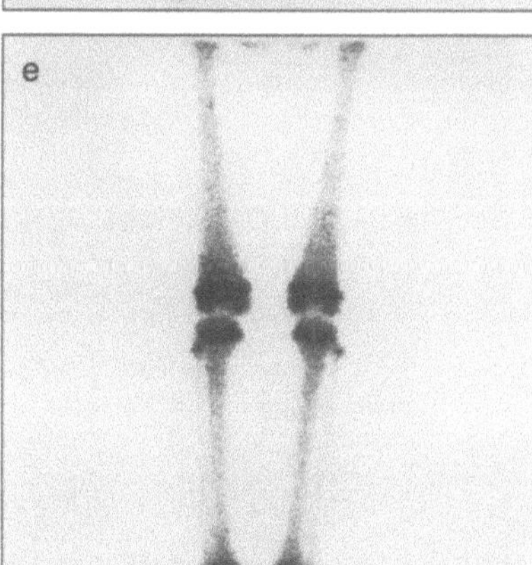

4.2.3.4 Myelofibrosis
(1 case; Fig. 4.71)

Case 4.71. An 8-year-old girl with myelofibrosis

Fig. 4.71a. Left lateral image of the skull shows abnormal increased uptake of isotope in both the frontal and parietal bones

Fig. 4.71b. Right lateral image of the skull shows less marked increased uptake of isotope in the frontal and parietal bones than on the left lateral view

Fig. 4.71c. Posterior image of the thorax, lumbar spine, pelvis and upper limbs. The epiphyseal plates in the proximal humeri are not well defined, nor are the growth plates in the upper femora clearly seen

Fig. 4.71d. Anterior image of the thorax and pelvis again shows poor definition of the epiphyseal plates. The normal hot anterior ends of the ribs are absent. Increased uptake of isotope is noted in the left hemipelvis, possibly due to rotation

Fig. 4.71e. Posterior image of the lower limbs shows loss of modelling of the distal femora associated with abnormal increased uptake of isotope extending from the epiphyseal plates into the diaphyses of the femora and proximal ends of the distal tibiae

Teaching Point
Myelofibrosis is uncommon in the paediatric age-group and is generally seen as a complication of certain therapies.

4.2.4 Other Tumours

4.2.4.1 Rhabdomyosarcoma
(1 Case; Fig. 4.72)

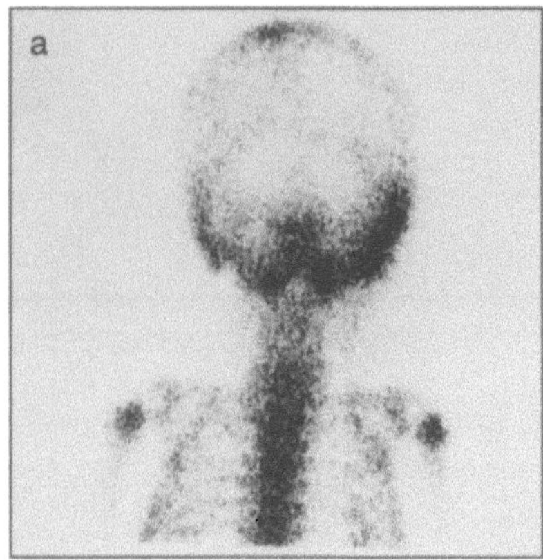

Case 4.72. A 1-year-old child with swelling on the right side of the face due to a rhabdomyosarcoma

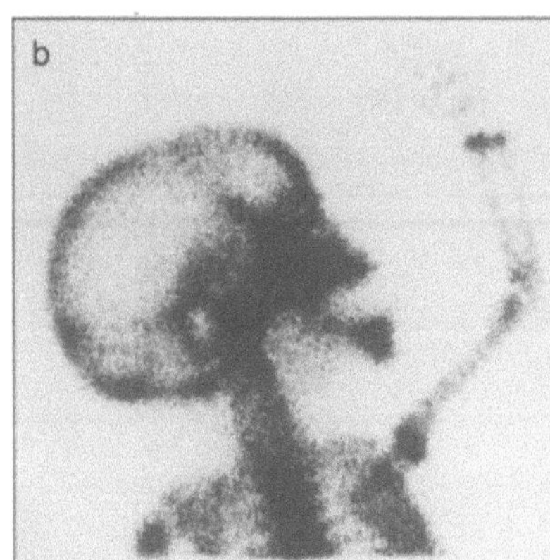

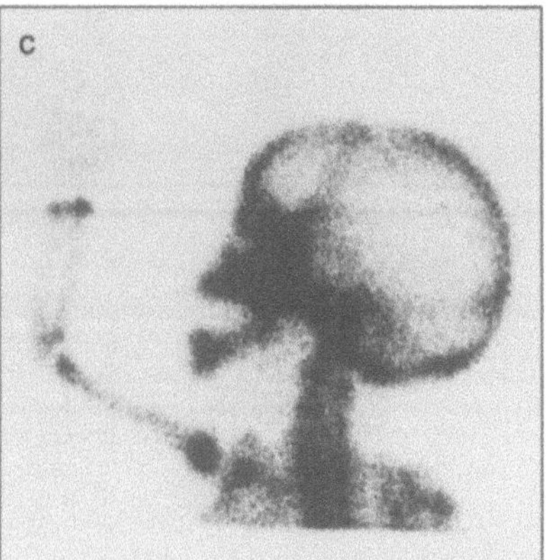

Fig. 4.72a. Posterior image of the skull shows abnormal increased uptake of isotope in the right parietal bone

Fig. 4.72b. Right lateral image of the skull shows abnormal increased uptake of isotope in the parietal bone

Fig. 4.72c. Left lateral image of the skull is normal

4.2.4.2 Germ Cell Tumour
(1 Case; Fig. 4.73)

Case 4.73. A 2-year-old boy presented with a large soft tissue swelling in the submandibular region which caused airway obstruction. Histology showed this to be a malignant germ cell tumour which involved the mandible

Fig. 4.73a. Anterior image of the face and thorax shows abnormal increased uptake of isotope on the right side of the mandible extending and crossing the mid-line

Fig. 4.73b. Left lateral image of the skull and left anterior oblique view of the thorax shows the abnormal increased uptake of isotope in the anterior portion of the mandible

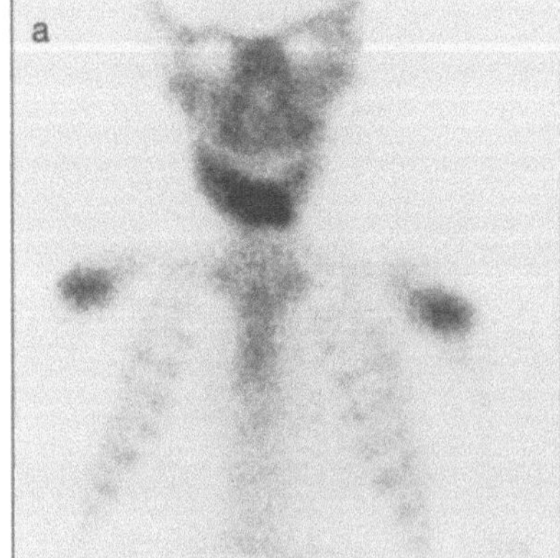

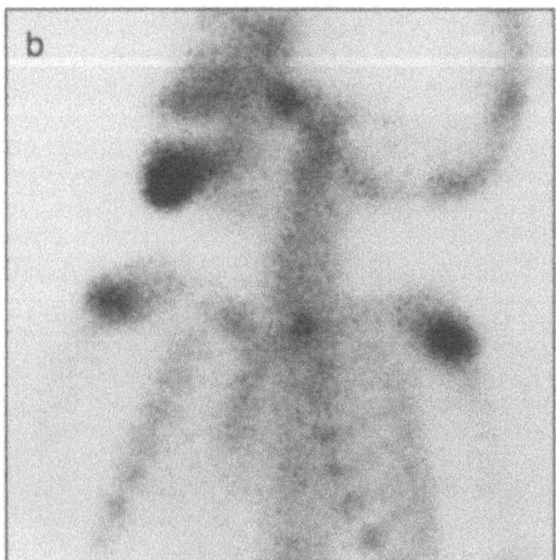

Teaching Point

This is an unusual tumour in an unusual site. Similar appearances may be seen in infection (see Case 2.21).

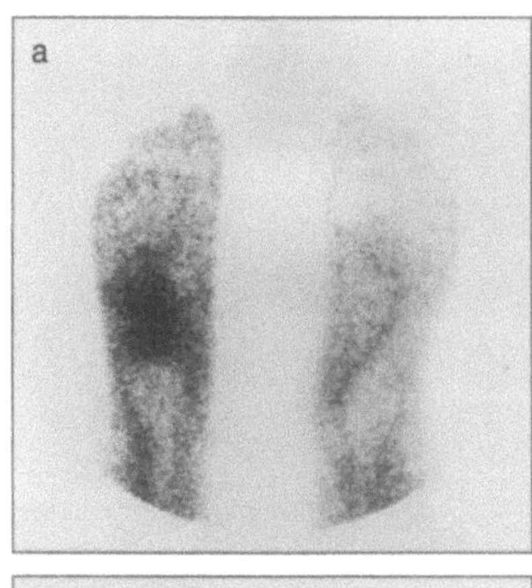

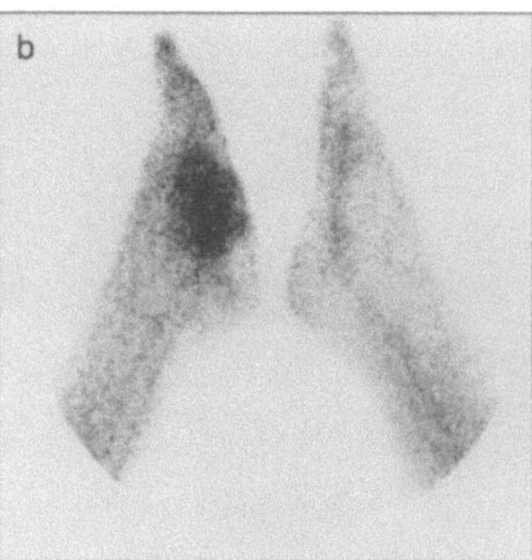

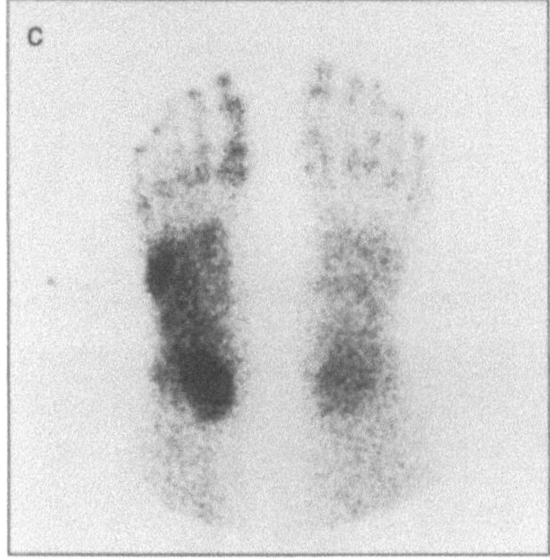

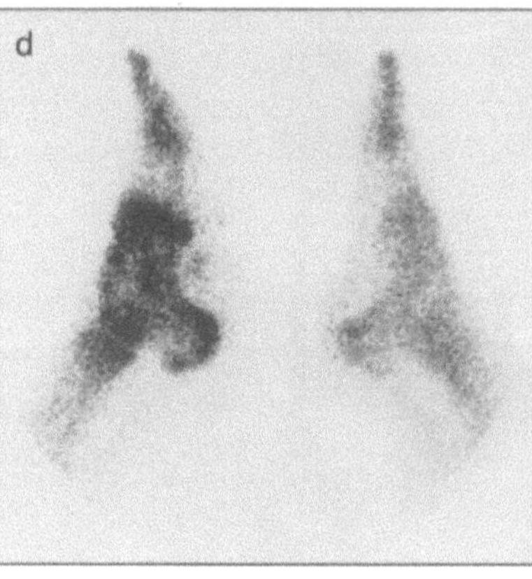

4.2.4.3 Synovioma
(1 Case; Fig. 4.74)

Case 4.74. A 21-year-old patient with pain in the right foot due to a malignant synovioma

Fig. 4.74a. Posterior blood pool image of the feet shows marked increased uptake of isotope in the small bones of the right foot

Fig. 4.74b. Blood pool lateral image of the feet confirms the increased uptake of isotope in the mid portion of the right foot

Fig. 4.74c. Posterior image of the feet shows generalised increased uptake of isotope throughout the right foot and ankle. In addition, there is focal abnormal increased uptake of isotope in the region of the lateral distal small bones, the site of the synovioma

Fig. 4.74d. Lateral image of the feet shows generalised increased uptake of isotope in the right foot. The synovioma is difficult to recognise on this view. Note abnormal isotope in the soft tissue of the right foot

Teaching Point

The generalised hyperaemia of the right foot was considered to be the reason for the increased uptake of isotope seen at 3 h. The diagnosis of a synovioma is not possible from the bone scan alone.

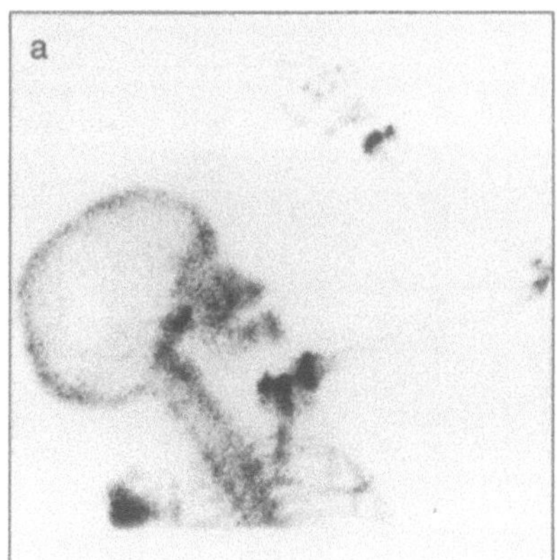

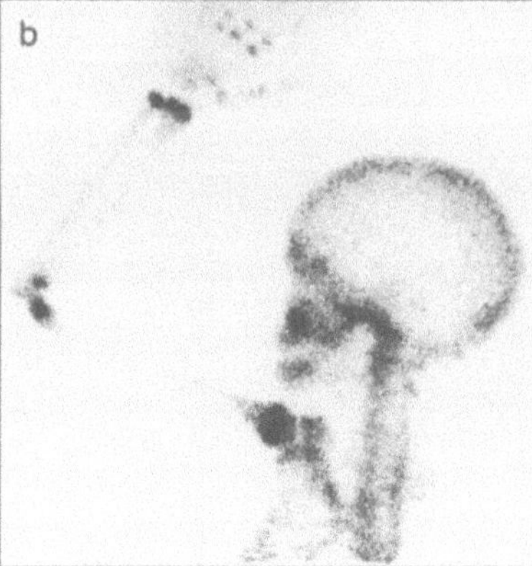

4.2.4.4 Soft Tissue Sarcoma
(2 Cases; Fig. 4.75, 4.76)

Case 4.75. A 7-year-old girl with swelling of the face due to a soft tissue fibrosarcoma

Fig. 4.75a. Right lateral image of the skull is normal

Fig. 4.75b. Left lateral image of the skull shows abnormal increased uptake of isotope in the maxilla. Bony involvement by the soft tissue sarcoma was confirmed on CT

Case 4.76. A 9-year-old girl with a swelling over the right shoulder due to a soft tissue sarcoma. The sarcoma was found to be infiltrating directly into the scapula

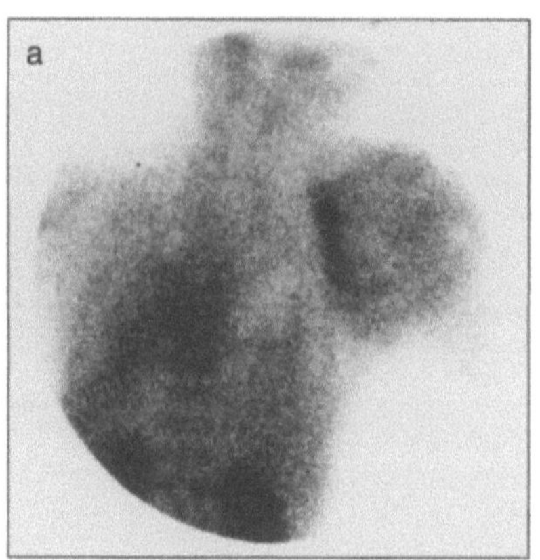

Fig. 4.76a. Blood pool posterior view of thorax shows marked increased uptake of isotope in the soft tissue swelling involving the right shoulder

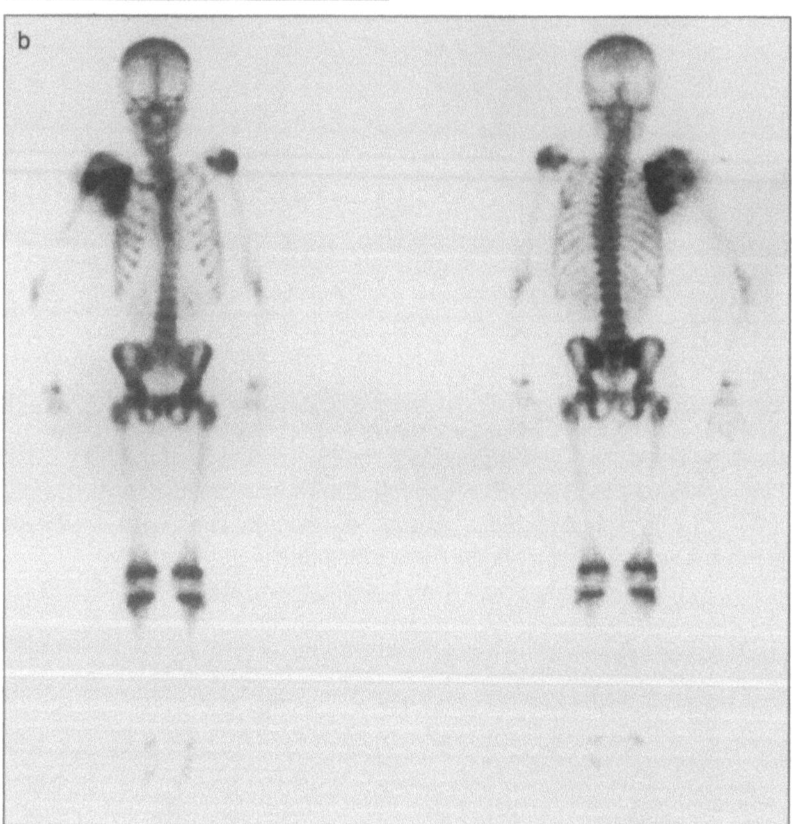

Fig. 4.76b. Whole body scans show intense abnormal increased uptake of isotope in the right scapula. There is also slight increased uptake of isotope in the right proximal humerus. The latter was a reflection of increased blood flow rather than tumour

Teaching Point
Compare this case to the child with an Ewing's sarcoma of the scapula (Case 4.29). This shows the sensitivity of bone scans but the non-specificity since the images are very similar.

4.3 Tumour Secondaries

4.3.1 Effect of Treatment
(1 Case; Fig. 4.77)

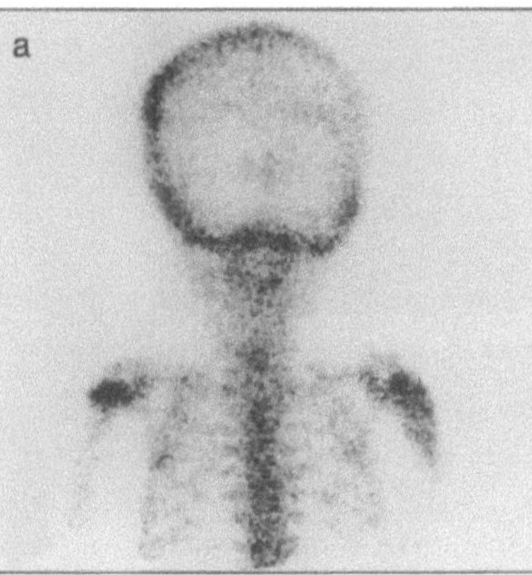

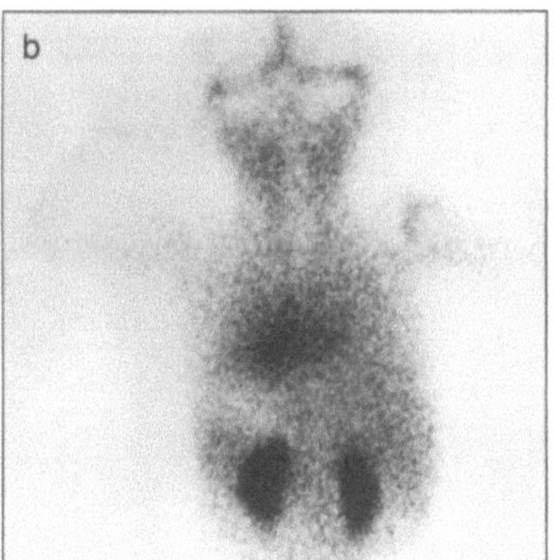

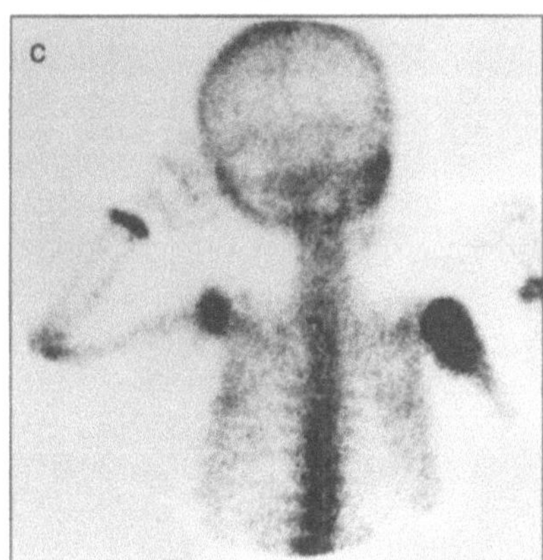

Case 4.77. A 2-year-old boy with osteogenic sarcoma of the right humerus. (This is the same patient as in Case 4.39)

Fig. 4.77a. Posterior image of the spine, skull and shoulders shows slight increased uptake in the right proximal humerus.

Following biopsy and 6 months of chemotherapy, the child underwent a follow-up study

Fig. 4.77b. Posterior blood pool image of the skull and thorax shows abnormal distribution of isotope in the region of the right upper humerus

Fig. 4.77c. Posterior image of the skull, spine and shoulders shows intense abnormal increased uptake of isotope in the right humerus

Teaching Point

This is an unusual response to biopsy or chemotherapy and suggests non-response of the tumour to the therapy. Also see Case 4.39.

4.3.2 Metastases
(3 Cases; Figs. 4.78–4.80)

Case 4.78. A 19-year-old boy who presented with a prostatic rhabdomyosarcoma with acute urinary retention. He was found to have disseminated disease at presentation and an urinary diversion was undertaken

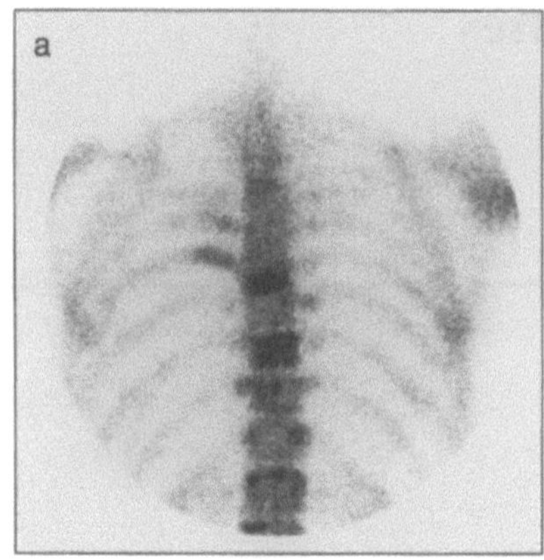

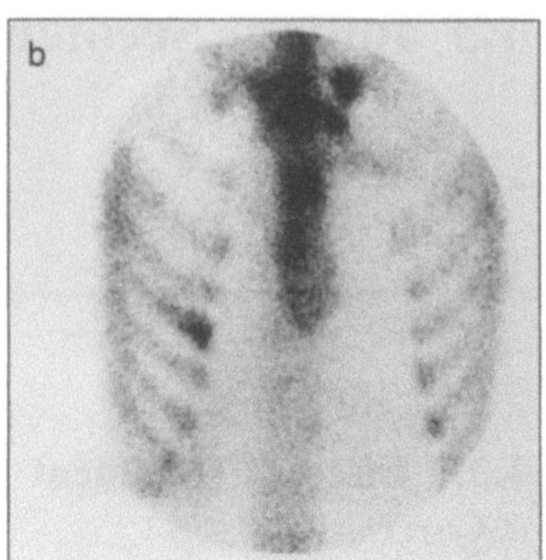

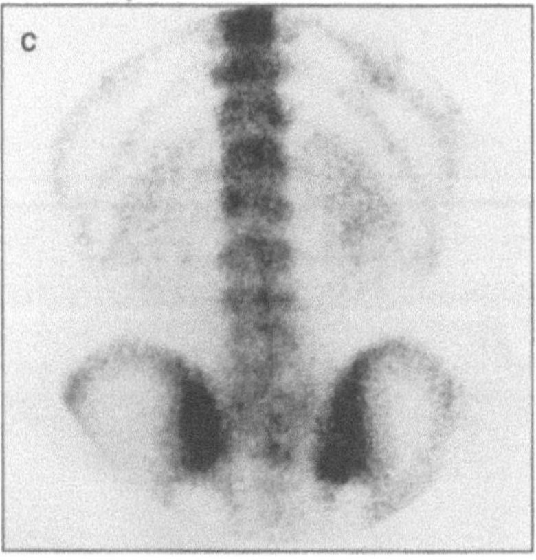

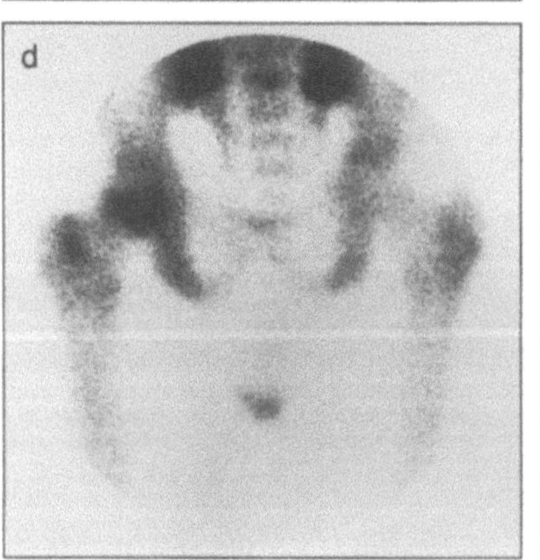

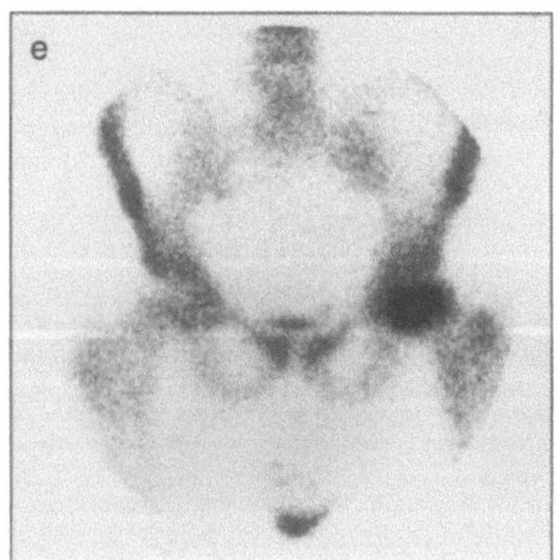

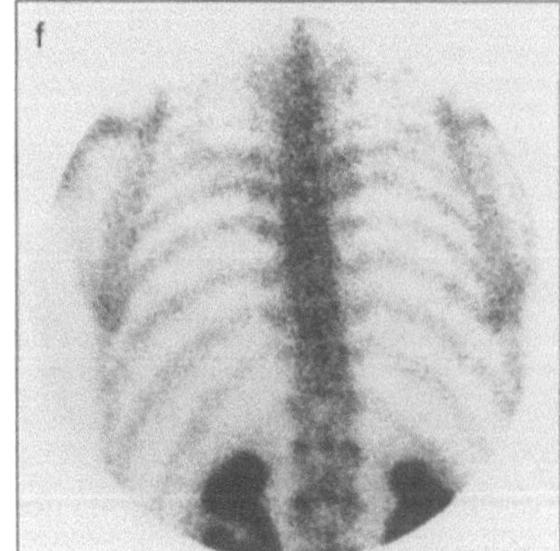

Fig. 4.78a. Posterior image of the thorax shows abnormal increased uptake of isotope in some of the mid dorsal vertebral bodies as well as in the posterior aspect of a few ribs on the left

Fig. 4.78b. Anterior image of the thorax shows abnormal increased uptake of isotope in the anterior end of one of the right ribs and the left sterno-clavicular joint

Fig. 4.78c. Posterior image of the dorsal spine and pelvis shows abnormal vertebral bodies with patchy increased uptake of isotope

Fig. 4.78d. Posterior image of the pelvis shows abnormal increased uptake of isotope in the left femoral head and shaft

Fig. 4.78e. Anterior image of the pelvis again shows the abnormal uptake in the left hip and femur.

Following chemotherapy and urinary diversion, a repeat scan was undertaken 7 months later. The skeleton is clear but the kidneys are now obstructed

Fig. 4.78f. Posterior image of the thorax shows that the vertebral bodies have improved significantly. The obstructed kidneys are seen

172

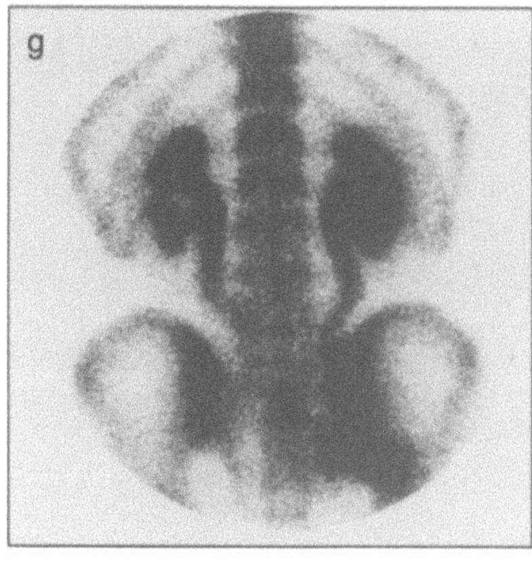 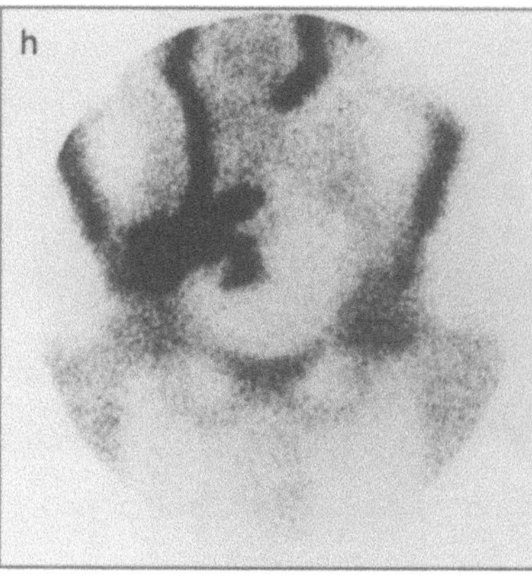

Fig. 4.78g. Posterior image of the spine and upper pelvis shows the vertebrae have returned to normal but the obstructed kidneys are seen

Fig. 4.78h. Anterior image of the pelvis still shows abnormal increased uptake of isotope in the left hip. The dilated ureters entering the urinary diversion are noted

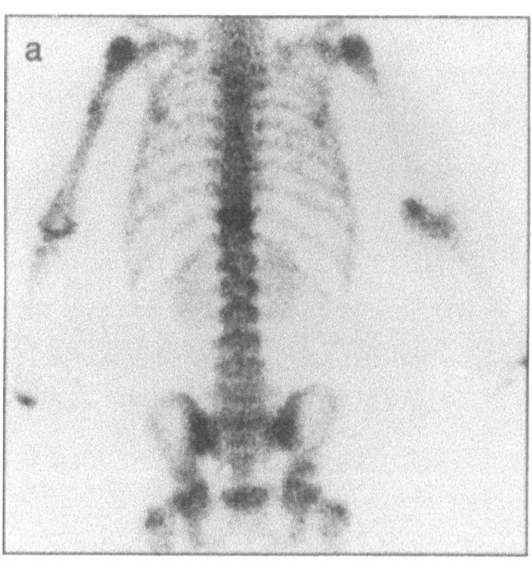 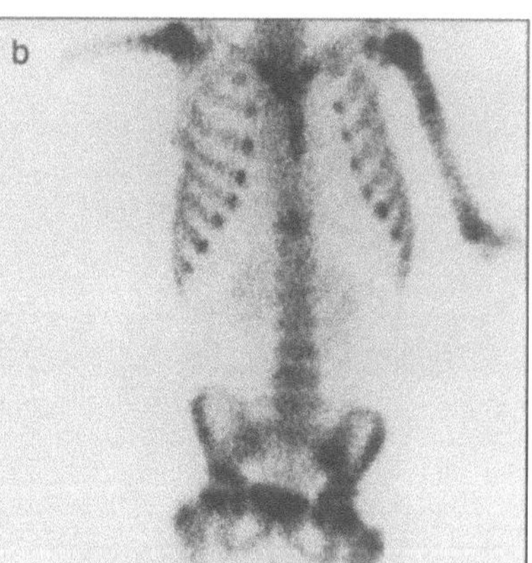

Case 4.79. A 5-year-old girl with a rhabdomyosarcoma of the vagina who presented with diffuse pain and was found to have secondaries

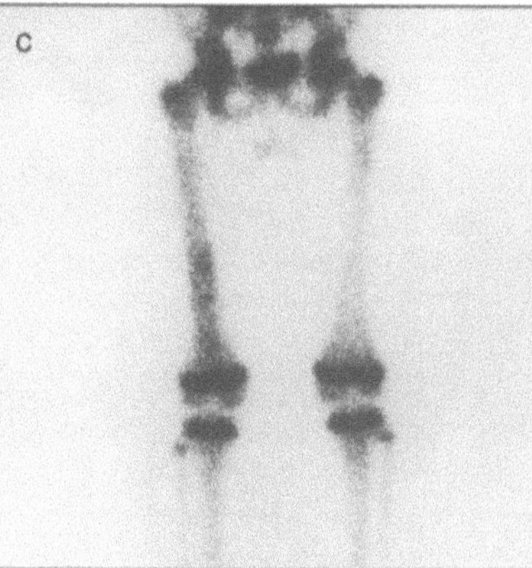

Fig. 4.79a. Posterior image of the thorax, upper limbs and pelvis shows abnormal increased uptake of isotope in the left humerus as well as in one of the lower dorsal vertebral bodies

Fig. 4.79b. Anterior image of the thorax and pelvis again shows the abnormal increased uptake of isotope in the left humerus and one lower dorsal vertebral body

Fig. 4.79c. Posterior image of the hips, femora and knees shows abnormal increased uptake of isotope in the shaft of the left femur

Technical Comment

The obliquity of the pelvis is the cause for the asymmetry between the sacro-iliac joints in Fig. 4.79b.

Teaching Point

Compare this to the child with Ewing's sarcoma and secondaries in tibia in Case 4.31.

Case 4.80. A 14-year-old boy who was found to have secondary deposits from a malignant melanoma

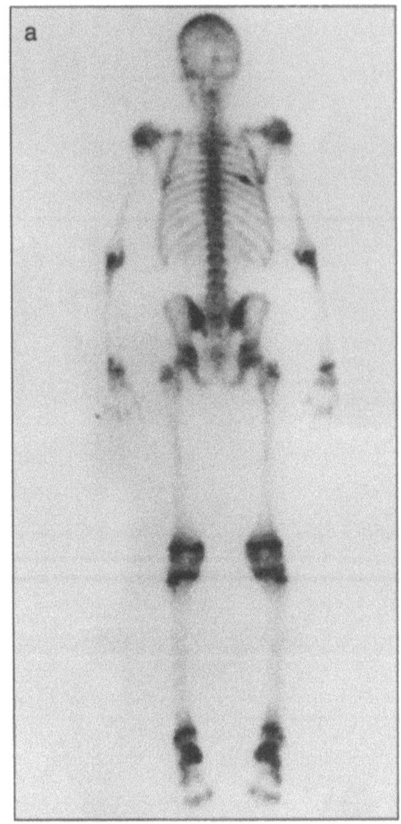

Fig. 4.80a. Posterior whole body scan shows abnormal increased uptake of isotope in the posterior aspect of the right sixth rib.

Follow-up scan 5 months later showed spread of the disease throughout the skeleton

Fig. 4.80b. Whole body scans show new areas of abnormal increased uptake of isotope in the right vault, the left iliac bone and right femur. Note the increased uptake of isotope in the kidneys. This was following chemotherapy

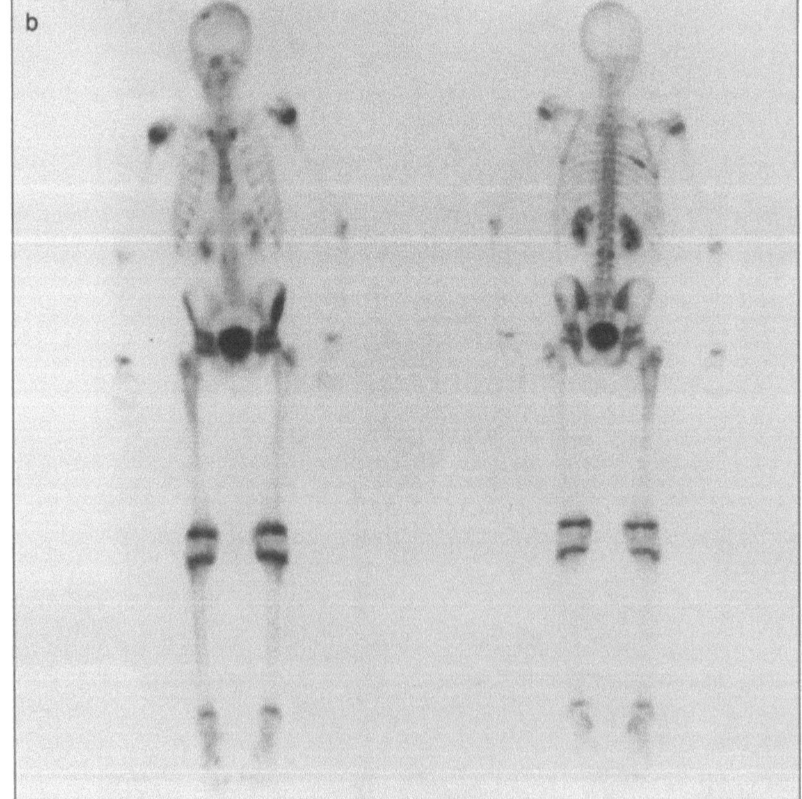

Teaching Point
Malignant melanoma is a very rare malignancy in childhood.

4.4 Langerhans' Histiocytosis
(7 Cases; Figs. 4.81–4.87)

Teaching Point
Langerhans' histiocytosis may provoke an osteoblastic response in the bone causing abnormal areas of increased uptake of isotope, according to the growth of the tumour; however, total absence of osteoblastic activity may result in photopenic areas.

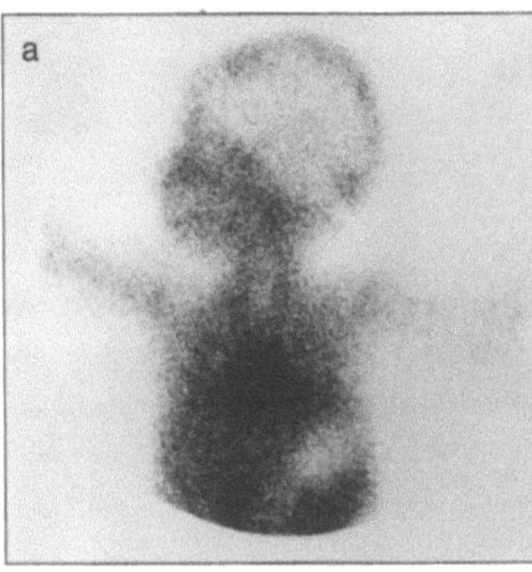

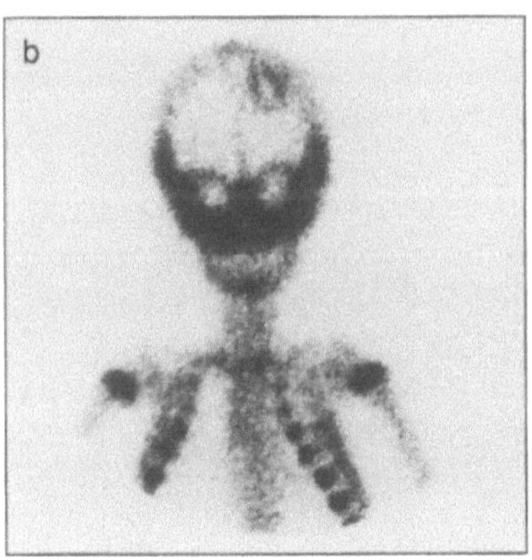

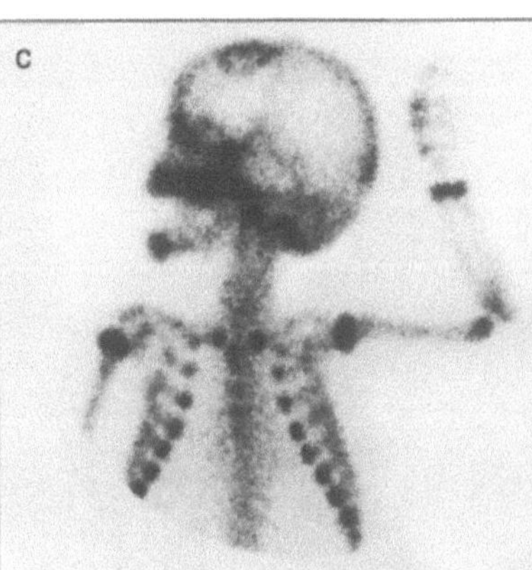

Case 4.81. A 6-month-old girl with Langerhans' histiocytosis

Fig. 4.81a. Blood pool left lateral skull image shows only slight abnormal increased uptake of isotope in the posterior aspect of the frontal bone. This is close to the anterior fontannel and without the later images difficult to interpret

Fig. 4.81b. Anterior image of the skull and thorax shows a circular area of increased uptake of isotope to the left of the mid line of the skull with a central photon-deficient area

Fig. 4.81c. Left lateral skull, anterior chest and left arm image shows a ring with osteoblastic activity and a central photon-deficient area in the skull. This is a mixed lesion typical for Langerhans' histiocytosis; the lesion was solitary

Teaching Point
Similar appearances to that seen in the skull may be seen following surgery (see Case 5.67).

Case 4.82. A 13-year-old girl who presented with recurrent ear infection on the right. The diagnosis was that of Langerhans' histiocytosis

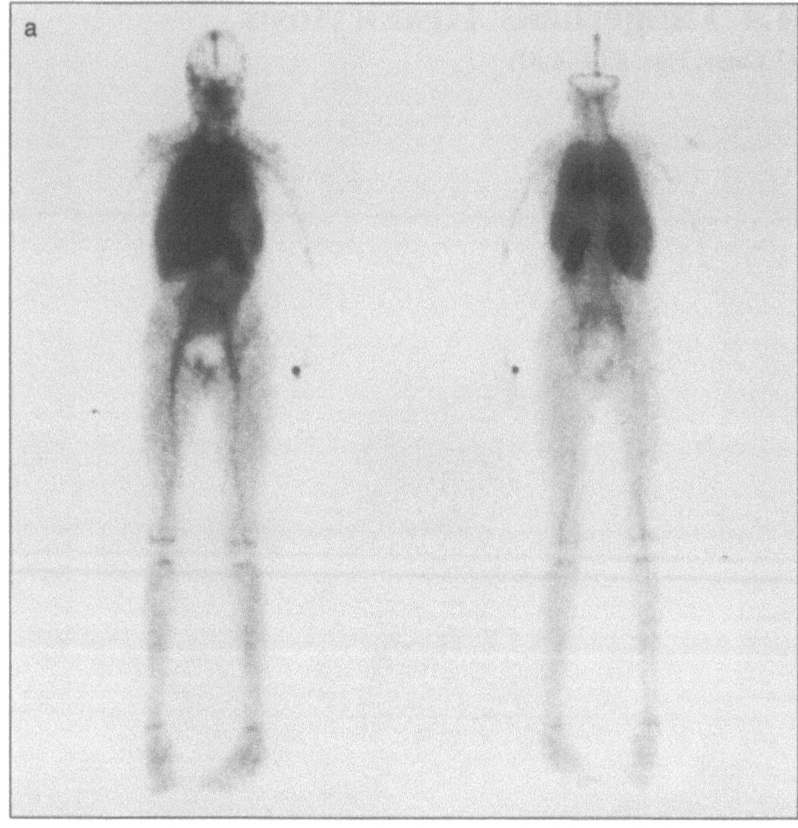

Fig. 4.82a. Blood pool whole body scans. There is asymmetry between the orbits and temporal bones on the two sides. This is best seen on the anterior view

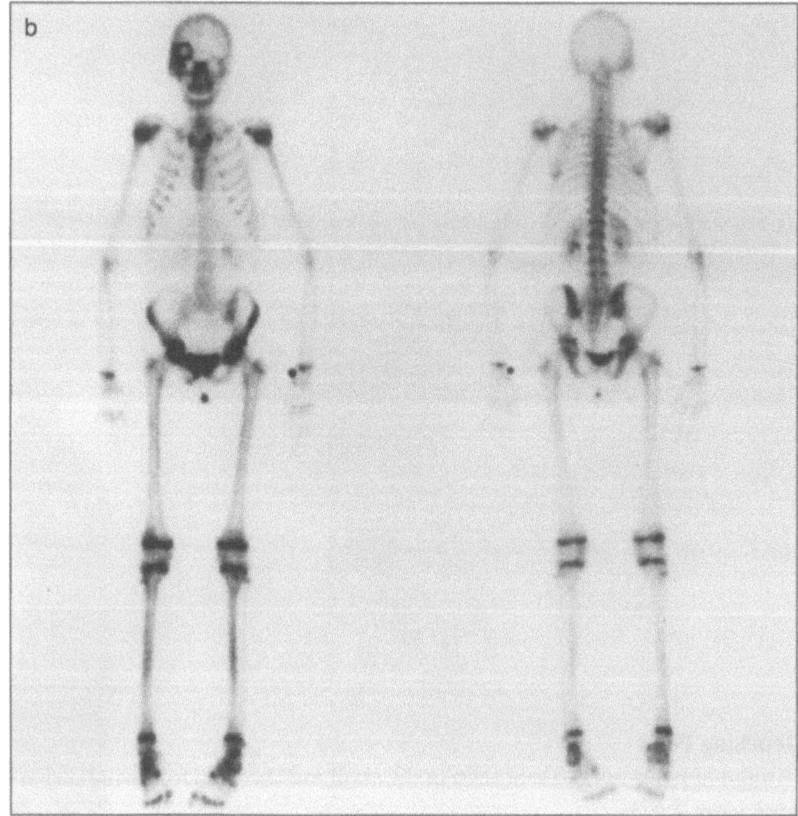

Fig. 4.82b. Whole body scans show abnormal increased uptake of isotope in the region of the right frontal and temporal bone, best seen on the anterior view

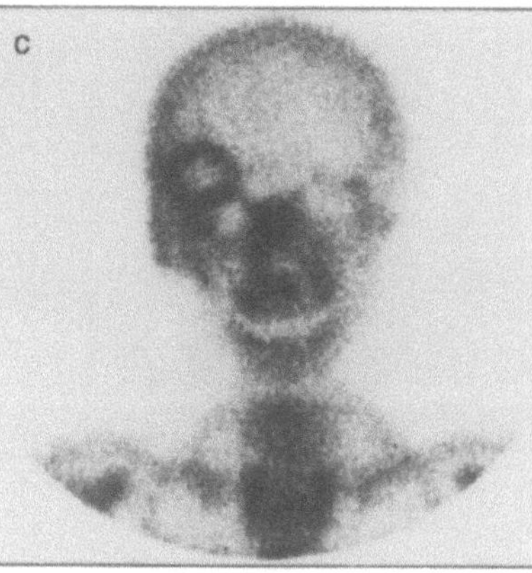

Fig. 4.82c. Anterior image of the skull shows the area of increased uptake of isotope with a central photon-deficient area extending from the superior orbital margin on the right into the frontal bone towards the temporal bone

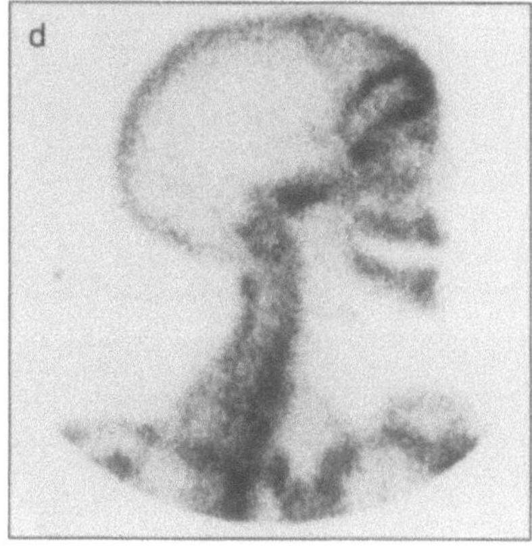

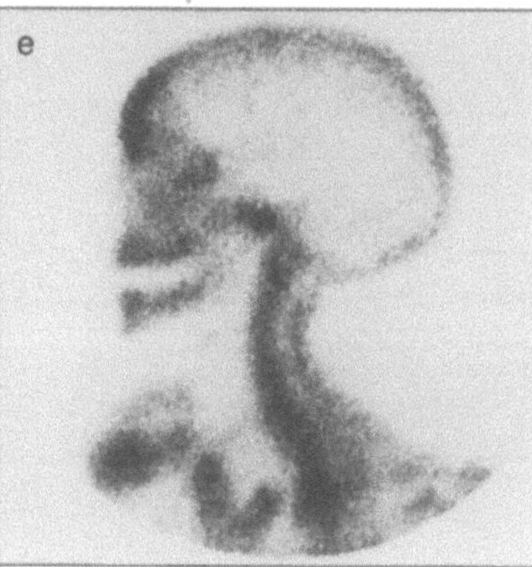

Fig. 4.82d. Right lateral image of the skull shows the extent of the bony involvement and the central photon-deficient area

Fig. 4.82e. Left lateral view of the skull shows minimal increased uptake of isotope in the region of the floor of the anterior fossa

Technical Comment: Note extravasation of isotope at the injection site adjacent to the left wrist in Figs. 4.82a,b.

Teaching Point: Similar appearances to that seen in the skull may be seen following surgery (see Case 5.67).

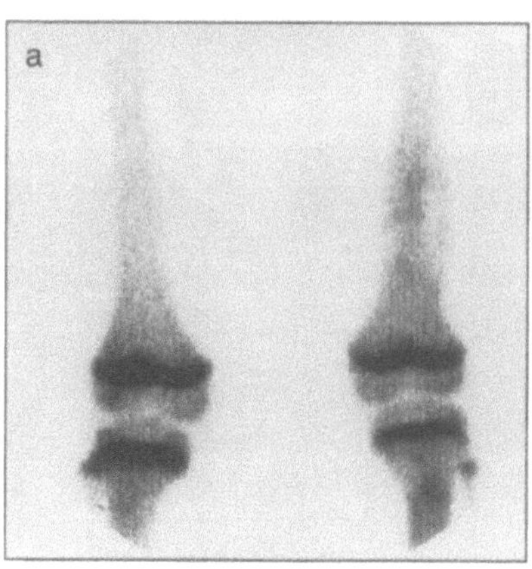

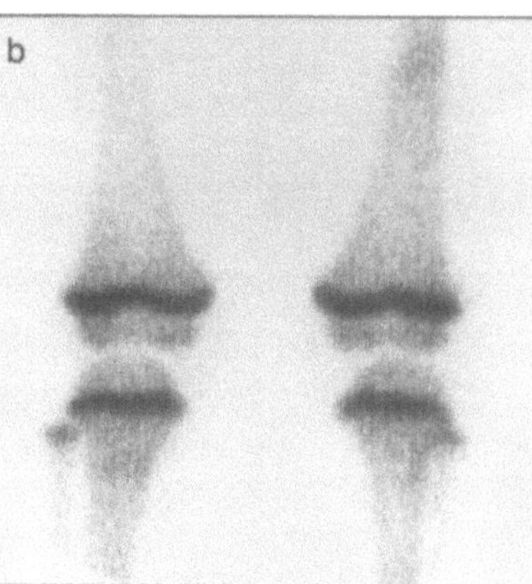

Case 4.83. A 4-year-old girl with active Langerhans' histiocytosis who developed new pain in the left thigh. There was evidence of extension of the disease as the cause of the pain

Fig. 4.83a. Anterior image of the lower femora and knees. There is abnormal increased uptake of isotope in the distal third of the left femur with an area of decreased uptake in this generalised area of increased uptake of isotope. There is a ghost outline of an expanded femoral shaft at this level

Fig. 4.83b. Anterior image of the knees. This image is 6 months after the previous bone scan and following chemotherapy. There has been consolidation of the lesion with only minimal increased uptake of isotope noted in the diaphysis of the left femur

Teaching Point: The abnormality shown in Fig. 4.83a is not diagnostic of Langerhans' histiocytosis, and a radiograph is essential to narrow the differential diagnosis.

Case 4.84. A 9-month-old girl with a swelling of the scalp due to Langerhans' histiocytosis. There was a solitary lesion in the skull

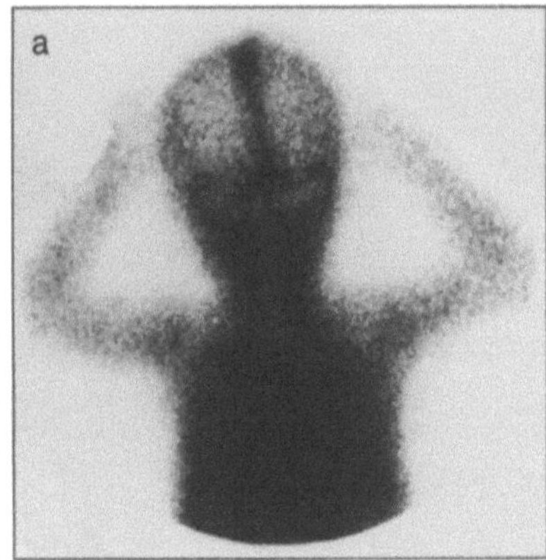

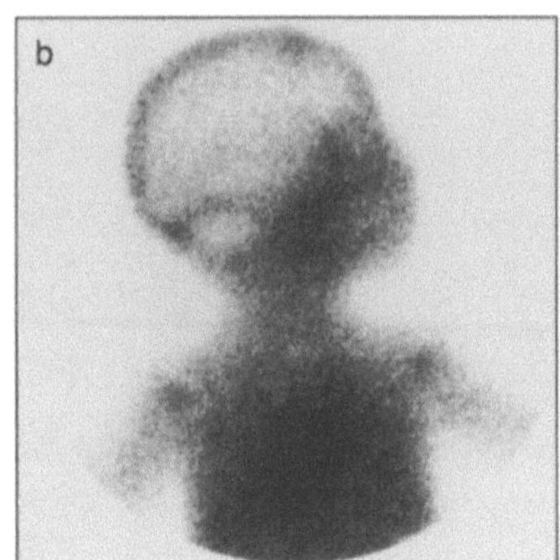

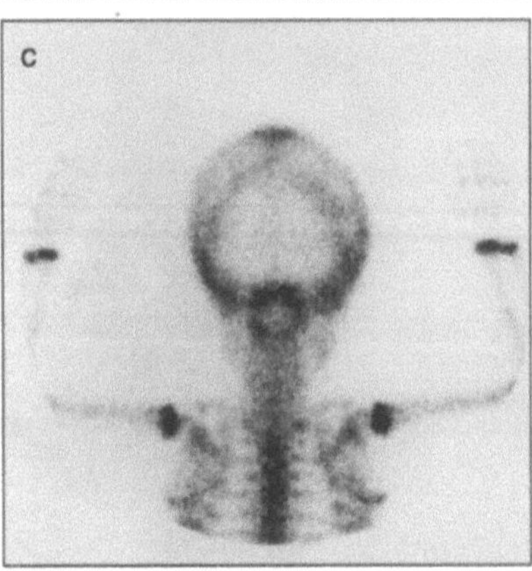

Fig. 4.84a. Blood pool posterior view of the skull and thorax is within normal limits. The sagittal sinus overlies the pathology

Fig. 4.84b. Blood pool image of the right lateral skull and posterior thorax shows slightly abnormal increased uptake of isotope in the posterior frontal bone

Fig. 4.84c. Posterior image of the skull, upper thorax and upper limbs suggests slightly increased uptake of isotope in the skull in the mid line. This site is difficult to interpret without the lateral image

Fig. 4.84d. Right lateral image of the skull and posterior thorax shows abnormal increased uptake of isotope in the posterior frontal bone, but on this occasion there is no translucent area within the lesion

Fig. 4.84e. Left lateral skull and posterior thorax. This is essentially normal

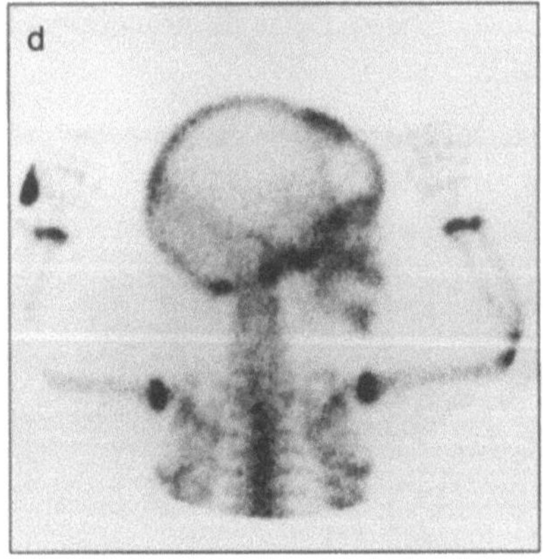

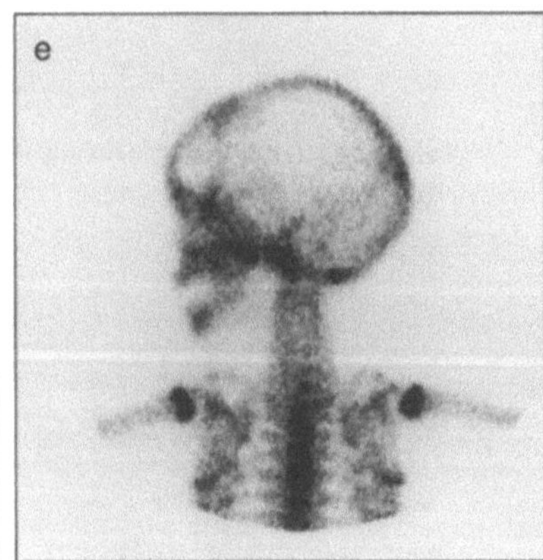

Teaching Point
Similar appearances to that seen in the skull may be seen following surgery (see Case 5.67).

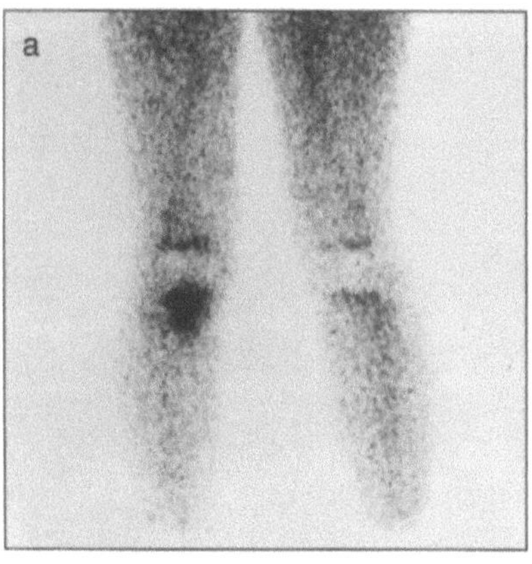

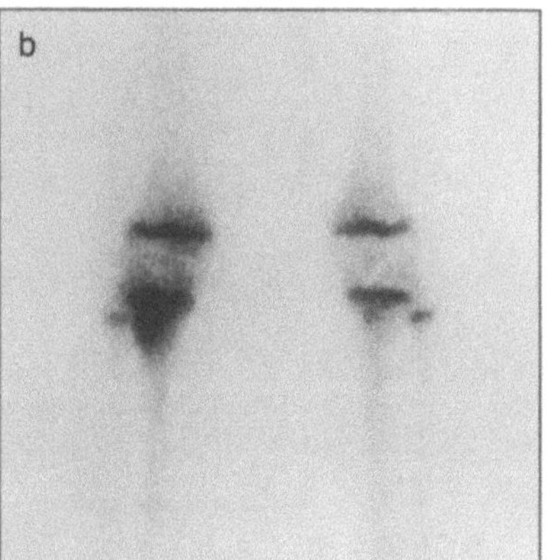

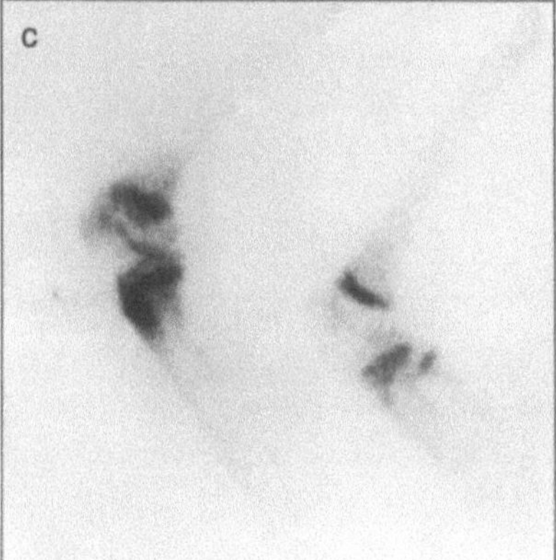

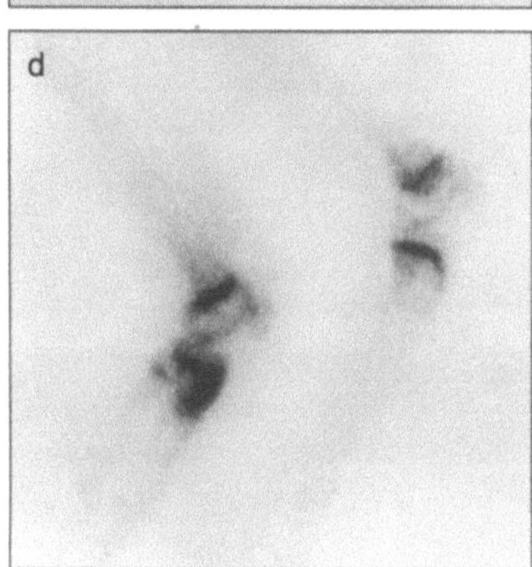

Case 4.85. A 13-year-old girl with a solitary lesion in the right upper tibia due to Langerhans' histiocytosis

Fig. 4.85a. Anterior blood pool image of the knees shows marked increased uptake of isotope in the upper right tibia

Fig. 4.85b. Anterior image of the knees shows marked increased uptake of isotope in the proximal lateral aspect of the right tibia, right up to the epiphyseal plate

Fig. 4.85c,d. Lateral images of the knees show that the abnormal uptake of isotope is anteriorly situated within the right tibia

Teaching Point
Similar appearances may be seen in infection (see Case 2.5) and osteo-genic sarcoma (see Case 4.49).

Case 4.86. A 10-year-old girl who was generally unwell with widespread Langerhans' histiocytosis

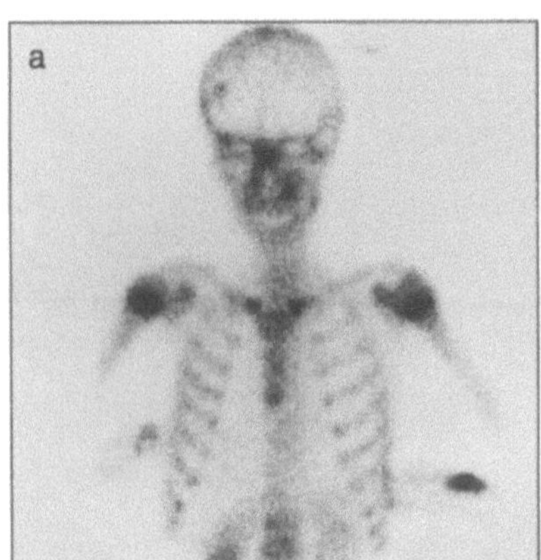

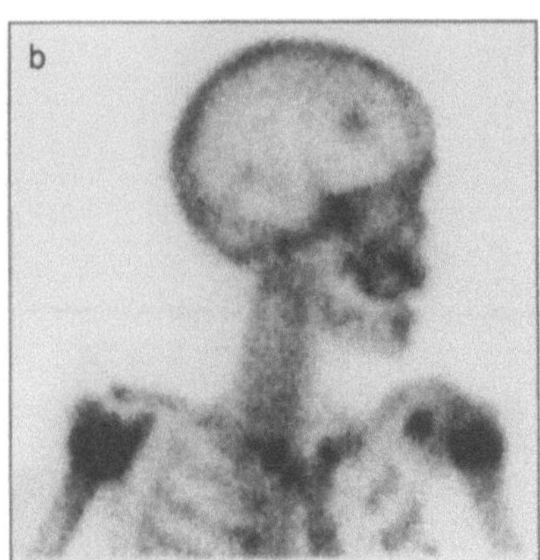

Fig. 4.86a. Anterior image of the skull and thorax shows focal abnormal increased uptake of isotope in the right frontal bone

Fig. 4.86b. Right lateral image of the skull shows the abnormal area of increased uptake of isotope

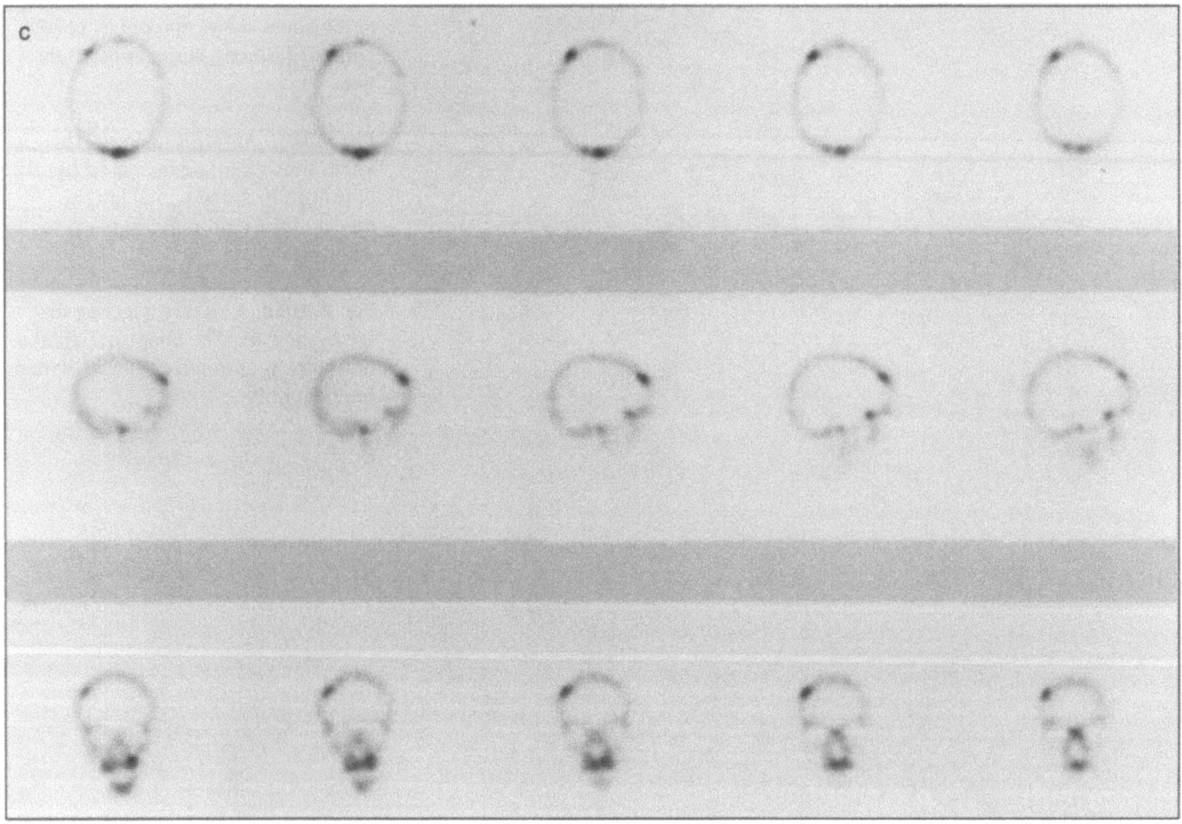

Fig. 4.86c. SPECT images in the transverse, sagittal and coronal planes localise the area of abnormal uptake of isotope in the vault

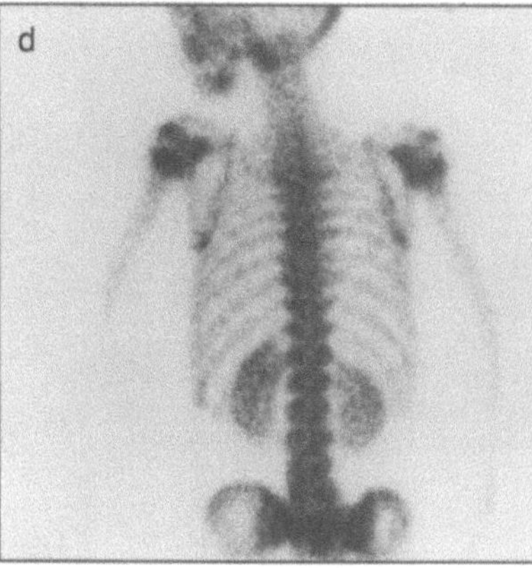

Fig. 4.86d. Posterior image of the spine fails to define any abnormality. Note the abnormal uptake of isotope in both kidneys

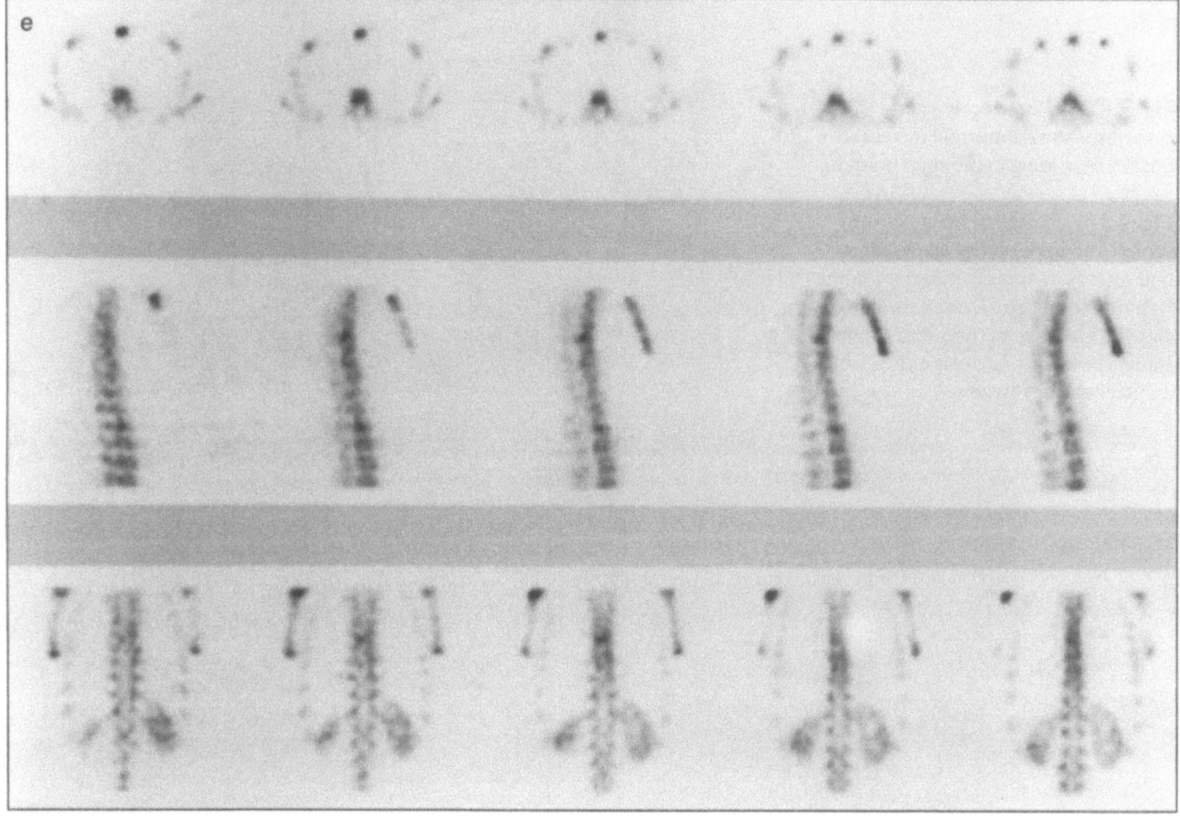

Fig. 4.86e. SPECT of the spine shows multiple focal areas of increased uptake of isotope on the sagittal, coronal and transaxial slices. There is also one vertebral body with decreased activity

Teaching Point

1. This is a case where the planar images of the spine are normal and the SPECT is abnormal. This case suggests that SPECT is required to exclude pathology in the spine.
2. Similar appearances to that seen in the skull may be seen following surgery (see Case 5.67).

Case 4.87. 13-year-old boy with active Langerhans' histiocytosis

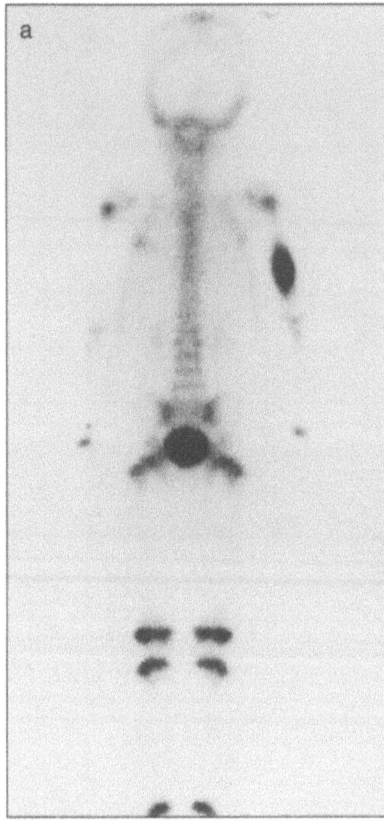
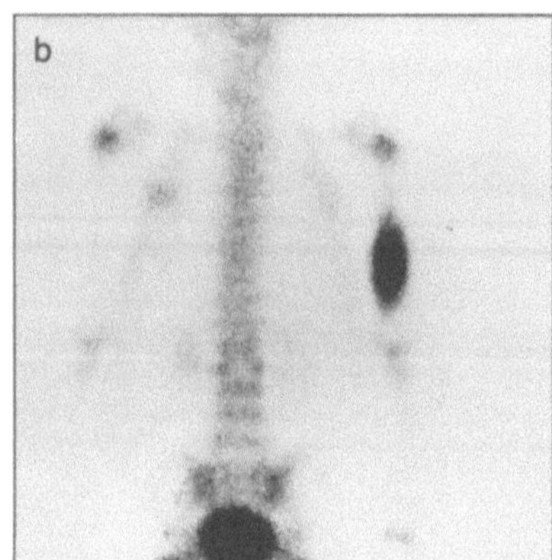

Fig. 4.87a. Whole body scan posterior view shows abnormal increased uptake of isotope in the right humerus

Fig. 4.87b. Posterior image of the thorax and upper limbs shows abnormal increased uptake of isotope in the right humerus. The L2 vertebral body shows absence of activity due to the Langerhans' histiocytosis not causing an osteoblastic response

Technical Comment

1. It is difficult to make out the vertebral abnormality on the whole body scan.
2. Highly specific activity is noted in the bladder. This child was unwell and refused to drink between the injection and the scan so that the urine was highly radioactive.

5 Trauma

5.1 Appearances at Common Sites

5.1.1 Skull and Face
(2 Cases; Figs. 5.1, 5.2)

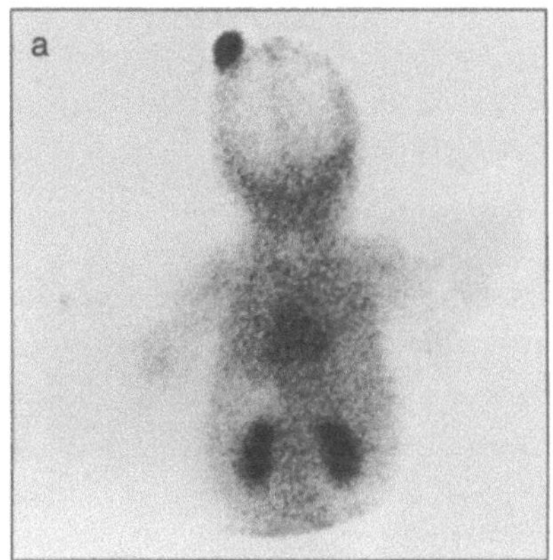

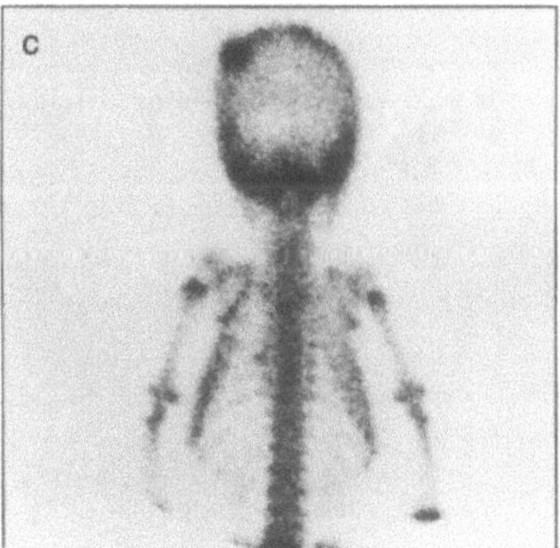

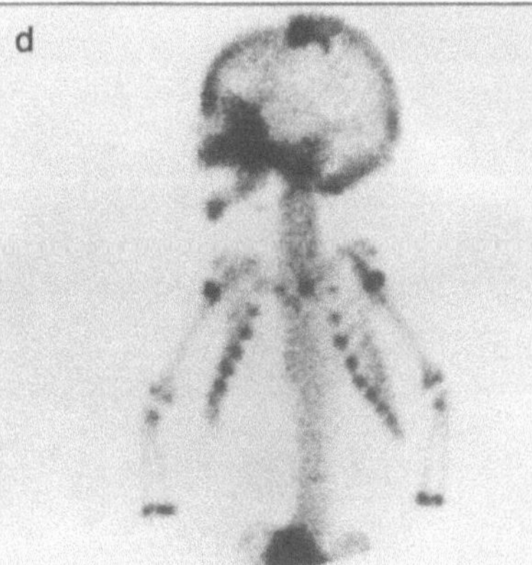

Case 5.1. A 2-month-old baby who had suffered from multiple repeated trauma (battered child). The skull radiograph (not demonstrated) showed a fracture on the left side but no fracture was seen on the bone scan

Fig. 5.1a. Posterior image of the blood pool phase shows intense focal increased uptake of isotope in the scalp

Fig. 5.1b. Left lateral blood pool phase shows abnormal uptake of isotope in the scalp

Fig. 5.1c. Posterior image of the skull, thorax and upper limbs. No fracture is seen. Abnormal uptake is noted in the skull vault

Fig. 5.1d. Left lateral image of the skull and anterior view of the thorax. The abnormal uptake is again seen. No fracture is seen

Technical Comment

The child was injected in the scalp and there was extravasation at the site of the injection. Injection of isotope should be distant from the site of suspected pathology.

Teaching Point

Bone scans have a very low sensitivity for detecting skull vault fractures.

Case 5.2. A 20-year-old patient who had injured his face whilst playing football. He was found to have a fracture of the right maxilla

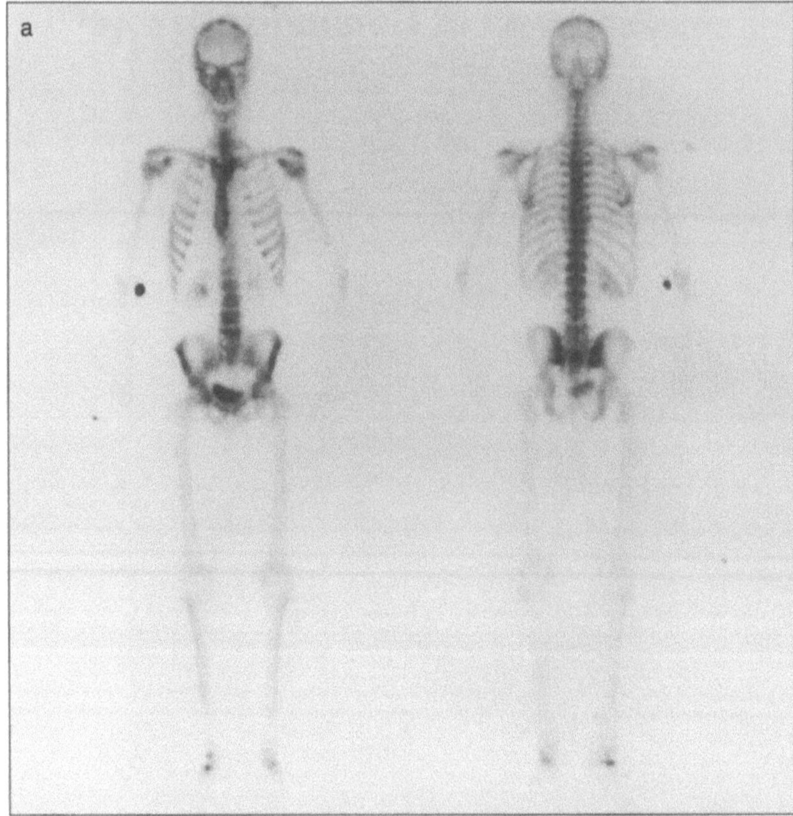

Fig. 5.2a. Whole body images show abnormal increased uptake of isotope most obvious on the anterior view in the region of the facial bones on the right. In the right ankle there is increased uptake due to previous trauma

Fig. 5.2b. Anterior image of the skull shows abnormal increased uptake of isotope in the region of the maxilla extending into the zygomatic arch

Fig. 5.2c. Right lateral image of the skull shows slightly increased uptake of isotope in the region of the anterior portion of the middle cranial fossa which is presumably due to the increased uptake in the overlying zygomatic arch

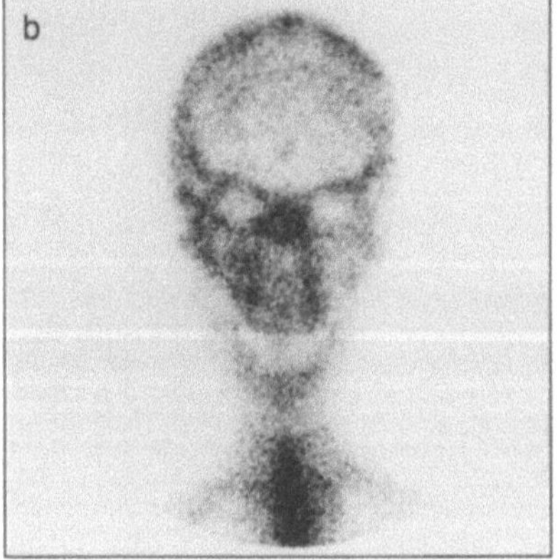

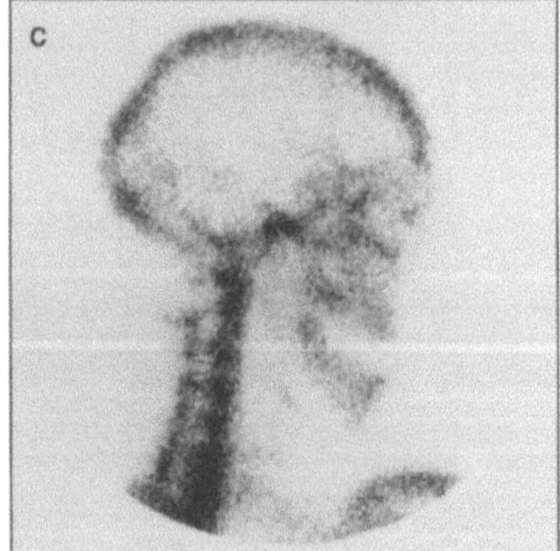

Technical Comment

Extravasation of isotope at the site of injection in the right elbow is noted.

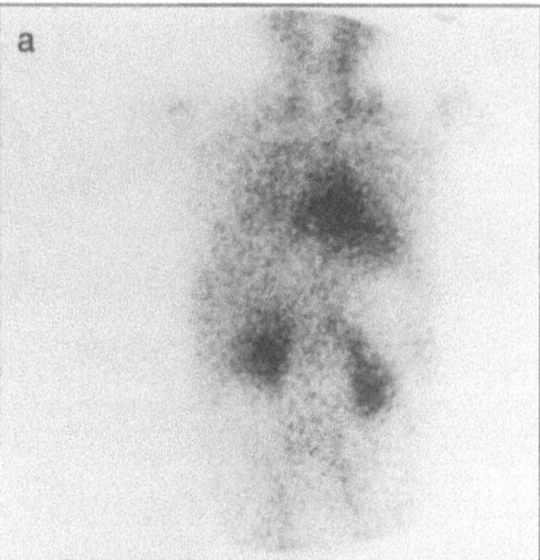

5.1.2 Thorax and Shoulder
(1 Case; Fig. 5.3)

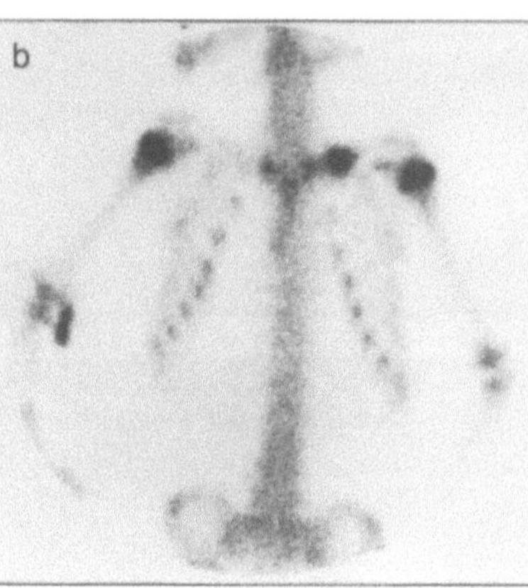

Case 5.3. A 3-year-old girl who presented with a swelling over the left clavicle due to a fracture, the cause of which was uncertain

Fig. 5.3a. Anterior blood pool image of the thorax shows abnormal increased uptake of isotope in the region of the left clavicle

Fig. 5.3b. Anterior image of the thorax and upper limbs shows focal, abnormal intense increase in uptake of isotope in the mid third of the left clavicle due to a healing fracture

Technical Comment

Note slight extravasation in the right elbow joint, the site of the injection of isotope.

Teaching Point

A similar appearance may be see with infection (see Case 2.28) or tumour (see Case 4.36). For fracture of the ribs see Case 7.26.

5.1.3 Upper Limbs
(3 Cases; Figs. 5.4–5.6)

Case 5.4. A 16-year-old boy who had suffered minor trauma and then had pain in the left wrist with a negative X-ray. He was found to have a fracture in the distal left radius

Fig. 5.4a. Blood flow images of the hands show increased blood flow to the left wrist and hand

Fig. 5.4b. Palmar blood pool image of the hands shows markedly increased uptake of isotope in the region of the left wrist

Fig. 5.4c. Palmar image of the hands shows intense abnormal increased uptake of isotope in the distal radius on the left.

A repeat bone scan was undertaken 4 weeks later

Fig. 5.4d. Blood flow images of the hands show slightly but definitely increased uptake of isotope on the left

Fig. 5.4e. Palmar blood pool image of the hands shows increased uptake of isotope in the left wrist

Fig. 5.4f. Palmar image of the hands shows abnormal increased uptake of isotope in the left distal radius. This has improved significantly when compared with the previous bone scan 1 month earlier

Teaching Point
Pain following minor trauma with a normal radiograph and focal intense abnormal increased uptake of isotope is strongly suggestive of a hairline fracture of the underlying bone. Pin hole views may be helpful to locate the exact site.

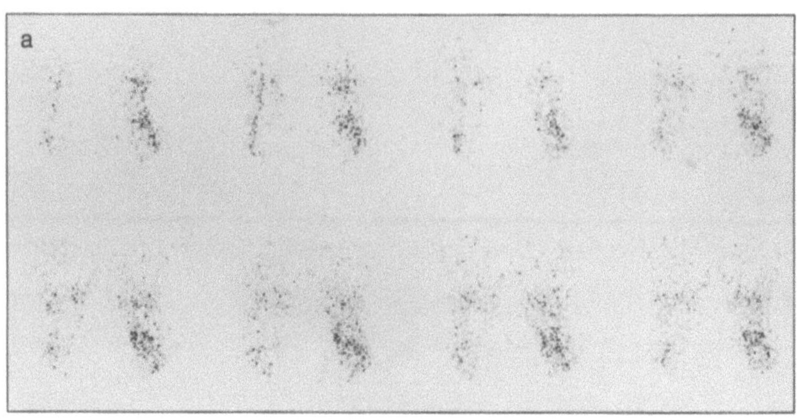

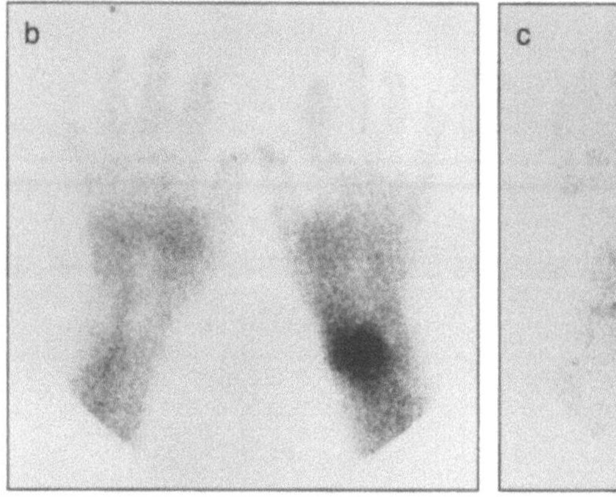

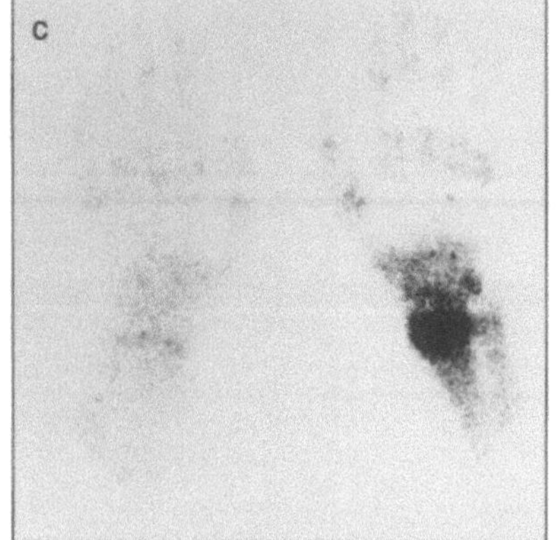

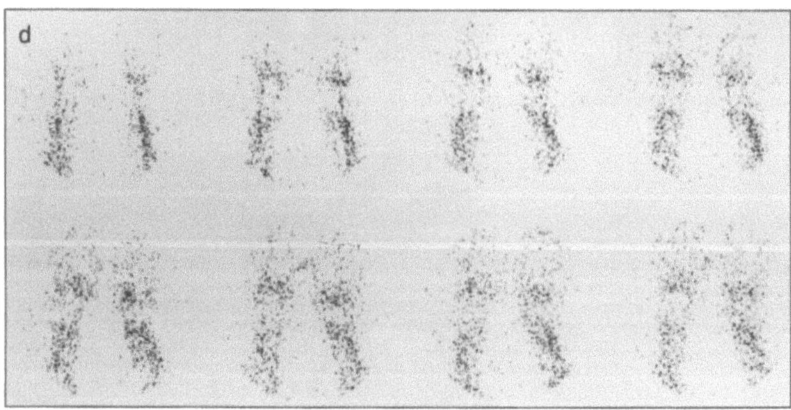

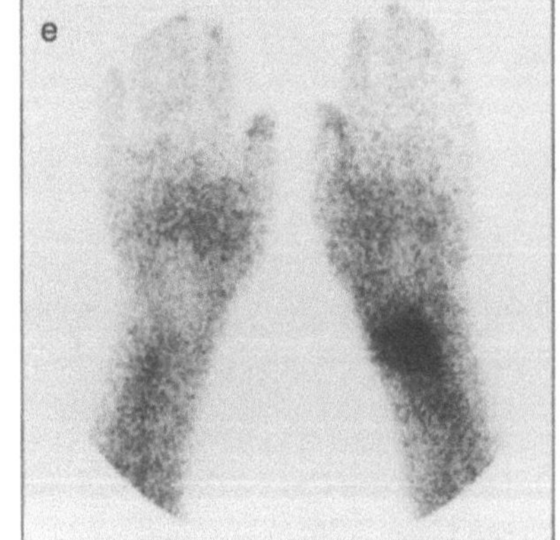

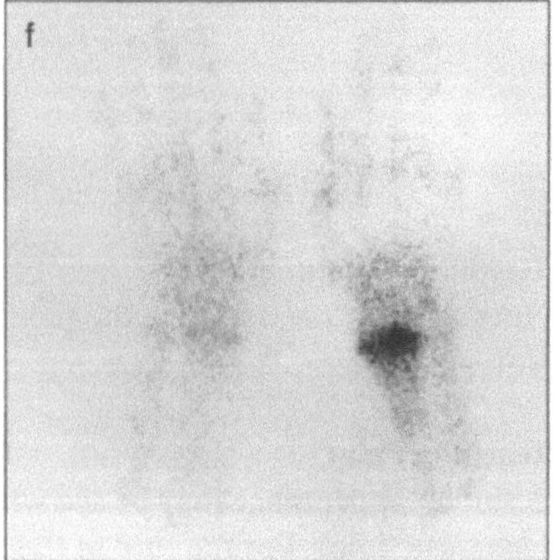

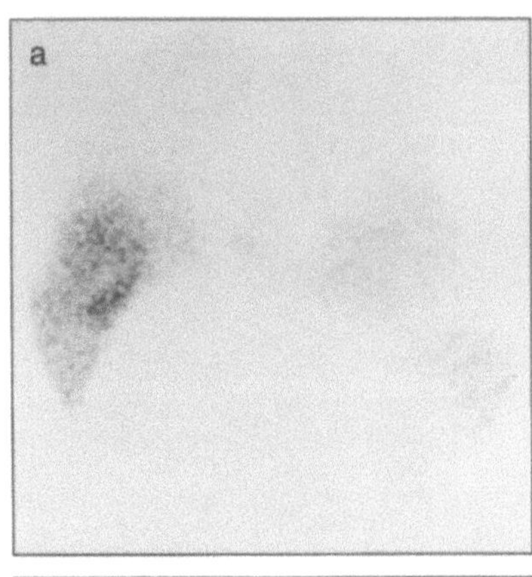 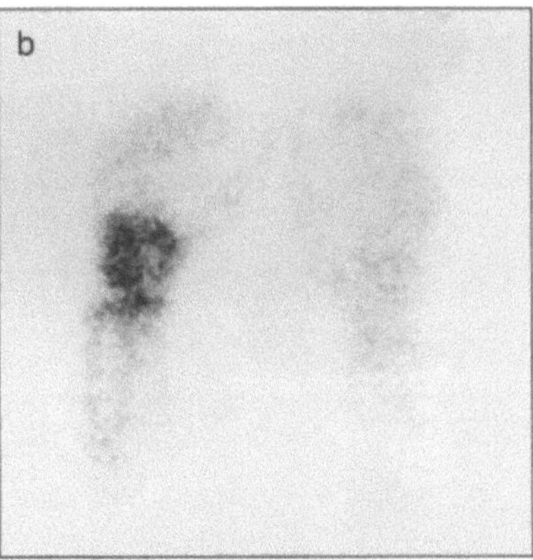

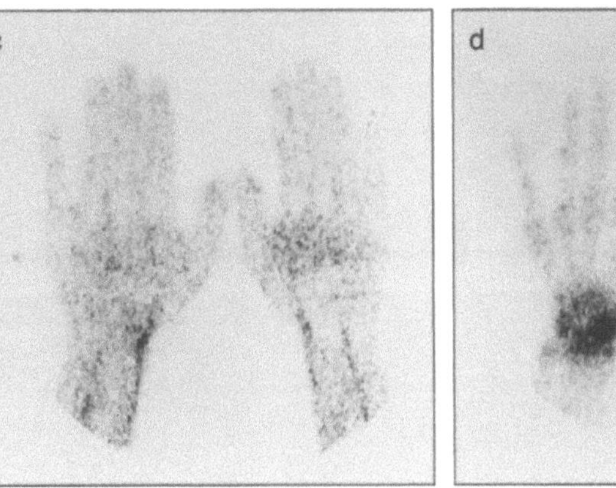 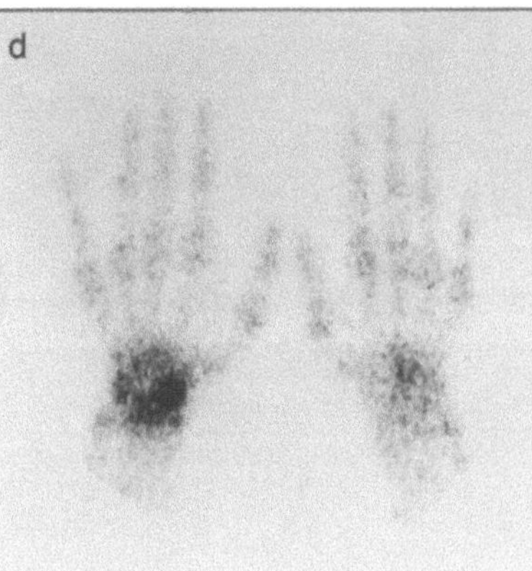

Case 5.5. A 22-year-old patient who fell onto the outstretched hand and suffered pain. He was found to have a fracture of the right navicular bone

Fig. 5.5a. Palmar blood pool image shows increased uptake of isotope in the right wrist

Fig. 5.5b. Palmar image of the hands shows generalised increased uptake of isotope in the right wrist with focal decreased activity on the radial aspect of the right wrist.

A follow-up bone scan was undertaken 8 months later for persisting pain in the wrist. This was due to poor union of the fracture

Fig. 5.5c. Palmar blood pool image of the hands shows slightly abnormal increased uptake of isotope in the right wrist on the radial aspect

Fig. 5.5d. Palmar image of the hands shows focal intense abnormal increased uptake of isotope in the right navicular bone

Technical Comment

Figure 5.5b is of relatively poor quality when compared to Fig. 5.5d. This is due to the high level of activity in the abnormal right wrist.

Teaching Point

On the first bone scan the site of fracture has less activity compared to the surrounding small bones in the wrist, suggesting impaired blood supply to the fractured bone. This may account for the long-term non-union and the changes seen on the follow-up bone scan.

Case 5.6. A 10-year-old girl with pain in the right hand for 1 week following minor trauma. The X-ray was normal. She was found to have fractures of the bone of the second and third metacarpal bones

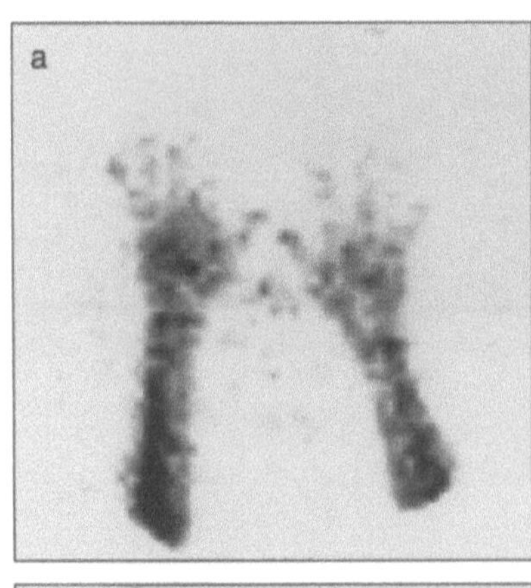

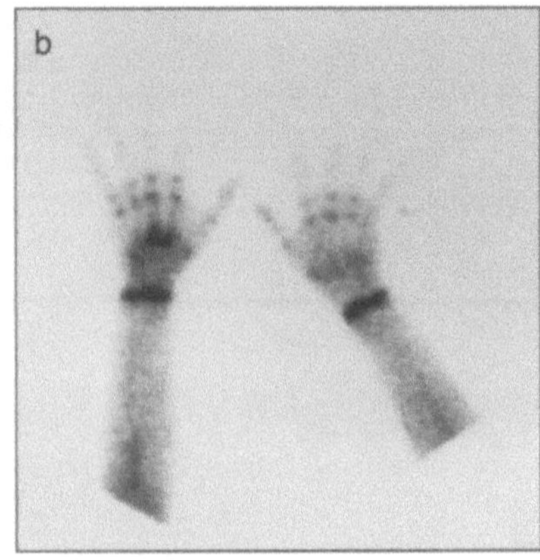

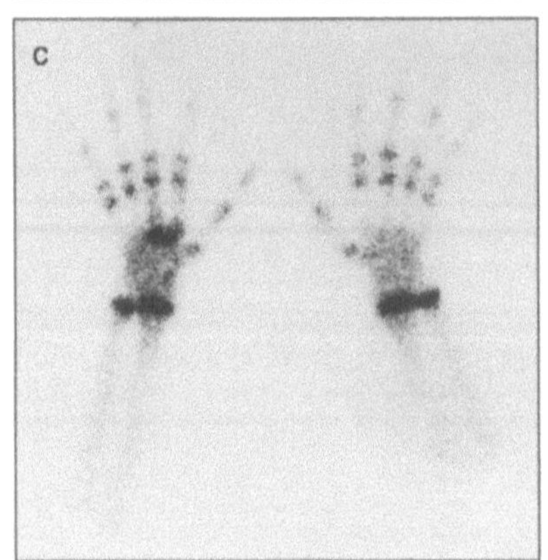

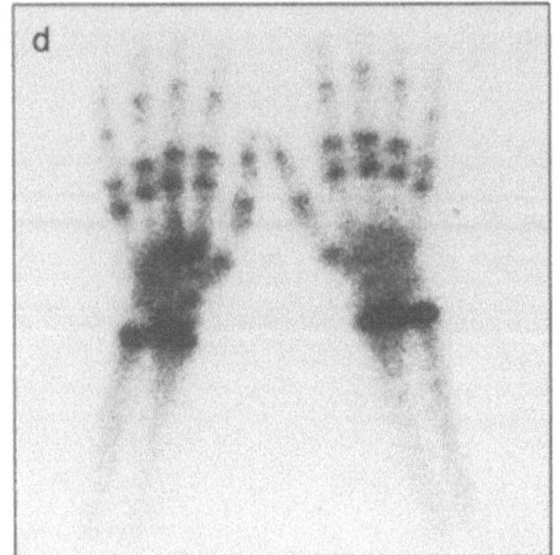

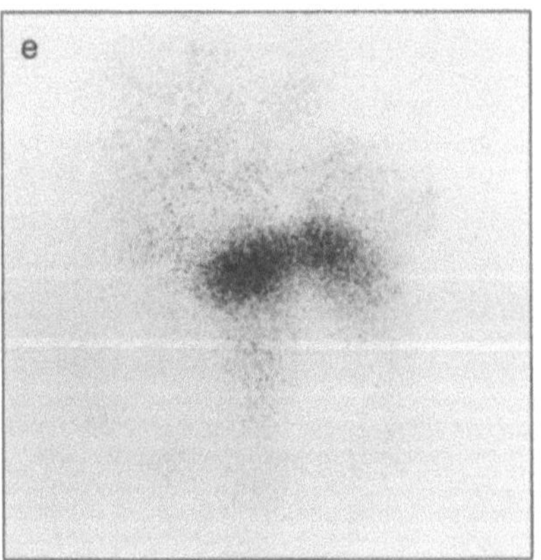

Fig. 5.6a. A blood flow image of the distal forearms and hands. This shows increased isotope on the right compared to the left

Fig. 5.6b. Palmar blood pool image of the hands shows increased uptake of isotope in the right second and third metacarpals with generalised increased uptake of isotope in the region of the right wrist

Fig. 5.6c. Non-magnified palmar view of the hands shows focal abnormal increased uptake of isotope in the region of the proximal ends of the second and third metacarpals

Fig. 5.6d. Magnified palmar view of the hands shows marked focal abnormal increased uptake of isotope in the region of the proximal second and third right metacarpals. There is slightly increased uptake of isotope throughout the right wrist

Fig. 5.6e. Pin hole palmar view of the right hand shows the focal abnormal increased uptake of isotope to be localised to the base of the second and third metacarpals

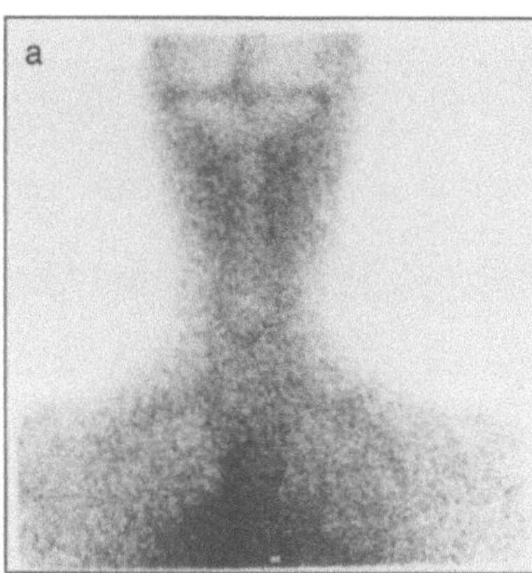

5.1.4 Spine
(7 Cases; Figs. 5.7–5.13)

Teaching Point

Confirmation and detailed anatomical extent of pathology, especially a fracture in the spine should be indentified with the addition of spot images using the high-resolution collimator and single photon emission computed tomography (SPECT).

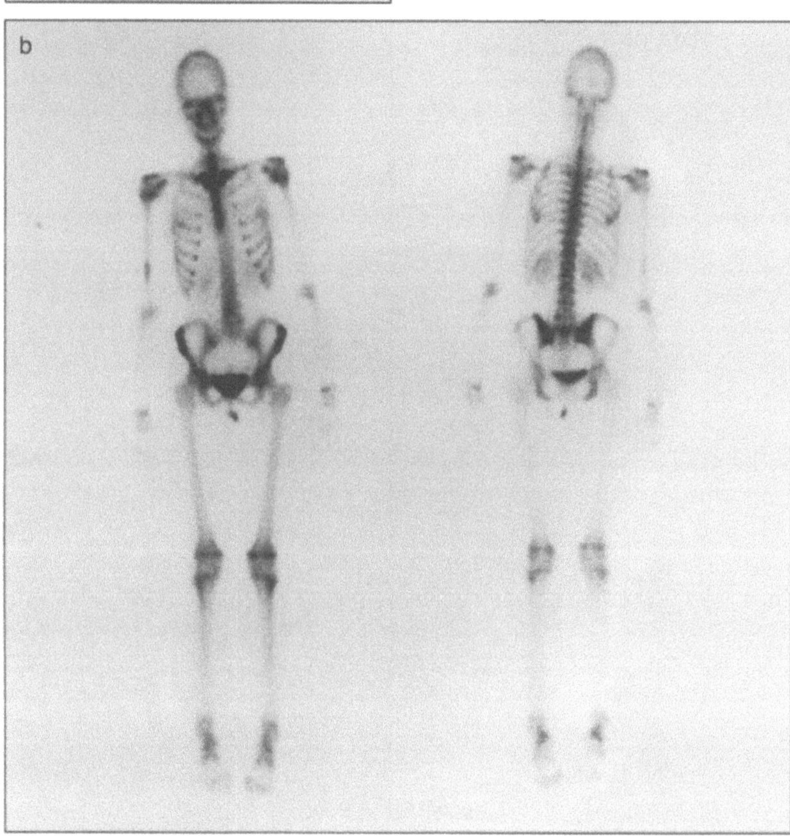

Case 5.7. A 15-year-old girl who had suffered trauma and was found to have a fracture of the seventh cervical vertebra and the right humerus

Fig. 5.7a. Blood pool posterior image of the cervical spine is unremarkable

Fig. 5.7b. Whole body scans show abnormal increased uptake of isotope at the level of C7, best seen on the posterior view. There is also increased uptake of isotope in the right humerus

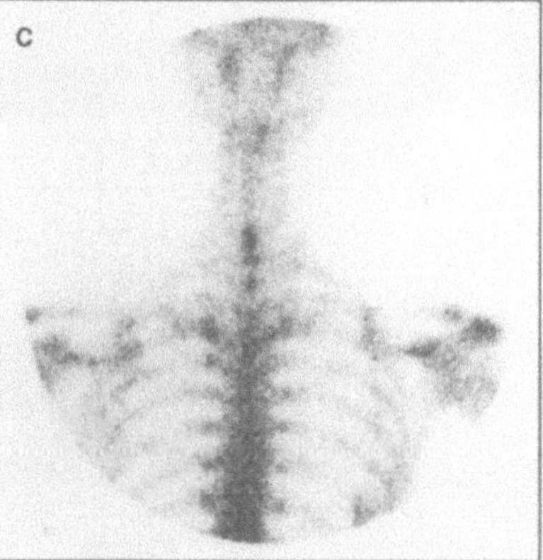

Fig. 5.7c. Posterior image of the cervical and dorsal spine shows the abnormal uptake of isotope at the level of C7 and also D1

Technical Comment

Note the improved resolution from the spot image when compared to the whole body scan.

Case 5.8. **An 8-year-old boy who had suffered trauma and was found to have fractures of the upper dorsal vertebrae**

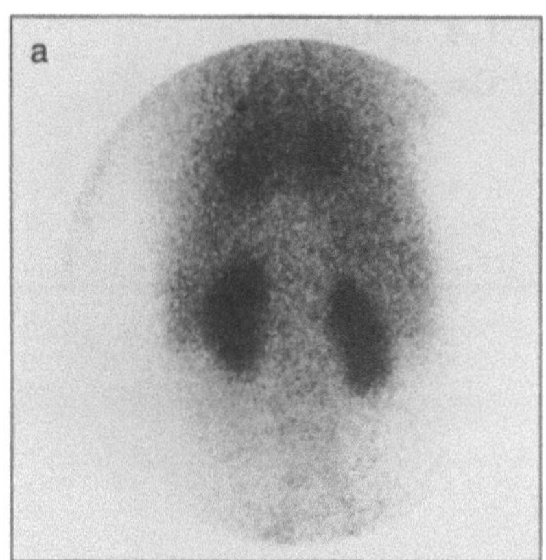

Fig. 5.8a. Posterior blood pool image of the spine is unremarkable

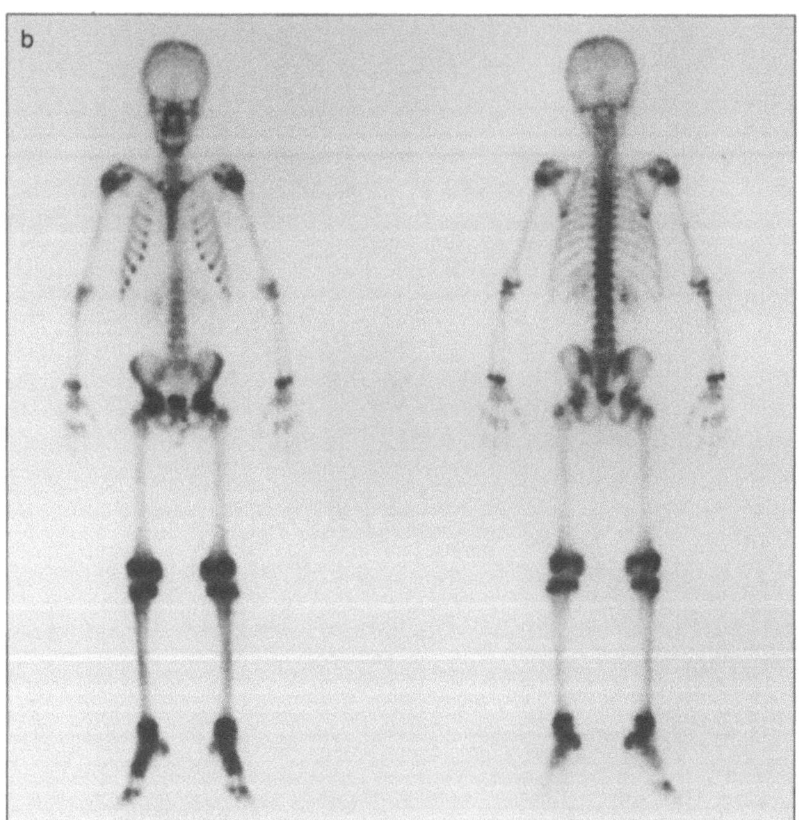

Fig. 5.8b. Whole body scans fail to show an abnormality in the upper dorsal vertebral level with confidence

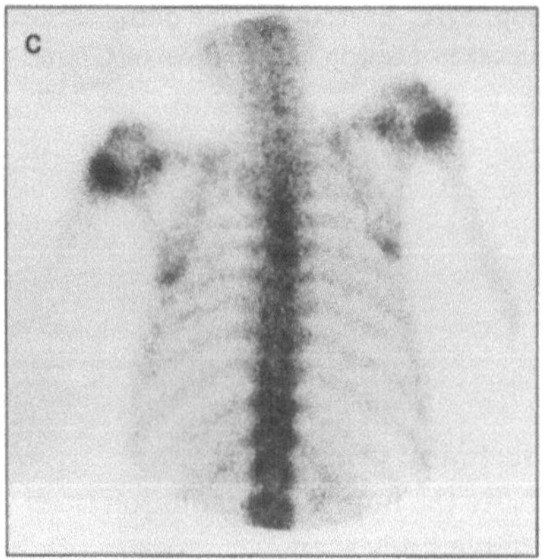

Fig. 5.8c. Posterior image of the dorsal spine shows abnormal increased uptake of isotope extending over three vertebral bodies in the upper dorsal region

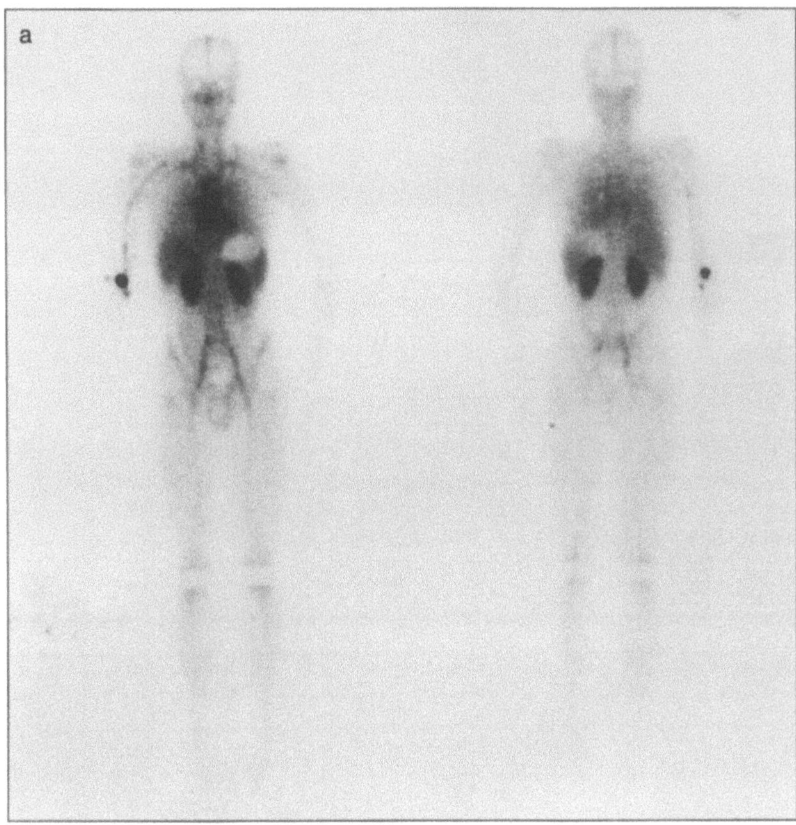

Case 5.9. A 16-year-old boy following a road traffic accident. He was found to have fractures of three vertebral bodies in the mid dorsal spine

Fig. 5.9a. Blood pool whole body images are not helpful in this case. Note extravasation at the site of the injection in the right elbow with isotope seen in the veins of the right upper limb

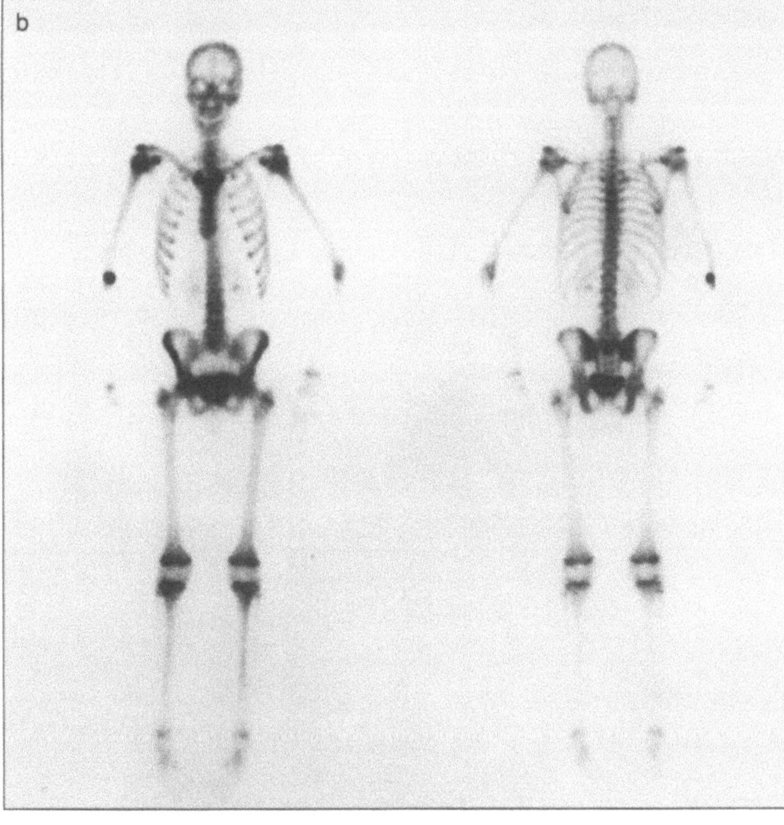

Fig. 5.9b. Whole body scans show abnormal increased uptake of isotope in three vertebrae in the mid dorsal spine. There is also abnormal uptake of isotope in one of the ribs posteriorly at the level of one fractured vertebral body. Again note the extravasation of isotope in the right elbow

Teaching Point
The high activity in the blood prevents adequate visualisation of the dorsal spine in the blood pool phase.

Case 5.10. A 10-year-old boy following a road traffic accident who suffered fractures of the mid dorsal spine

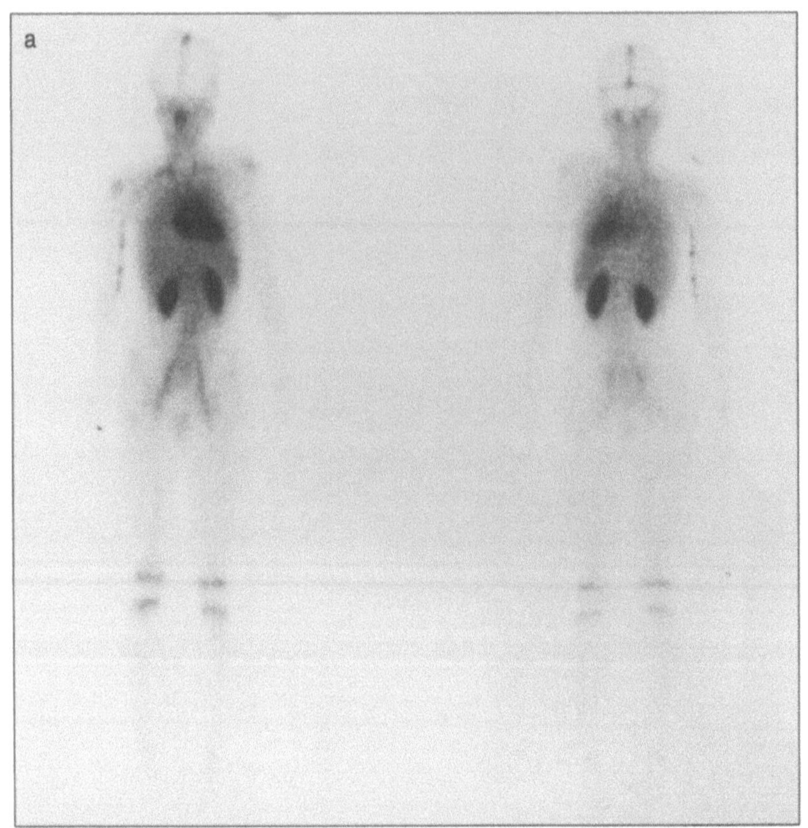

Fig. 5.10a. Whole body blood pool images are normal. Note hold-up of the isotope in the veins of the right upper limb following the injection of isotope in the right cubital fossa

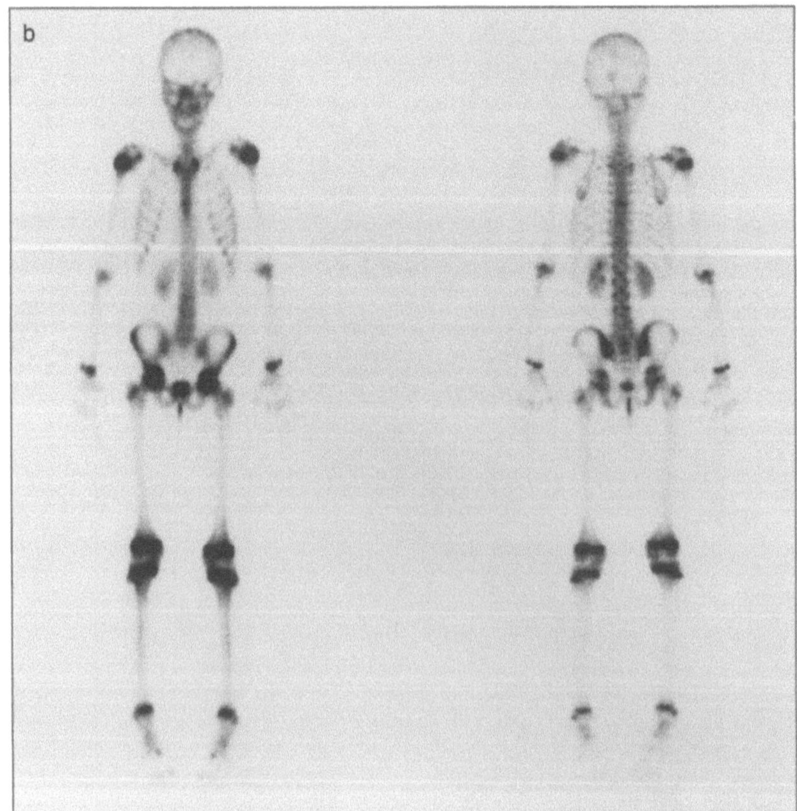

Fig. 5.10b. Whole body images show focal abnormal increased uptake of isotope in the mid dorsal spine. Note the unusual appearances of the kidneys which have retained the tracer. The cause for this was not ascertained

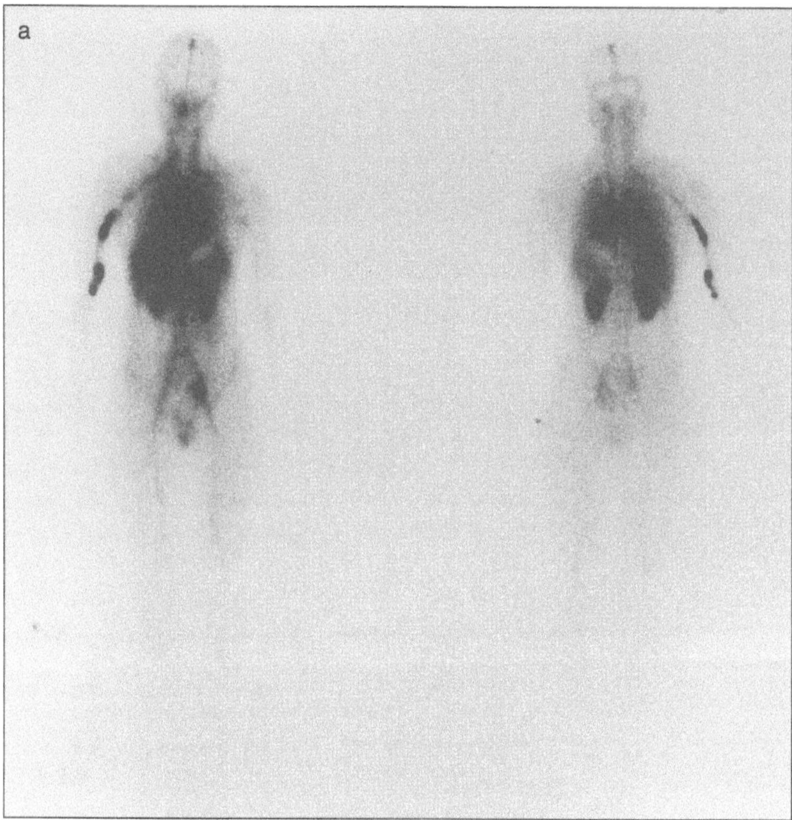

Case 5.11. A 16-year-old girl who had been involved in a road traffic accident and had suffered fractures of the lower dorsal spine

Fig. 5.11a. Blood pool whole body images are unremarkable. Isotope is noted in the veins of the right arm. The injection was made in the right cubital fossa

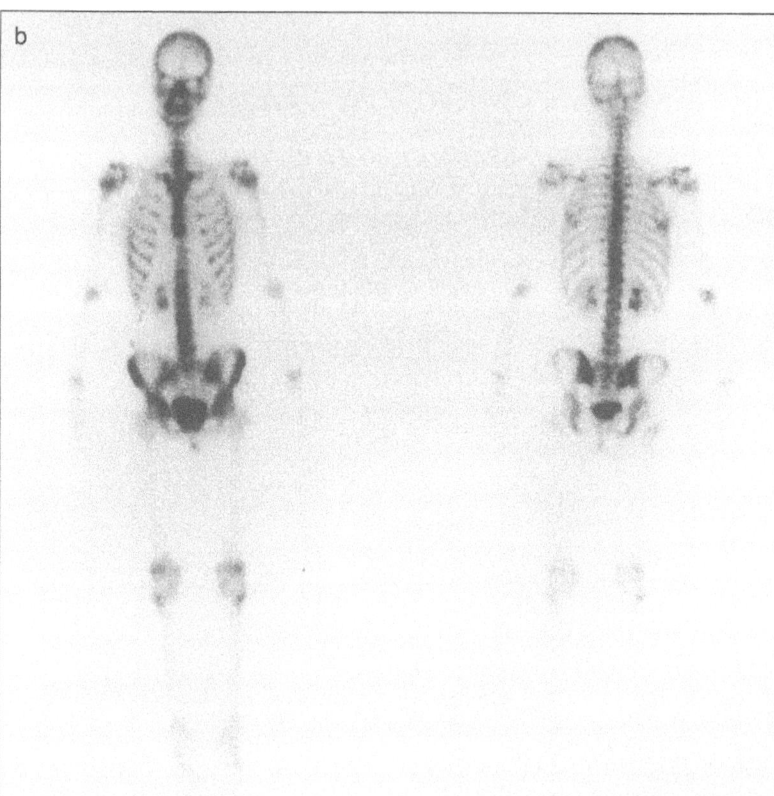

Fig. 5.11b. Whole body scans show abnormal increased uptake of isotope in the lower dorsal vertebral bodies. There is asymmetry of the sacro-iliac joints on both the anterior and posterior views but this is not constant and is thought to be due to the patient's positioning and not trauma

Case 5.12. A 3-year-old girl who had suffered direct trauma to her back and was found to have a fracture of the fourth lumbar vertebra

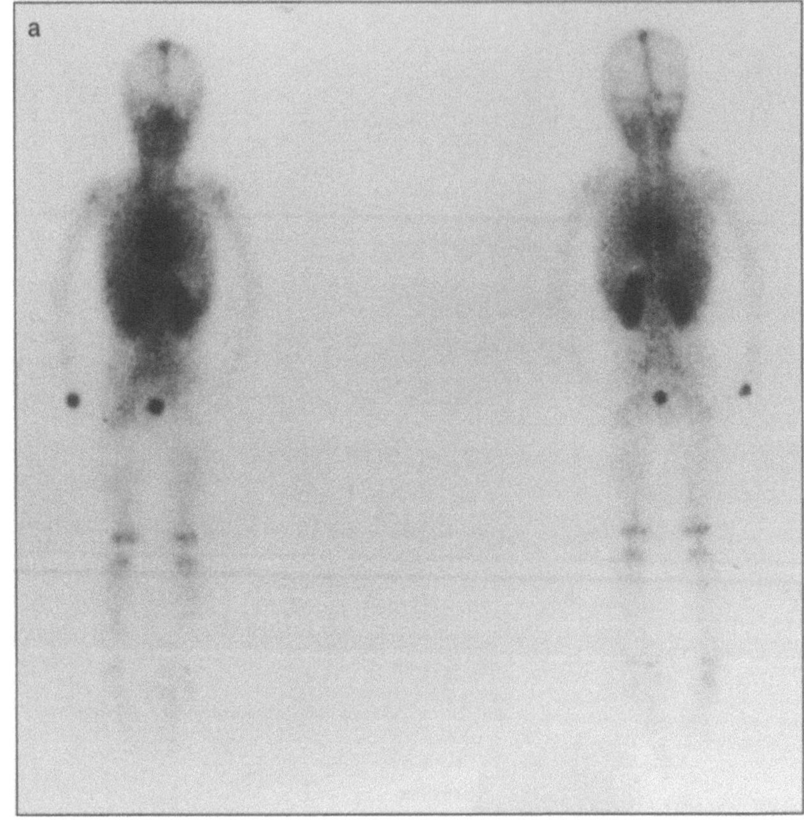

Fig. 5.12a. Whole body blood pool images are unremarkable. Note the extravasation of isotope in the region of the right wrist, the site of the injection

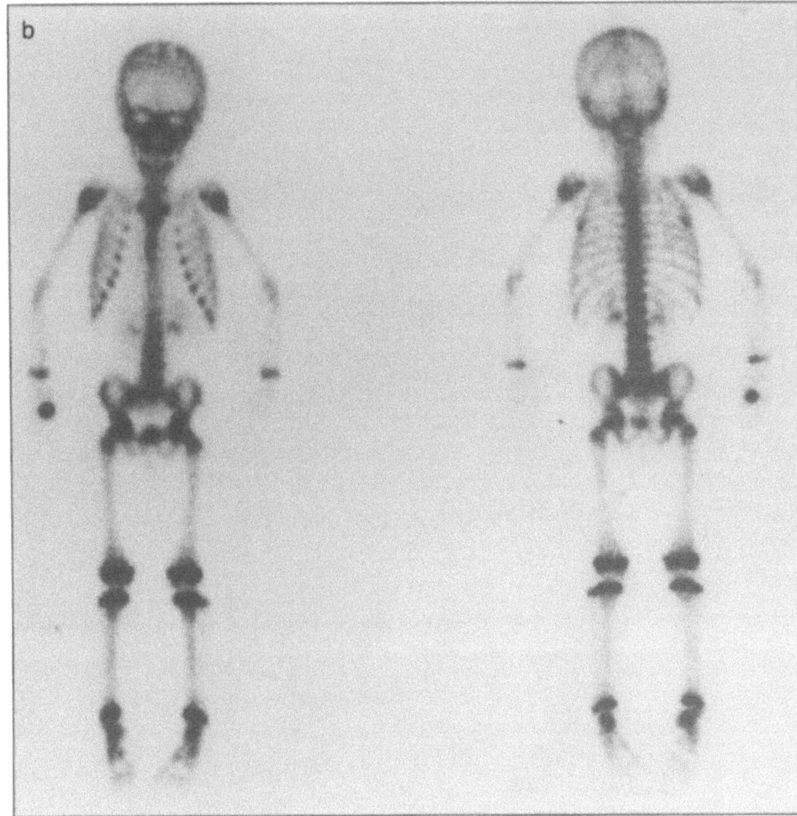

Fig. 5.12b. Whole body images are normal. Note the extravasation in the right hand again

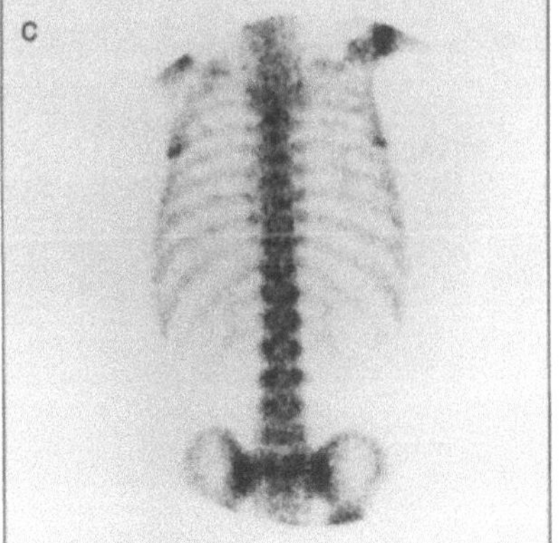

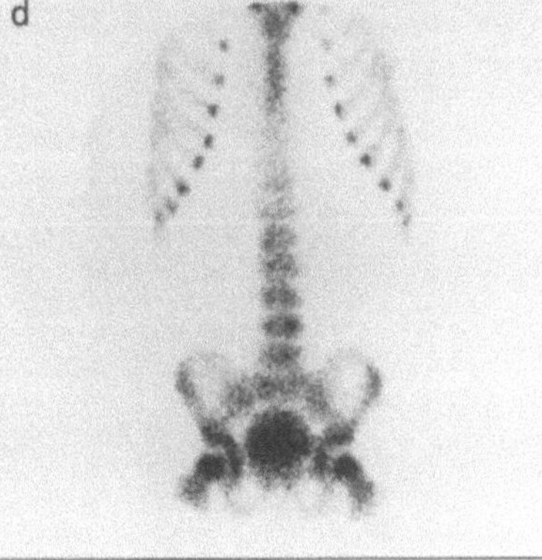

Fig. 5.12c. Posterior image of the dorsal and lumbar spine is unremarkable

Fig. 5.12d. Anterior image of the thorax, lumbar spine and pelvis shows focal abnormal increased uptake of isotope on the left side of the body of L4, the site of the fracture

Teaching Point
Pathology of the lower lumbar spine can sometimes be better seen on the anterior view than on the posterior view.

Case 5.13. Pain in the back on and off for 2 years in this boy aged 7 years. He was active on the sports field and undertook ballet dancing daily. The final diagnosis was a stress fracture at the level of L5

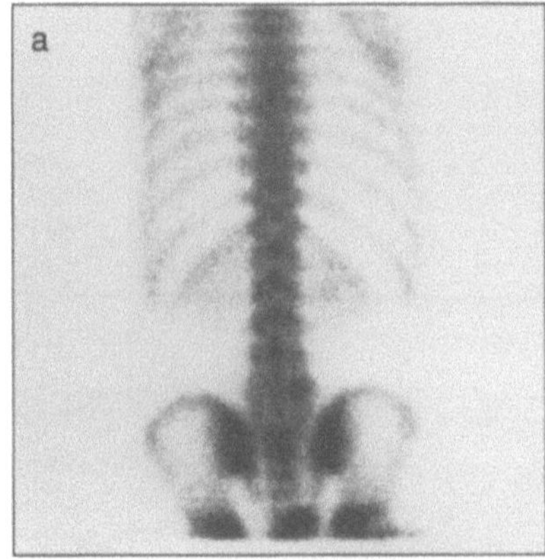

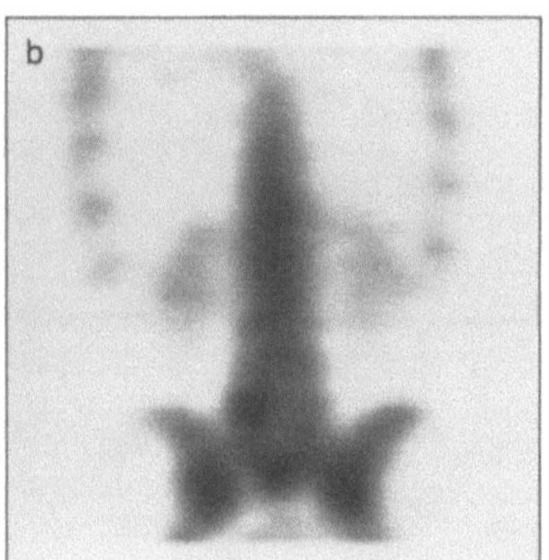

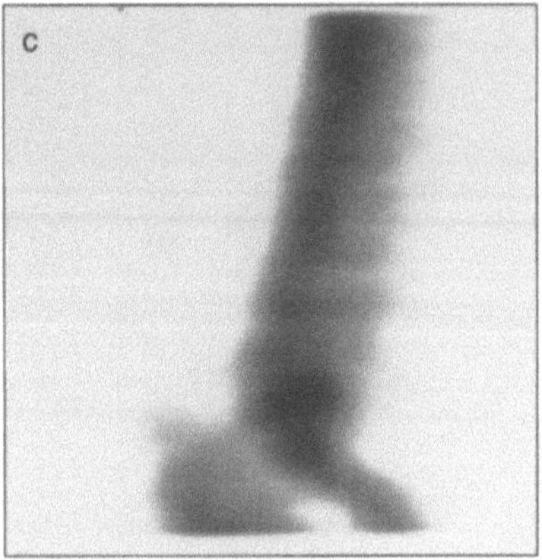

Fig. 5.13a. Posterior view of the lower dorsal spine, lumbar spine and upper pelvis shows focal abnormal increased uptake of isotope on the right side of L5

Fig. 5.13b. Coronal SPECT image shows focal abnormal increased uptake of isotope localised to the right side of the body of L5

Fig. 5.13c. The sagittal section shows this focal abnormal increased uptake of isotope in the posterior aspect of the body of L5 extending into the neural arch

Fig. 5.13d. Transaxial slice at the L5 level shows focal abnormal uptake in the region of the posterior aspect of the body of L5 extending into the neural arch. The computed tomography (CT) scan showed a thin sclerotic line in this area. The child was treated in a brace and the pain went away. Final diagnosis was that of a stress fracture

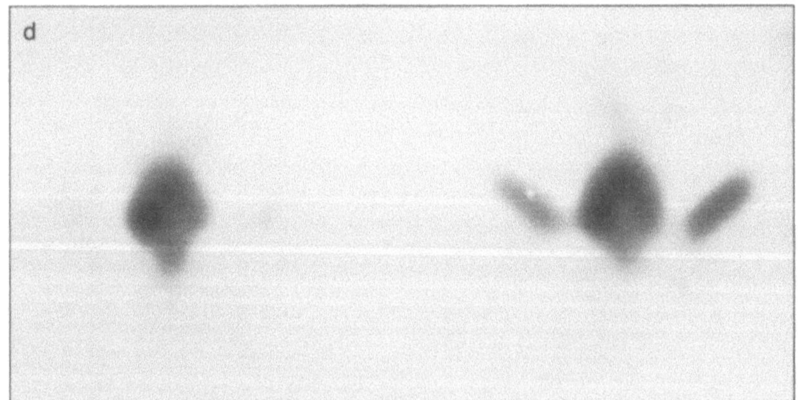

Teaching Point

Note the similarity between this and the appearances of a primary benign bone tumour, e.g. osteoid osteoma. Compare to Cases 4.9 and 4.10. Also see Cases 4.12 and 4.13 in the section on "Osteoblastoma", Case 4.24 in "Aneurysmal Bone Cysts" and Case 2.38 in "Infection". This shows the sensitivity but non-specificity of bone scans. Also see "Spondylolisthesis" (chapter 5.2.3).

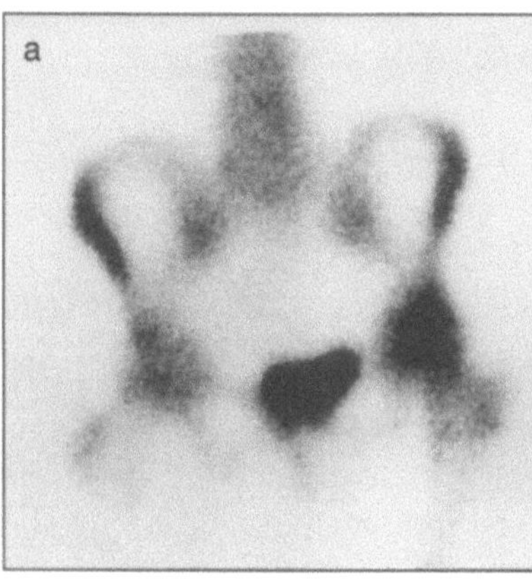

5.1.5 Femur
(1 Case; Fig. 5.14)

Case 5.14. A 10-year-old girl who had suffered trauma 4 months prior to the bone scan. The radiographs had shown subluxation of the left femoral head which was also flat. At surgery, there was a fracture of the femoral neck with subluxation of the hip joint

Fig. 5.14a. Anterior image of the pelvis shows abnormal increased uptake of isotope throughout the left hip joint

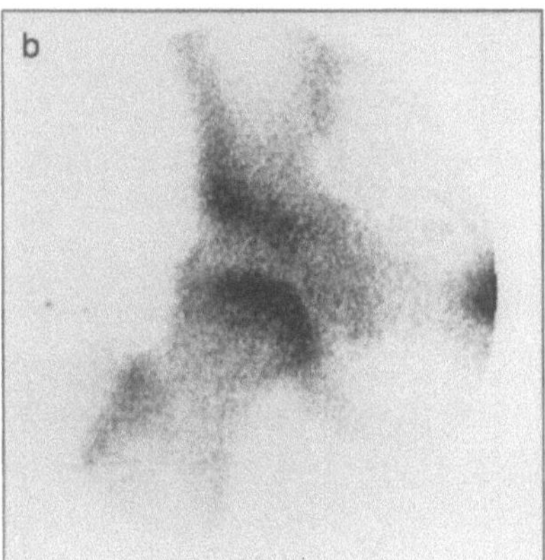

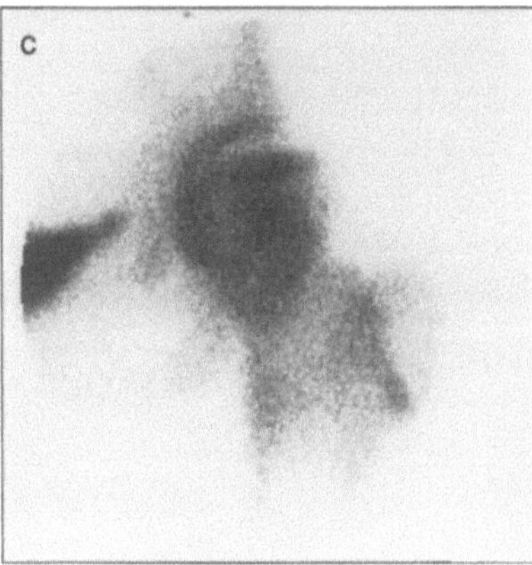

Fig. 5.14b. Pin hole view of the right hip is normal

Fig. 5.14c. Pin hole view of the left hip shows flattening of the femoral capital epiphysis as well as abnormal increased uptake of isotope in the neck of the femur, the site of the fracture

5.1.6 Fibula
(1 Case; Fig. 5.15)

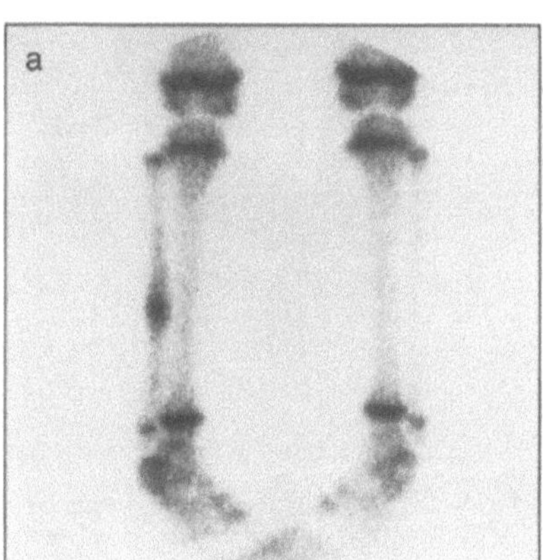

Case 5.15. A 2-year-old girl who was limping after minor trauma. She was found to have a fracture of the left fibula

Fig. 5.15a. Posterior image of the lower limbs shows focal abnormal increased uptake of isotope in the mid shaft of the left fibula

Teaching Point

The appearances seen had a differential diagnosis, which include malignant tumour (see Case 4.32) and stress fracture (see Case 5.22).

5.1.7 Feet
(3 Cases; Figs. 5.16–5.18)

Case 5.16. An 8-year-old boy who had been playing football and had suffered an injury to the right ankle. There was no evidence of a fracture at any stage but avulsion of the lateral ligament of the ankle had occurred

Fig. 5.16a. Blood pool whole body images show abnormal increased uptake of isotope on both sides of the right ankle joint. Note extravasation at the site of the injection in the right hand

Fig. 5.16b. Whole body images show increased uptake of isotope in the right ankle compared to the left. Extravasation in the wrist is again noted

Technical Comment
There is slight movement of the skull, causing blurring of the skull images on both anterior and posterior views.

Teaching Point
1. Despite the fact that no fracture had occurred, the increased uptake of isotope in the small bones of the foot is presumably related to the extensive soft tissue injury causing the intense hyperaemia.
2. Similar appearances could be seen with infection.

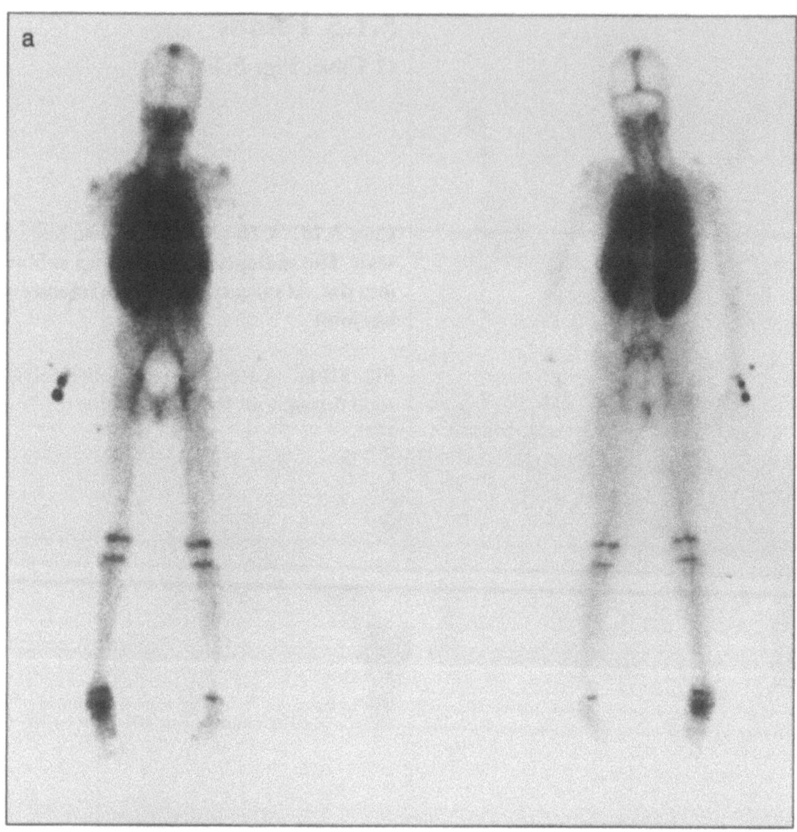

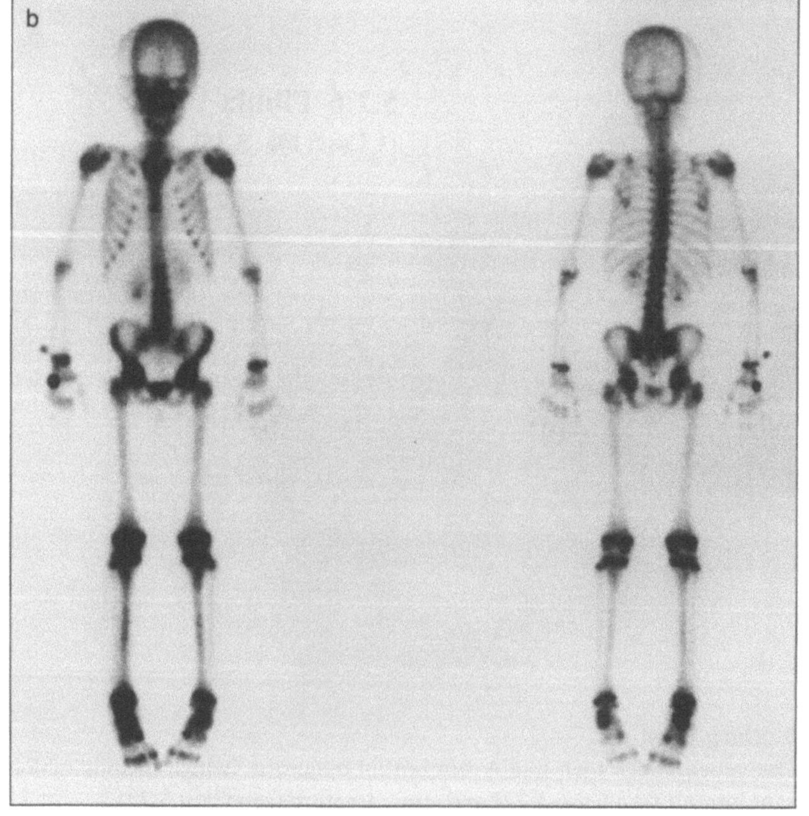

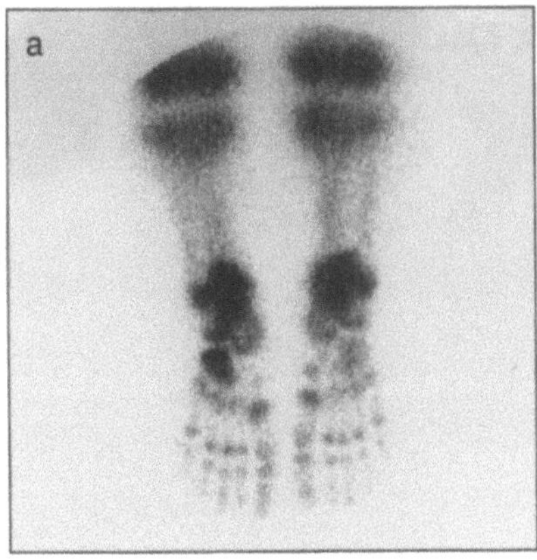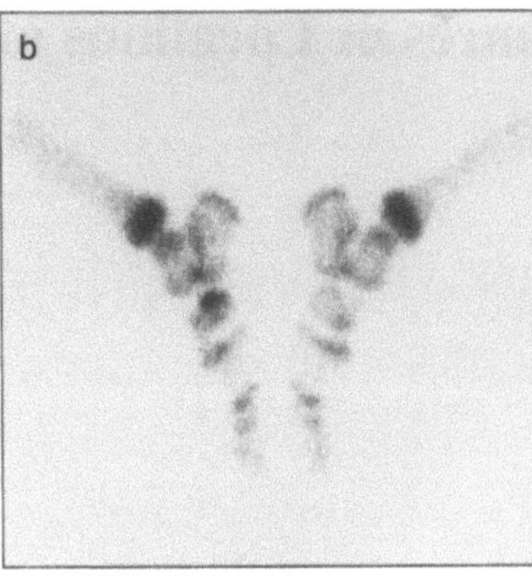

Case 5.17. 3-year-old girl who had pain in the right foot following trauma. She was found to have a fracture of the right cuboid bone

Fig. 5.17a. Plantar image of the feet shows abnormal increased uptake of isotope in the lateral aspect of the small bones of the right foot

Fig. 5.17b. Lateral image of the feet. The abnormal increased uptake of isotope is again noted on the right

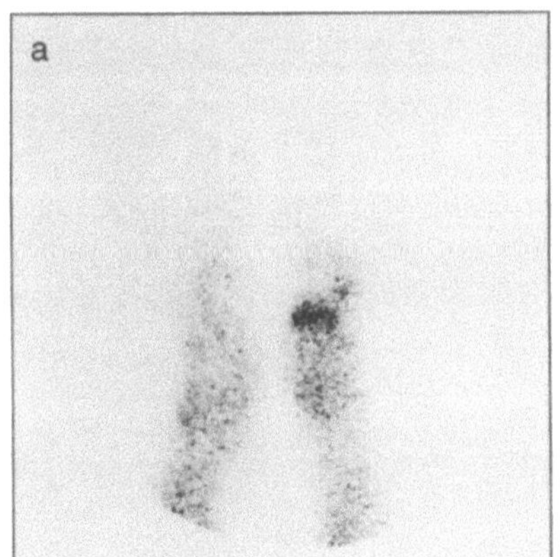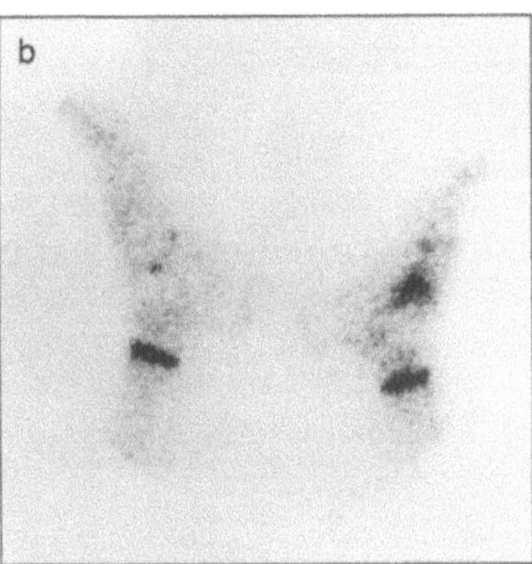
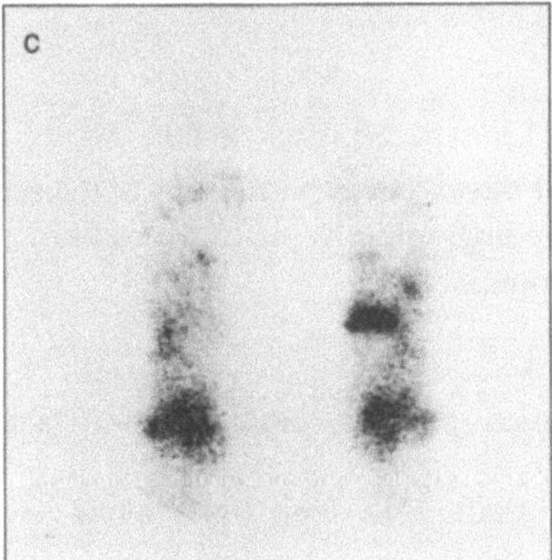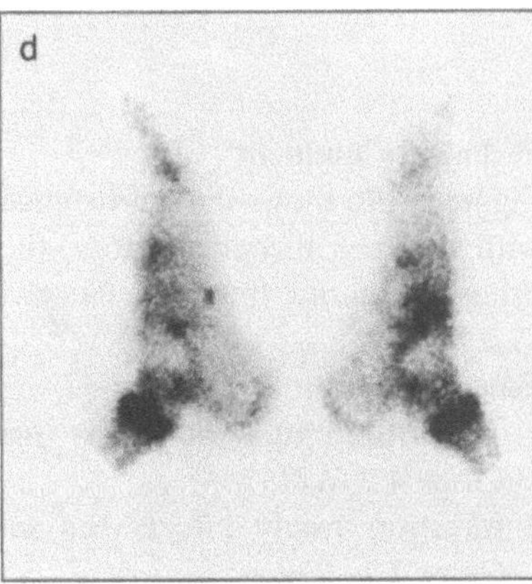

Case 5.18. A 10-year-old boy who had suffered trauma and was found to have a fracture of the medial cuneiform bone of the left foot

Fig. 5.18a. Blood pool plantar image of the feet shows abnormal increased uptake of isotope in the mid portion of the left foot

Fig. 5.18b. Blood pool lateral image of the feet shows abnormal increased uptake of isotope in the small distal bones on the left

Fig. 5.18c. Plantar image of the feet shows intense abnormal increased uptake of isotope in the distal medial small bones of the foot on the left

Fig. 5.18d. Lateral image of the feet confirms the position of the abnormal increased uptake of isotope on the left

5.2 Unusual Appearances or Locations of Fractures

5.2.1 Stress Fracture
(5 Cases; Figs. 5.19–5.23)

Case 5.19. A 7-year-old girl who had pain in the right tibia. The final diagnosis was that of a stress fracture

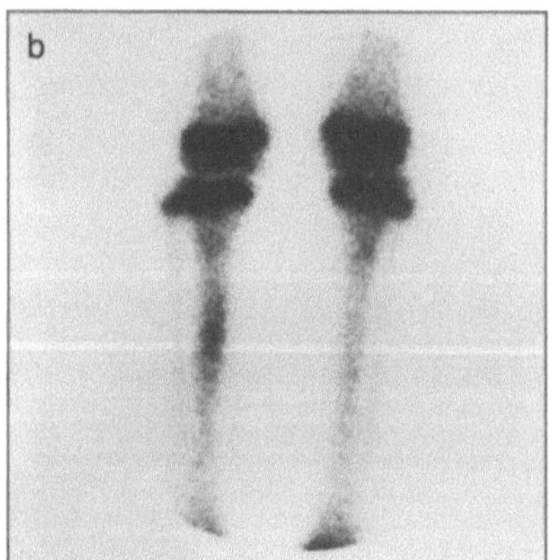

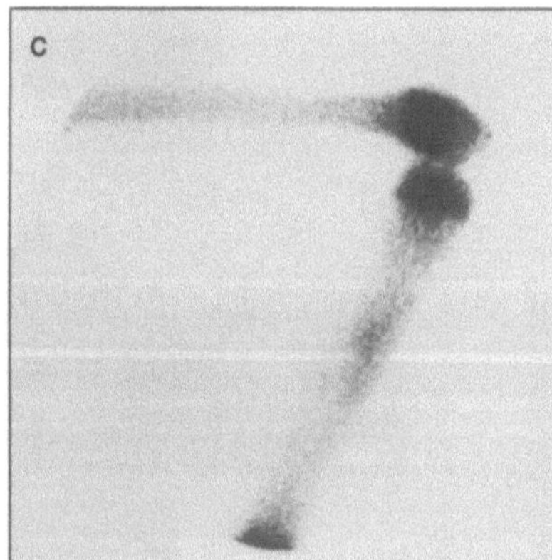

Fig. 5.19a. Anterior blood pool image of the tibiae shows slightly increased uptake on the medial aspect of the mid shaft of the right tibia

Fig. 5.19b. Anterior image of the knees and lower limbs shows focal abnormal increased uptake of isotope in the mid shaft of the right tibia with surrounding slight hyperactivity

Fig. 5.19c. Lateral image of the right knee and tibia shows the focal abnormal area of increased uptake of isotope in the anterior aspect of the right tibia

Technical Comment

Figure 5.19b shows the importance of the excellent positioning of the feet with the toes turned inwards, the radiographically neutral position, in order to separate the fibula clearly from the tibia.

Teaching Point

1. The differential diagnosis includes primary bone tumours (see Cases 4.7, 4.8).
2. Infection rarely affects the mid shaft of a long bone alone (see Cases 2.1–2.3).

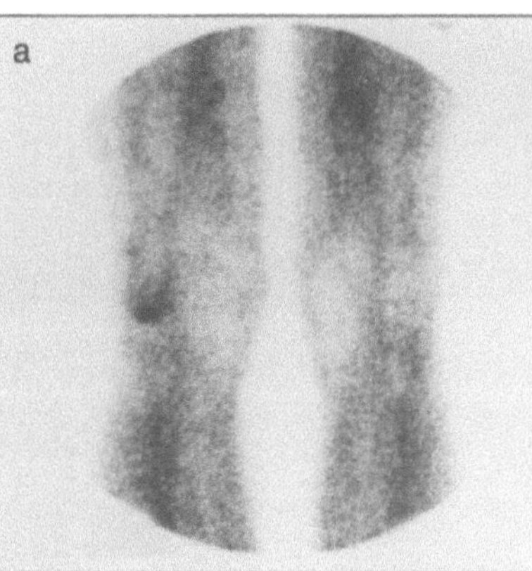

Case 5.20. A 21-year-old patient who had suffered minor trauma to the knees. The radiographs showed periosteal reactions and the final diagnosis was thought to be due to stress fractures

Fig. 5.20a. Blood pool image of the knees, anterior view. There is focal abnormal increased uptake of isotope in the lower right lateral femoral condyle

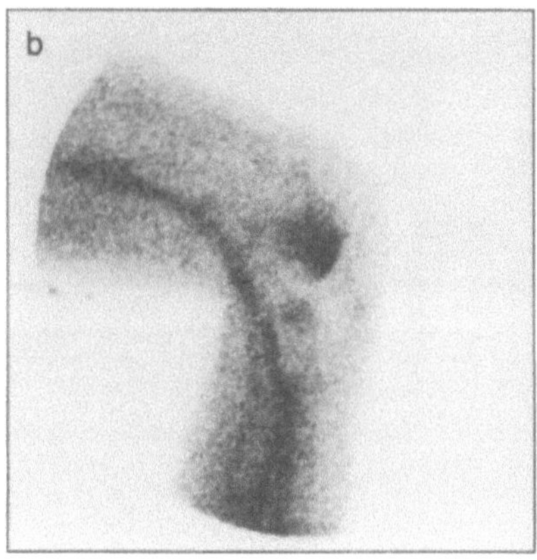

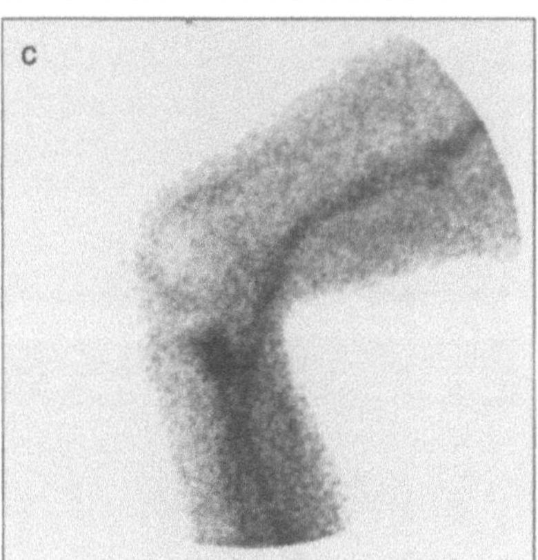

Fig. 5.20b. Right lateral blood pool image of the right knee shows increased uptake in the distal femur

Fig. 5.20c. Left lateral blood pool image of the left knee shows focal abnormal increased uptake of isotope in the region of the head of the fibula

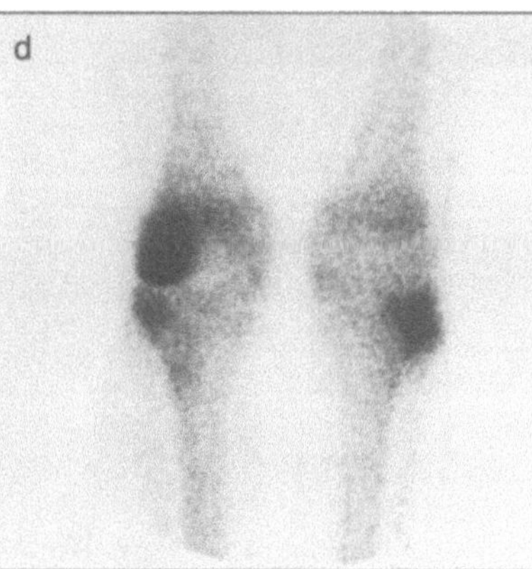

Fig. 5.20d. Anterior image of the knees shows focal areas of abnormal increased uptake of isotope in the right lateral femoral condyle and heads of both fibulae

Fig. 5.20e. Right lateral image of the right knee shows focal abnormal uptake of isotope in the femoral condyle and the head of the fibula

Fig. 5.20f. Left lateral image of the left knee shows focal abnormal uptake of isotope in the head of the fibula

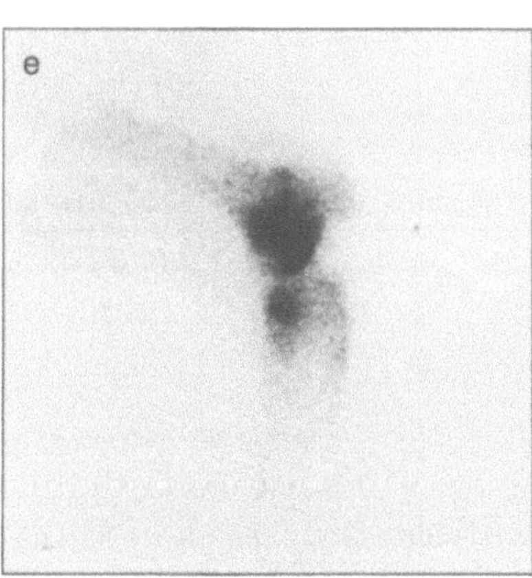

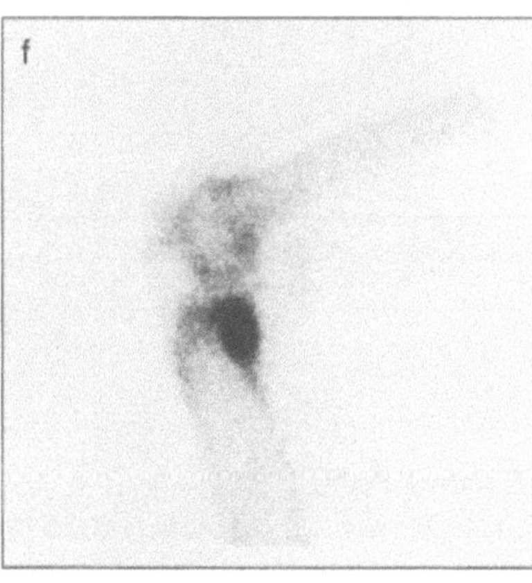

Teaching Point
There is a high probability that the focal areas of abnormal increased uptake of isotope, which were associated with periosteal reactions, were due to bilateral small fractures.

Case 5.21. A 21-year-old patient with pain in the right tibia. This was due to a stress fracture

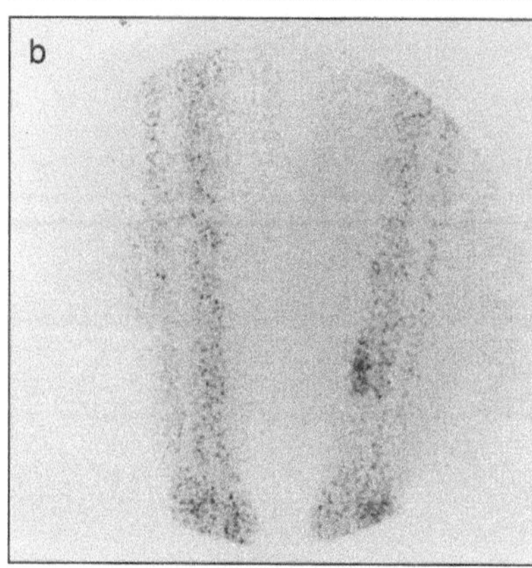

Fig. 5.21a. Posterior blood pool image of the lower limbs shows focal abnormal increased uptake of isotope in the lower third of the right tibia

Fig. 5.21b. Posterior image of the tibiae shows a focal abnormal increased uptake of isotope in the lower third of the shaft of the right tibia

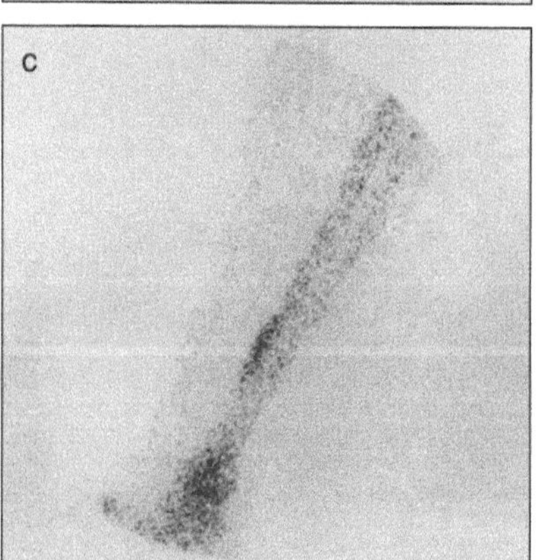

Fig. 5.21c. Right lateral image of the right tibia shows the focal increased uptake of isotope to be posteriorly located

Teaching Point
These are the typical features of a stress fracture. Similiar appearances may be seen with benign bone tumours (see also Cases 4.7 and 4.8).

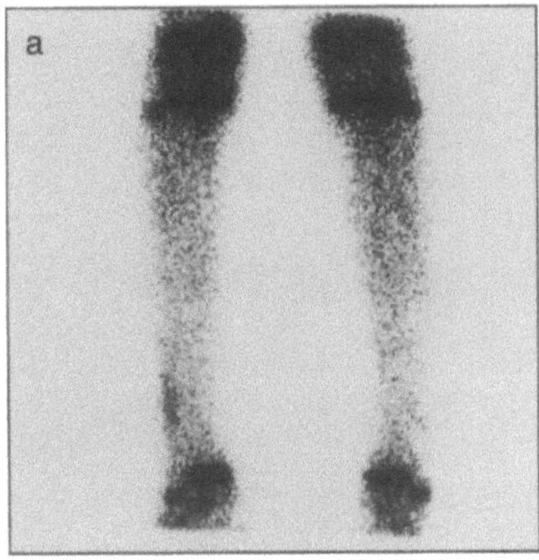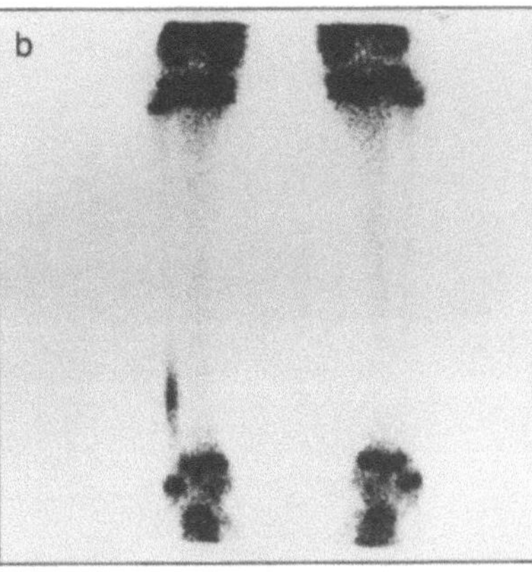

Case 5.22. A 6-year-old boy who complained of pain in the left leg for a week after playing football. He later developed a periosteal reaction from a stress fracture of the lower fibula

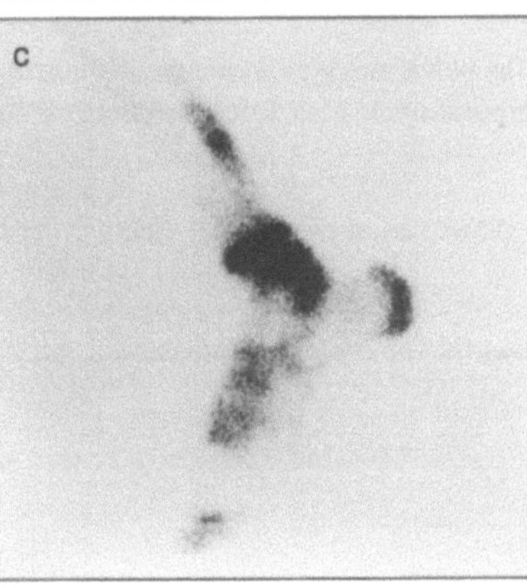

Fig. 5.22a. Posterior blood pool image of the lower legs shows increased uptake of isotope in the lateral aspect of the left leg above the ankle

Fig. 5.22b. Posterior image of the lower legs shows focal abnormal increased uptake of isotope in the lower third of the shaft of the left fibula

Fig. 5.22c. Lateral image of the left leg, ankle and foot confirms the increased uptake of isotope in the left fibula

Technical Comment

Note the radiographically neutral position in Fig. 5.22a,b, which allows differentiation between the fibula and tibia.

Teaching Point

Similar appearances may be seen in Ewing's sarcoma (see Case 4.32) and a traumatic fracture (see Case 5.15).

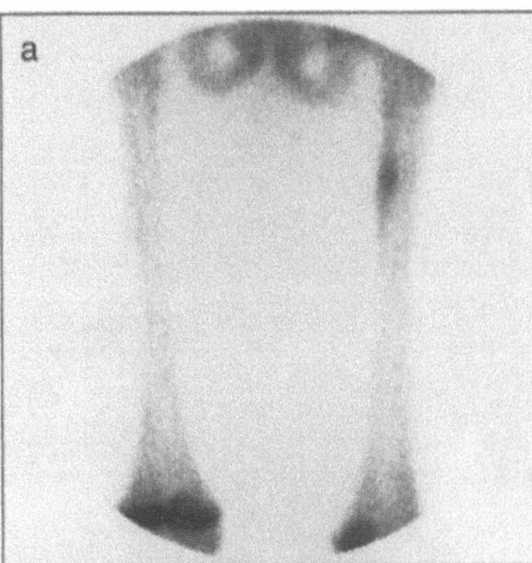

Case 5.23. An 8-year-old boy who complained of pain 15 days after minor trauma. The final diagnosis was that of a stress fracture of the left upper femoral shaft

Fig. 5.23a. Anterior image of the femora shows focal abnormal increased uptake of isotope in the upper third of the shaft of the left femur

Teaching Point

Similar appearances would be seen with an osteoid osteoma (see Case 4.4).

5.2.2 Slipped Femoral Capital Epiphysis
(1 Case; Fig. 5.24)

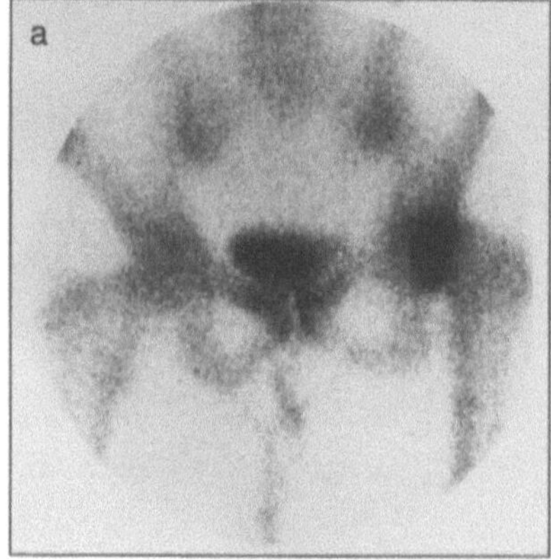
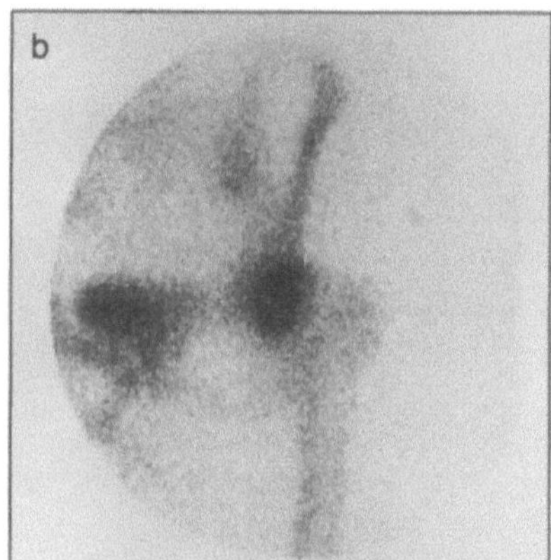
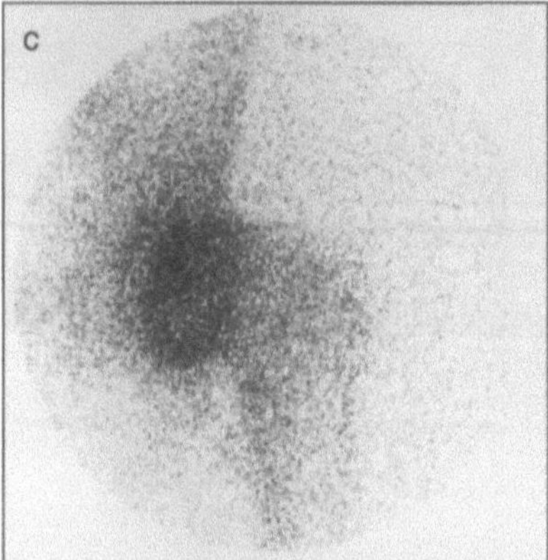

Case 5.24. A 14-year-old girl with pain in the left hip due to slipped femoral capital epiphysis

Fig. 5.24a. Anterior blood pool image of the pelvis and hips shows focal abnormal increased uptake of isotope in the left femoral neck with foreshortening of the femur

Fig. 5.24b. Anterior image of the left hip shows loss of the normal architecture of the hip joint

Fig. 5.24c. Pin hole view of the left hip shows the slip of the femoral capital epiphysis infra-medially

5.2.3 Spondylolisthesis
(4 Cases; Figs. 5.25–5.28)

> **Teaching Point**
> 1. Confirmation and detailed anatomical extent of pathology in the spine should be identified with the addition of spot images using the high-resolution collimator and SPECT.
> 2. Bone scans are sensitive on the detection of a fracture in the spine, but cannot distinguish between fracture with or without displacement (see also Case 5.13).
> 3. Other causes of similar appearances include infection (see Cases 2.31, 2.44) and benign bone tumour (see Case 4.24).

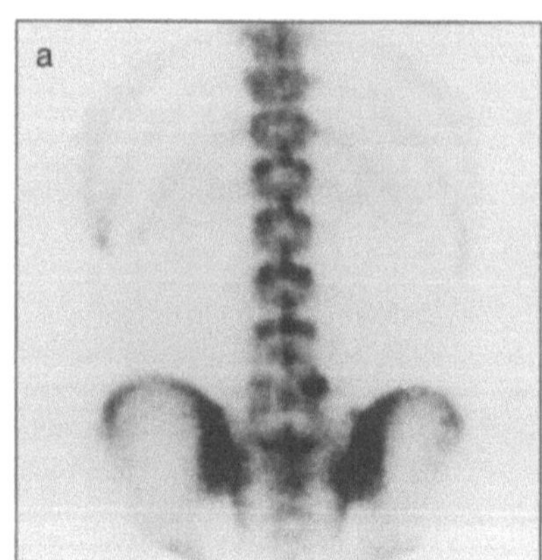
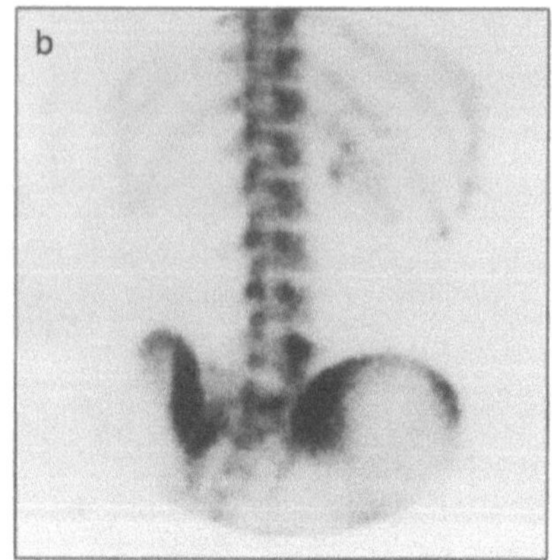

Case 5.25. A 14-year-old boy with pain on the right side of the lower back. There was a spondylolisthesis with a fractured pars interarticularis at the L4/5 level

Fig. 5.25a,b. Posterior and right posterior oblique images of the lumbar spine and pelvis show intense abnormal increased uptake of isotope on the right at the level of L5, the site of the fractured pars interarticularis

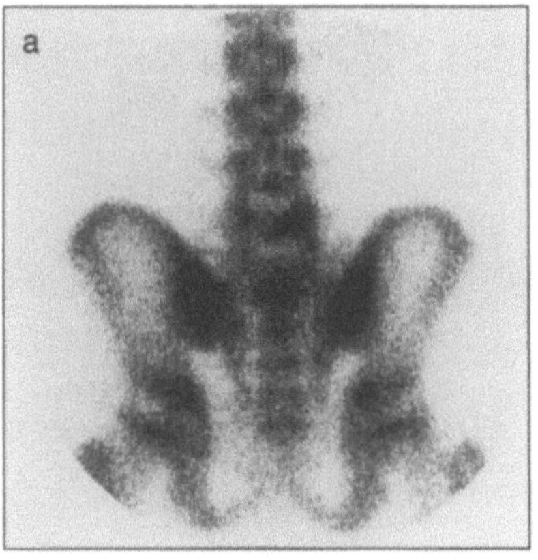

Case 5.26. A 12-year-old boy with pain in the back due to spondylolisthesis

Fig. 5.26a. Posterior image of lumbar spine and pelvis shows focal abnormal increased uptake of isotope at the level of L5 on the right

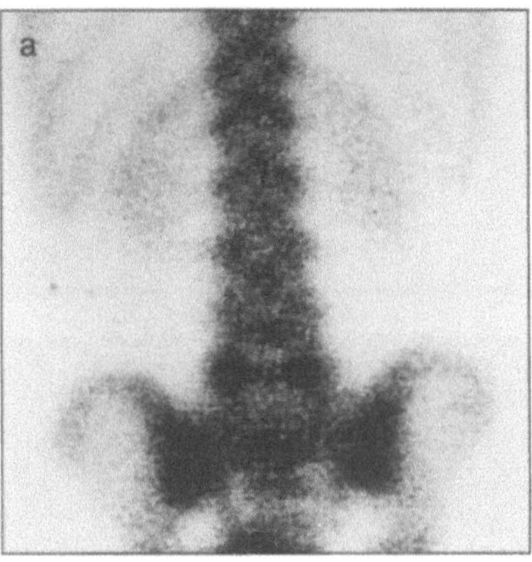

Case 5.27. A 13-year-old boy with pain in the back who was found to have spondylolisthesis with a fracture of the pars interarticularis

Fig. 5.27a. Posterior image of the spine and upper pelvis shows focal abnormal increased uptake of isotope in the region of the pedicles on both sides at the level of L5

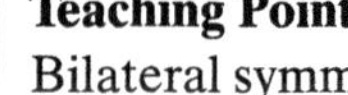

Teaching Point
Bilateral symmetrical changes can be seen with spondylolisthesis.

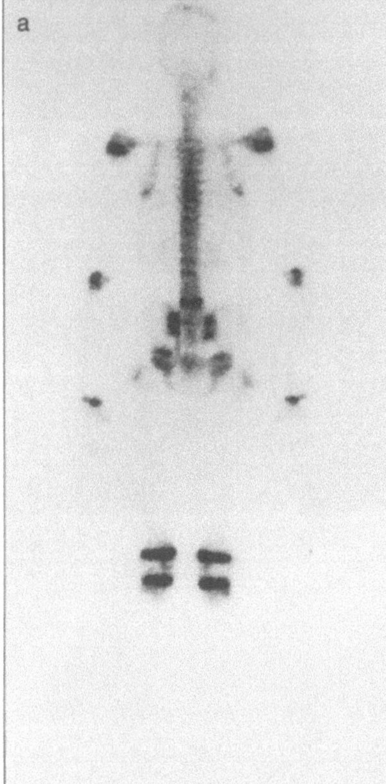

Case 5.28. A 12-year-old girl with pain in the back due to spondylolisthesis at L5

Fig. 5.28a. Posterior whole body scan shows focal abnormal increased uptake of isotope mainly on the right at the level of L5

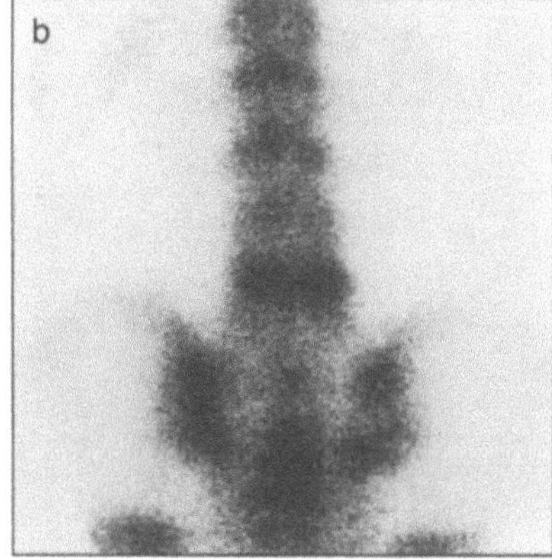

Fig. 5.28b. Posterior image of the lower lumbar spine and upper pelvis shows abnormal increased uptake of isotope at the level of L5 bilaterally, typical of bilateral spondylolisthesis

5.2.4 Trauma Secondary to Cold Exposure
(1 Case; Fig. 5.29)

Case 5.29. 15-year-old boy who had suffered trauma on the sports field and applied ice packs to the right foot. The first scan was done some hours after the cold ice bags had been applied intensely

Fig. 5.29a. Plantar blood pool image of the feet shows little perfusion to the right foot and ankle

Fig. 5.29b. Lateral blood pool image of the feet. Little activity is seen in the epiphyseal plate of the distal right tibia and fibula, but little else

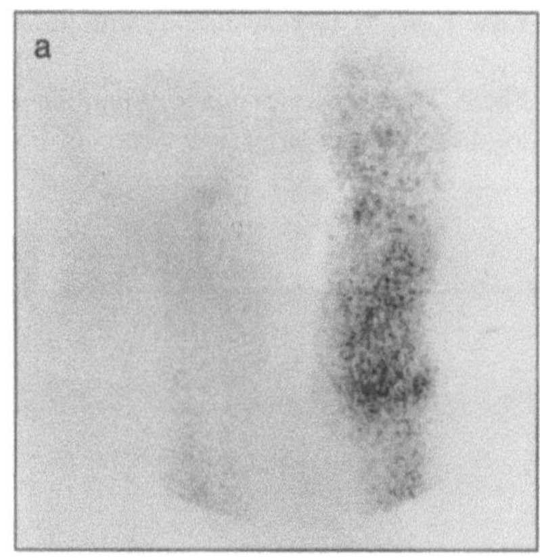
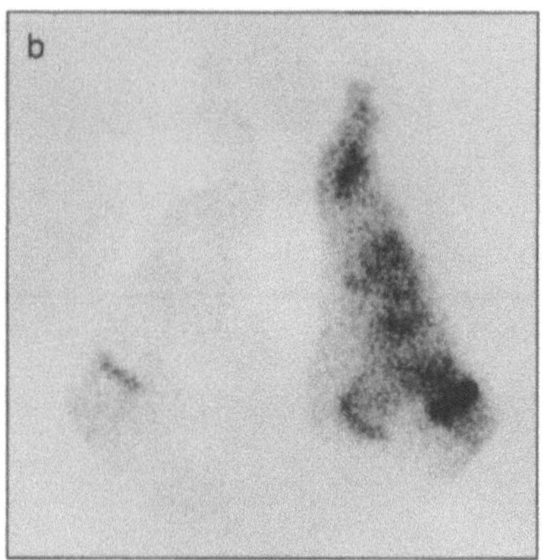
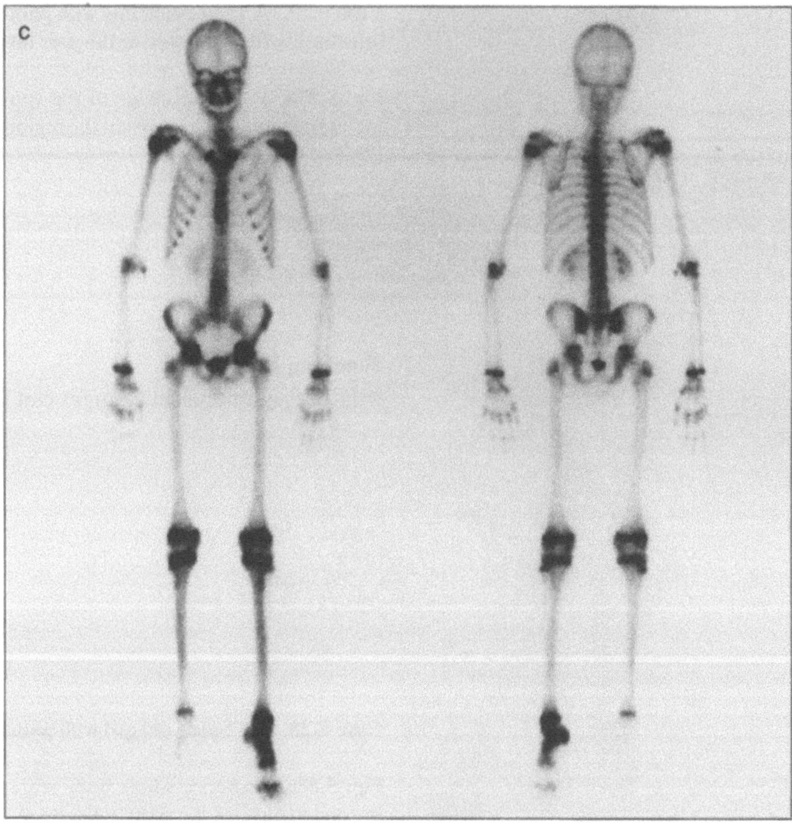

Fig. 5.29c. Whole body images. The right foot shows virtually total absence of activity with decreased activity in the distal tibial epiphyseal plate

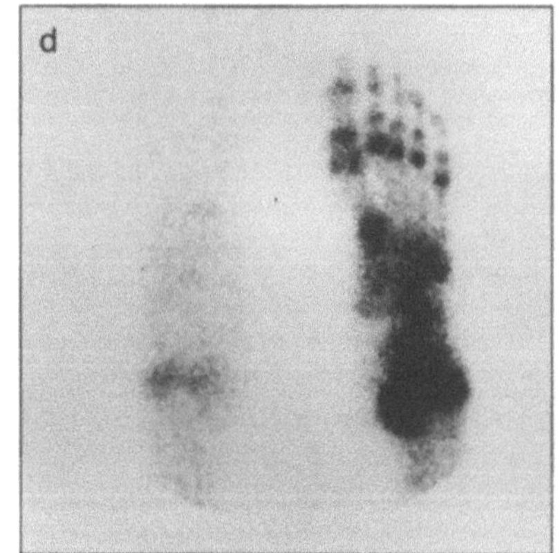
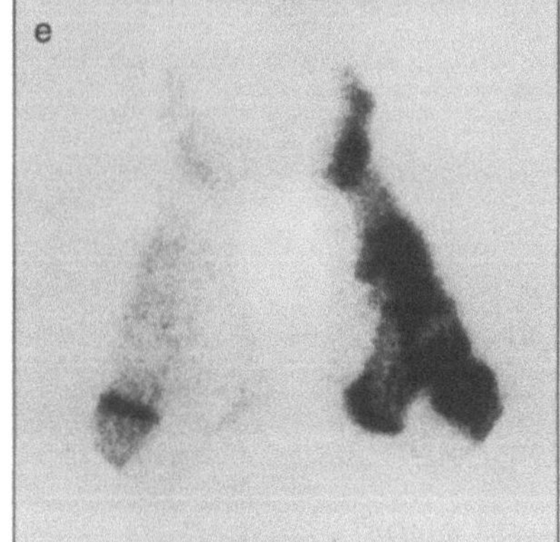

Fig. 5.29d,e. Plantar and lateral images of the feet show little activity in the epiphyseal plate of the distal right tibia and fibula, but little else.

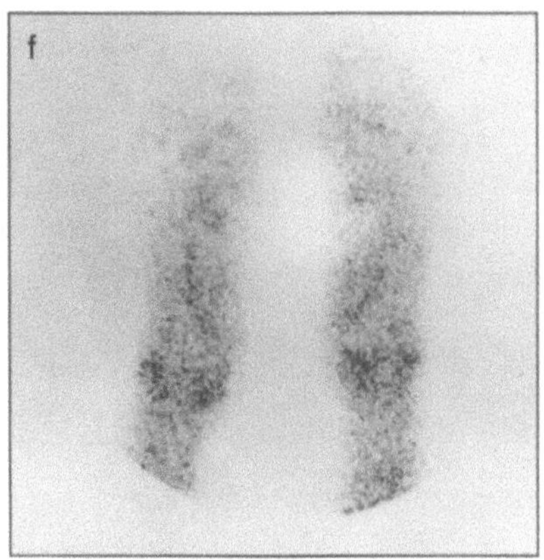

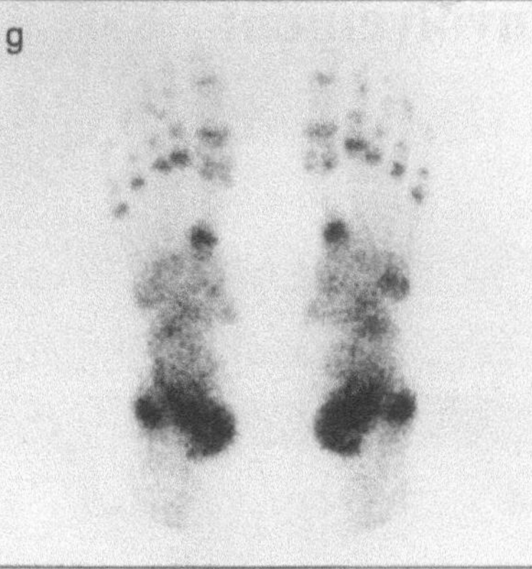

A follow-up scan was done 1 week later, when the boy was symptom free

Fig. 5.29f. Plantar blood pool image of the feet is normal

Fig. 5.29g. Plantar image of the feet shows equal distribution in the two feet

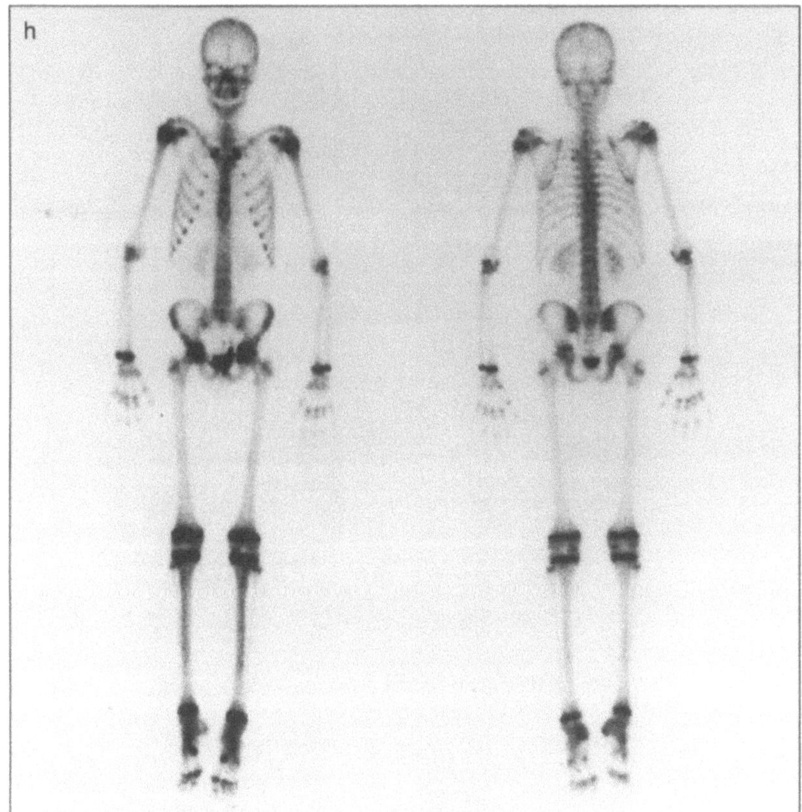

Fig. 5.29h. Whole body scan is unre-markable

Teaching Point

The severe prolonged cold caused decreased perfusion and metabolism in the right foot, which returned to normal 1 week later.

5.3 Diffuse Skeletal Involvement

5.3.1 Polytrauma
(6 Cases; Figs. 5.30–5.35)

Case 5.30. A 20-year-old patient who was unfortunate to have a tree fall on top of him. He suffered multiple fractures mainly to the head and face, the left shoulder and the spine

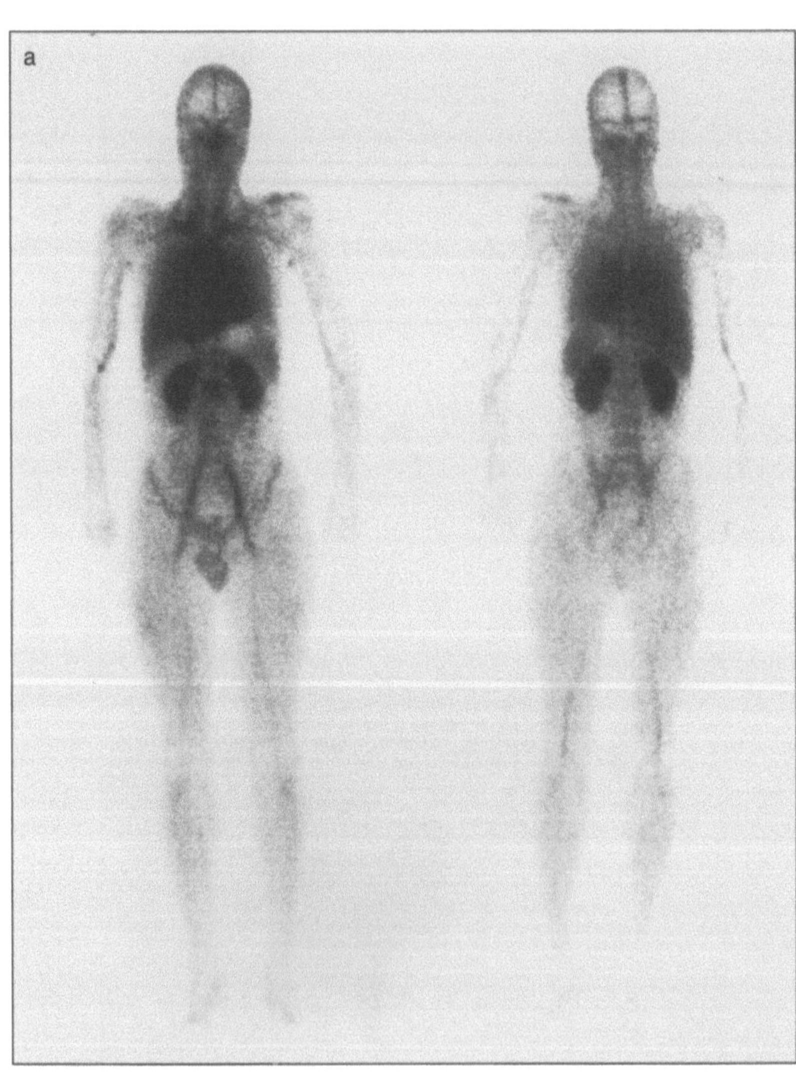

Fig. 5.30a. Blood pool whole body images show abnormal increased uptake of isotope in the region of the left shoulder

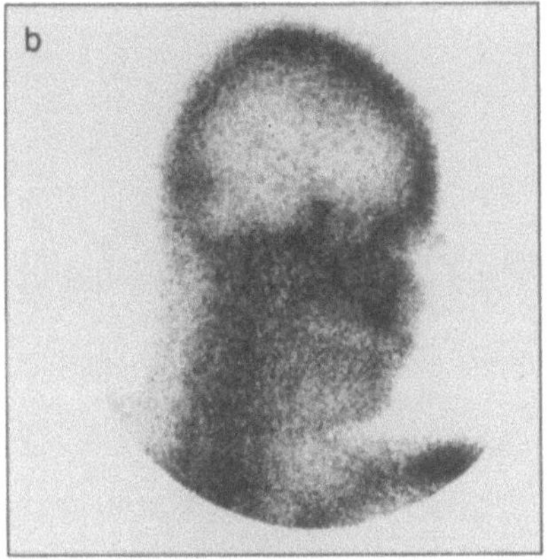 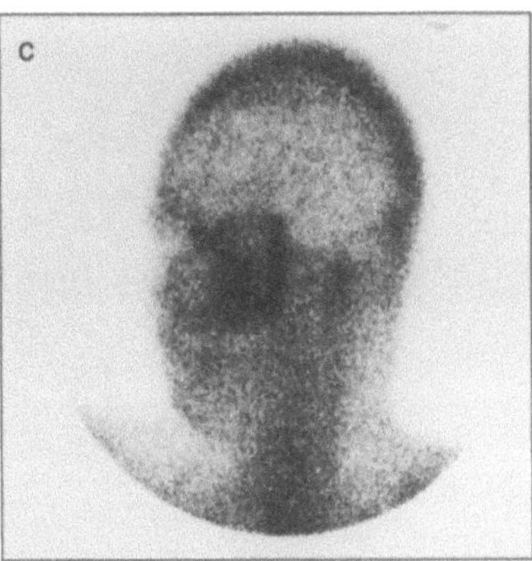

Fig. 5.30b. Blood pool right lateral image of the skull shows abnormal increased uptake of isotope in the anterior portion of the maxilla

Fig. 5.30c. Blood pool left lateral image of the skull shows marked increased activity in the posterior portion of the maxilla

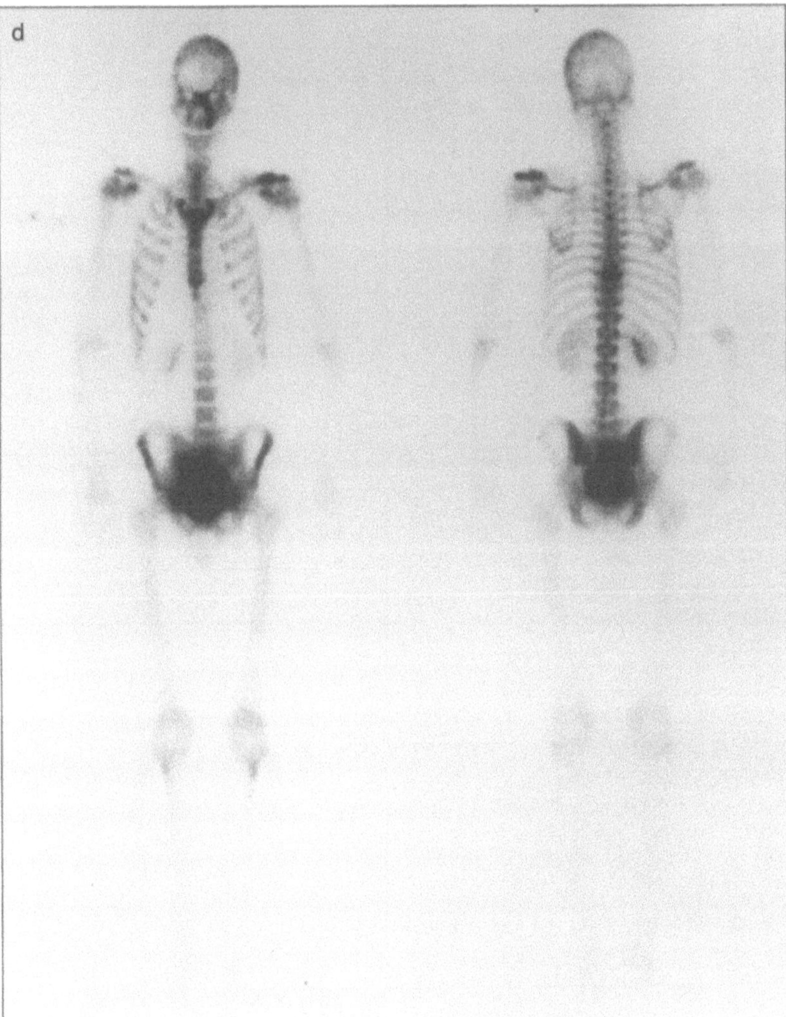

Fig. 5.30d. Whole body scans show abnormal increased uptake of isotope in the left shoulder joint as well as in the lower dorsal spine and the facial bones on the left

Case 5.31. A 7-year-old girl who fell from the first floor and suffered multiple fractures

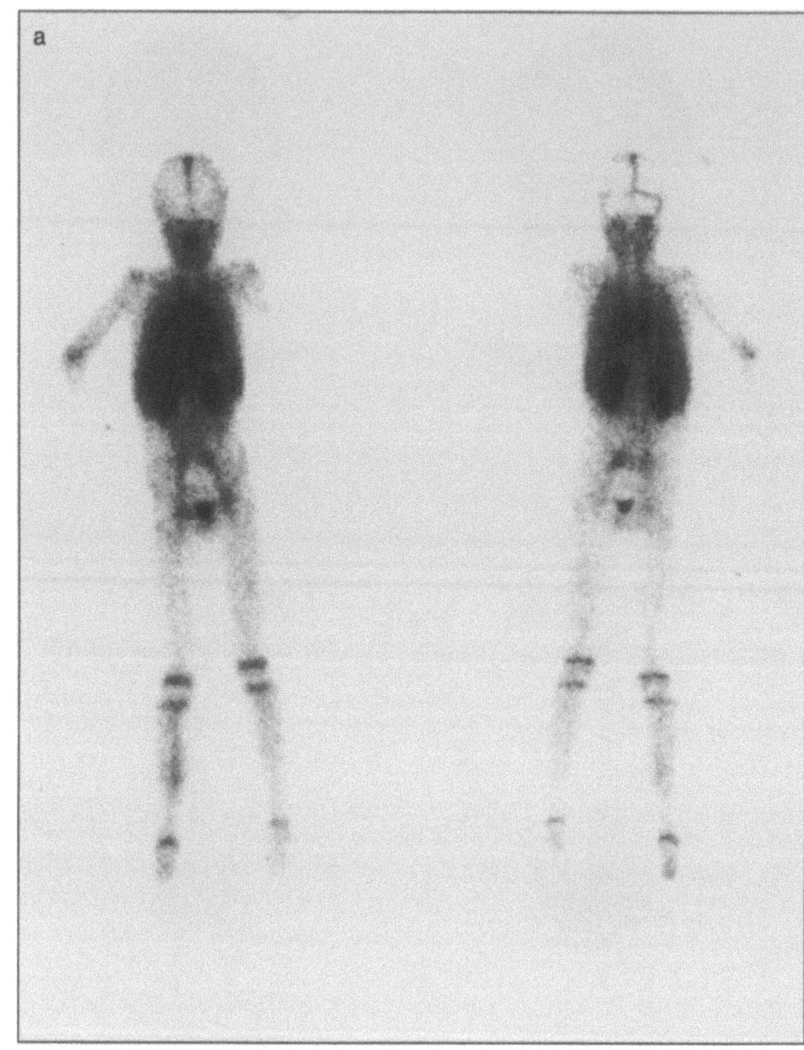

Fig. 5.31a. Blood pool whole body images show abnormal increased uptake of isotope in the right arm as well as in the right tibia, the right foot and the left sacro-iliac joint

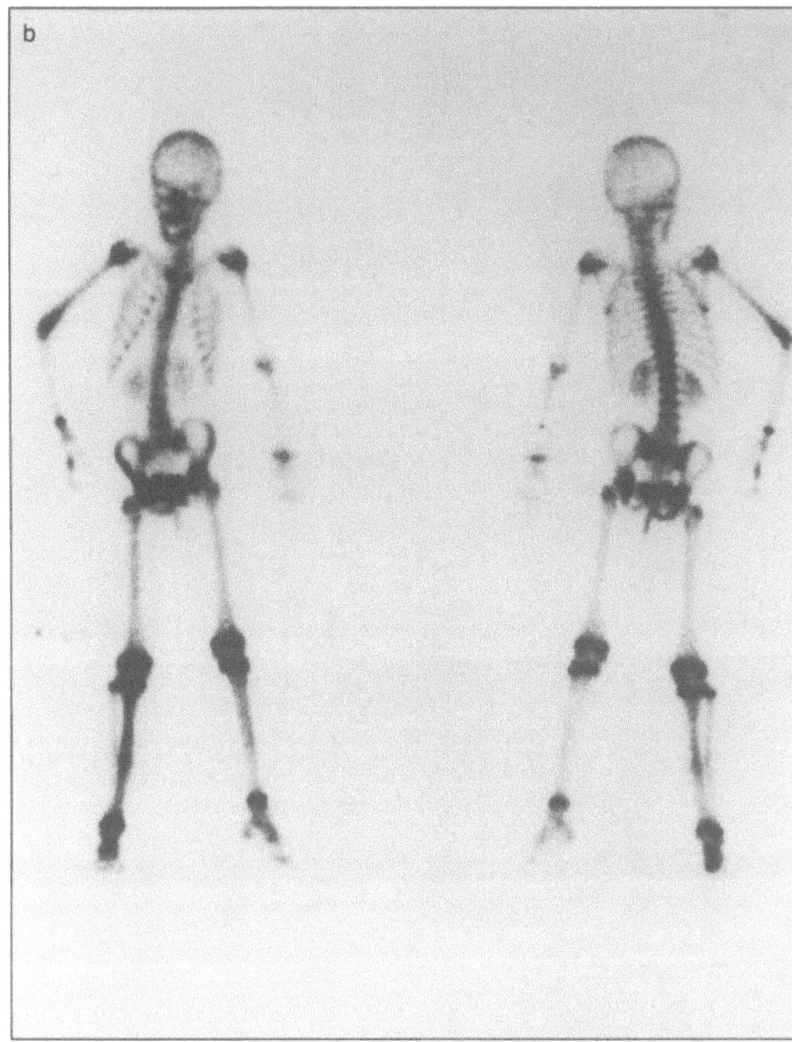

Fig. 5.31b. Whole body scans show abnormal increased uptake of isotope in the distal right humerus, right wrist and right tibia. There is a scoliosis concave to the left. Asymmetry of the pelvis is noted

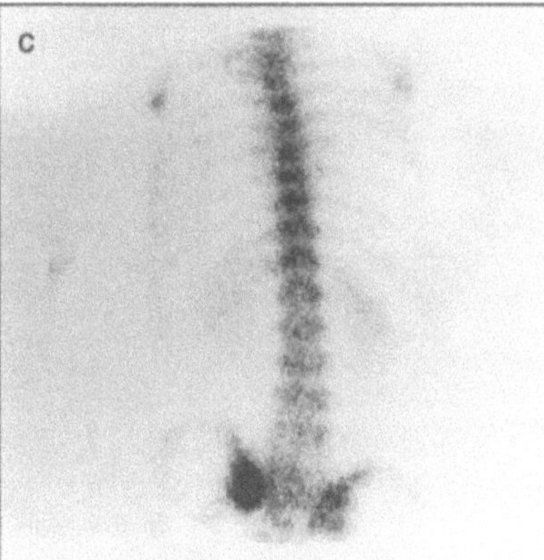

Fig. 5.31c. Posterior image of the lumbar spine and pelvis shows abnormal increased uptake of isotope in the dorsal spine and in the left sacro-iliac joint

Case 5.32. A 22-year-old patient who had been involved in a road traffic accident. Multiple fractures of the right femur and tibia were found as well as a fracture of the left clavicle. There was occlusion of the left femoral artery

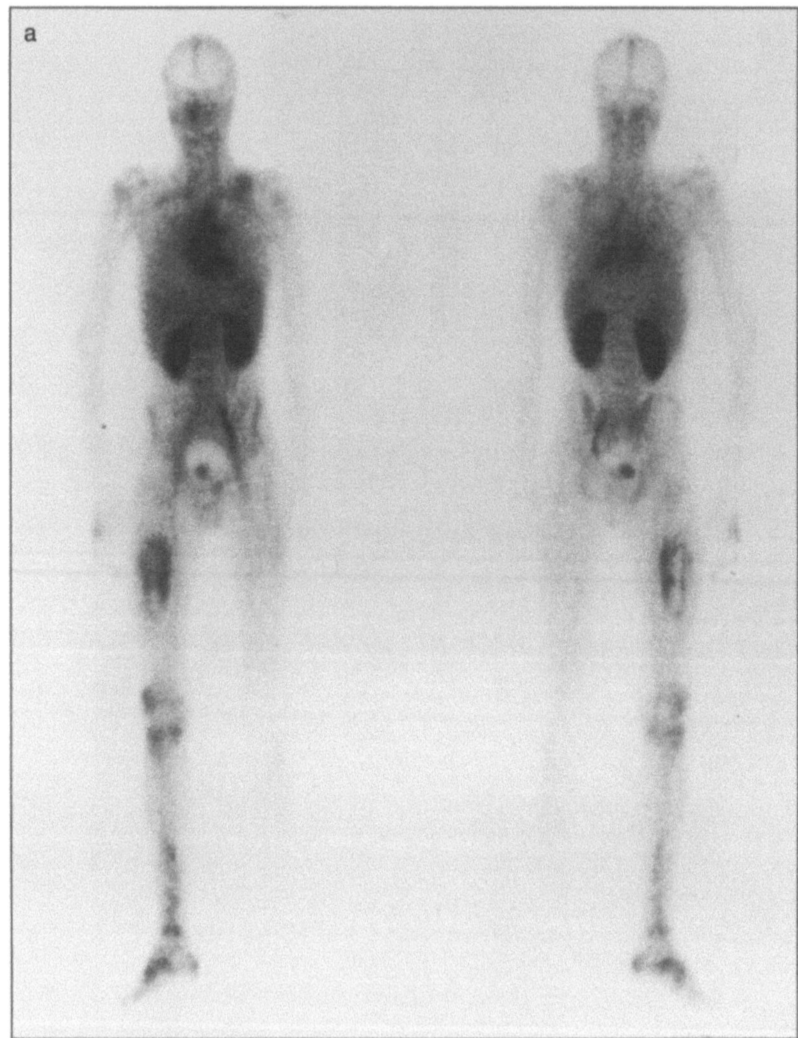

Fig. 5.32a. Whole body blood pool images show abnormal increased uptake of isotope in the right femur and right distal tibia as well as in the right foot. There is increased uptake of isotope in the left clavicle and the right hand and a decreased uptake of nearly the whole left leg

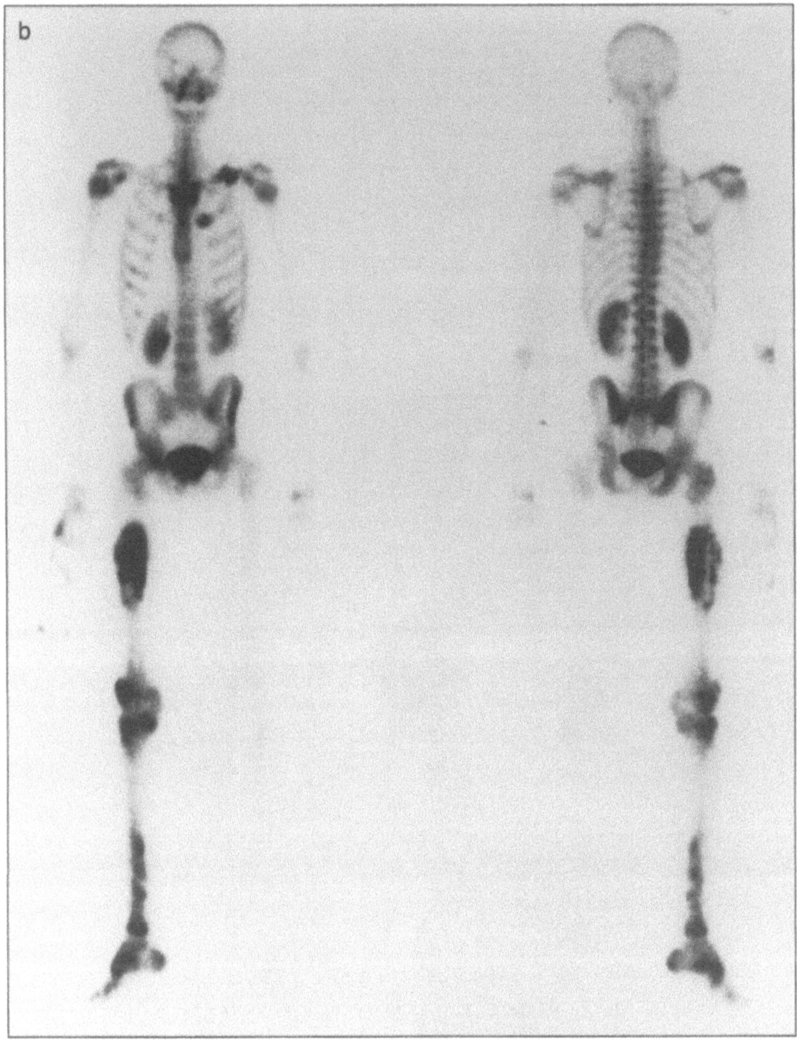

Fig. 5.32b. Whole body images show intense abnormal uptake of isotope in the mid portion of the right femur as well as in the distal right tibia. The right knee is difficult to assess because of the positioning of the foot. Abnormal increased uptake of isotope is also noted in the left clavicle, best seen on the anterior view. Increased uptake of isotope is also noted in the right hand, multiple ribs, the right elbow and the facial bones. The kidneys retain the tracer. No bony uptake is seen in the left leg, secondary to the occlusion of the left femoral artery

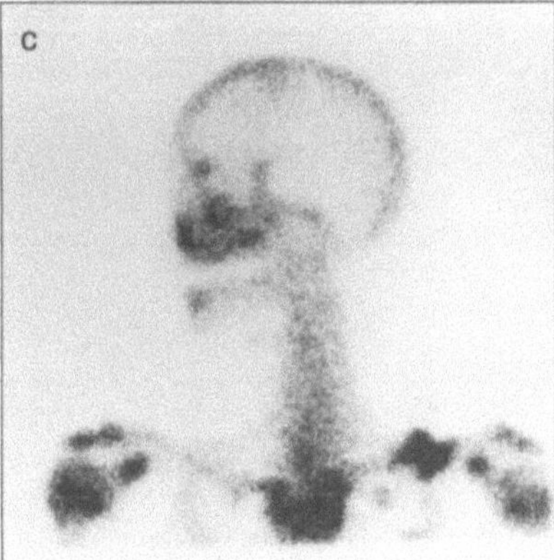

Fig. 5.32c. Left lateral image of the skull and clavicles. The fractured facial bones and the fracture in the left clavicle are seen to better advantage

Teaching Point

The reason for the abnormal retention of isotope by the kidneys is uncertain, but the possibility that the kidneys suffered ischaemia was highly likely.

Case 5.33. **A 16-year-old boy who had suffered a motor cycle accident and had undergone an amputation of the left arm. He was found to have had multiple fractures of the left femur and left tibia and a fracture of the left foot as well as of the left scapula**

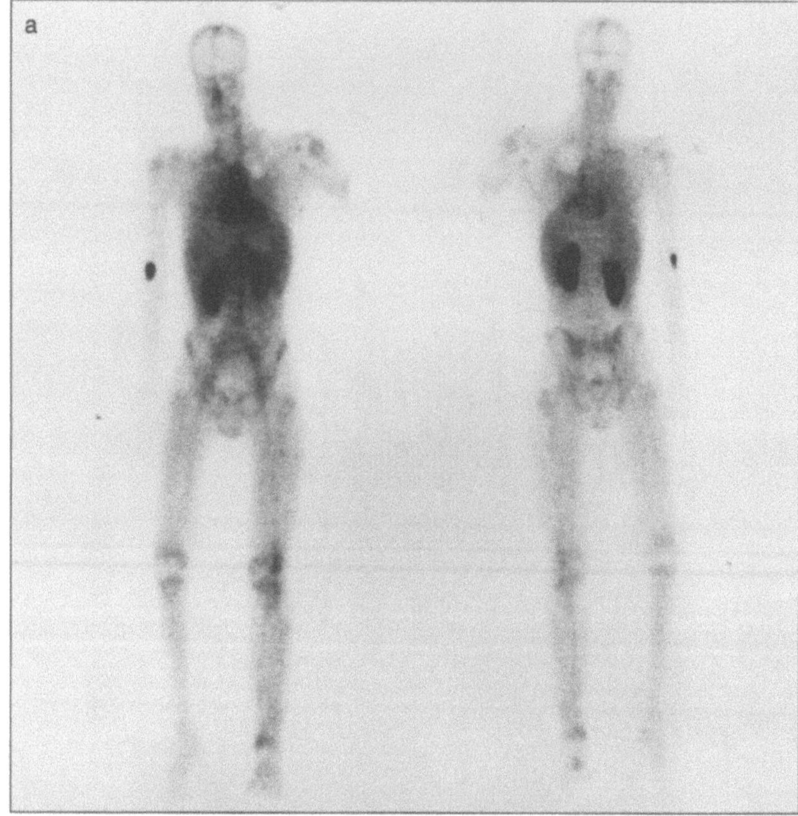

Fig. 5.33a. Whole body blood pool images show abnormal increased uptake of isotope around the left knee and ankle. A photon-deficient area is noted in the chest above the heart on the left on both the anterior and posterior views. This was due to a lung haematoma

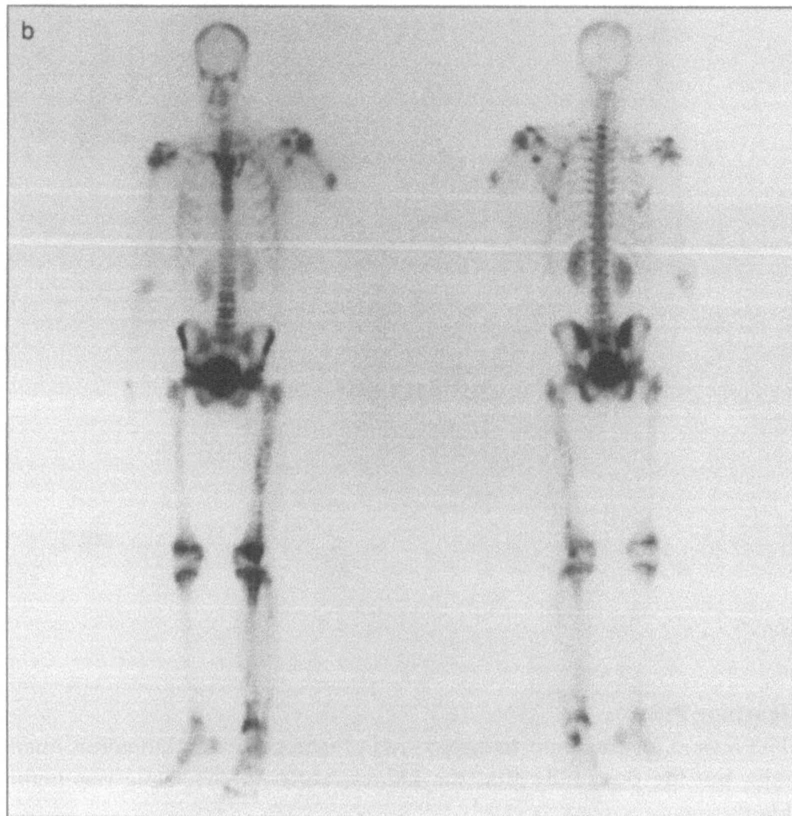

Fig. 5.33b. Whole body images show abnormal uptake of isotope in the upper dorsal spine, the upper left dorsal ribs, the left scapula and the left femur as well as in the left knee and tibia. The left sternoclavicular joint and the left calcaneus show also increased uptake of isotope. Increased uptake of isotope at the amputation site of the left arm is seen. There is retention of tracer by the kidneys

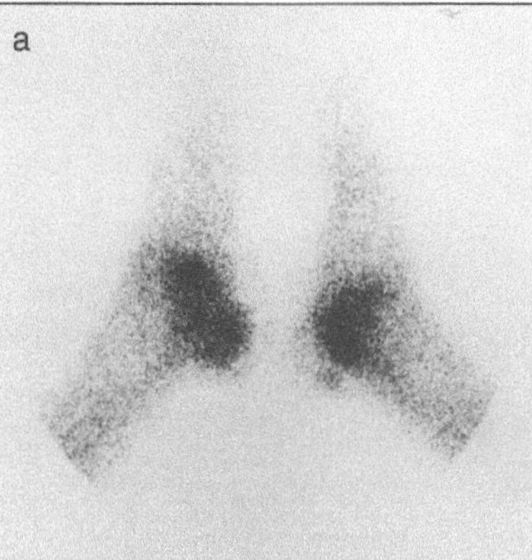

Case 5.34. A 20-year-old female who jumped off a bridge and suffered multiple fractures of the calcaneus and cuboid on both sides as well as the radius on the left, the upper lumbar spine and the ribs. Prior to the bone scan, surgery with insertion of rods in the spine was performed (same patient as in Case 5.63).

Fig. 5.34a. Lateral blood pool image of the feet shows abnormal increased uptake of isotope in the calcaneus on both sides

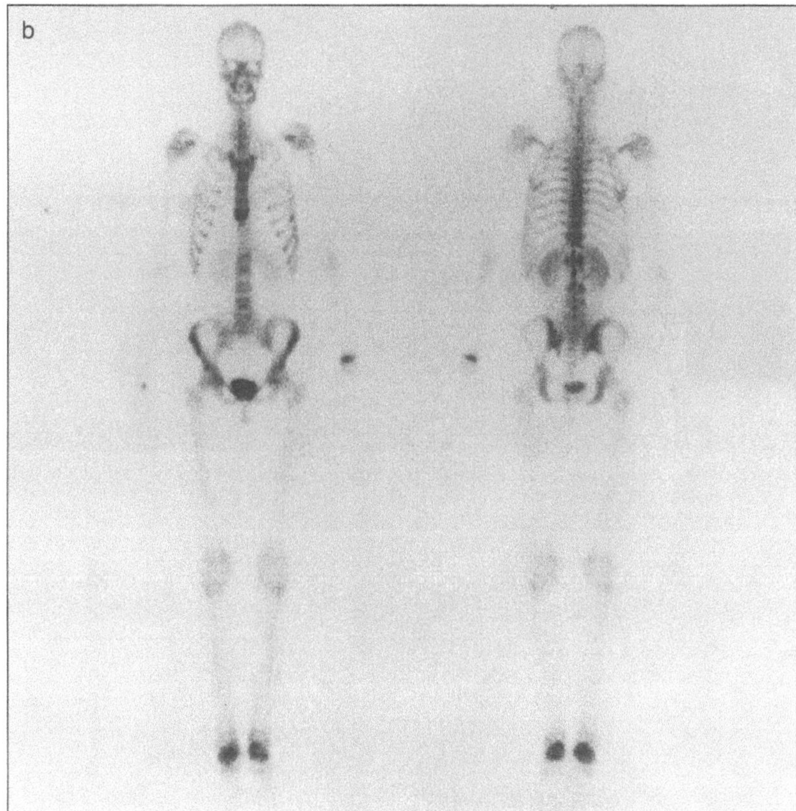

Fig. 5.34b. Whole body images show absent activity in the mid lumbar spine and increased activity in the lower sternum and the lower ribs left ventro-laterally. There is increased activity in the feet bilaterally. Retention of tracer by the kidneys is noted

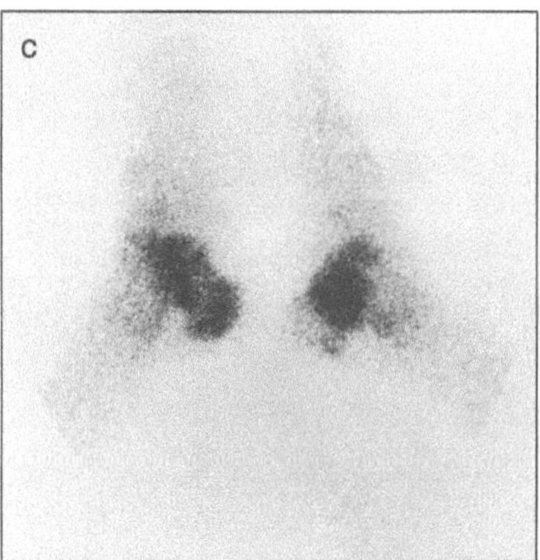

Fig. 5.34c. Lateral image of the feet shows abnormal increased uptake of isotope in the calcaneus and cuboid on both sides

Case 5.35. An 11-year-old girl who had been involved in a motor traffic accident and suffered multiple fractures. The bone scan was undertaken 4 weeks following the accident

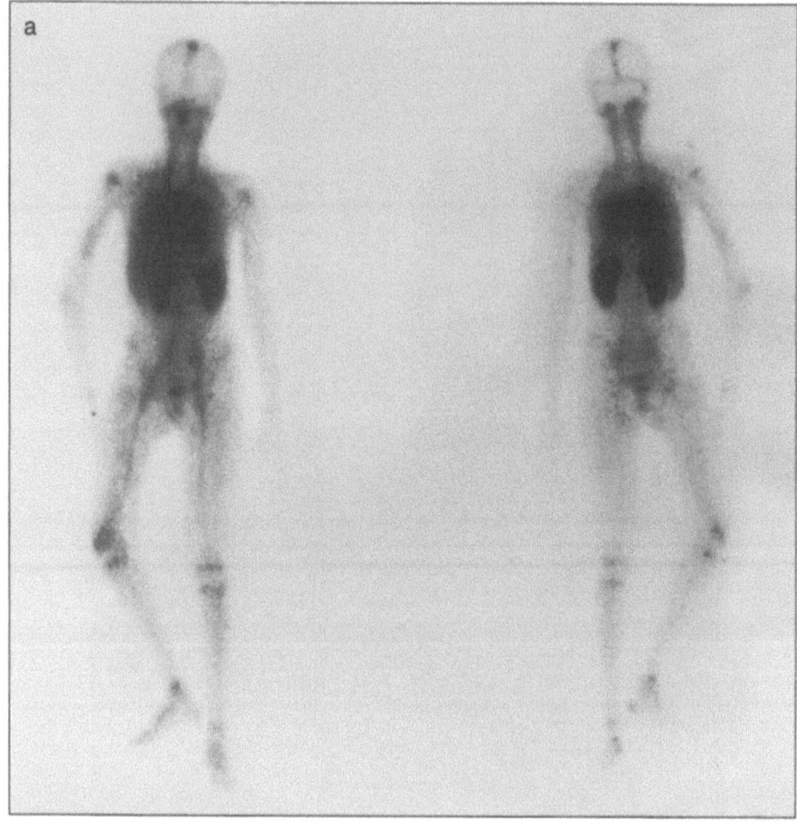

Fig. 5.35a. Blood pool whole body images show abnormal positioning of the right hip and knee with increased distribution of isotope in the distal right femur and right humerus

Fig. 5.35b. Whole body images show abnormal increased uptake of isotope in the right shoulder joint, the right humerus and the left clavicle as well as in the distal right femur. Marked asymmetry between the hips is noted. This is of no significance and related to the positioning of the child who had a fixed flexion deformity of the right lower limb

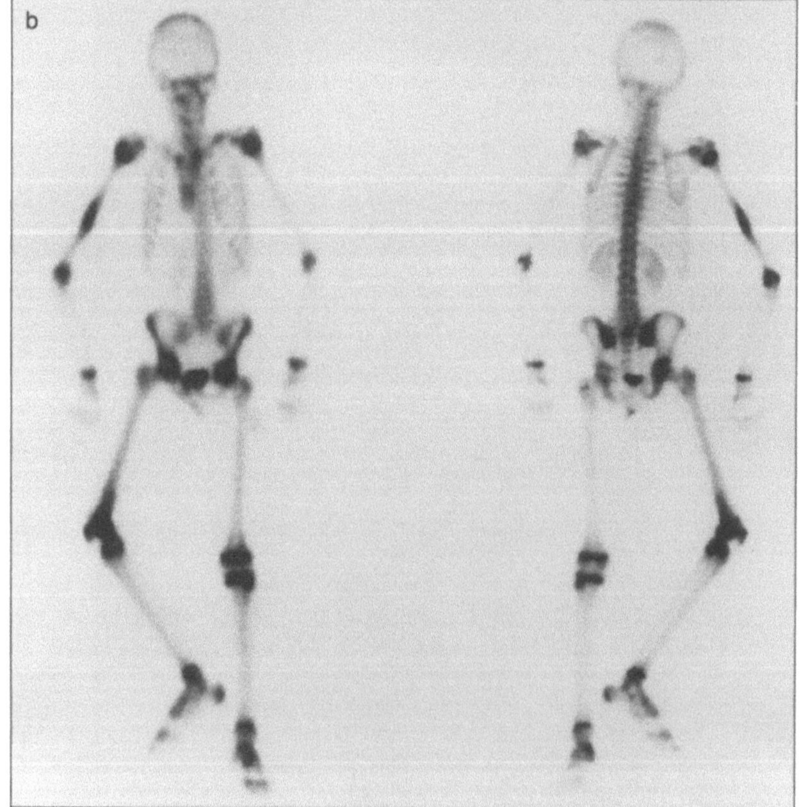

Technical Comment
The sternum is difficult to evaluate on the anterior view due to the obliquety of the position of the child.

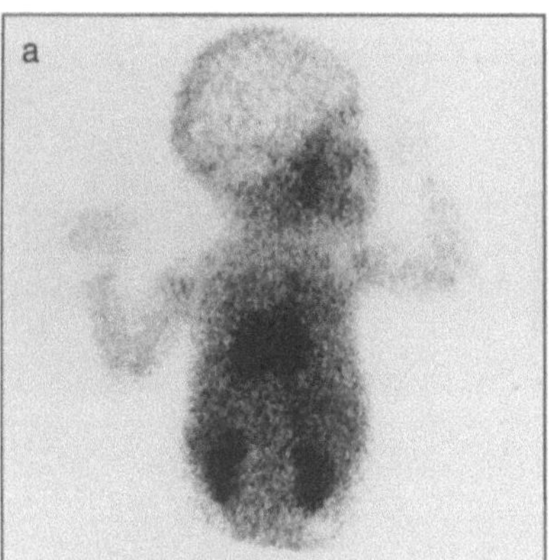

5.3.2 Battered Child
(8 Cases; Figs. 5.36–5.43)

Case 5.36. A 2-month-old battered baby boy

Fig. 5.36a. Blood pool posterior view of thorax, abdomen, upper limbs and right lateral skull. No obvious abnormality is seen

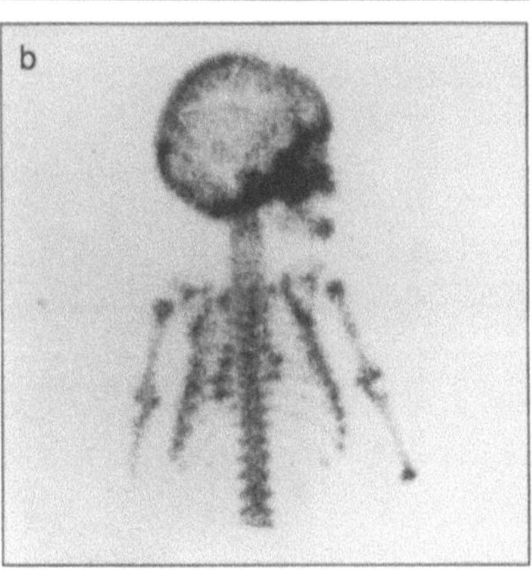

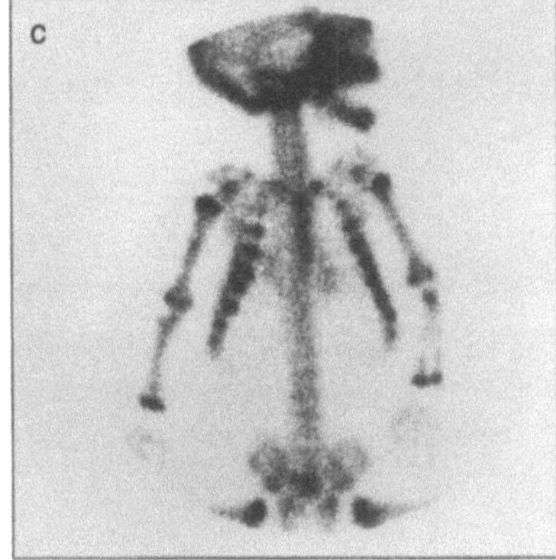

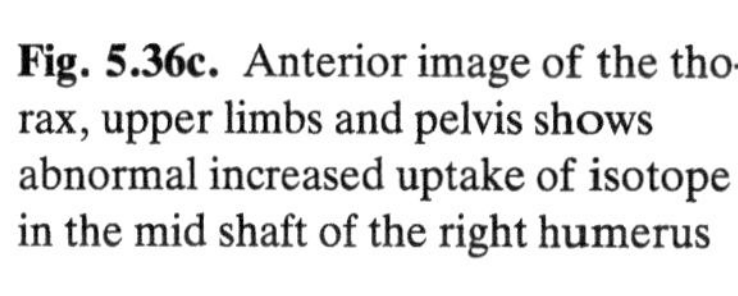

Fig. 5.36b. Posterior image of the spine, thorax, upper limbs and right lateral skull. There is increased uptake of isotope in the mid shaft of the right humerus. Abnormal increased uptake of isotope is noted in four posterior ribs on the left and in two on the right

Fig. 5.36c. Anterior image of the thorax, upper limbs and pelvis shows abnormal increased uptake of isotope in the mid shaft of the right humerus

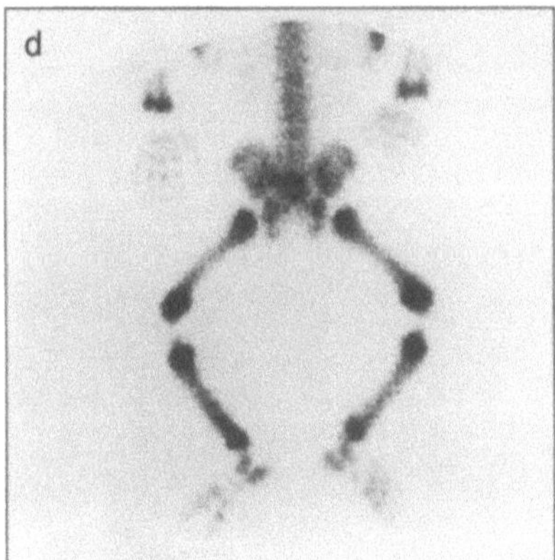

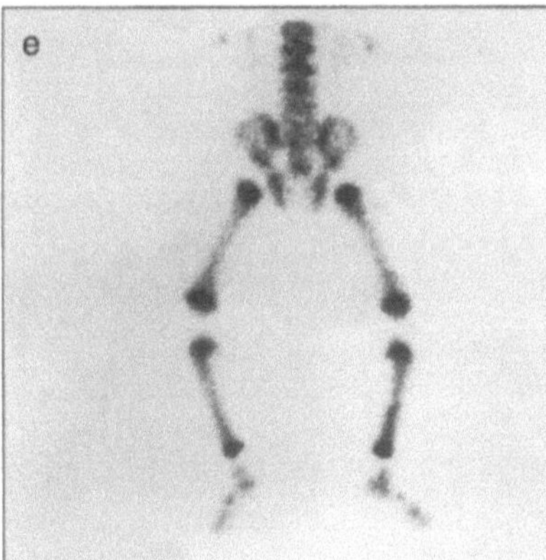

Fig. 5.36d. Anterior image of the pelvis and lateral lower limbs shows abnormal increased uptake of isotope in the right tibia or fibula

Fig. 5.36e. Posterior image of the pelvis and lower limbs shows the abnormal increased uptake of isotope in the distal right tibia or fibula

Technical Comment
1. The normal increased activity in the costochondral junctions (clearly seen in Fig. 5.36c) is the cause of the high rib activity laterally seen in Fig. 5.36b. These normal high areas of activity are a potential pitfall.
2. The postitioning of the knees and feet in Figs. 5.36d and e precludes differentiation between abnormal activity in the tibia and fibula. This poor positioning has resulted in inadequate visualisation of the tibia and fibula.

Case 5.37. A 5-month-old baby girl
who was found to be battered. No
fractures were identified at any stage.
There was an subdural haematoma
which took up the bone tracer

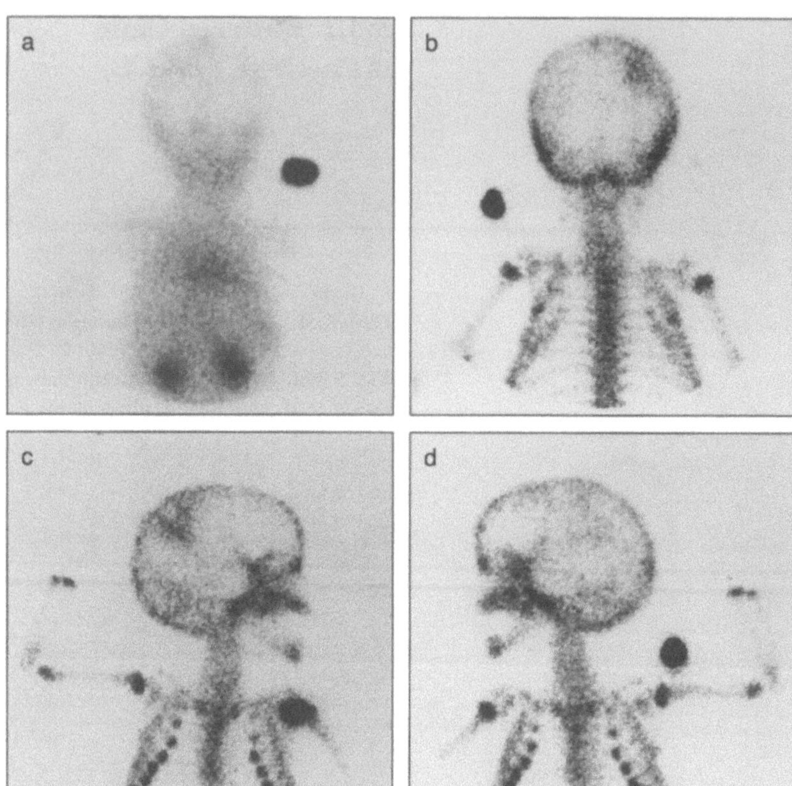

Fig. 5.37a. Blood pool anterior view
of skull, chest and upper abdomen
fails to reveal any abnormality

Fig. 5.37b. Posterior image of the
skull and thorax shows abnormal
increased uptake of isotope in the
region of the right parietal bone

Fig. 5.37c. Right lateral image of the
skull and anterior chest shows abnormal increased uptake of isotope
overlying the parietal bone

Fig. 5.37d. Left lateral image of the
skull and anterior chest is normal

Technical Comment

In all four images there is an artefact due to isotope on the side of the
patient, caused by the injection system. In Fig. 5.37c it overlies the left
shoulder.

Teaching Point

1. It is unusual for a haematoma to take up the isotope, but this appearance
   would be most unusual for a fracture of the skull.
2. For brain uptake of isotope see Case 8.33.

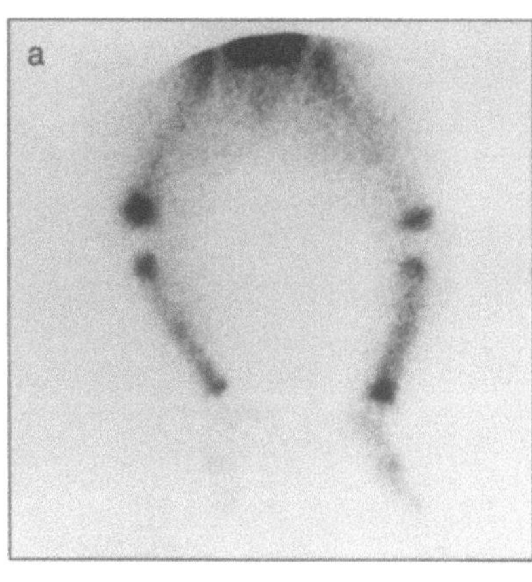 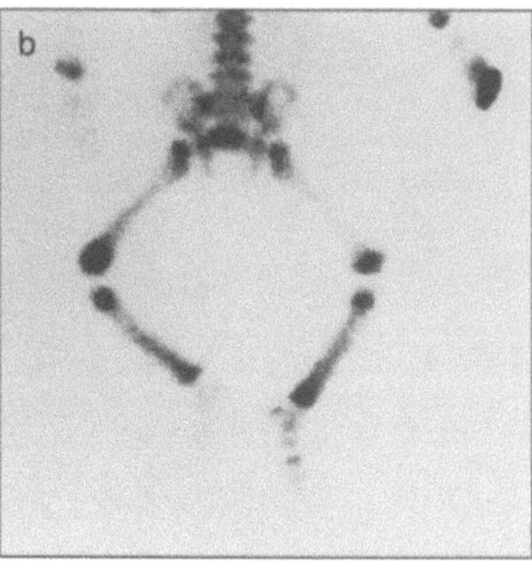

Case. 5.38. A 5-month-old baby boy with multiple fractures due to repetitive trauma (battered child)

Fig. 5.38a. Posterior blood pool image of the lower limbs shows increased uptake of isotope at the distal end of the left femur compared to the right. The distal right tibia shows increased uptake compared to the left. There is very poor blood flow to the left foot

Fig. 5.38b. Posterior image of the lumbar spine and pelvis with the lower limbs in a lateral projection. Increased uptake of isotope is noted in the distal left femur and distal right tibia, due to fractures. Poor accumulation of isotope is noted in the left foot, caused by a haematoma

Technical Comment

The lateral positioning of the lower limbs precludes full evaluation of the tibia and fibula.

Teaching Point

Similar appearances could be due to multifocal infection (see Chap. 2.2.4 "Acute Multifocal Osteomyelitis").

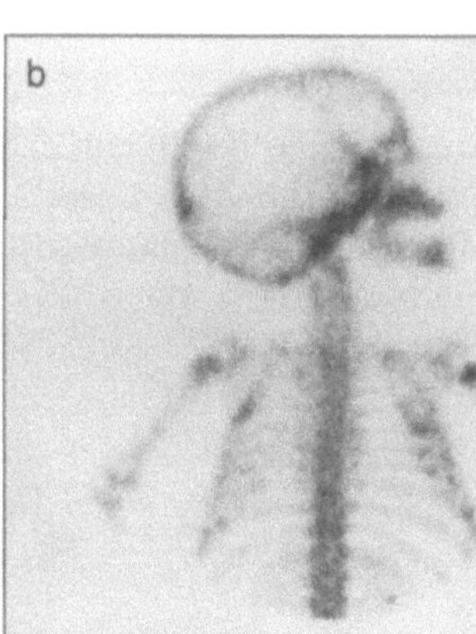

Case 5.39. 8-month-old girl who was a battered child

Fig. 5.39a. Posterior blood pool image of the upper abdomen, thorax, skull and upper limbs. There is slightly increased blood flow in the right shoulder. Note the extravasation at the site of the injection in the right hand

Fig. 5.39b. Posterior image of the thorax and upper limbs and right lateral skull. Note the increased uptake in the proximal right humeral epiphysis due to a fracture in this area

Technical Comment

Note the appearances of the ribs on the right. This is normal and due to shine through from the hot costochondral junctions.

Case 5.40. A 10-month-old girl who was found to be a battered child

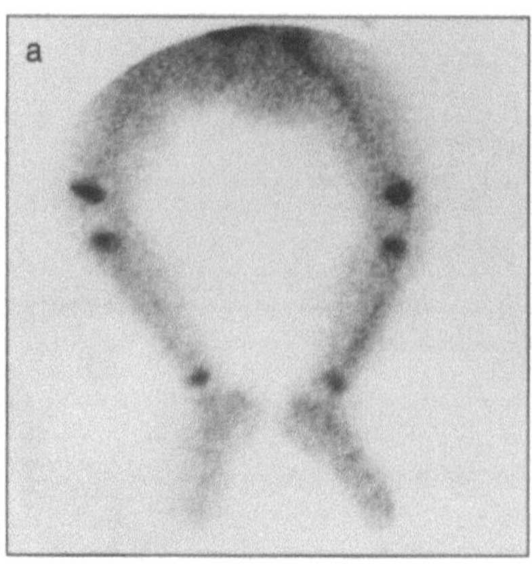

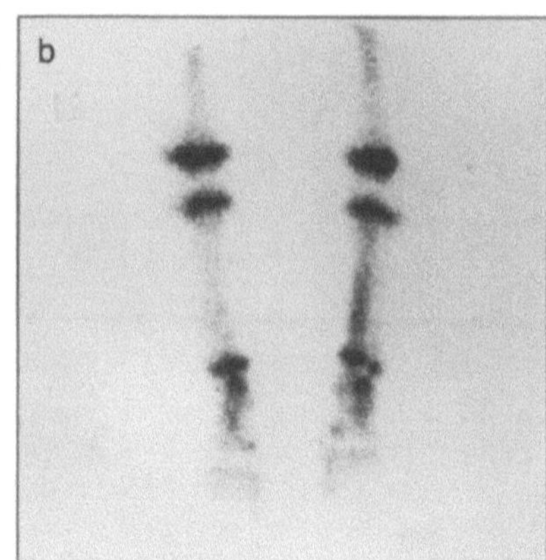

Fig. 5.40a. Lateral blood pool image of the lower legs shows increased uptake throughout the right lower limb

Fig. 5.40b. Posterior image of the lower limbs shows increased uptake of isotope in the distal two thirds of the right tibia due to a fracture

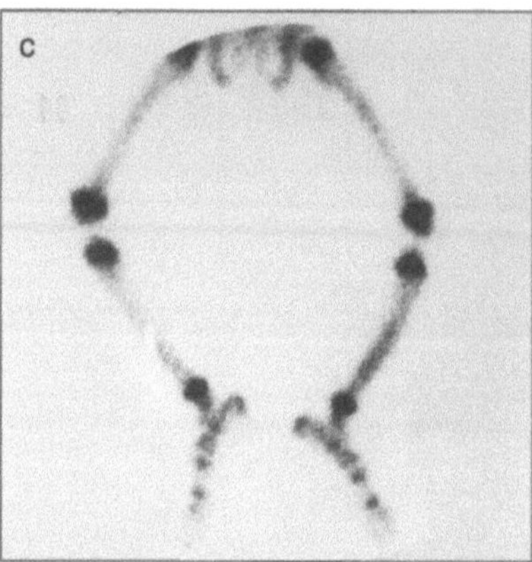

Fig. 5.40c. Lateral image of the lower limbs shows abnormal increased uptake in the right tibia

Teaching Point

In some cases it may be difficult to distinguish between a fracture of the leg and an osteomyelitis (see Cases 2.1–2.3.); however, with infection, the well-defined hot growth plate is lost. Secondaries in the tibia should also be considered (see Case 4.31).

Case 5.41. A 10-month-old girl who had multiple fractures due to battered child

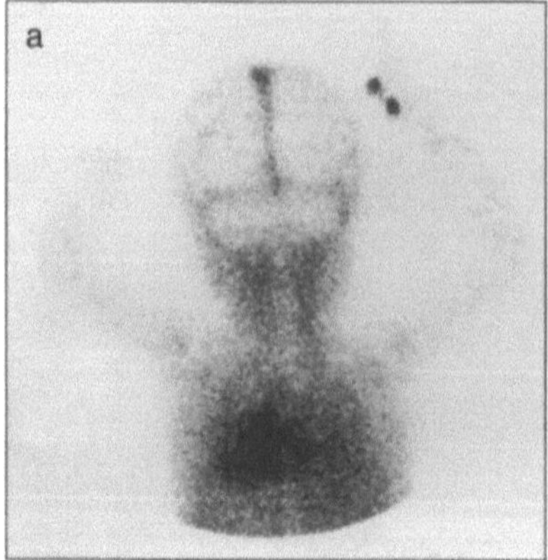

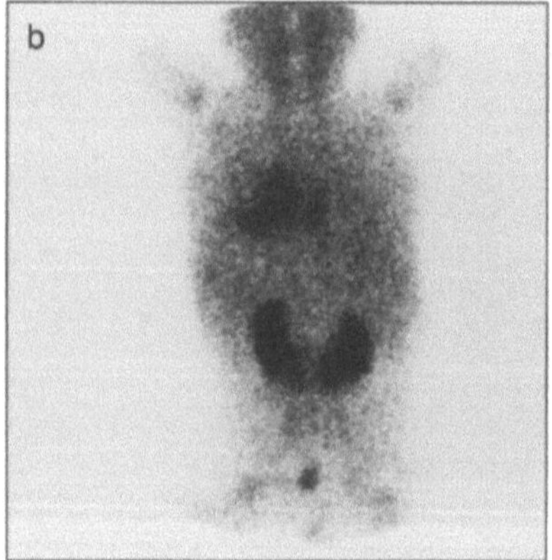

Fig. 5.41a. Posterior blood pool image of the skull, thorax and upper limbs fails to reveal any abnormality. Note the extravasation of isotope in the right hand

Fig. 5.41b. Posterior blood pool image of the thorax and abdomen. The kidneys are clearly seen to be malrotated and joined in the center due to a horseshoe kidney

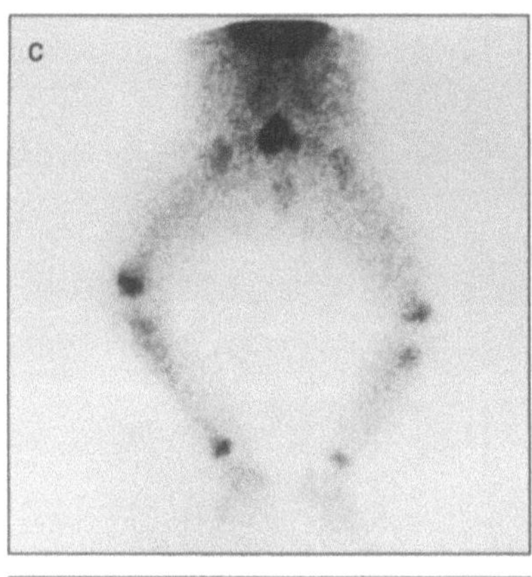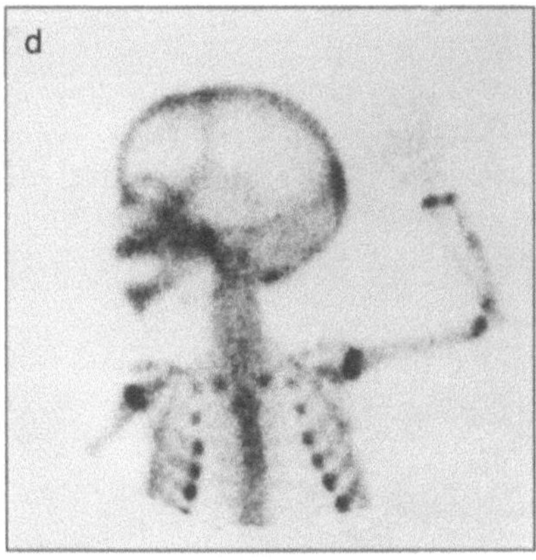

Fig. 5.41c. Posterior blood pool image of the lower limbs shows increased uptake of isotope in both the distal left femoral and tibial epiphyseal plate

Fig. 5.41d. Anterior image of the thorax and left lateral view of the skull and left arm shows abnormal increased uptake of isotope in the left ulna

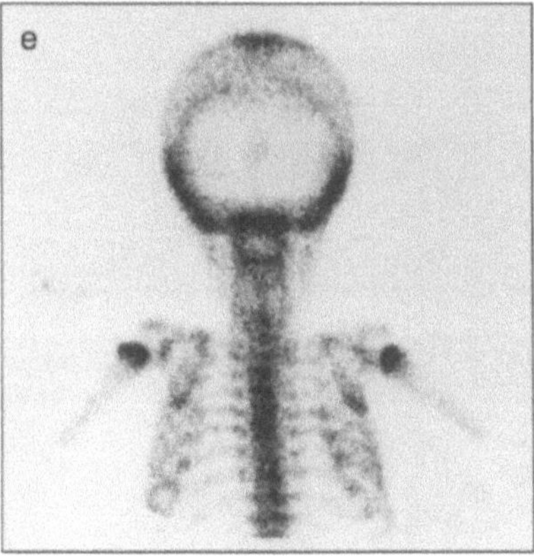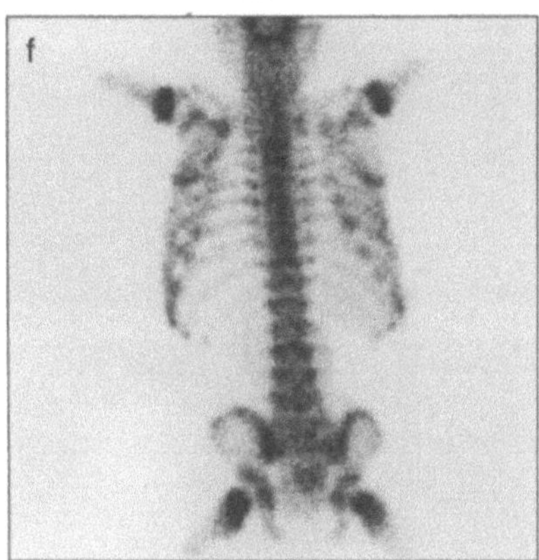

Fig. 5.41e. Posterior image of the skull and thorax shows abnormal increased uptake of isotope in the posterior ribs mainly on the right

Fig. 5.41f. Posterior image of the dorsal and lumbar spine and pelvis shows the abnormal ribs on the right to better advantage

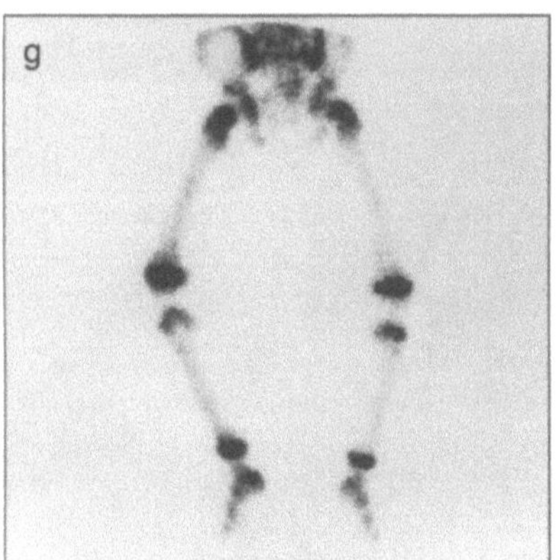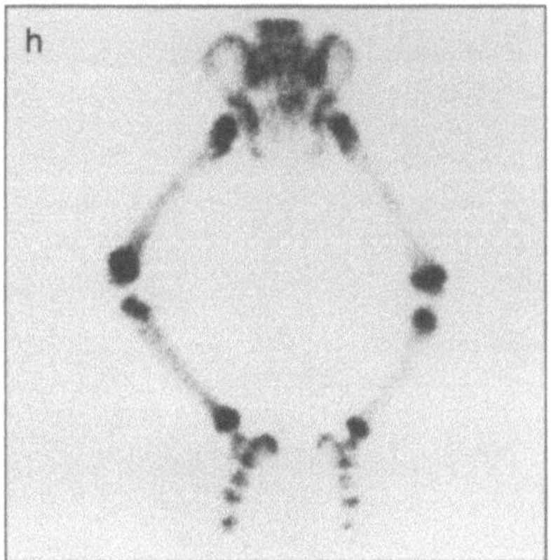

Fig. 5.41g. Posterior image of the pelvis and lower limbs shows abnormal increased uptake of isotope in the epiphyseal plate of the distal left femur and the distal left tibia as well as marked decreased uptake of isotope in the proximal epiphyseal plate of the left tibia. Fractures were found at these sites

Fig. 5.41h. Posterior image of the pelvis and lateral view of the lower limbs and feet. In addition to the previous abnormalities seen in Fig. 5.41g, the left foot shows generalised increased uptake of isotope compared to the right. However, no fracture was seen in the foot

Technical Comment

Note the poor positioning of the lower limbs in Fig. 5.41g. This does not allow adequate evaluation of the lower limbs.

Teaching Point

It may be difficult to distinguish on the posterior view of the thorax a rib fracture from shine through from the anterior costochondral junctions, and oblique views are helpful.

Case 5.42. A 2-year-old battered girl

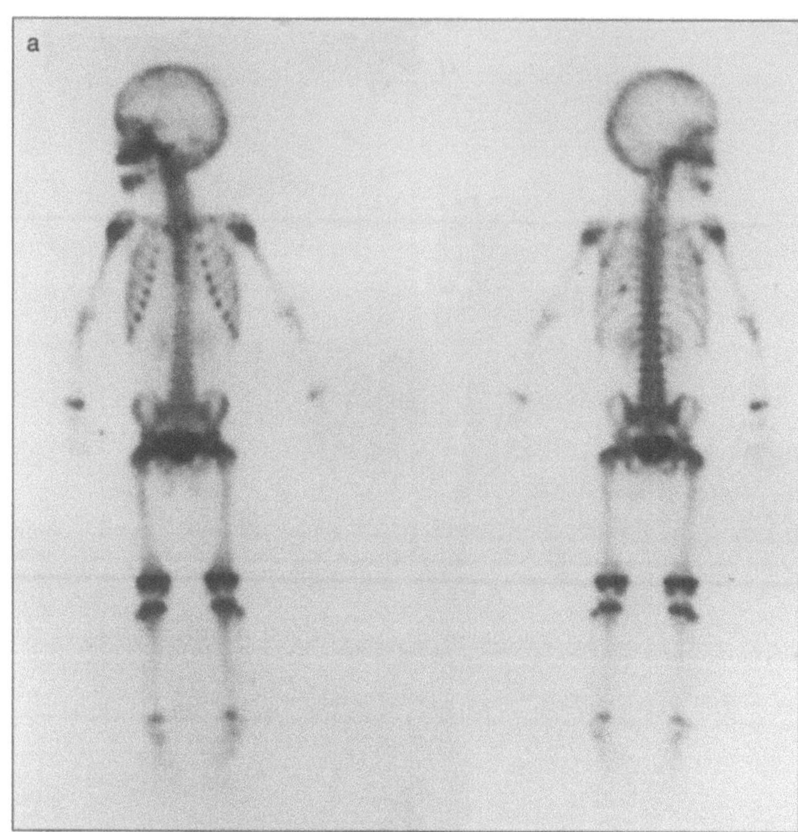

Fig. 5.42a. Whole body scans show abnormal increased uptake of isotope in the posterior aspect of one of the left lower ribs on the posterior view. There is also increased uptake of isotope in the distal right forearm

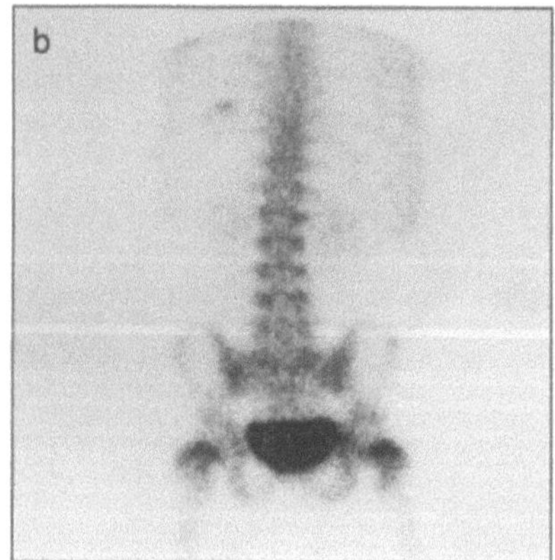

Fig. 5.42b. Posterior image of the lower dorsal and lumbar spine and pelvis shows increased uptake of isotope in the posterior left lower ribs

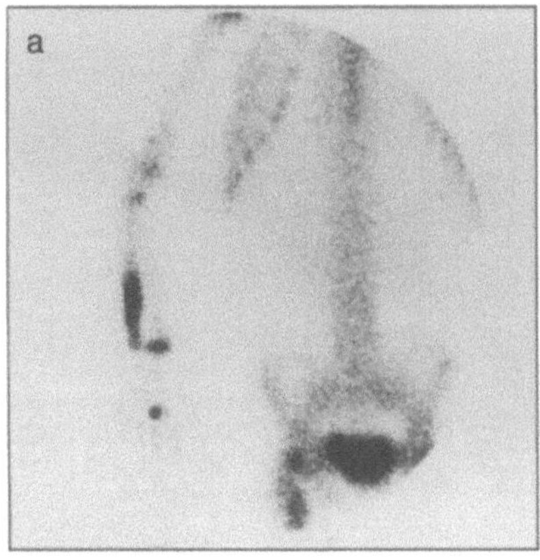
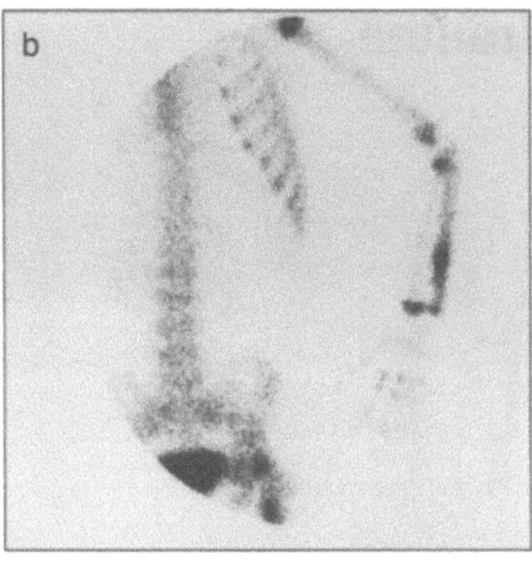
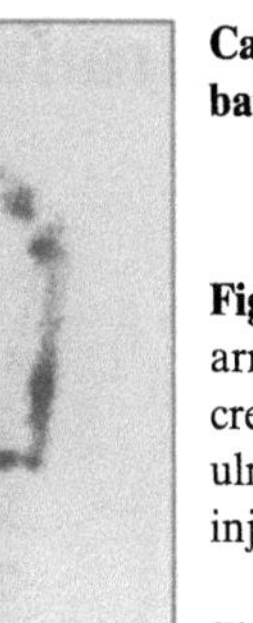

Case 5.43. A 2-year-old boy who was battered

Fig. 5.43a. Anterior image of the right arm and thorax shows abnormal increased uptake of isotope in the distal ulna. Note extravasation due to the injection site in the right hand

Fig. 5.43b. Anterior image of the left arm and thorax shows diffuse abnormal increased uptake of isotope in the ulna

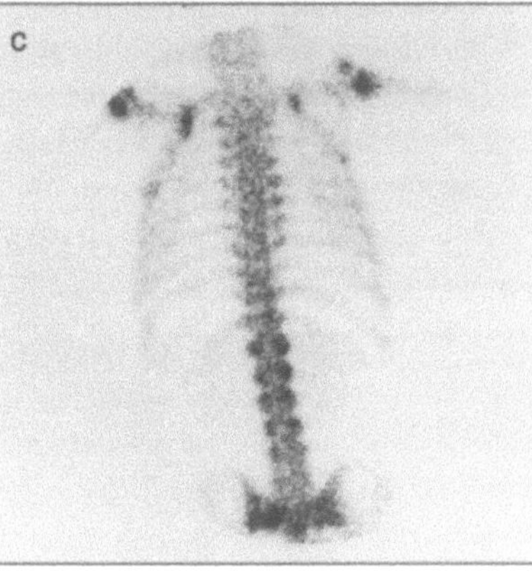

Fig. 5.43c. Posterior image of the spine and pelvis shows abnormal increased uptake of isotope in the posterior aspect of the right sixth, seventh, eigth and ninth ribs, the lumbar spine and the upper left sacro-iliac joint

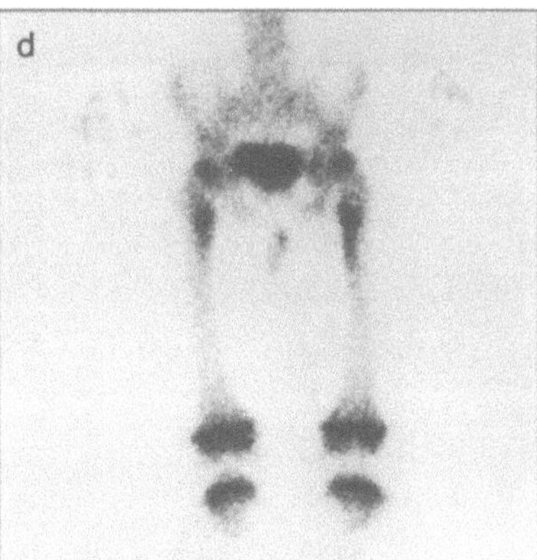

Fig. 5.43d. Anterior image of the pelvis, femora and knees shows abnormal increased uptake of isotope in the proximal shafts of both femora

Teaching Point

The abnormal distal thirds of the ulnae should be easily recognized as pathological and not due to extravasation of isotope at the injection site. It is rare to inject children in the mid forearm region. If in doubt, oblique and/ or lateral views will readily distinguish which is the case.

5.4 Complicaton of Trauma

5.4.1 Pseudarthrosis
(4 Cases; Fig. 5.44–5.47)

Case 5.44. A 6-year-old boy who had suffered trauma which required surgery for a fractured femur. No union was noted at the site of the fracture. The clinical question now arose as to whether osteomyelitis existed within this femur. The result of the bone scan suggested that there was no infection within the bone but pseudarthrosis. (Same child as in Case 5.68)

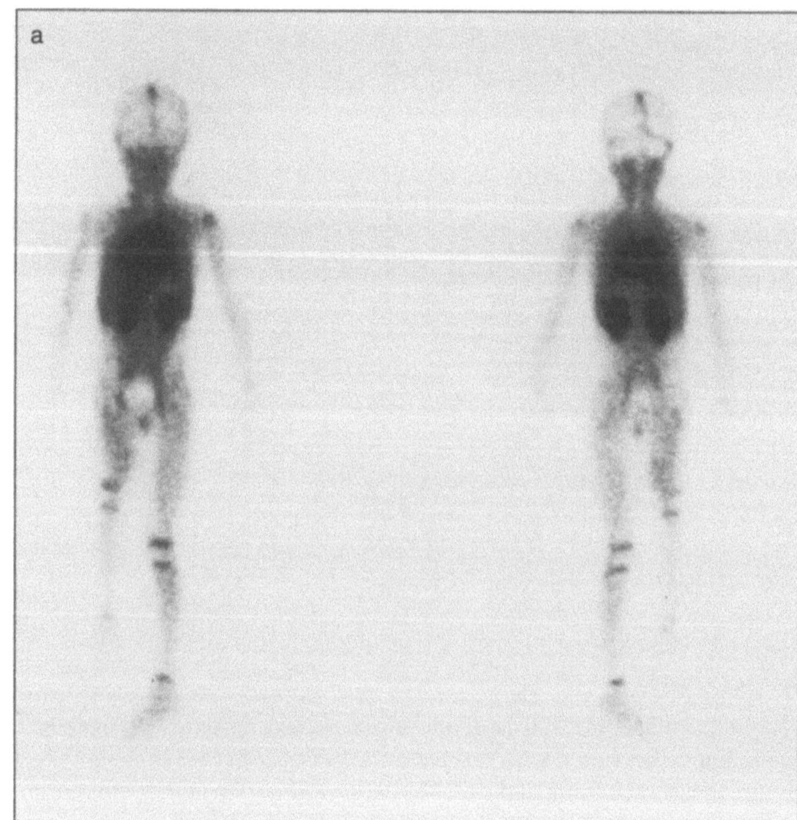

Fig. 5.44a. Blood pool whole body scans show abnormal increased uptake of isotope in the region of the right thigh. The right leg is shorter than the left. Note the photon-deficient area in the region of the bladder. This was due to a full bladder prior to the injection of the isotope

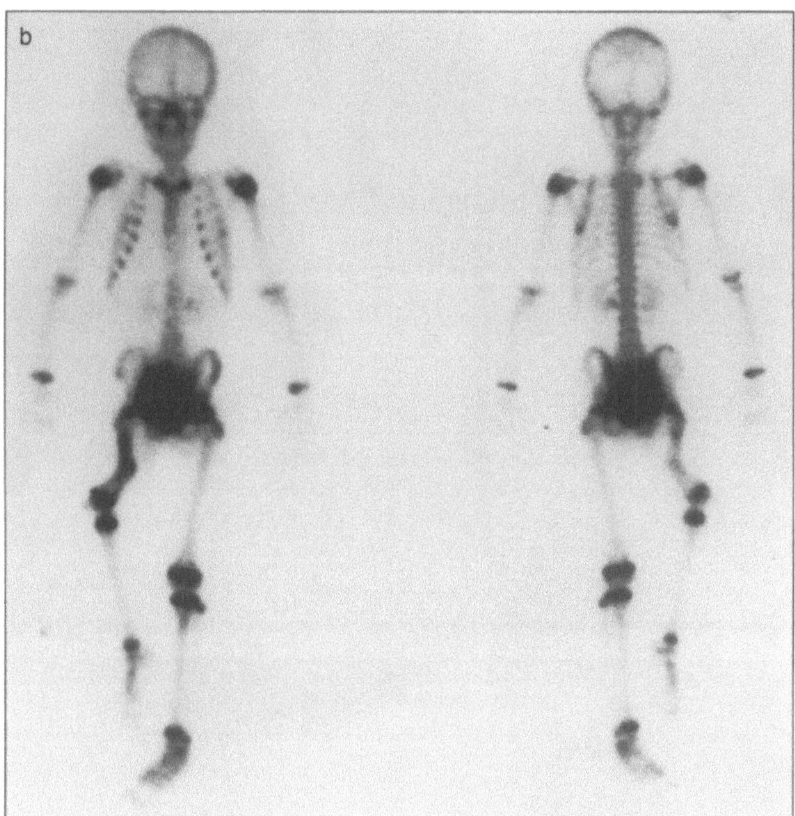

Fig. 5.44b. Whole body images. The abnormal short right femur is noted with increased uptake in the shaft of the femur

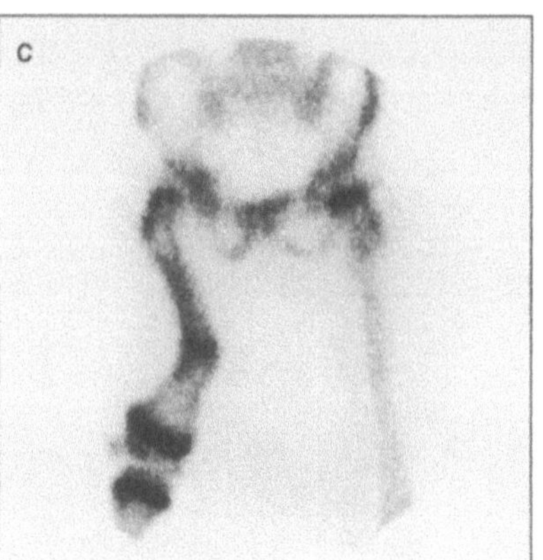

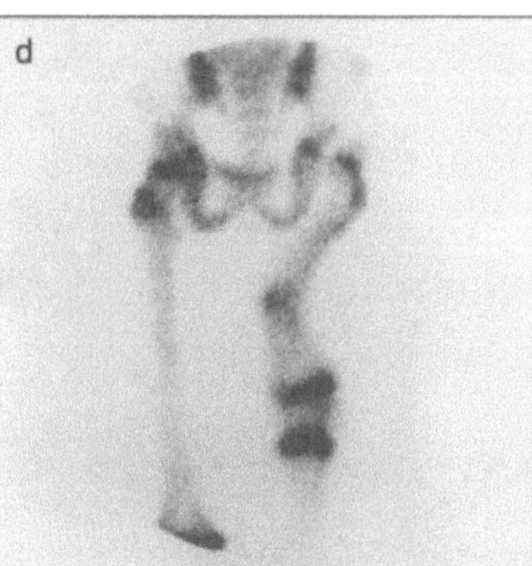

Fig. 5.44 c. Anterior image of the pelvis and femur shows abnormal increased uptake of isotope in the right short femur, confined to the mid portion of the femur with focal increased uptake at the junction of the middle and distal thirds, the site of the pseudarthrosis

Fig. 5.44d. Posterior image of the pelvis and upper femora shows increased uptake of isotope in the deformed short right femur but there is no focal area, over and above the site of the pseudarthrosis, to suggest active infection

Case 5.45. An 18-year-old girl with osteogenesis imperfecta. Following surgery for a fracture, there appeared to be non-union radiologically. (Same patient as in Case 7.27)

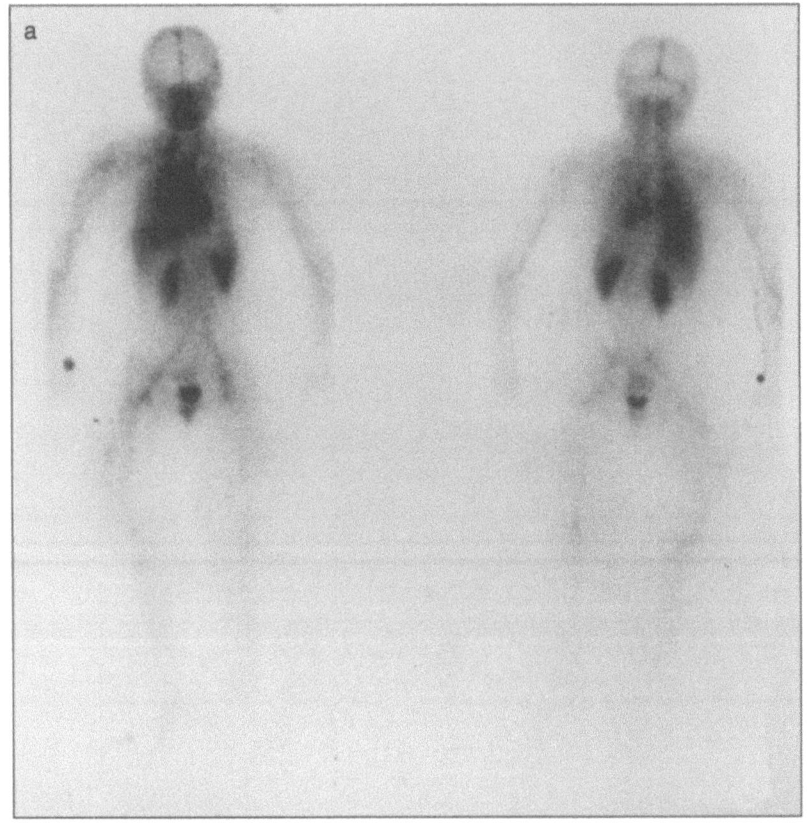

Fig. 5.45a. Blood pool whole body images show rather poor blood flow to the skeleton. Note the extravasation of isotope in the right hand, the site of injection

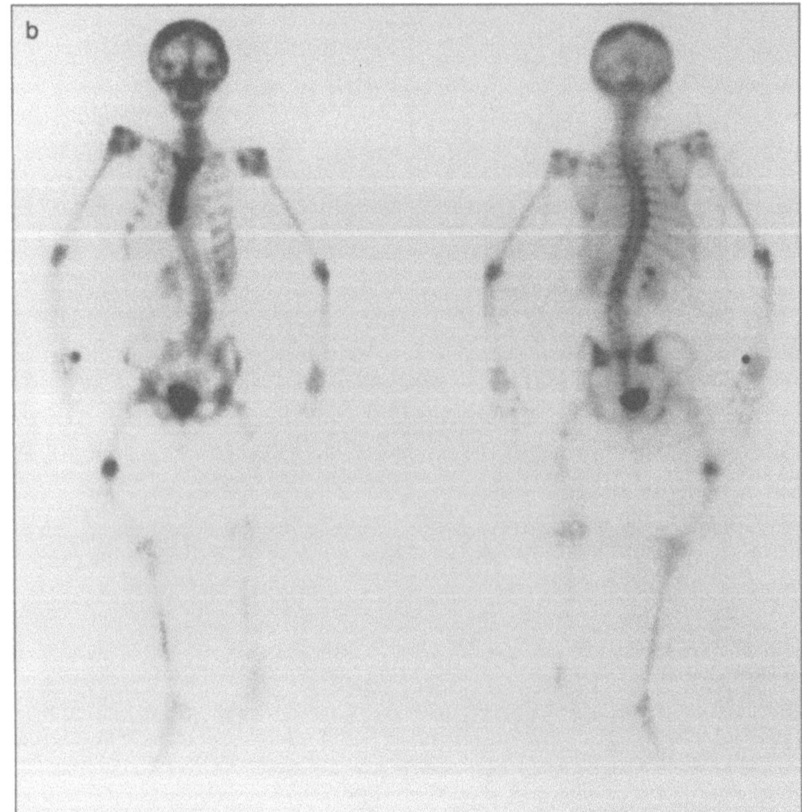

Fig. 5.45b. Whole body scans show poor uptake by the epiphyseal plates throughout the skeleton. All the long bones are deformed. Focal abnormal increased uptake of isotope is noted in the mid shaft of the right femur due to a pseudarthrosis. The scoliosis of both dorsal and lumbar spine is well shown

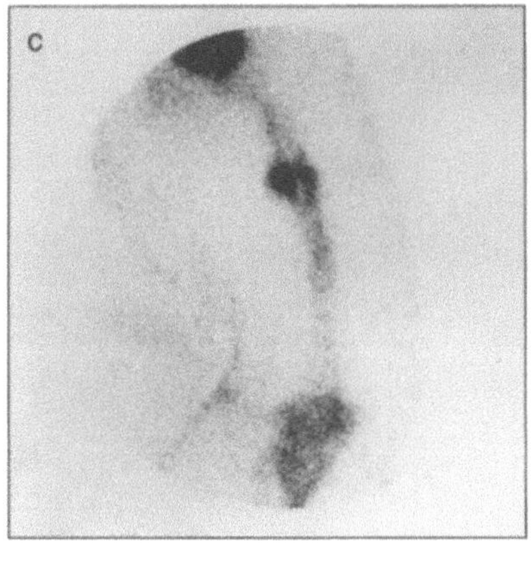 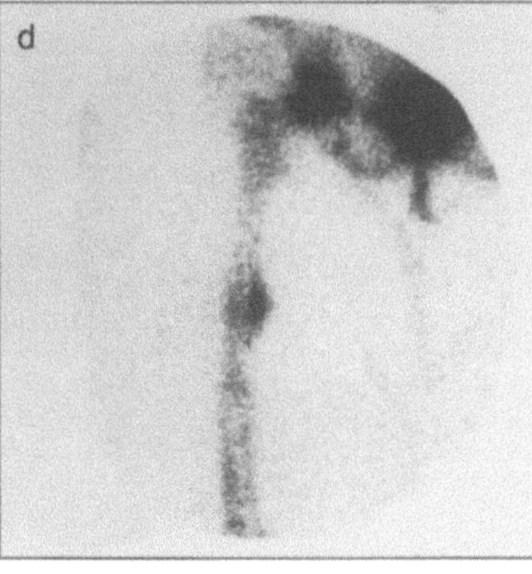

Fig. 5.45c. Posterior oblique image of the right femur shows focal increased uptake in the shaft of the femur, in the region of the pseudarthrosis on X-ray.

The child underwent a follow-up bone scan 9 months later after a lithotrypsy

Fig. 5.45d. Anterior image of the right femur shows focal abnormal increased uptake of isotope in the mid shaft

Teaching Point
Also see Case 7.7 (patient with ostegenesis imperfecta).

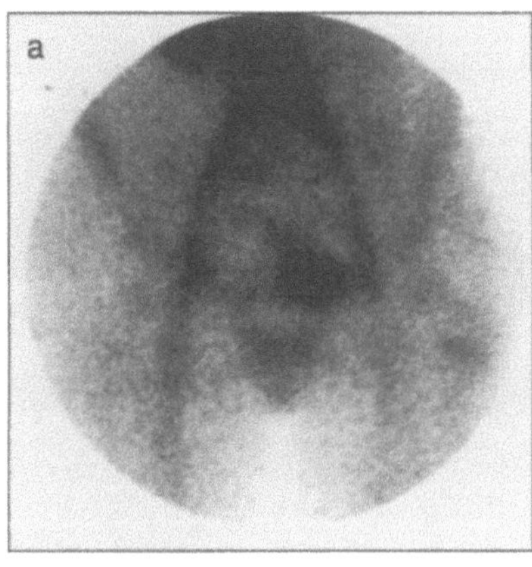 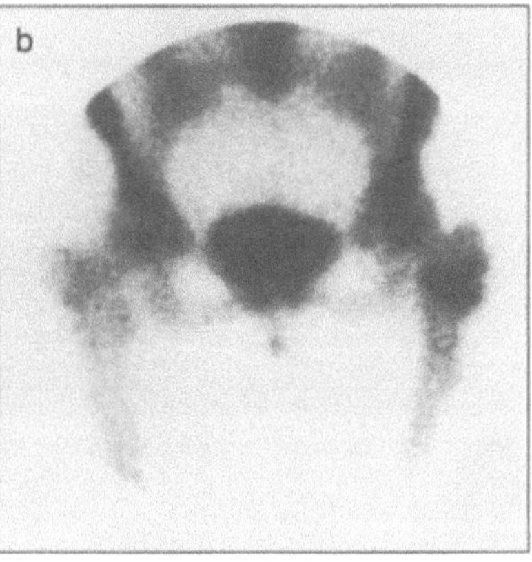

Case 5.46. A 16-year-old girl who had undergone a rotational osteotomy of the left femur 6 months before

Fig. 5.46a. Anterior blood pool image of the pelvis shows increased uptake of isotope in the region of the left proximal femur

Fig. 5.46b. Anterior image of the pelvis and upper femora shows focal abnormal increased uptake of isotope in the proximal shaft of the left femur, the site of the rotational osteotomy

Teaching Point
The appearances of the increased uptake in the femoral shaft are not specific for a pseudarthrosis. This final diagnosis can only be made by taking the history together with the length of time following surgery and the radiographic appearances.

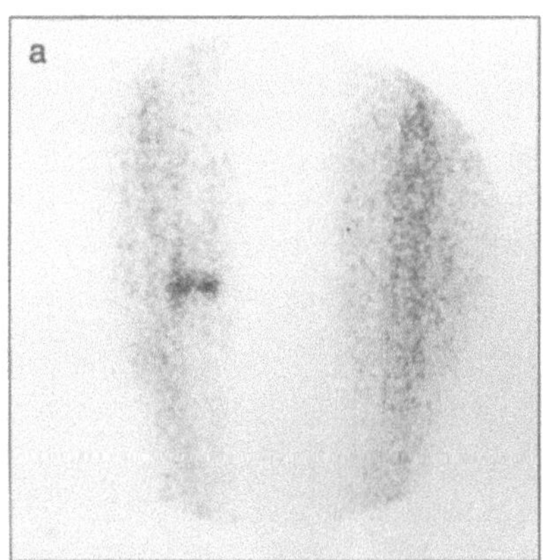 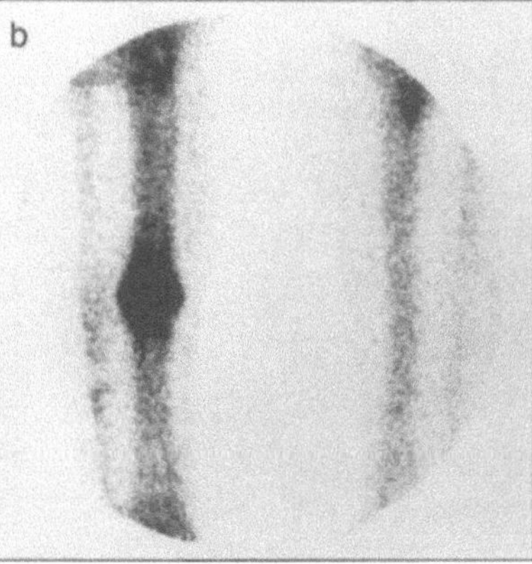

Case 5.47. A 19-year-old boy who had failed to show healing following surgery. A pseudarthrosis of the right tibia was present on X-ray

Fig. 5.47a. Anterior blood pool image of the legs shows abnormal increased uptake of isotope in the mid shaft of the right tibia. The remainder of the right calf shows decreased blood flow

Fig. 5.47b. Anterior view of the tibiae and fibulae. There is marked increased uptake of isotope in the mid shaft of the right tibia, the site of the pseudarthrosis

5.4.2 Infection with Trauma
(1 Case; Fig. 5.48)

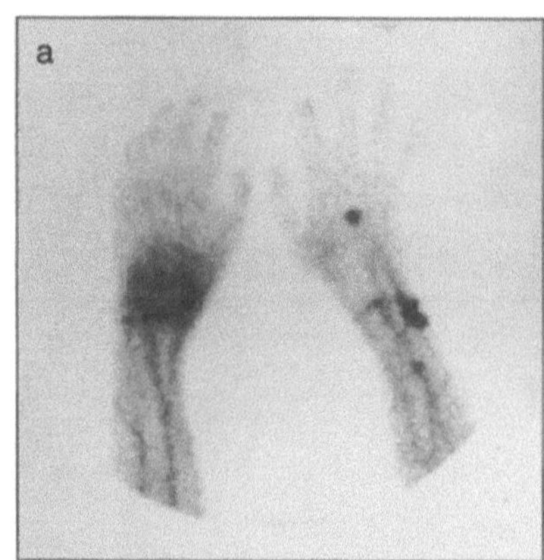

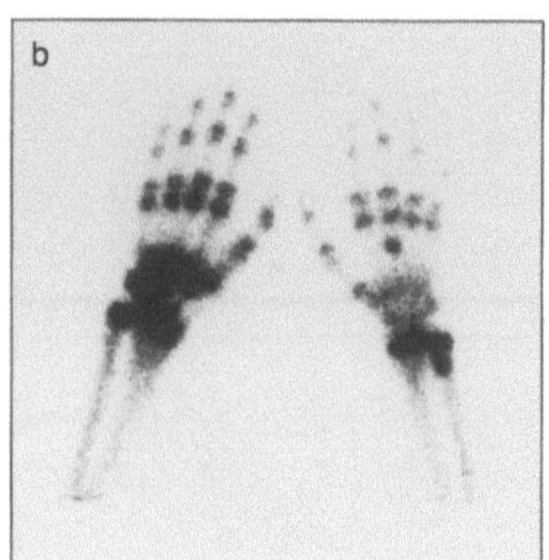

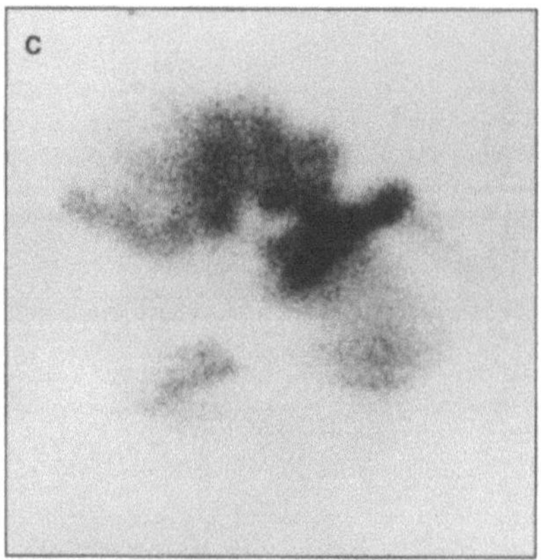

Case 5.48. A 10-year-old boy who had suffered a horse bite of the right hand. He developed cellulitis with an abscess and avascular necrosis of the os naviculare of the right wrist

Fig. 5.48a. Palmar blood pool image of the hands shows marked increased uptake of isotope in the region of the right wrist joint. Note extravasations of the isotope at the site of injection in the left hand

Fig. 5.48b. Palmar image of the hands shows increased uptake throughout the epiphyses of the hand as well as in the small bones of the wrist. Focal abnormal increased uptake of isotope was noted over the middle metacarpal of the left hand at the injection site

Fig. 5.48c. Pin hole palmar view of the right wrist shows focal absence of activity on the radial side of the wrist.

A follow-up bone scan was undertaken 4 months later

Fig. 5.48d. Blood pool image of the hands shows now only slight increased uptake of isotope in the right wrist and decreased uptake of isotope in the epiphyseal plate of radius, ulna and small joints

Fig. 5.48e. Palmar image of the hands. There is now a decreased uptake in the distal radial and ulna epiphyseal plates. The right wrist shows decreased uptake of isotope especially in the region of the naviculare

Fig. 5.48f. Pin hole dorsal view of the right hand shows that the os naviculare has not recovered

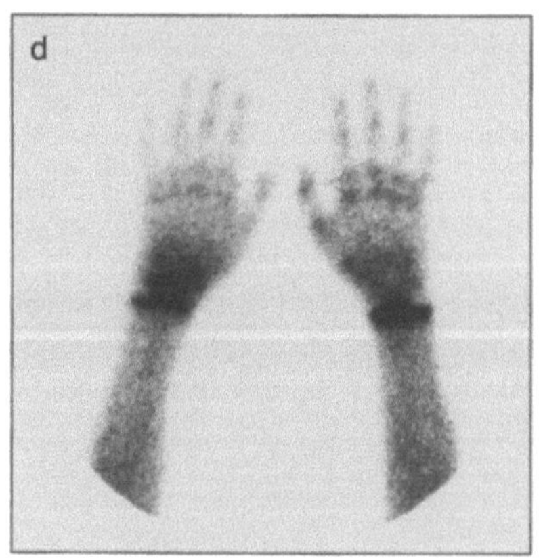

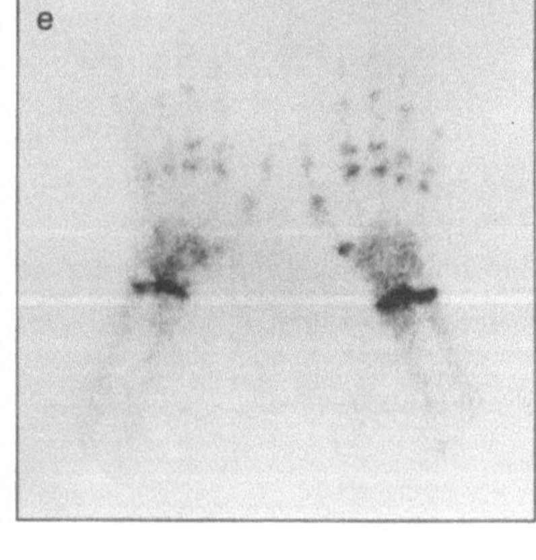

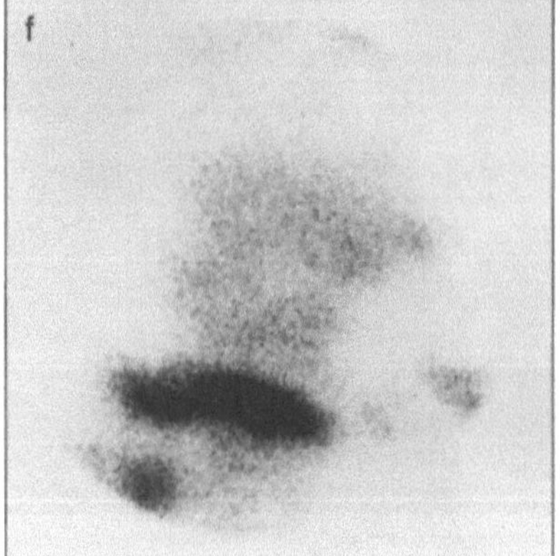

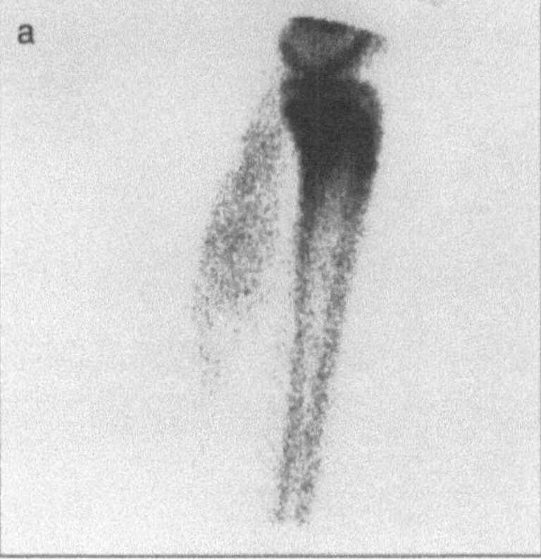

5.4.3 Soft Tissue Damage
(1 Case; Fig. 5.49)

Case 5.49. A 14-year-old girl who suffered pain of the knee following minor trauma. No fracture was seen. This trauma caused damage to the soft tissue only

Fig. 5.49a. Lateral image of the upper tibia shows a normal tibia with abnormal uptake of isotope in the upper third of the calf. A follow-up bone scan 2 months later was normal (not illustrated)

Teaching Point

The abnormal uptake of isotope in the soft tissue represents damage to the tissue. This could either be due to a haematoma or damage to the muscle.

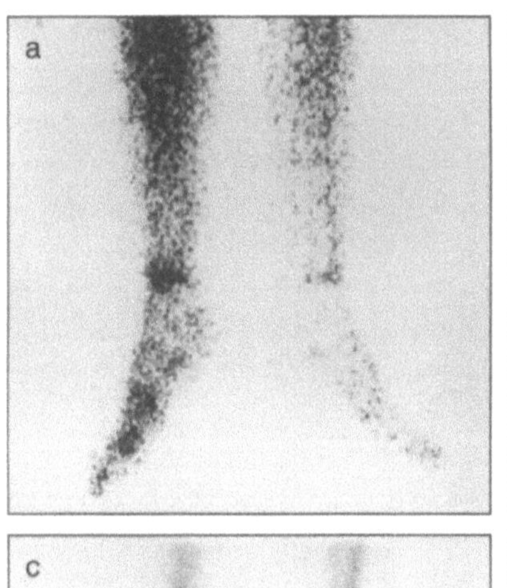

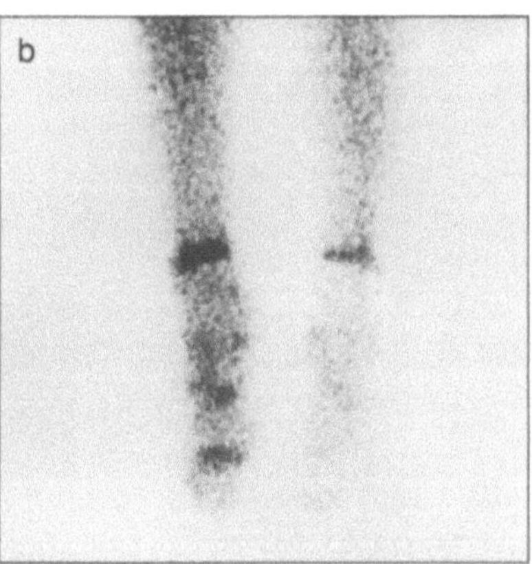

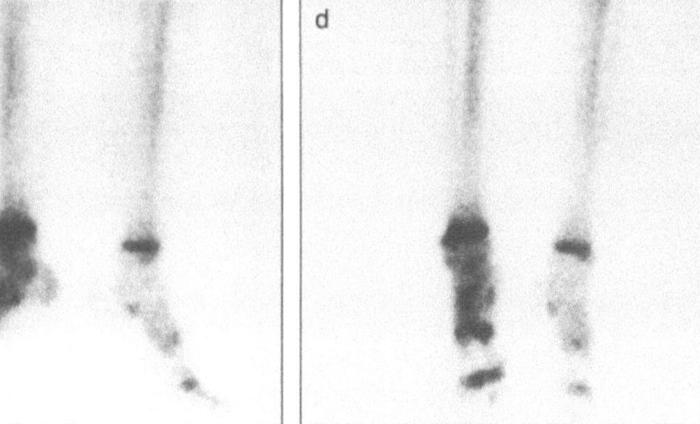

5.4.4 Reflex Sympathetic Dystrophy – Sudeck's Atrophy
(3 Cases; Figs. 5.50–5.52)

Case 5.50. A 13-year-old boy with a limp and pain in the left foot due to reflex sympathetic dystrophy

Fig. 5.50a. Lateral image in the blood pool phase of the calves, ankles and feet shows decreased activity throughout the left leg

Fig. 5.50b. Anterior blood pool image of the feet and ankles shows decreased activity in the epiphyseal plates as well as throughout the remainder of the distal calf, ankle and foot on the left

Fig. 5.50c. Lateral image of the feet shows reduced activity throughout the left leg and foot

Fig. 5.50d. Anterior image of the tibiae, ankles and feet shows reduced activity in the left tibia, left ankle and left foot

Teaching Point

The reduced activity in the two phase bone scan is well described and probably represents the later phase of disease. Compare this to Case 5.52.

Case 5.51. An 8-year-old girl who had pain in the left foot and had stopped using the foot due to reflex sympathetic dystrophy following minor trauma

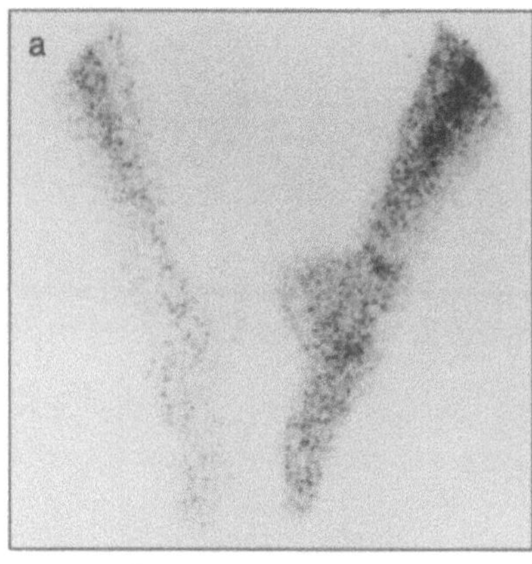
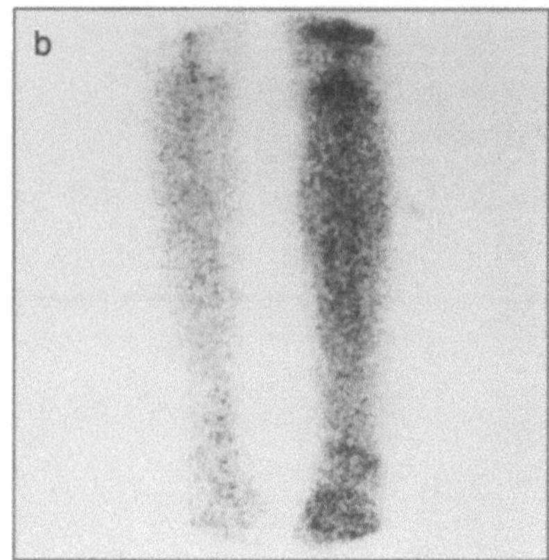

Fig. 5.51a. Blood pool lateral image of the feet shows decreased flow to the left ankle and foot

Fig. 5.51b. Posterior blood pool image of the calves and ankles shows reduced activity throughout the left leg

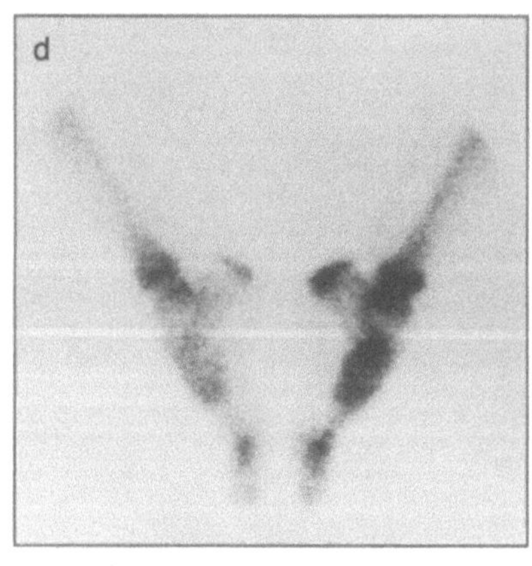

Fig. 5.51c. Posterior blood pool image of the knees shows decreased isotope throughout the left femur, knee and tibia

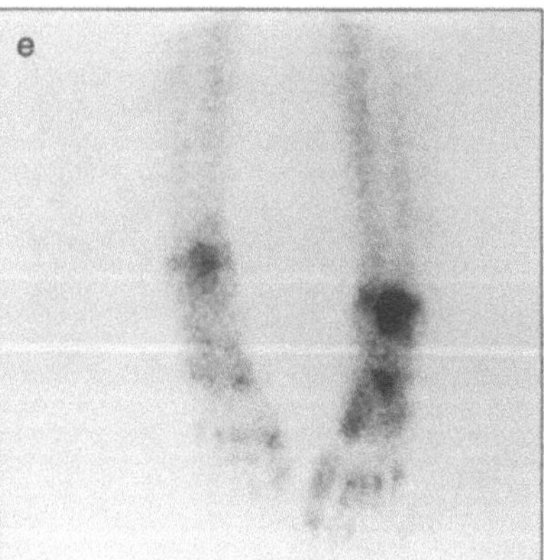

Fig. 5.51d. Lateral image of the feet shows reduced uptake of isotope throughout the bones of the left foot

Fig. 5.51e. Posterior image of the ankles and feet shows decreased activity throughout the left foot

Fig. 5.51f. Posterior image of the knees shows decreased activity in all the bones and the growth plates on the left

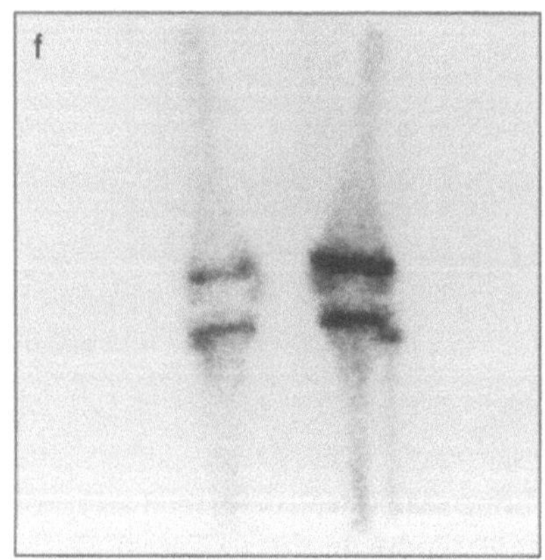

Teaching Point

1. The reduced activity in the two phase bone scan is well described and probably represents the later phase of the disease. Compare this to the next case (Case 5.52).
2. Similar appearances may be seen from disuse arthropathy (see Case 7.33).

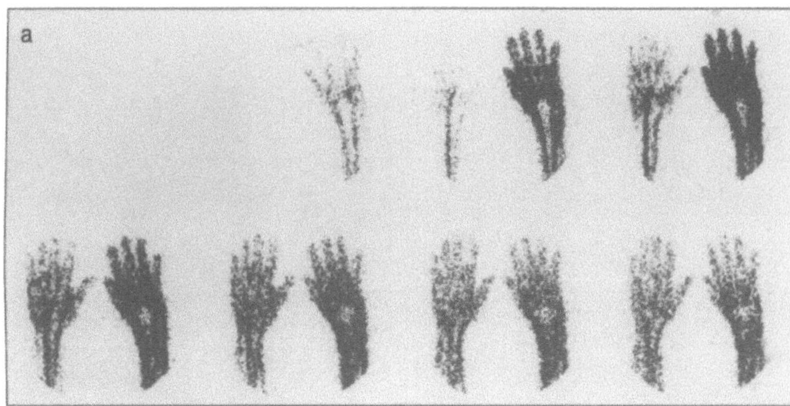

Case 5.52. A 22-year-old female who had pain in the left hand following trauma due to reflex sympathetic dystrophy

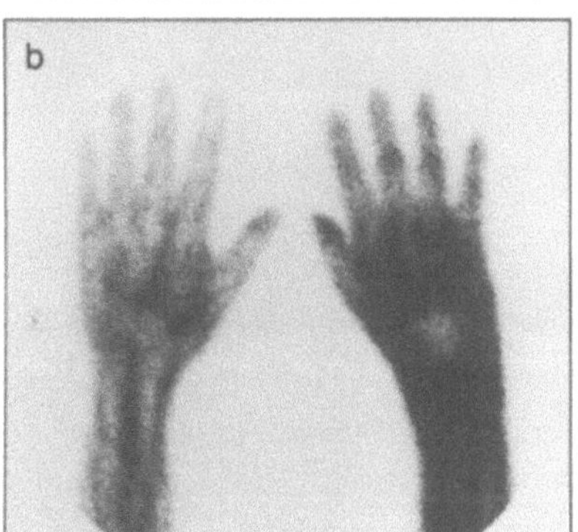

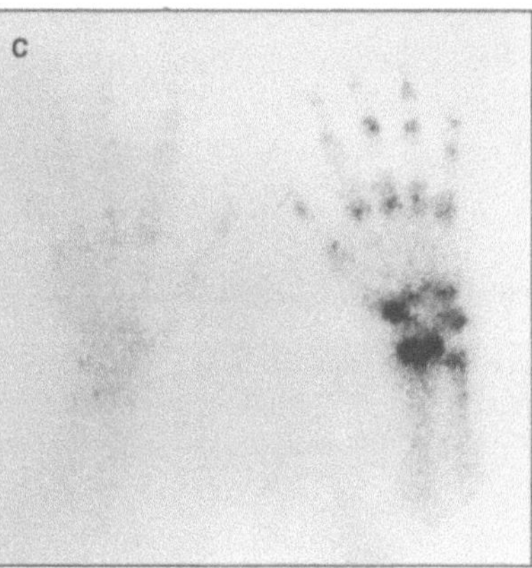

Fig. 5.52a. Blood flow images of the hands show marked disparity between the two forearms and hands with the left showing increased blood flow, especially in the finger joints, compared to the right

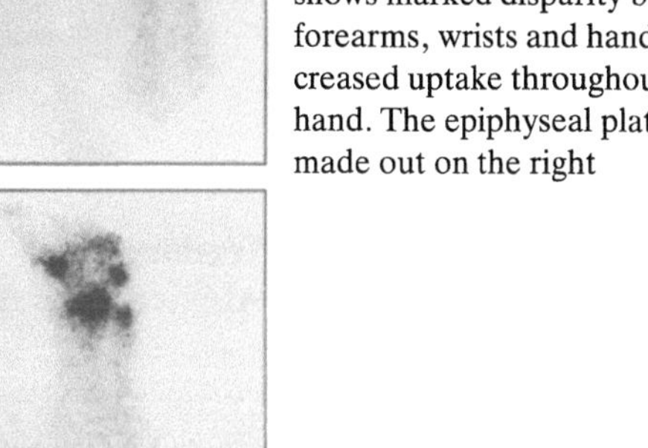

Fig. 5.52b. Palmar blood pool image of the hands shows disparity between the forearms and hands with the left showing increased isotope compared to the right

Fig. 5.52c. Palmar image of the hands shows marked disparity between the forearms, wrists and hands with increased uptake throughout the left hand. The epiphyseal plates cannot be made out on the right

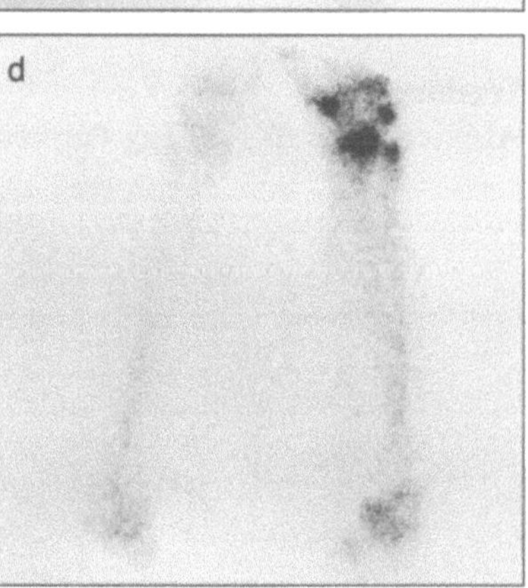

Fig. 5.52d. Posterior image of the forearms shows increased uptake throughout the left forearm

Teaching Point

1. The blood flow and blood pool images allow the diagnosis of reflex sympathetic dystrophy to be made with confidence. The focal abnormal increased uptake of isotope noted in the wrist on the late images is not typical of the syndrome and suggests localised trauma to the small bones of the wrist.

2. Compare these blood pool images with those of the previous two cases (Cases 5.50, 5.51), which show the less common appearances of reduced activity thought to be the late phase of this disease.

5.4.5 Necrosis of Bone
(1 Case; Fig. 5.53)

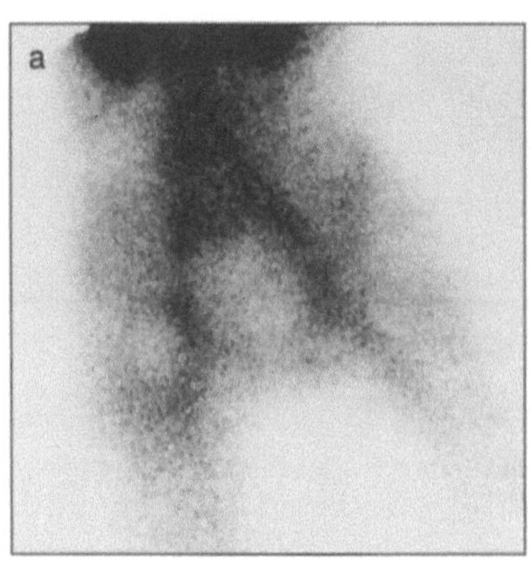
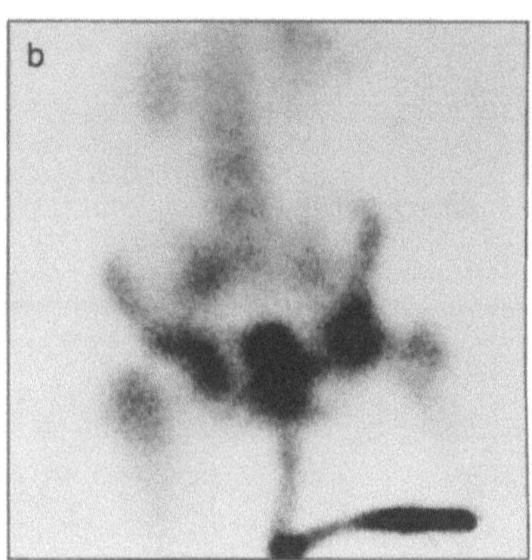

**Case 5.53. A 12-year-old girl suffe-
ring from a traumatic avascular necrosis of the head of the right femur**

Fig. 5.53a. Anterior blood pool
image of the pelvis shows absent activity in the region of the right hip

Fig. 5.53b. Anterior view of the pelvis shows a normal left hip. On the
right there is total absence of activity
of the femoral head and neck. Note
the bladder is on catheter drainage
with isotope seen in the bladder catheter

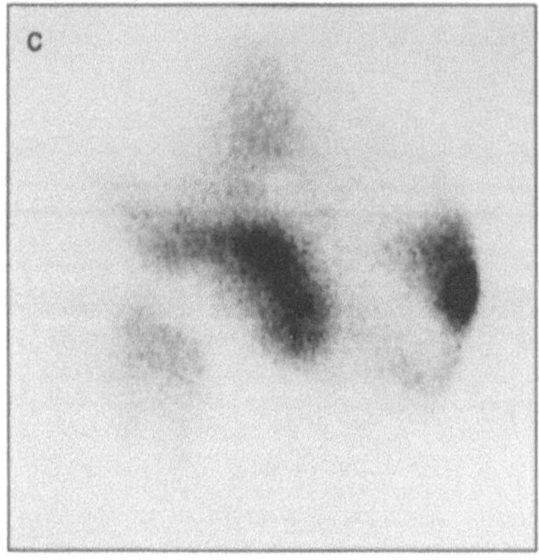

Fig. 5.53c. Pin hole view of the right
hip shows total absence of activity in
the femoral head and neck on the
right

Teaching Point
Also see Chap. 6.1, "Legg-Perthes' Disease".

5.4.6 Growth Arrest
(1 Case; Fig. 5.54)

**Case 5.54. A 10-year-old girl who suf-
fered trauma to her left knee. Final
diagnosis was partial fusion of the
distal left femoral growth plate**

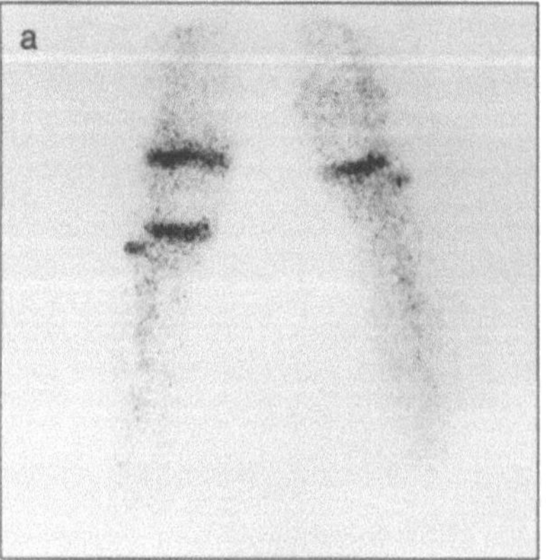
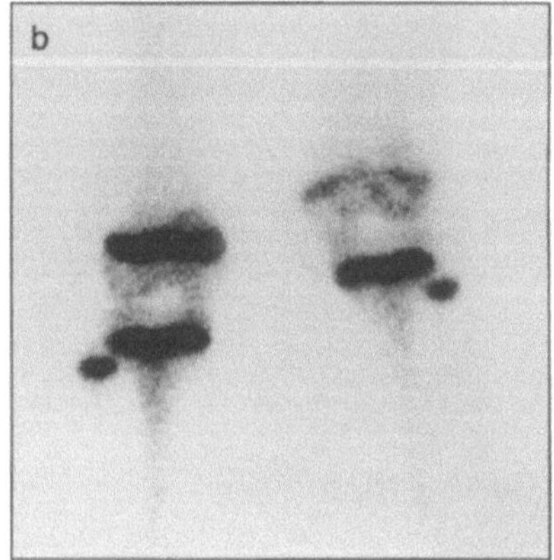

Fig. 5.54a. Anterior blood pool
image shows poor uptake of isotope in
the distal femoral growth plate of the
left knee

Fig. 5.54b. Anterior view of the knee
shows a normal right knee. On the left
in the distal femoral growth plate
there is reduced uptake compared to
the right

Teaching Point
See Cases 2.58, 7.35 and 7.36.

5.5 Bone Response to Underlying Pathology

5.5.1 Pathological Fracture
(1 Case; Fig. 5.55)

> **Teaching Point**
> Fractures may also occur in benign bone cysts (see Chap. 4.1.4.2, "Fractures in a Simple Bone Cyst").

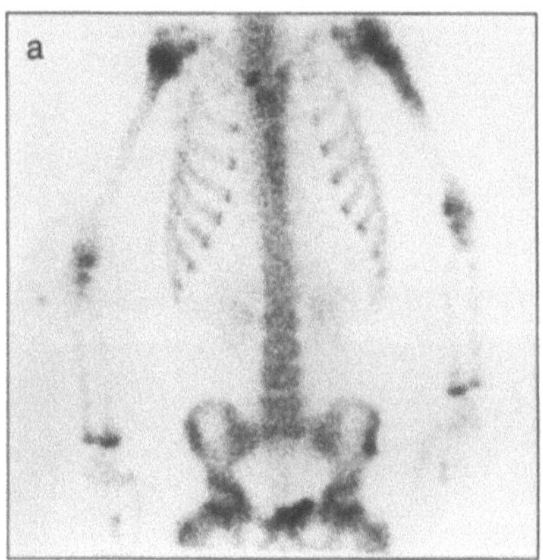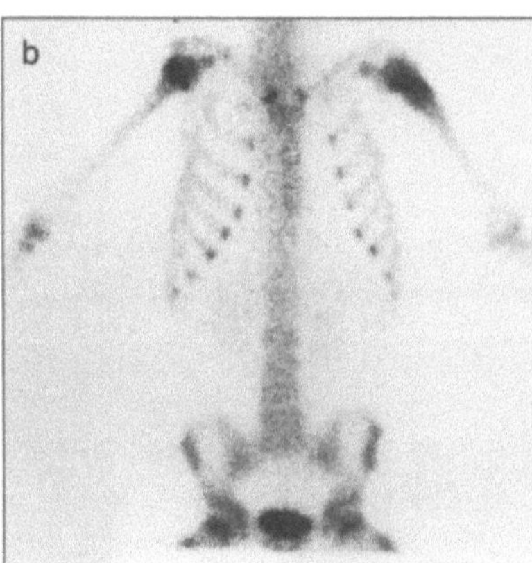

Case 5.55. Ewing's sarcoma of the upper left humerus in an 8-year-old boy

Fig. 5.55a. Anterior image of the thorax and upper limbs shows increased activity in the upper left humerus which cannot be separated from the adjacent epiphyseal plate.

Following treatment, the child presented 2 years later with a pathological fracture through the upper humerus

Fig. 5.55b. Anterior view of the thorax and upper limbs shows abnormal increased uptake in the left humerus extending into the mid shaft of the humerus

Teaching Point
The appearances are due to a combination of therapy of the tumour and a pathological fracture. It is not possible to distinguish between these two simply on the bone scan.

5.2.2 Response to Pressure

(2 Cases; Figs. 5.56, 5.57)

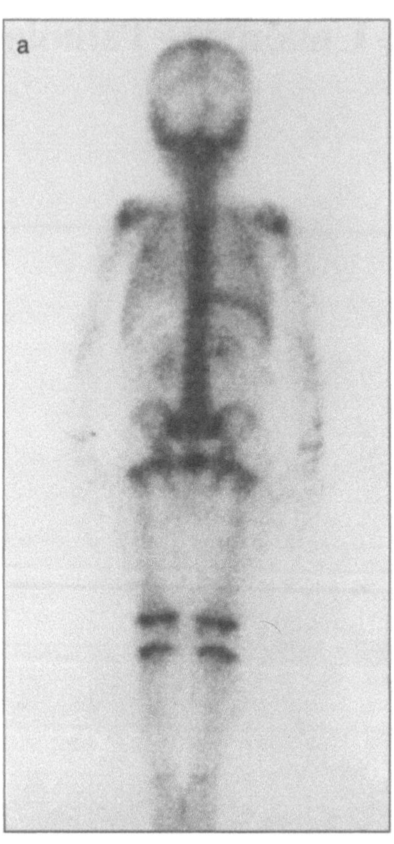

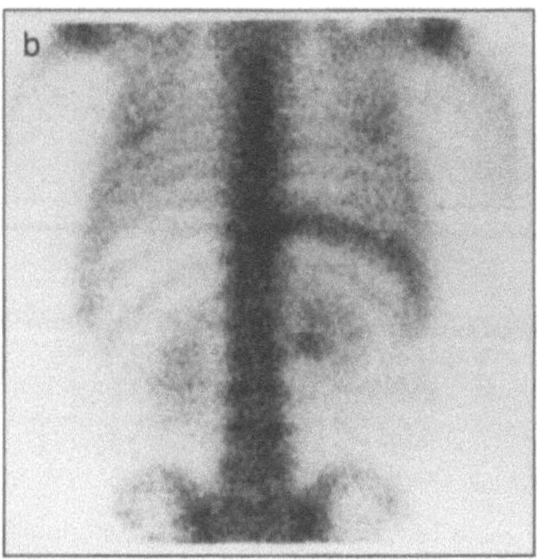

Case 5.56. A 3-year-old boy with a mass in the right side of the chest which had been present for 2 years. The mass was a lipoma on biopsy

Fig. 5.56a. Whole body scan posterior view. There is abnormal increased uptake of isotope in the ribs on the right

Fig. 5.56b. Posterior image of the dorsal and lumbar spine and the thoracic cage shows increased uptake of isotope throughout the right ribs simply due to pressure of the benign slow-growing lipoma

Teaching Point
Similar appearances may be see due to other masses (see Cases 4.28, 4.30, 4.31, 4.40).

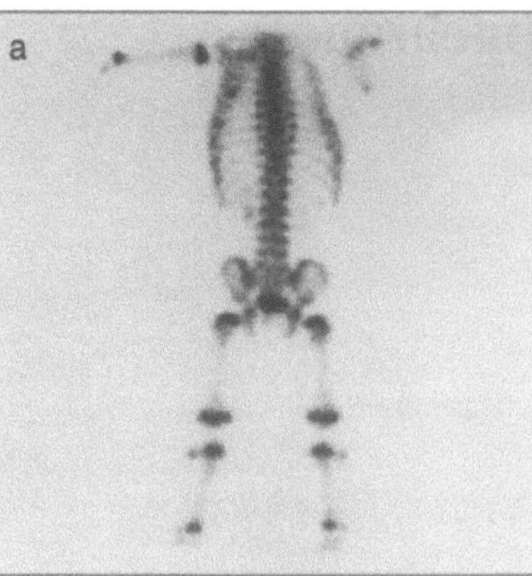

Case 5.57. A 6-week-old boy who had a large mass in the right hemithorax due to a primitive neuroectodermal tumour (PNET). The tumour was not infiltrating the ribs

Fig. 5.57a. Posterior view of the dorsal and lumbar spine, pelvis and lower limbs shows marked decreased uptake of isotope in the posterior and axillary portions of the upper ribs on the right. There is displacement of the right scapula

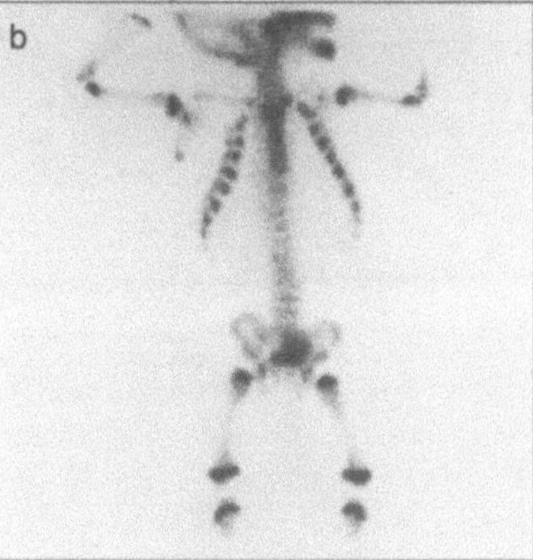

Fig. 5.57b. Anterior view of the thorax, abdomen, pelvis and upper limbs shows displacement of the right shoulder

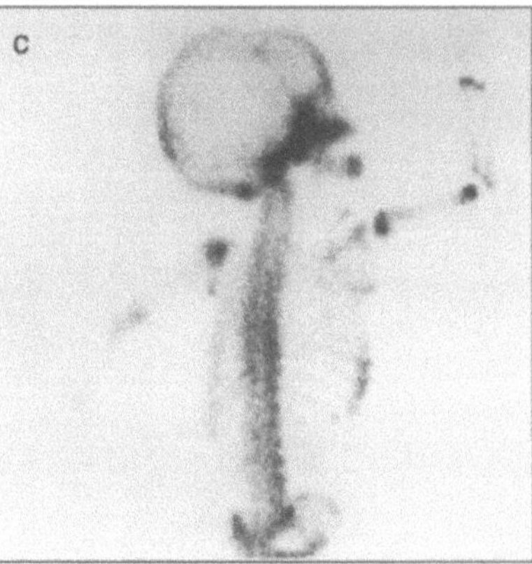

Fig. 5.57c. Right posterior oblique view of the thorax, lumbar spine and right arm shows virtually no activity in the upper seven ribs with significant decreased activity in the right scapula as well

Teaching Point
The effect of the mass lesion may be either an osteoblastic response with increased activity on the bone scan or an ostcoclastic response with decreased activity as seen in this young infant. Also see Cases 4.30, 4.31 and 4.40.

5.6 Post-operative Appearances

(19 Cases; 5.58–5.76)

Case 5.58. A 2-year-old girl who had a malignant tumour of the right humerus. Amputation of the right upper limb had been carried out

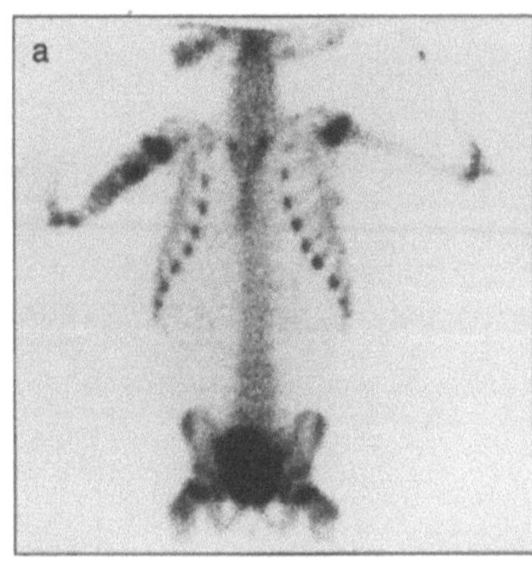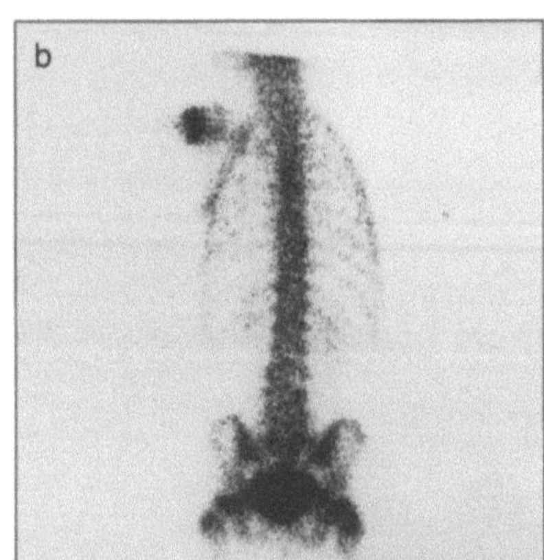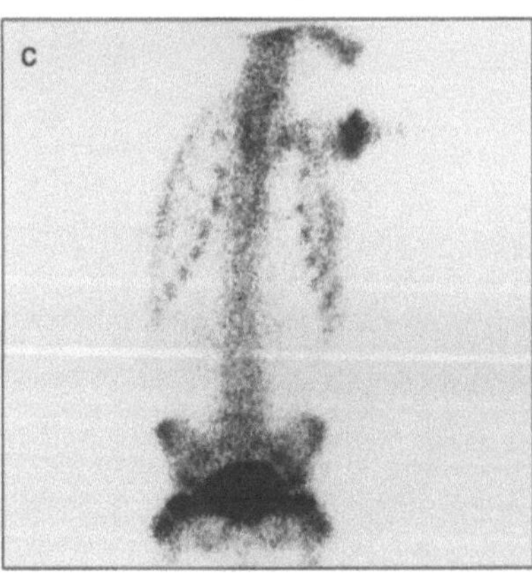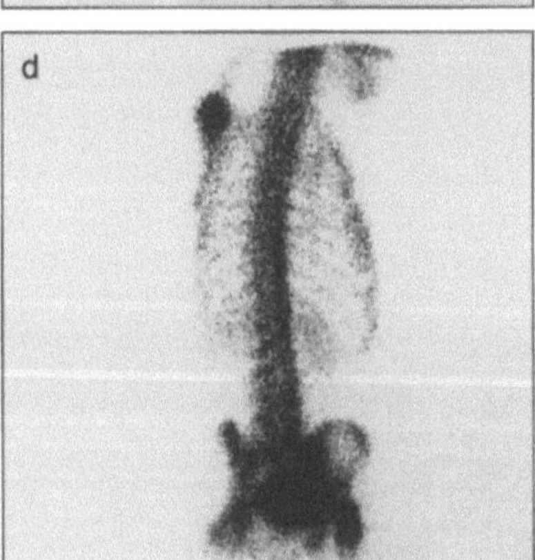

Fig. 5.58a. Pre-operative scan. Anterior image of the upper limbs, thorax and pelvis shows patchy increased uptake in the right humerus

Fig. 5.58b. Posterior image of the dorsal and lumbar spine, thorax and pelvis. The right arm is missing

Fig. 5.58c. Anterior image of the thorax. The right arm is missing

Fig. 5.58d. Right posterior oblique image of the thorax, lumbar spine and pelvis shows lack of the right shoulder girdle and right arm

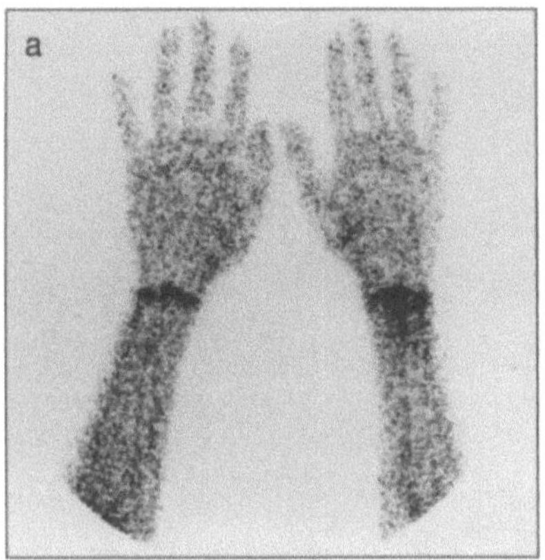 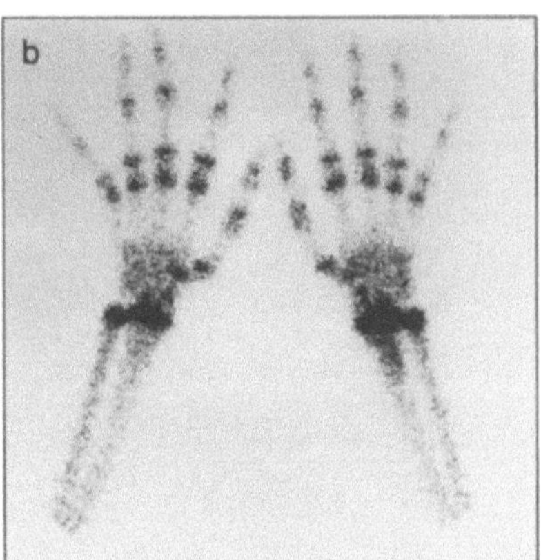

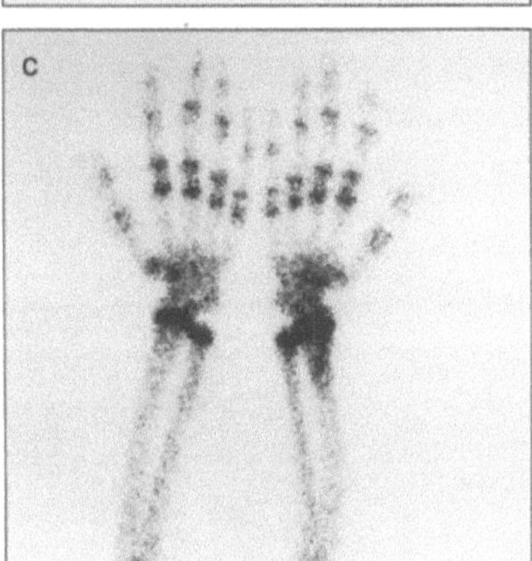

Case 5.59. A 9-year-old boy who had a mesenchymoma of the liver with secondaries in the right forearm. Following minor trauma, a pathological fracture through the distal left radius was noted. Bone chips had been placed into the pathological fracture prior to the undertaking of the bone scan

Fig. 5.59a. Blood pool image of the hands and wrists shows increased uptake of isotope in the left distal radius

Fig. 5.59b. Palmar image of the hands shows abnormal increased uptake of isotope in the distal left radial diaphysis extending to involve the epiphyseal plate

Fig. 5.59c. Posterior view of the forearms, wrists and hands shows abnormal increased uptake of isotope in the distal left radius extending to the epiphyseal plate. The small bones of the left wrist also show a slightly increased uptake of isotope compared to those on the other side

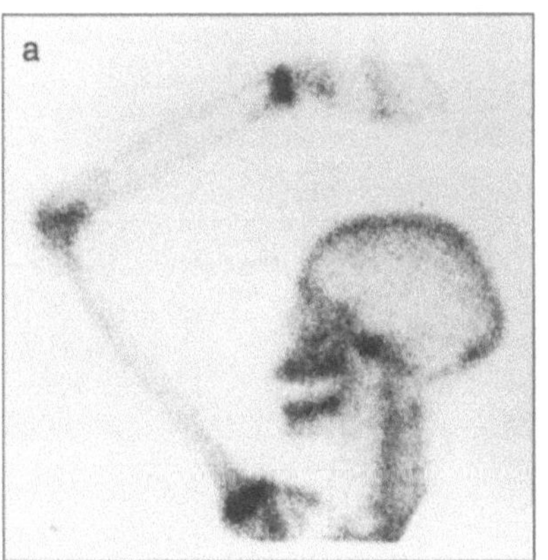 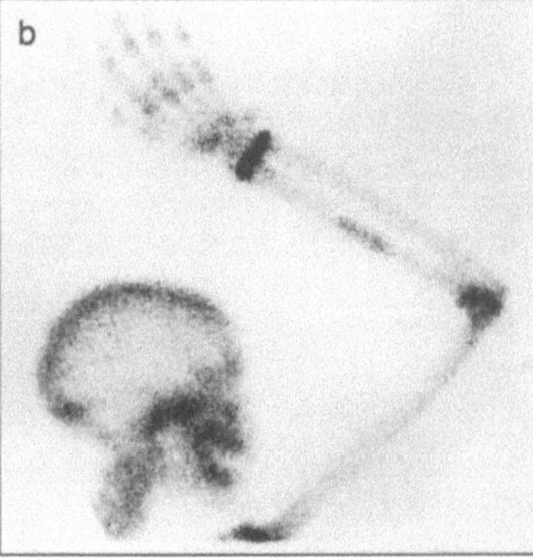

Case 5.60. A 13-year-old boy who had suffered from acute lymphatic leukaemia but was in remission. There was a past history of a fracture of the right radius which has been treated with open reduction and a plate and screws had been applied. He now represented with backache

Fig. 5.60a. Left lateral image of the skull and left arm is normal

Fig. 5.60a. Right lateral view of the skull and right arm shows abnormal increased uptake of isotope in the mid shaft of the right radius, the site of the plate and screws, which were still in place

Case 5.61. A 14-year-old girl who had undergone heart and lung transplantation

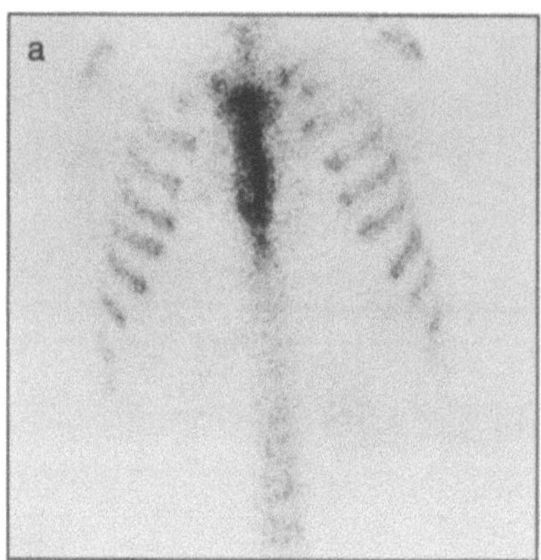

Fig. 5.61a. Anterior view of the thorax shows increased uptake of isotope in a straight line in the middle of the sternum. This was following the surgery

Case 5.62. A 16-year-old boy who had undergone surgery on the sternum for pectus excavatum 6 months prior to the scan

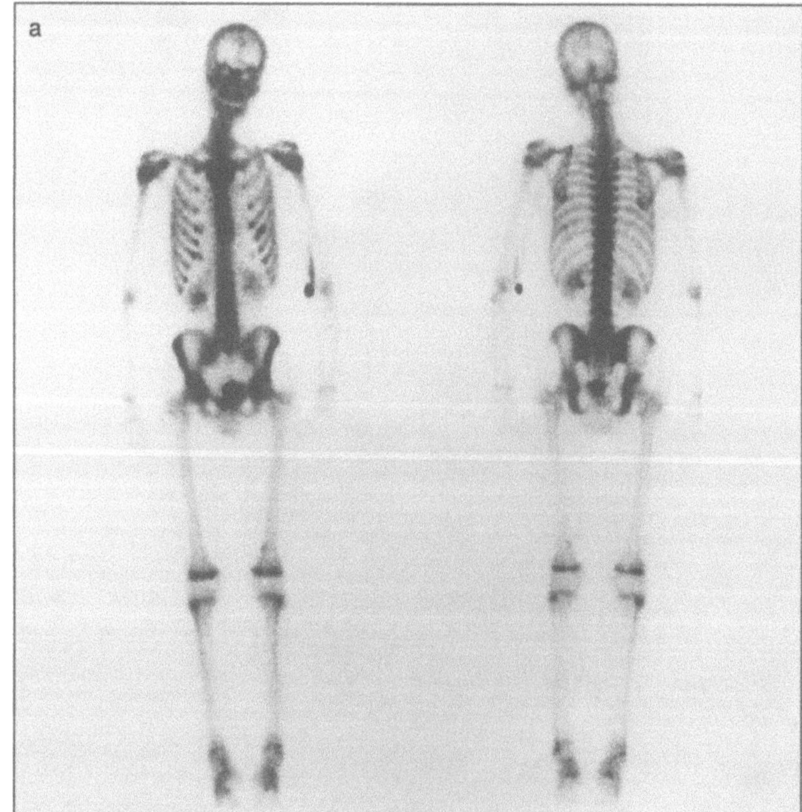

Fig. 5.62a. Whole body scan shows abnormal increased uptake of isotope in the anterior ends of the left fourth and fifth ribs as well as in the anterior ends of the right fourth and sixth rib. These were due to the surgical procedure

Technical Comment
Extravasation in the left cubital fossa is noted from the injection of tracer.

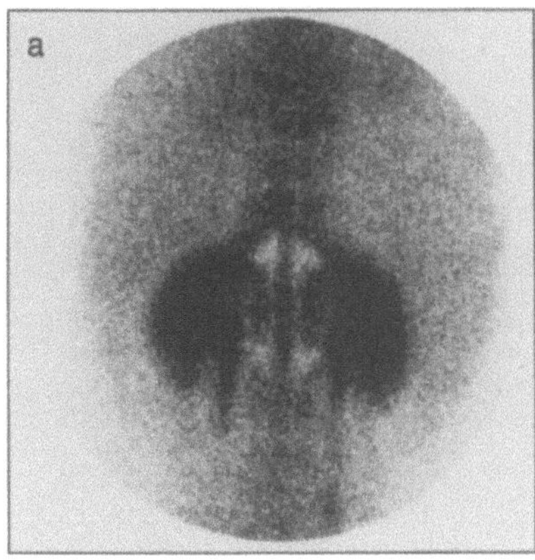

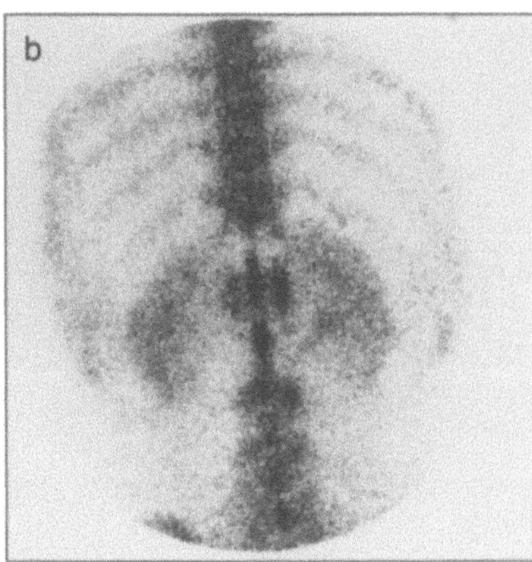

Case 5.63. A 20-year-old female who jumped off a bridge and suffered a fracture in the lower spine. Prior to the bone scan surgery with insertion of rods had occurred in the spine. (This is the same patient as in Case 5.34)

Fig. 5.63a. Posterior blood pool image of the spine. There is absent activity in the spine at the level of the kidneys, the site of the surgery

Fig. 5.63b. Posterior image of the lumbar spine. There is total absence of activity at L1 with marked decreased activity at L3. L2 shows focal increased activity

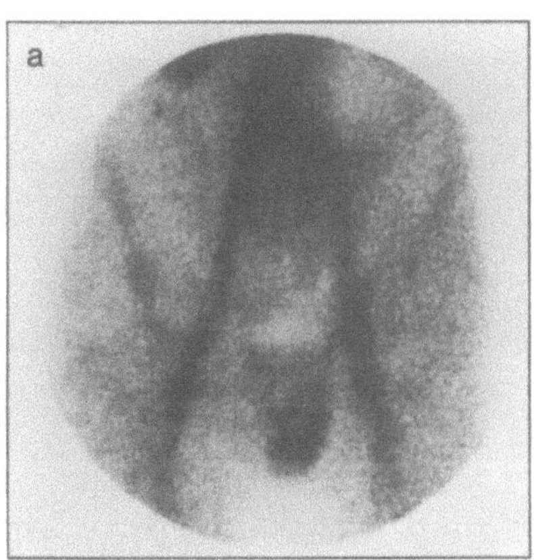

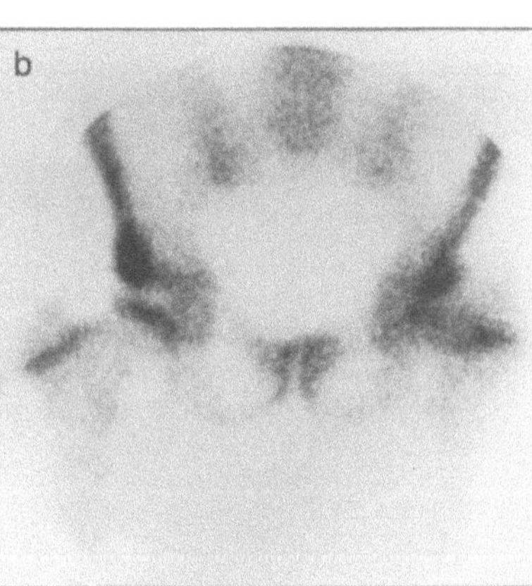

Case 5.64. A 15-year-old boy with Legg-Perthes' disease on the left. Surgery on the right hip involved placement of bone chips in the roof of the right acetabulum (Salter osteotomy)

Fig. 5.64a. Anterior blood pool image of the pelvis shows a small area of increased uptake of isotope in the region of the right anterior inferior iliac crest

Fig. 5.64b. Anterior view of the pelvis shows abnormal increased uptake of isotope in the region of the right inferior iliac crest, the site of surgery. The left hip is abnormal due to the known Legg-Perthes' disease

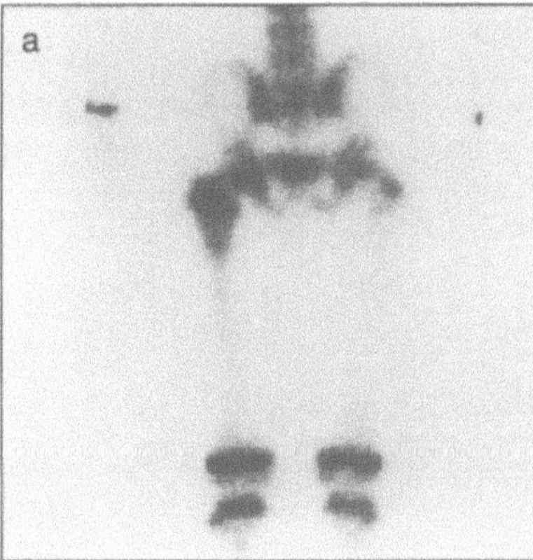

Case 5.65. A 5-year-old boy who had fractured the left femur; internal fixation had occurred 6 weeks prior to the scan. The surgeon was interested to know whether avascular necrosis of the left femoral head had occurred. The answer was no

Fig. 5.65a. Posterior image of pelvis and femora shows abnormal increased uptake of isotope in the region of the left femoral neck and upper shaft. The left femoral head is clearly seen to have normal activity, thus excluding the diagnosis of an avascular femoral head

Case 5.66. A 12-year-old boy who had undergone surgery 6 weeks prior to the scan for a fracture of the left femur where pins and a plate had been inserted. The surgeon wished to know whether the head of the femur was viable. The bone scan suggested that it was. Follow-up proved this to be correct

Fig. 5.66a. Anterior blood pool image of the pelvis shows slightly increased uptake in the left hip compared to the right

Fig. 5.66b. Posterior blood pool image of the pelvis shows increased uptake of isotope in the region of the left hip

Fig. 5.66c. Anterior image of the pelvis shows increased uptake of isotope in the left hip; the right is normal

Fig. 5.66d. Posterior image of the pelvis shows abnormal increased uptake of isotope in the left hip. In Fig. 5.66c and d, increased uptake in the left upper femoral shaft is noted

Fig. 5.66e. Pin hole view of the right hip is normal

Fig. 5.66f. Pin hole view of the left hip shows increased activity in the acetabular roof as well as in the neck of the femur. The head of the femur is clearly seen and has more activity when compared to the right pin hole image, thus confirming the viability of the femoral head.

A follow-up bone scan was obtained 6 weeks after the first bone scan

Fig. 5.66g. Anterior image of the pelvis shows abnormal increased uptake of isotope in the left femoral head and also in the shaft of the left femur

Fig. 5.66h. Posterior image of the pelvis shows abnormal increased uptake of isotope in the left femoral head and also in the shaft of the left femur

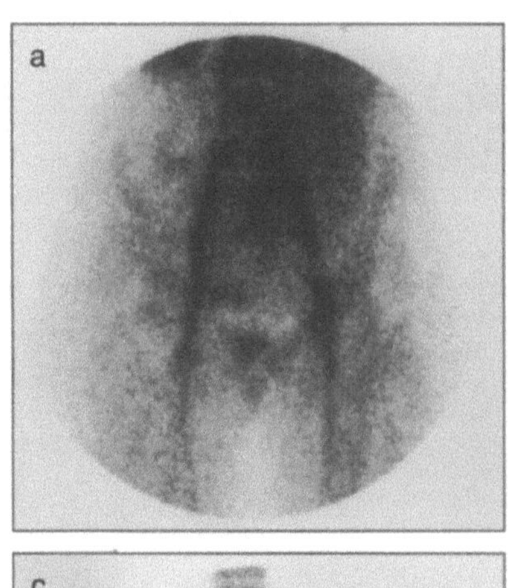
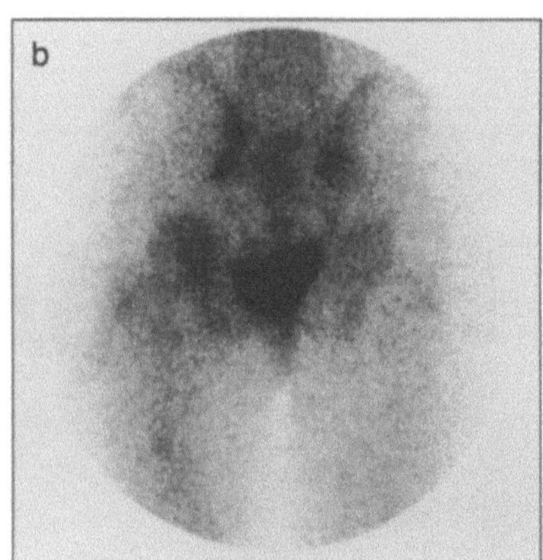
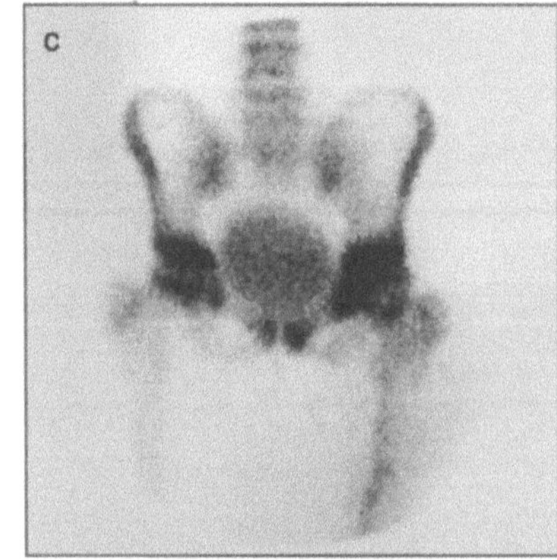
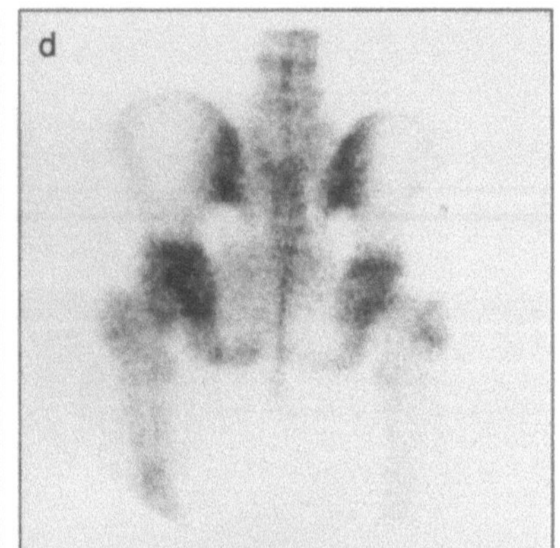
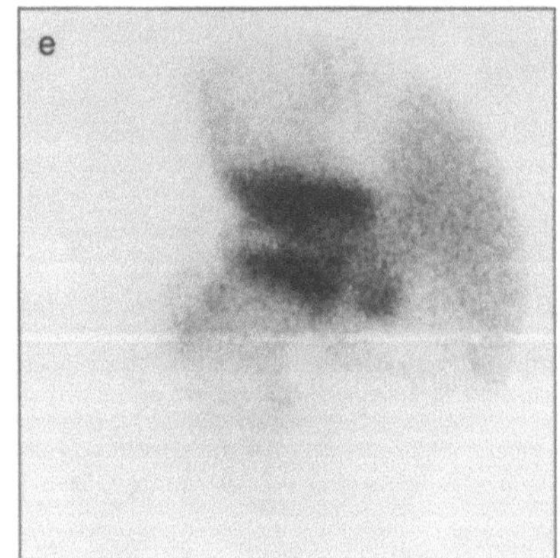
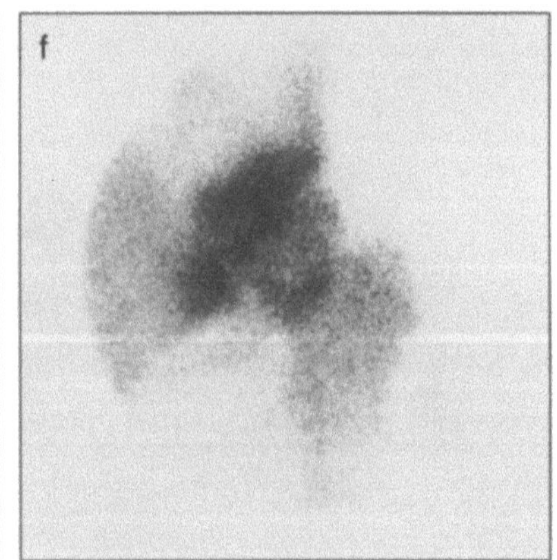
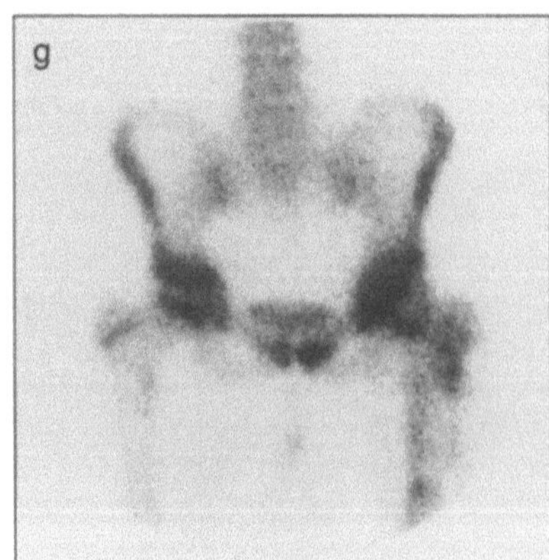
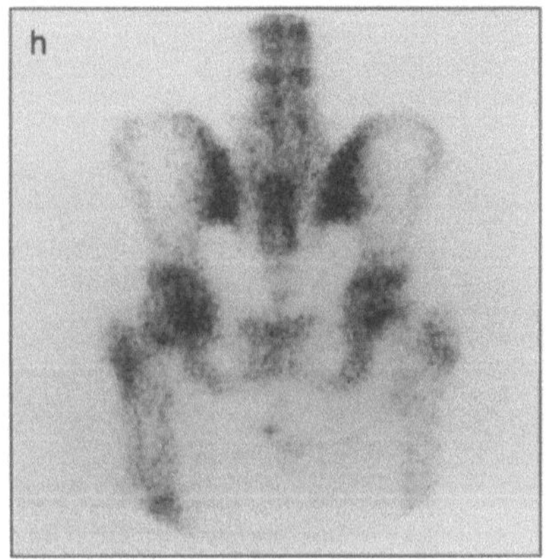

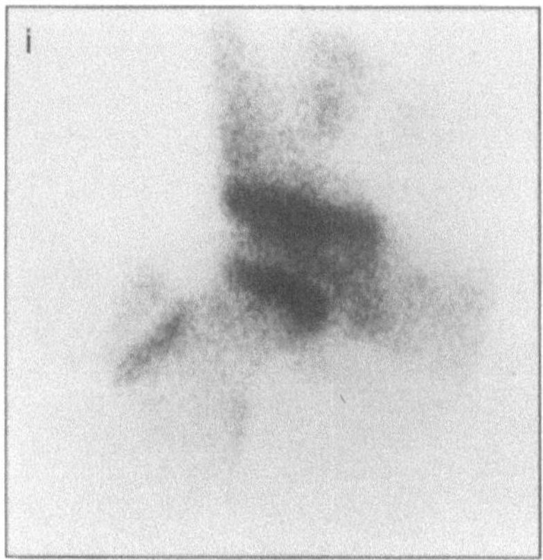

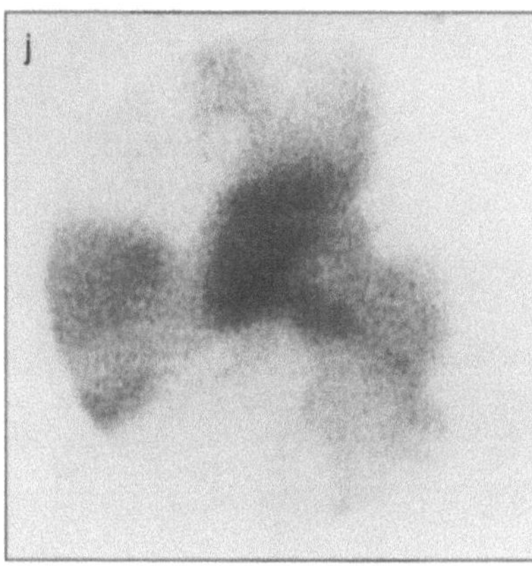

Fig. 5.66i. Pin hole view of the right hip is normal

Fig. 5.66j. Pin hole view of the left hip again confirms the activity in the femoral head which is increased compared to the normal side and also shows marked increased activity in the femoral neck due to repair

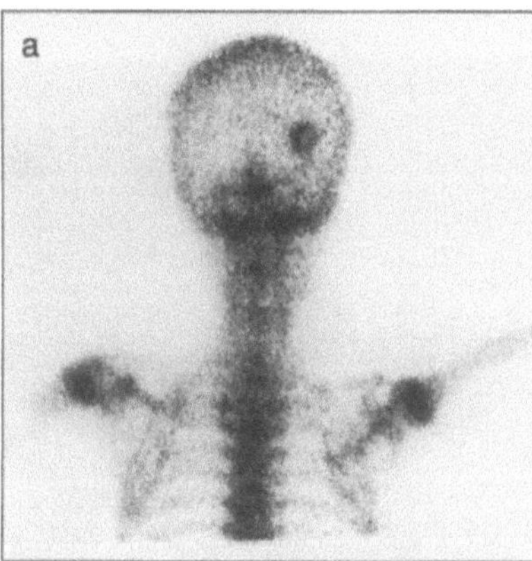

Case 5.67. This 7-year-old girl presented with headache, vomiting and was found to have papilledema due to a posterior brain fossa tumour. The bone scan was undertaken following surgical removal of the tumour looking for bone metastases

Fig. 5.67a. Posterior view of the skull shows increased uptake of isotope in the right skull vault with activity in the centre

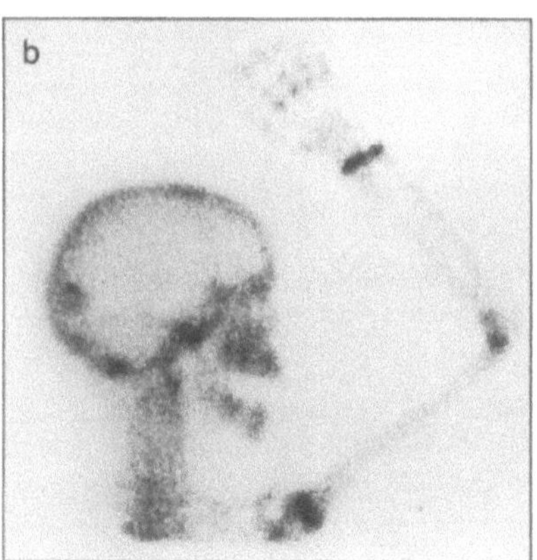

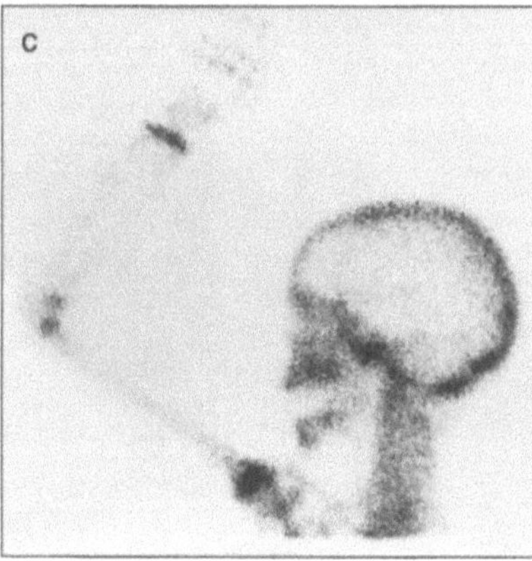

Fig. 5.67b. Right lateral view of the skull shows focal absent uptake of isotope in the central portions surrounded by a room of increased activity. These appearances are simply following the surgery

Fig. 5.67c. Left lateral view of the skull is normal

Teaching Point

Similar appearances may be seen with Langerhans' histiocytosis (see Cases 4.81–4.82, 4.84, 4.86).

Case 5.68. A 6-year-old boy who had suffered trauma which required surgery for a fractured femur. No union was noted at the site of the fracture. The clinical question now arose as to whether osteomyelitis existed within this femur. The result of the bone scan suggested that there was no infection within the bone. (Same child as in Case 5.44)

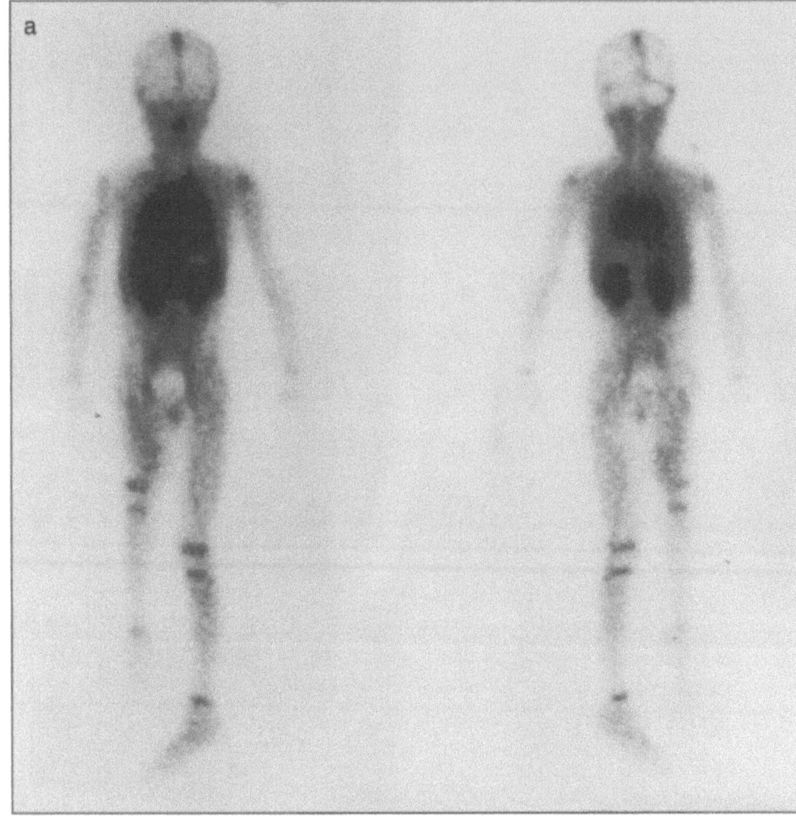

Fig. 5.68a. Blood pool whole body scans show abnormal increased uptake of isotope in the region of the right thigh. The right leg is shorter than the left. Note the photon-deficient area in the region of the bladder; this was due to a full bladder prior to the injection of the isotope

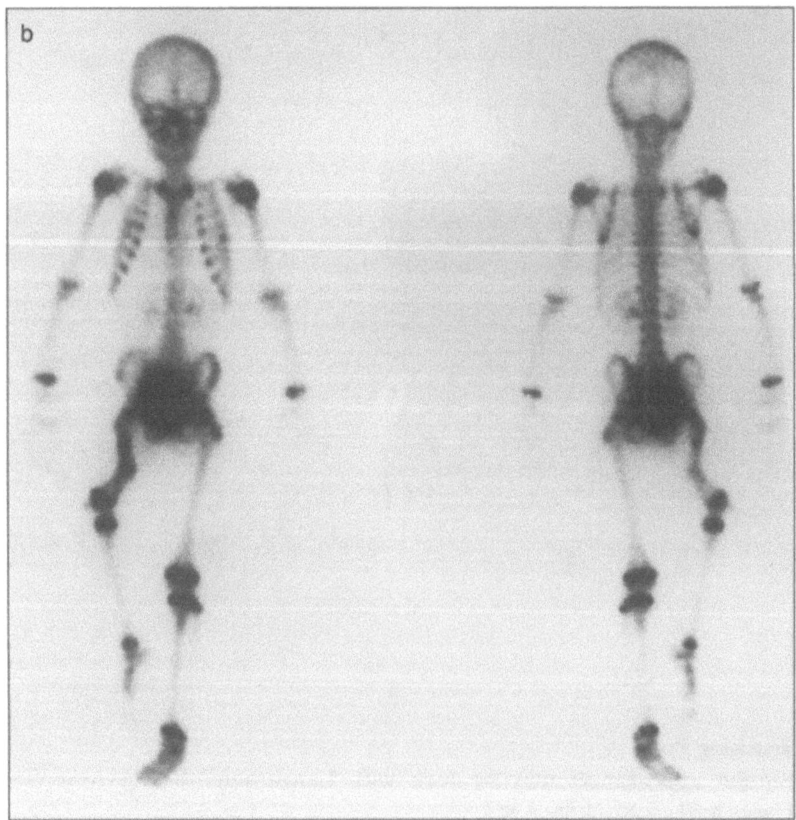

Fig. 5.68b. Whole body images. The abnormal short right femur is noted with increased uptake in the shaft of the femur

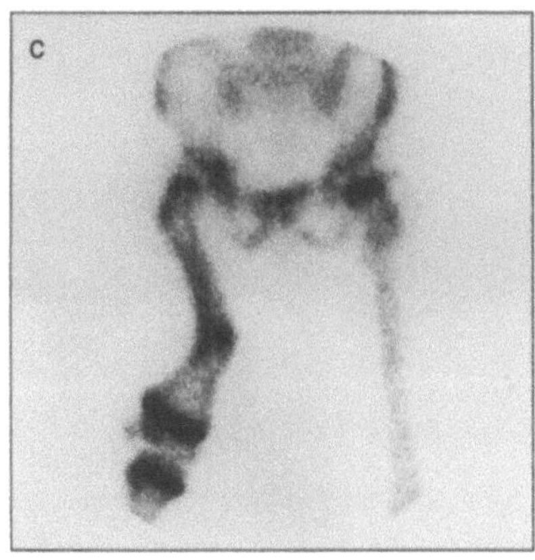

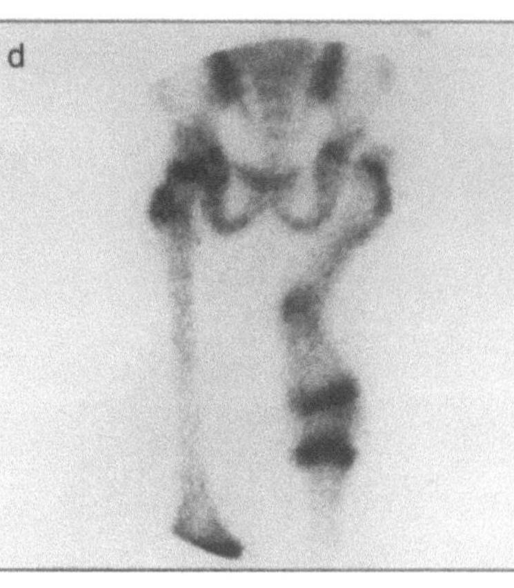

Fig. 5.68c. Anterior image of the pelvis and femora shows abnormal increased uptake of isotope in the right short femur, confined to the mid portion of the femur with focal increased uptake at the junction of the middle and distal thirds, the site of the pseudarthrosis

Fig. 5.68d. Posterior image of the pelvis and upper femora shows increased uptake of isotope in the deformed short right femur, but there is no focal area over and above the site of the pseudarthrosis to suggest active infection

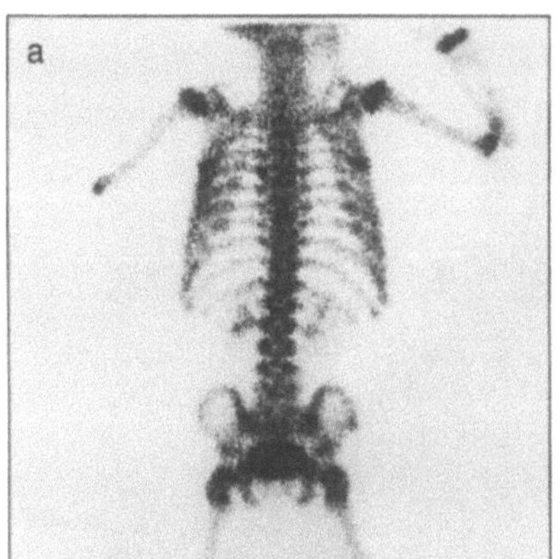

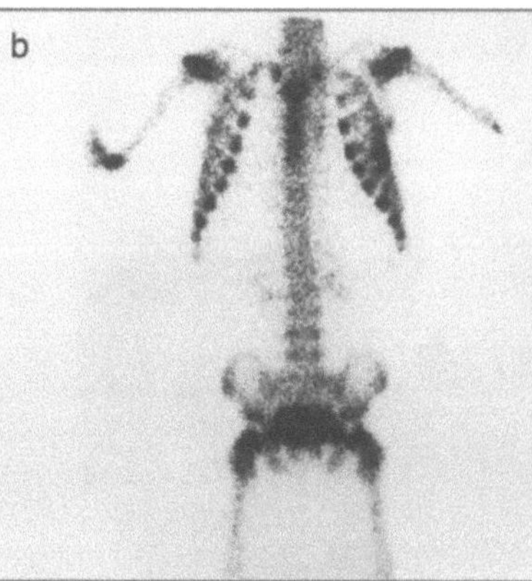

Case 5.69. A 1-year-old boy who had undergone thoracotomy for a ganglioneuroblastoma. He developed a periosteal reaction along the ribs on chest radiograph. There was no evidence of infection

Fig. 5.69a. Posterior view of thorax, dorsal and lumbar spine and pelvis shows abnormal increased uptake of isotope in the axillary portion of the ribs on the left

Fig. 5.69b. Anterior view of the thorax, spine and pelvis. The abnormal activity in the anterior and axillary portions of the lower ribs on the left is noted

Case 5.70. A 7-year-old boy who had been battered for some time. Surgery on the right femur revealed pus in the femur. The bone scan was obtained following this surgery

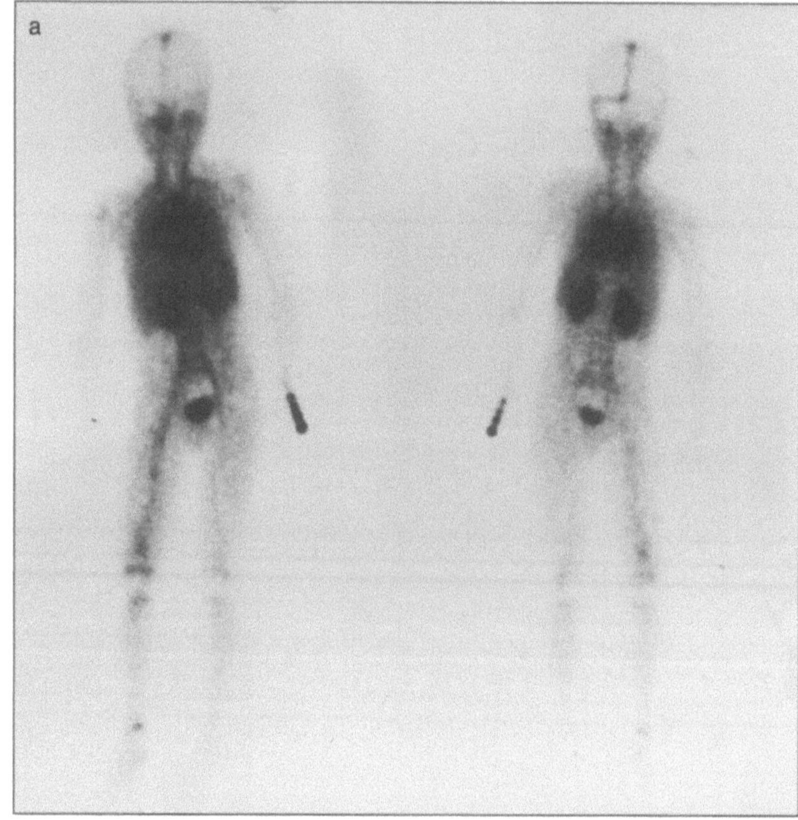

Fig. 5.70a. Whole body blood pool scans show abnormal increased uptake of isotope throughout the entire right lower limb. Note accumulation of isotope in the injection line on the left hand

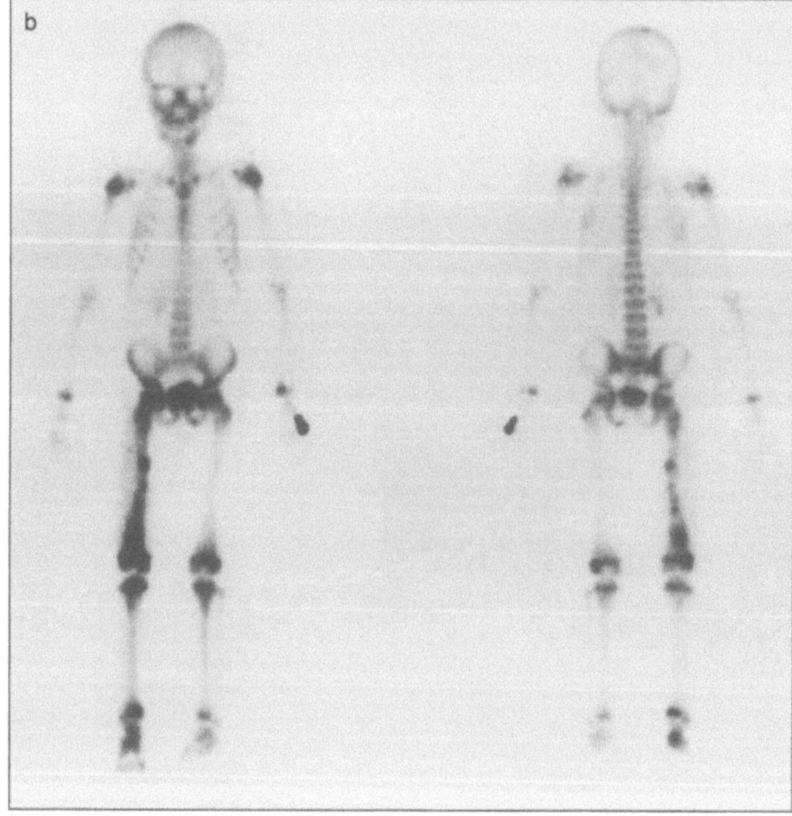

Fig. 5.70b. Whole body images show abnormal increased uptake of isotope in the right femur. This is non-homogeneous with focal areas of intense increased uptake. Increased uptake of isotope was also noted in the distal right tibial growth plate and the entire right foot. Note isotope in the injection line on the left hand at the site of the injection

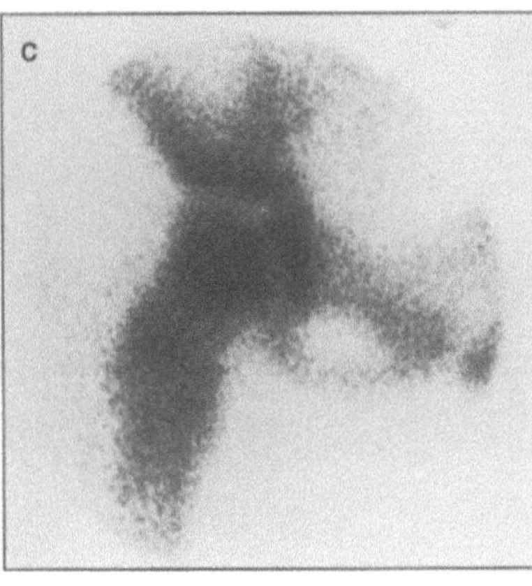

Fig. 5.70c. Pin hole image of the right hip shows increased activity throughout the femoral head and neck extending into the shaft, thus excluding the diagnosis of avascular necrosis of the femoral head

Teaching Point

The abnormality in the right femur is non-specific and does not allow differentiation between the two types of trauma (battering and surgical trauma) and the infection which was discovered.

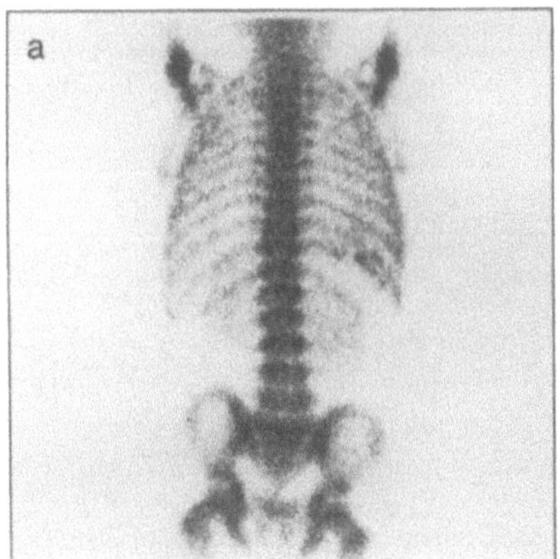

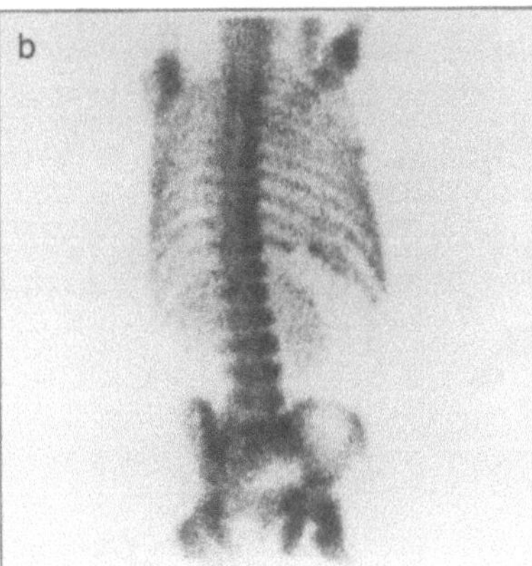

Case 5.71. Ewing's sarcoma of the rib in a 4-year-old boy. The bone scan was carried out following surgical resection of the tumour

Fig. 5.71a. Posterior image of the thorax, spine and pelvis. There is increased uptake of isotope in the right 11th rib laterally with a short area of absent activity more posteriorly

Fig. 5.71b. Right posterior oblique image of the ribs shows the small area with absent activity adjacent to the focal abnormal increased activity

Teaching Point

The absent activity is related to the previous surgery. The area of increased activity could be secondary to the surgery or local recurrence of tumour. The bone scan alone cannot distinguish between these two conditions.

Case 5.72. **A 13-year-old boy who had suffered osteochondritis dissecans of the left knee and had undergone surgery on the knee. The bone scan was undertaken following surgery**

Fig. 5.72a. Anterior blood pool image of the knees shows marked increased uptake of isotope throughout the left knee involving both the femur and tibia

Fig. 5.72b. Anterior image of the knees shows abnormal increased uptake of isotope in both femoral condyles of the left knee as well as the left patella. There is also abnormal increased uptake of isotope in the tibial metaphysis extending down into the diaphysis.

A follow-up bone scan was undertaken 8 months later

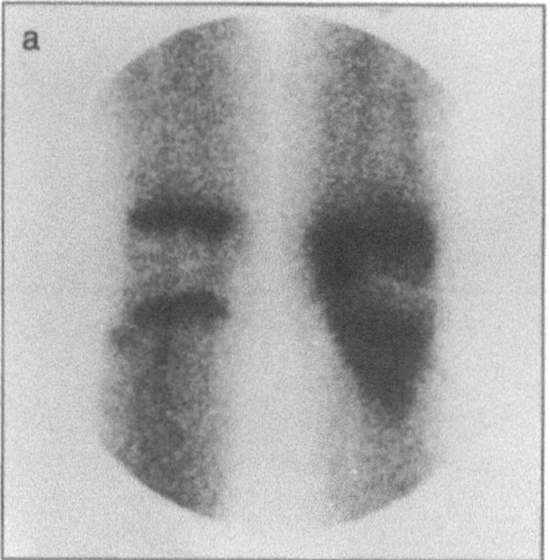

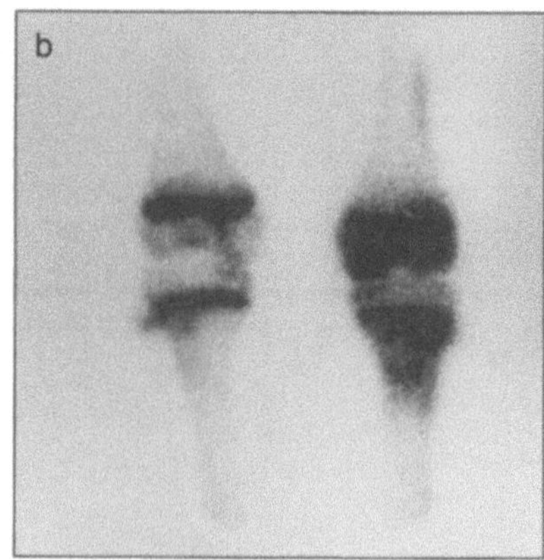

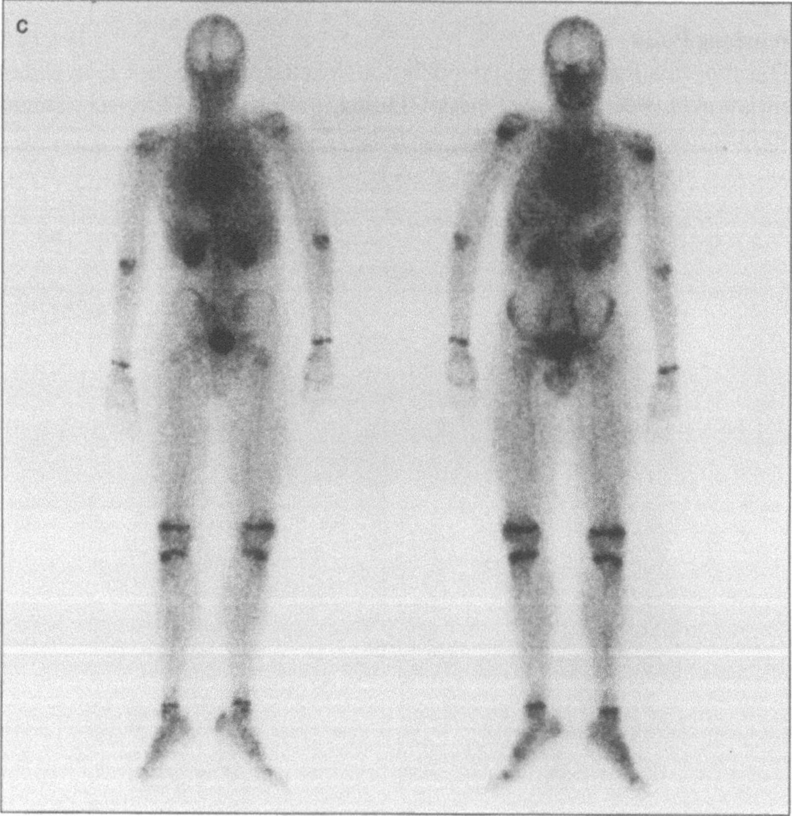

Fig. 5.72c. Blood pool whole body images show minimal increased uptake of isotope around the left femoral condyles

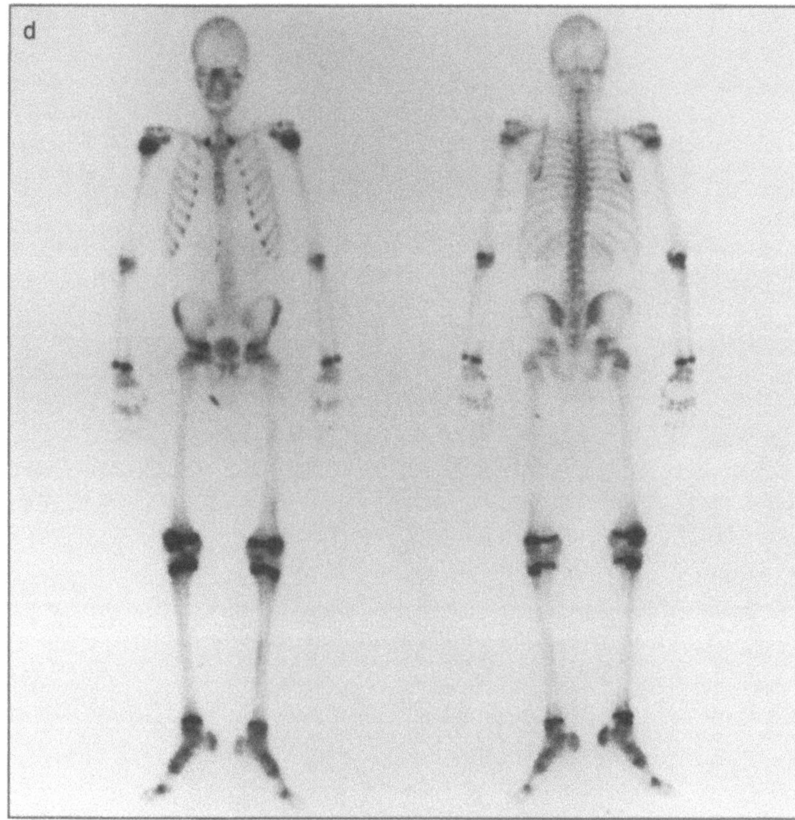

Fig. 5.72d. Whole body images show that the left knee has returned virtually to normality

Case 5.73. A 17-year-old boy with osteogenic sarcoma in the right femur following chemotherapy and amputation. Follow-up scans were obtained 8 months later. (Same patient as in Case 4.49)

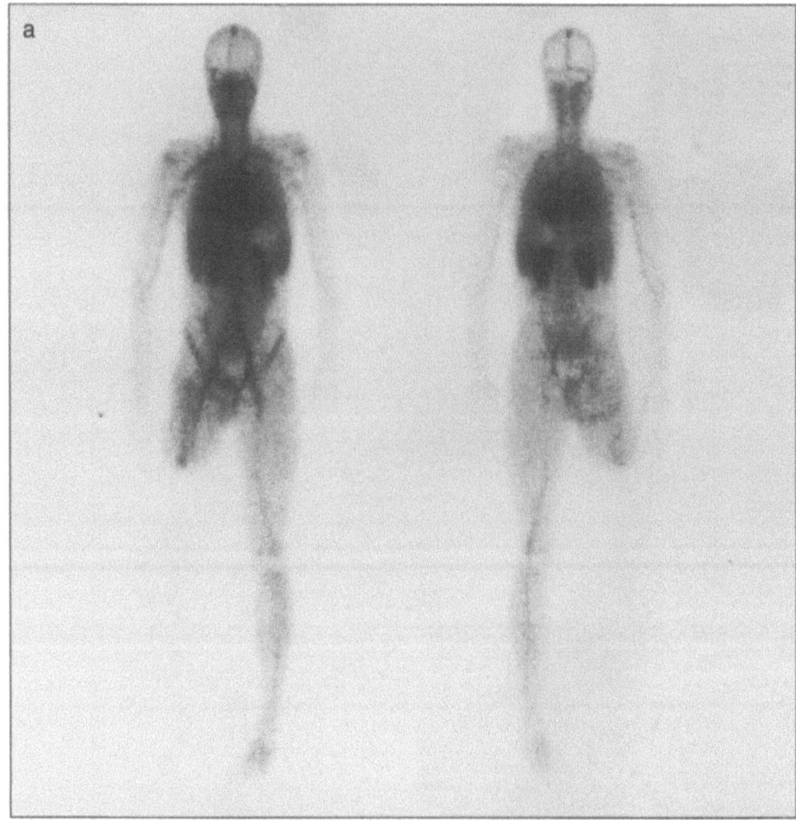

Fig. 5.73a. Whole body blood pool images show increased uptake of isotope around the distal end of the amputation site of the femur

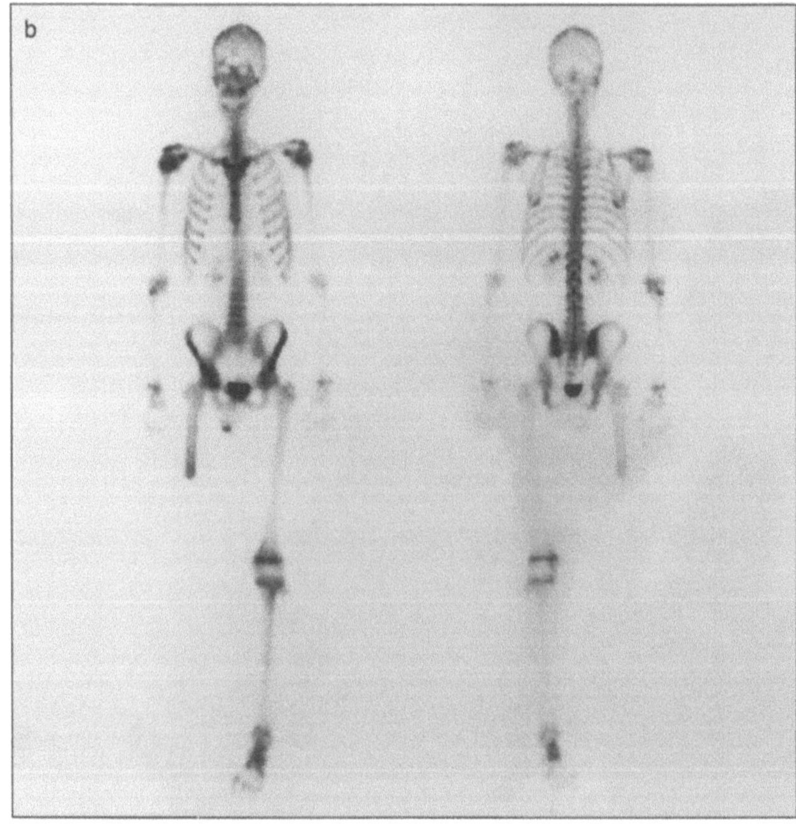

Fig. 5.73b. Whole body images show increased uptake in the distal right femur presumed to be caused by the artificial limb. These appearances were noted on subsequent follow-up scans over a period of a further 2 years but no metastasis was noted at this site

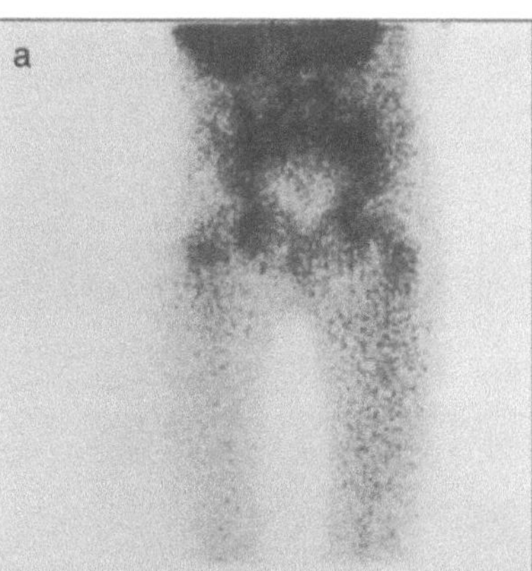

Case 5.74. A 6-year-old boy with a stage IV neuroblastoma who presented with a pathological fracture of the left femoral neck which was surgically treated with a total hip replacement

Fig. 5.74a. Posterior blood pool image of pelvis and femora shows a slightly increased uptake in the region of the left upper femur

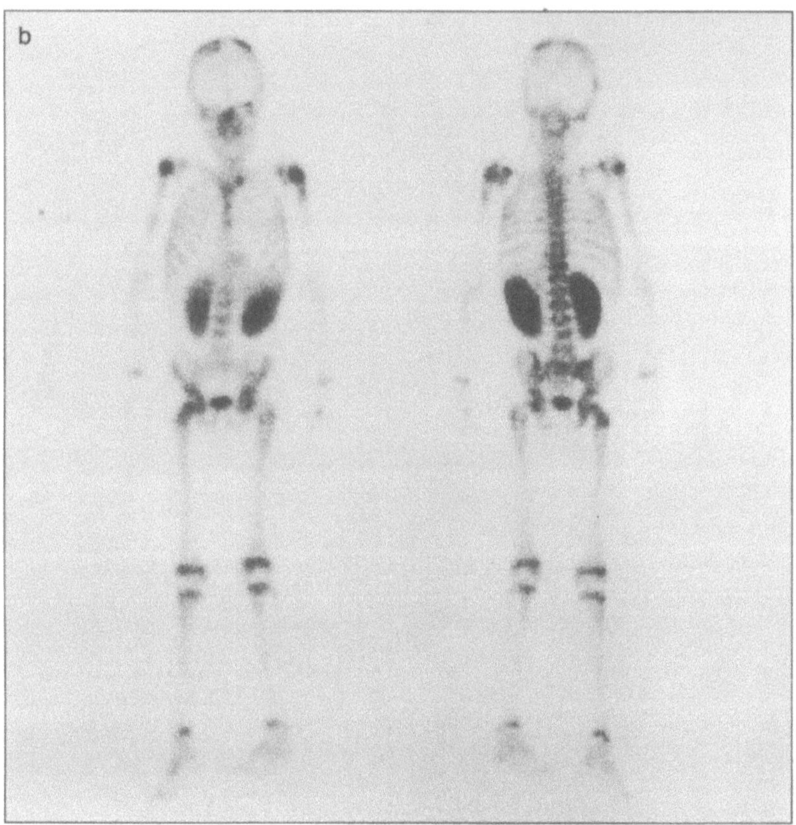

Fig. 5.74b. Whole body images show increased uptake of isotope in multiple areas of the whole skeleton. There is a photon-deficient area in the left femoral neck from the prosthesis. Retention of tracer in both kidneys is noted. There is displacement of the upper pole of the left kidney due to the primary tumour, which shows a slightly increased uptake of isotope

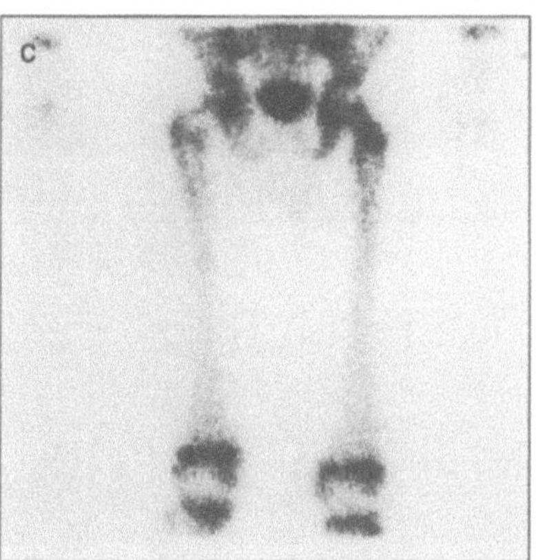

Fig. 5.74c. Posterior image of pelvis and femora shows a photon-deficient area in the left upper femur

Case 5.75. A 15-year-old girl with a PNET tumour of the ileum after hemipelvectomy with an artificial hemipelvis and a total replacement of the left hemipelvis. (This is the same child as in Case 4.55)

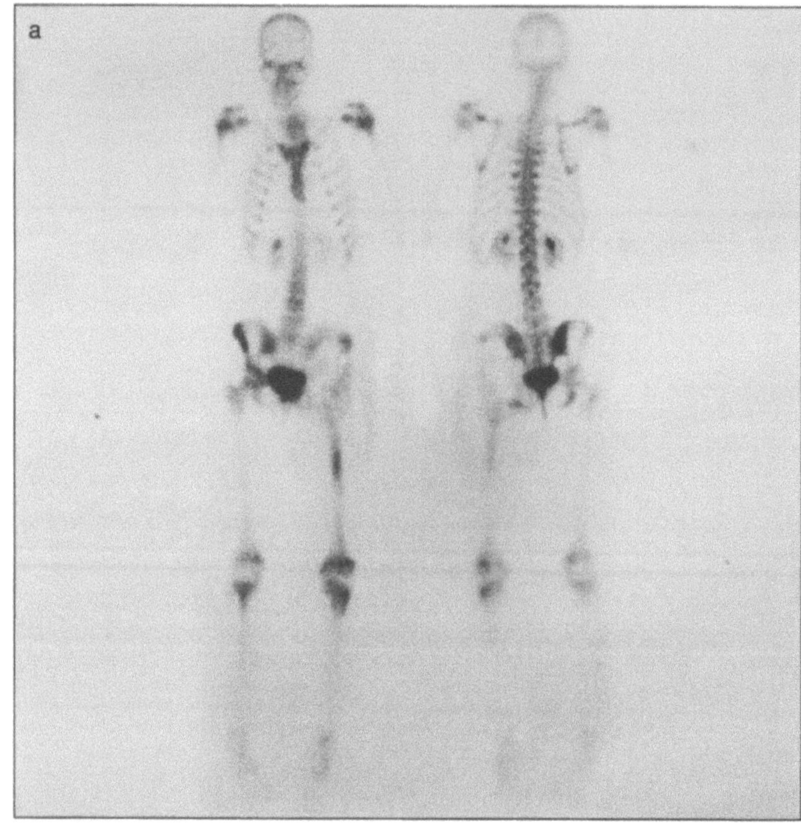

Fig. 5.75a. Whole body images show a photon-deficient area in the region of the left hemipelvis and the left upper femur. There is increased uptake of isotope in the mid shaft of the left femur due to surgery

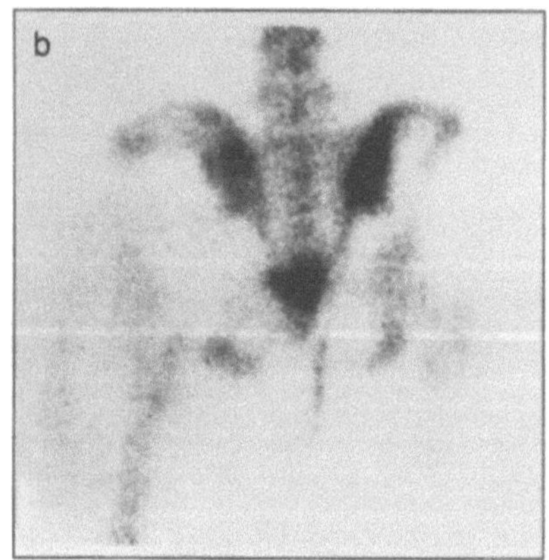

Fig. 5.75b. Posterior image of the pelvis again shows the photon-deficient area throughout the left hemipelvis

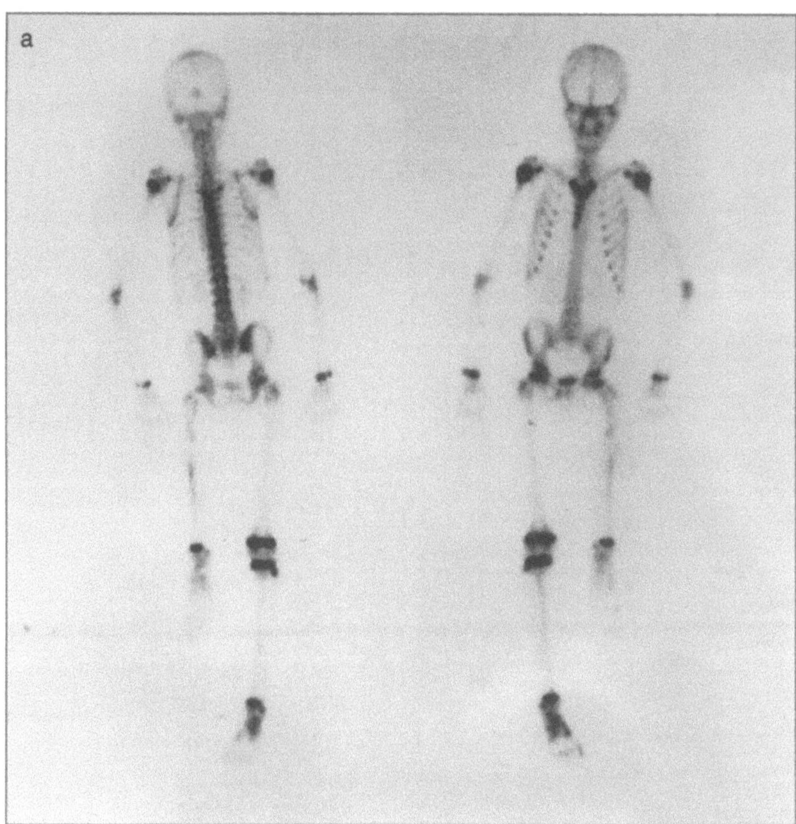

Case 5.76. A 9-year-old boy with an osteogenic sarcoma of the left knee after reverse osteotomy of the left foot

Fig. 5.76a. Whole body scans show the shortened left leg after the reverse osteotomy with patchy increased uptake throughout the "new" left femur

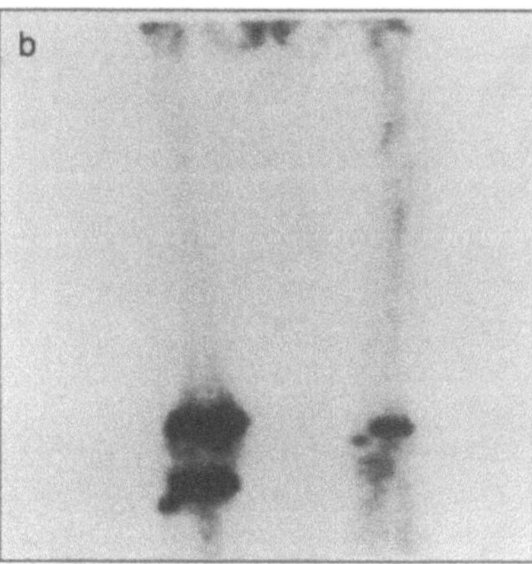

Fig. 5.76b. Anterior view of femora and knees again shows the shortened left femur with patchy increased uptake. The left foot is seen to articulate with the femur

5.7 Effect of Radiotherapy
(1 Case; Fig. 5.77)

Case 5.77. A 5-year-old boy with a Wilm's tumour. Recurrence of the tumour had been diagnosed 2 years before the bone scan. Following the diagnosis of recurrence, radiotherapy had been applied to the tumour. The field included the lumbar spine

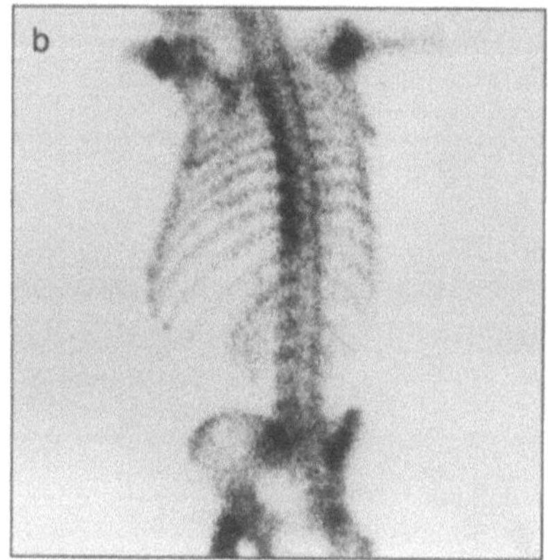

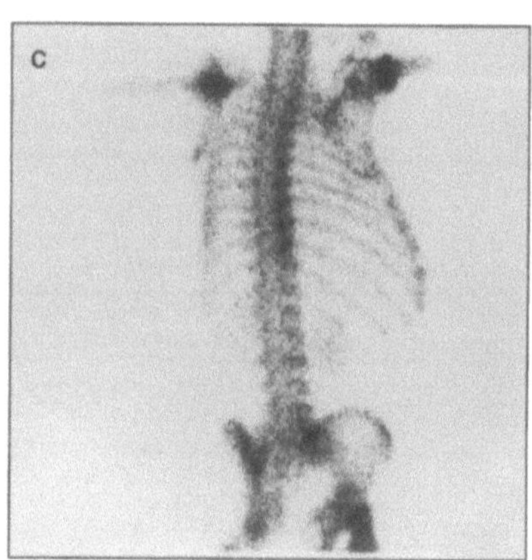

Fig. 5.77a. Posterior image of the spine and pelvis shows decreased uptake of isotope in the lumbar spine

Fig. 5.77b. Left posterior oblique image of the spine, thorax and pelvis shows decreased uptake of isotope throughout the lumbar spine

Fig. 5.77c. Right posterior oblique image of the thorax, spine and pelvis again shows the diffuse decreased uptake of isotope throughout the lumbar spine. This is the field of radiotherapy

Teaching Point
Also see Case 4.65.

6 Osteochondritis Dissecans – Avascular Necrosis

6.1 Legg-Perthes' Disease

(9 Cases; Figs. 6.1–6.9)

Case 6.1. 3-year-old boy who presented with pain in the right hip and was found to have bilateral Legg-Perthes' disease

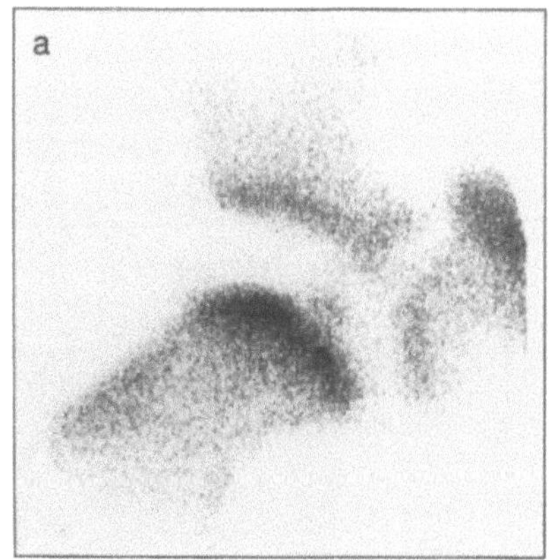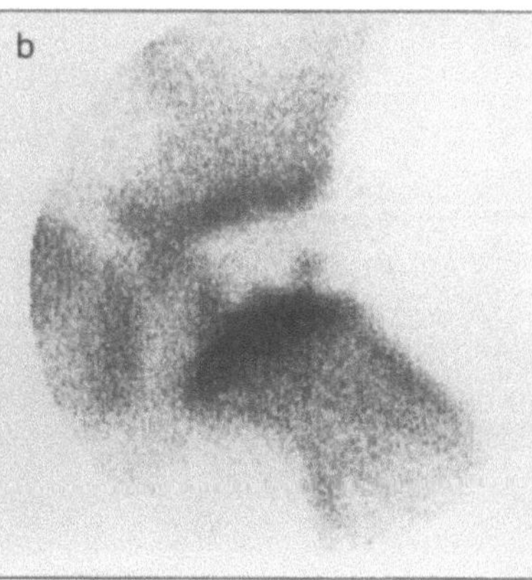

Fig. 6.1a. Pin hole view of the right hip shows total absence of activity in the lateral two thirds of the femoral head

Fig. 6.1b. Pin hole view of the left hip shows absence of activity in the femoral head. This is not complete as there is a small area of activity seen in the lateral third immediately above the epiphyseal plate. This suggests that the left sided Legg-Perthes' disease was in the early phase of healing

Case 6.2. A 6-year-old boy with left-sided Legg-Perthes' disease

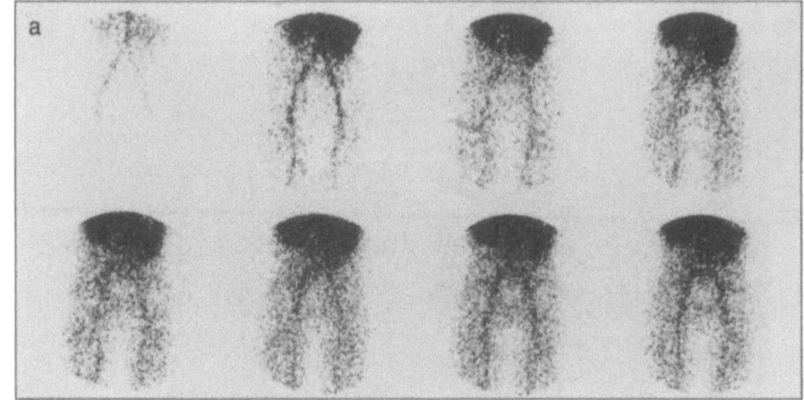

Fig. 6.2a. Blood flow anterior views fail to reveal any abnormality

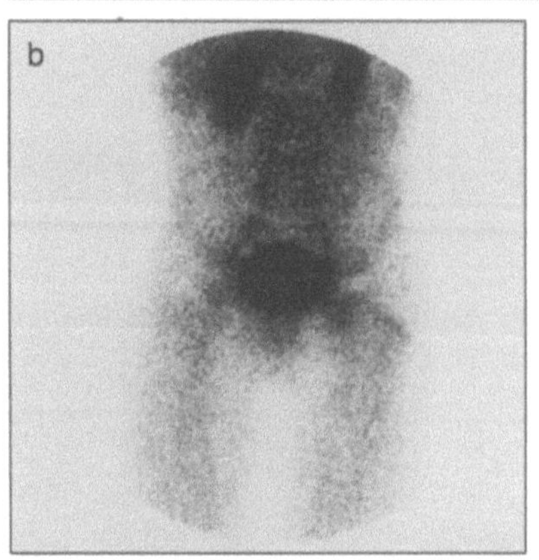

Fig. 6.2b. Anterior blood pool image of the pelvis shows decreased isotope in the left hip compared to the right

Fig. 6.2c. Anterior view of the lumbar spine, pelvis and upper femora shows decreased uptake of isotope in the left femoral head

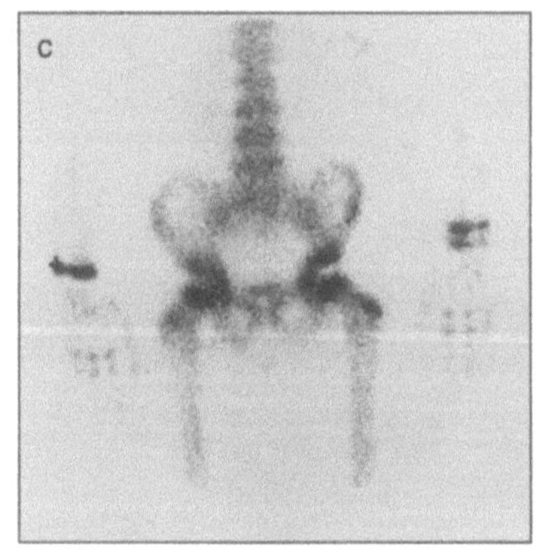
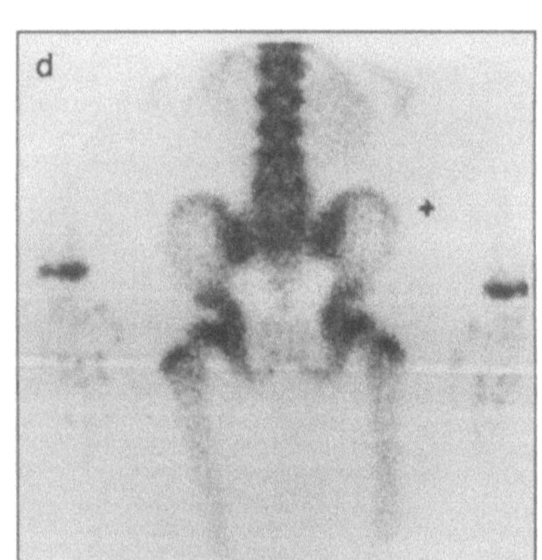

Fig. 6.2d. Posterior view of the lumbar spine, pelvis and upper femora shows focal decreased uptake of isotope in the head of the left femur

Fig. 6.2e. Anterior pin hole view of the right hip is within normal limits

Fig. 6.2f. Anterior pin hole view of the left hip shows total absence of activity in the lateral and medial aspect of the left femoral head

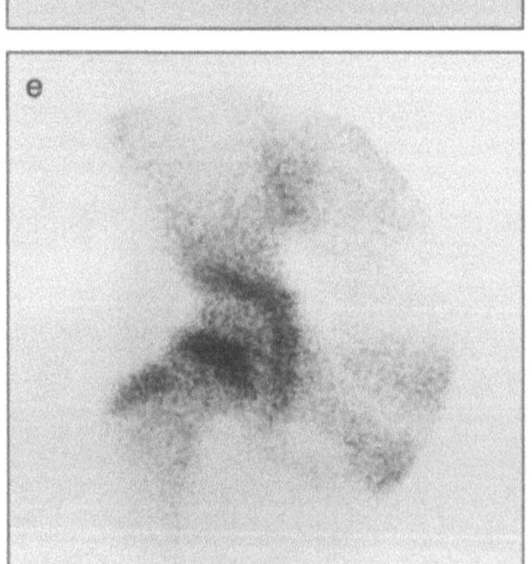
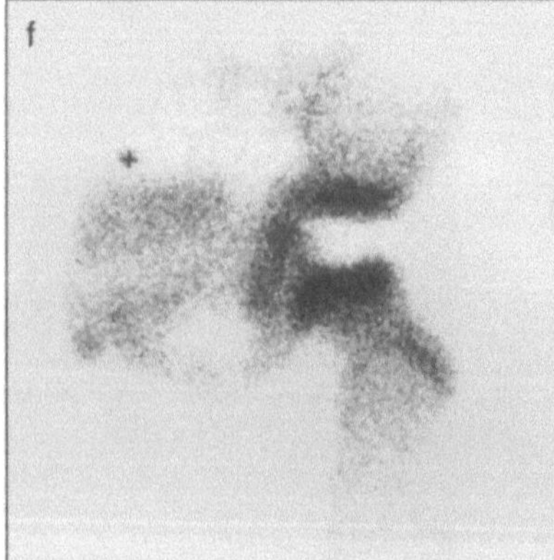

Technical Comment

Figure 6.2b (the blood pool phase) was taken rather late (5 min), and isotope in the bladder makes assessment of the hip joints more difficult.

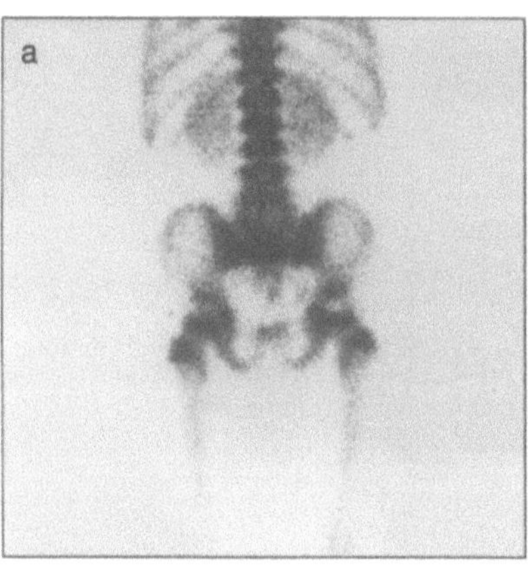

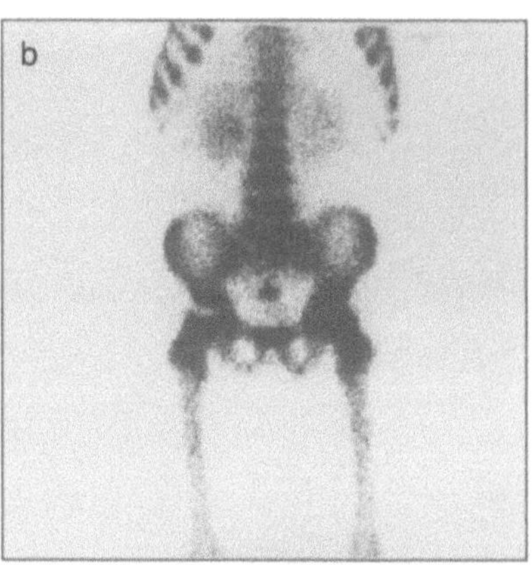

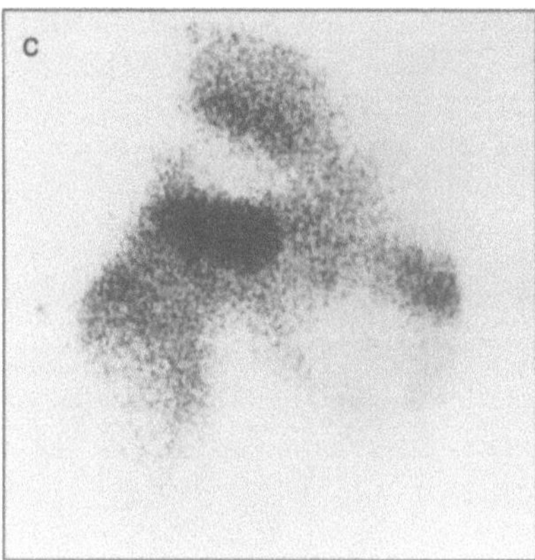

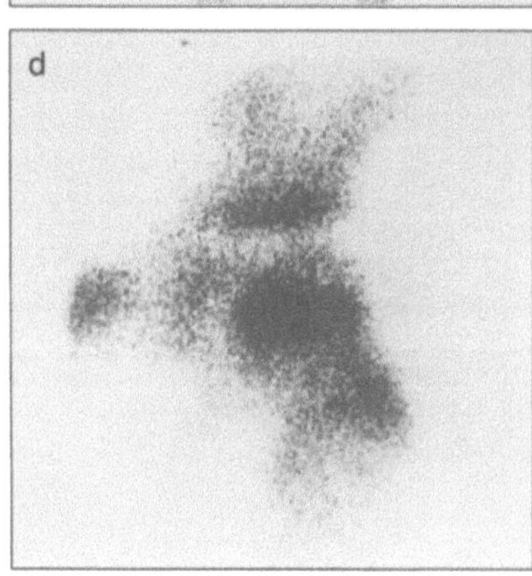

Case 6.3. A 5-year-old boy with Legg-Perthes' disease of the right hip

Fig. 6.3a. Posterior image of the hips shows decreased activity in the right femoral head

Fig. 6.3b. Anterior image of the lumbar spine, pelvis and upper femora shows decreased activity in the right femoral head. Note activity in the centre of the pelvis. This could represent activity in the bladder or contamination

Fig. 6.3c. Pin hole view of the right hip shows decreased activity in most of the head, with minimal activity seen on the lateral aspect immediately above the epiphyseal plate. This is the first sign of the healing phase of Perthes' disease

Fig. 6.3d. Pin hole view of the left hip is normal

Case 6.4. A 5-year-old boy with Legg-Perthes' disease of the left hip

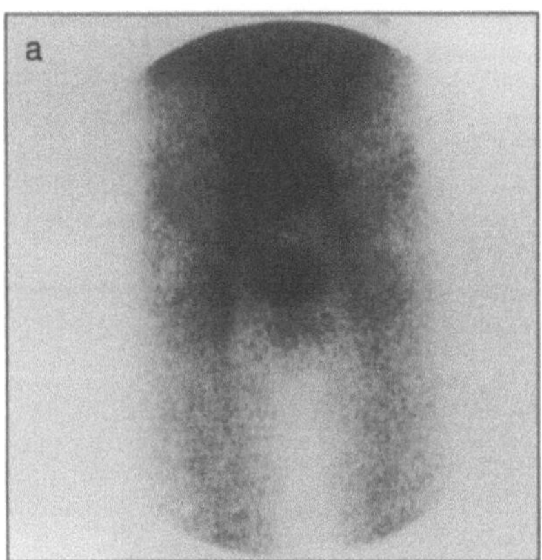

Fig. 6.4a. Blood pool anterior image of the hips shows only slight reduction of activity in the region of the left hip compared to the right

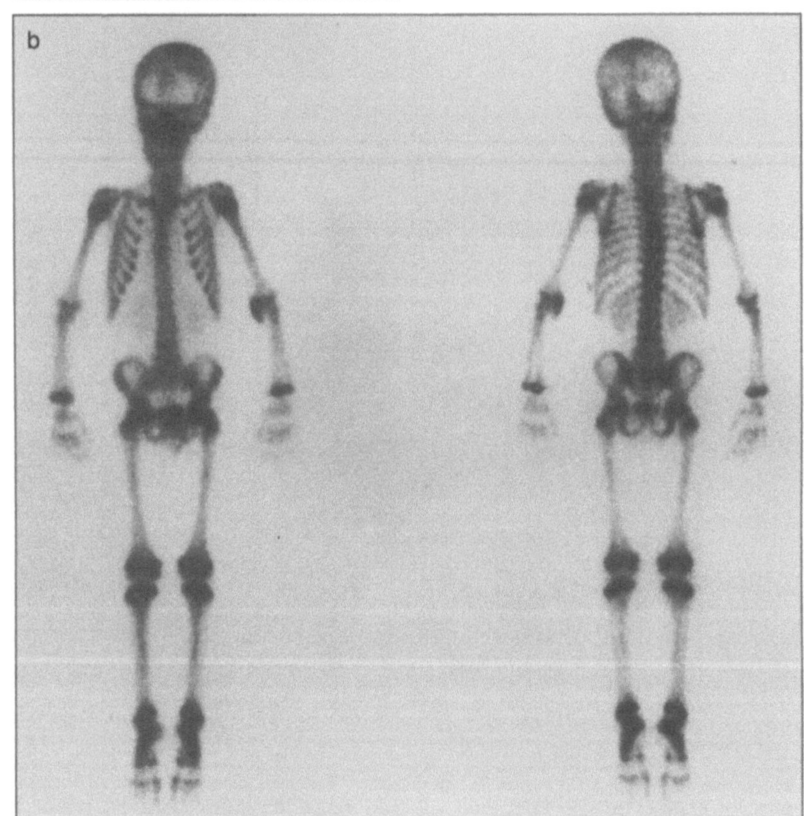

Fig. 6.4b. Whole body scans. The posterior view suggests decreased activity in the left hip. Extravasation of isotope in the left elbow is noted

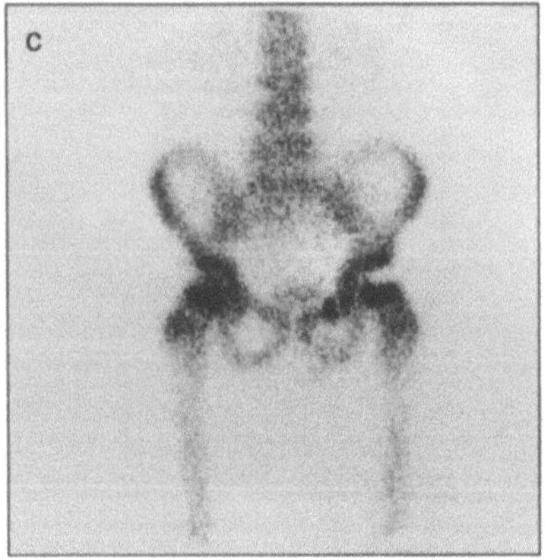

Fig. 6.4c. Anterior image of the lumbar spine, pelvis and upper femora shows decreased activity in the left femoral head

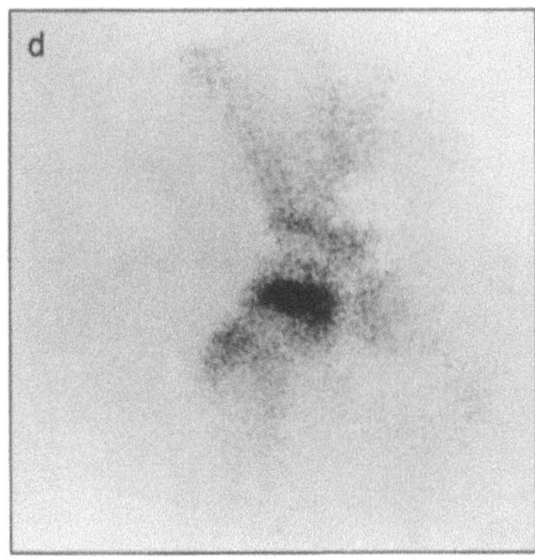

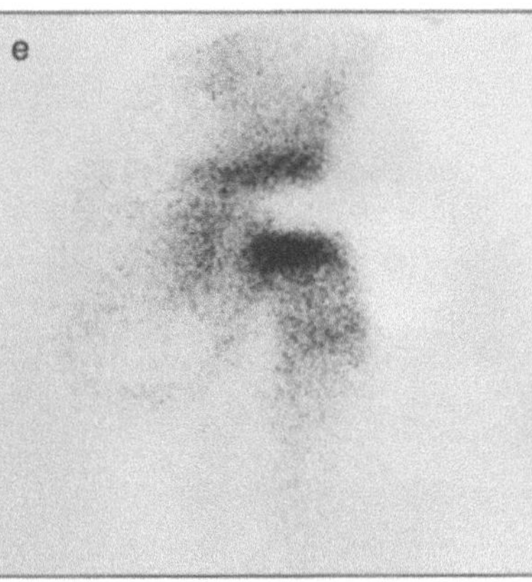

Fig. 6.4d. Anterior pin hole view of the right hip is normal

Fig. 6.4e. Anterior pin hole image of the left hip shows total absence of activity in the lateral two thirds of the femoral head.

The child had a follow-up scan 11 months later after a rotational osteotomy

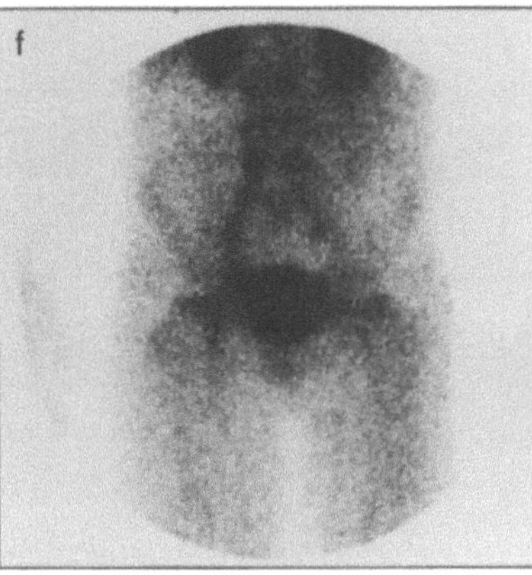

Fig. 6.4f. Blood pool anterior view of the pelvis and femora shows increased activity in the region of the left hip

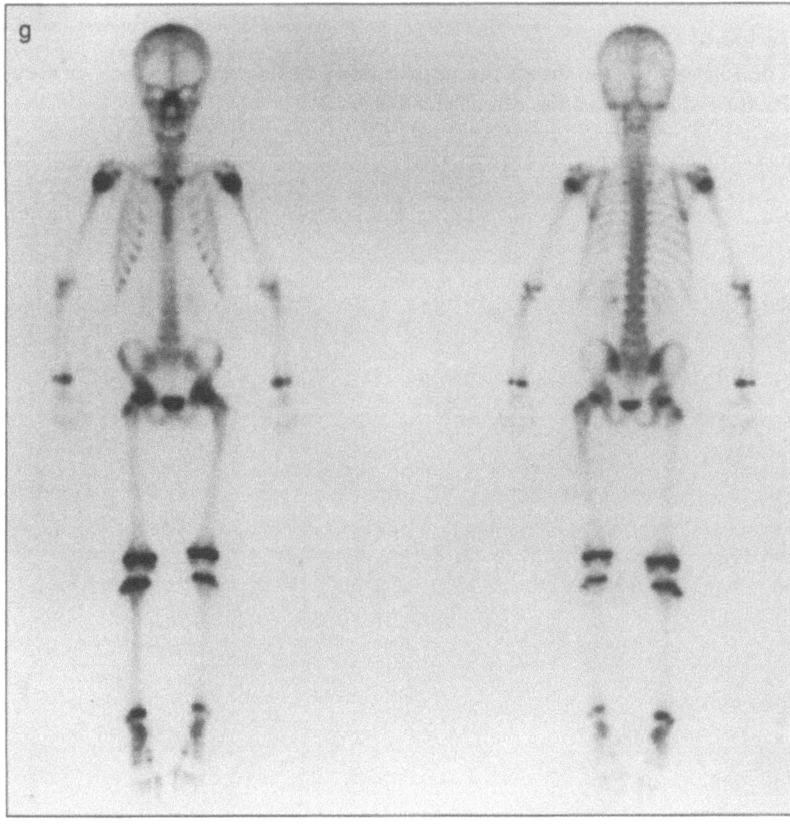

Fig. 6.4g. Whole body scans show slight increased uptake of isotope in the left femoral head extending into the proximal shaft best seen on the posterior view. There is a diffuse decreased uptake of isotope in the left knee and ankle presumably due to immobilisation
(continued on p. 262)

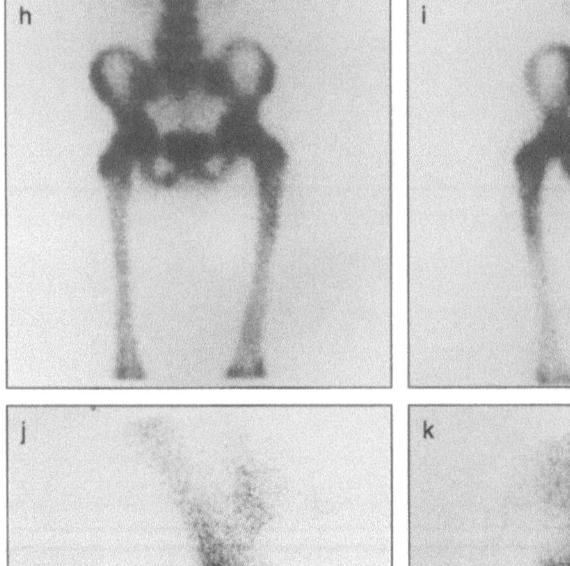

Fig. 6.4h. Anterior image of the pelvis and femora shows increased uptake of isotope in the upper shaft of the left femur

Fig. 6.4i. Posterior image of the pelvis and femora shows increased uptake in the left femoral neck and shaft

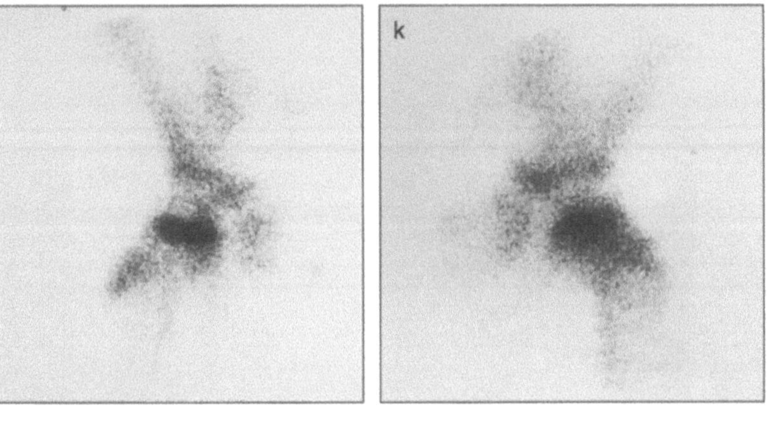

Fig. 6.4j. Anterior pin hole image of the right hip. This remains normal

Fig. 6.4k. Anterior pin hole view of the left hip shows increased uptake of isotope in the epiphyseal plate and neck of the femur with activity now seen in the femoral capital epiphysis

Technical Comment

The follow-up scan shows the appearances of the healing phase of Legg-Perthes' disease and the effect of surgery.

Case 6.5. A 7-year-old boy with pain in the right hip for 14 days due to Legg-Perthes' disease

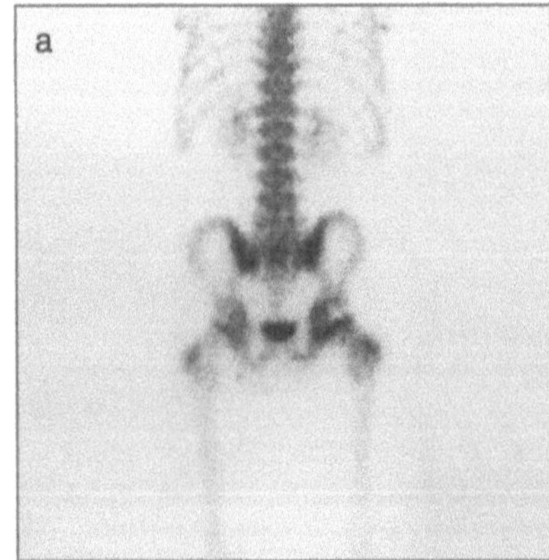
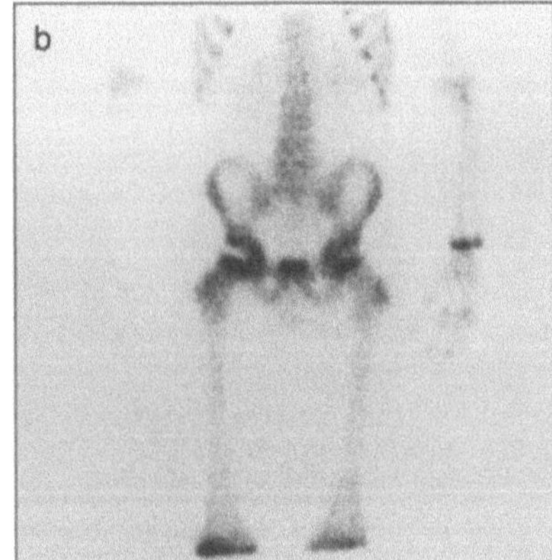

Fig. 6.5a. Posterior image of the pelvis shows absent activity in the right femoral head

Fig. 6.5b. Anterior view of the pelvis and femora shows absent activity in the lateral aspect of the right femoral head

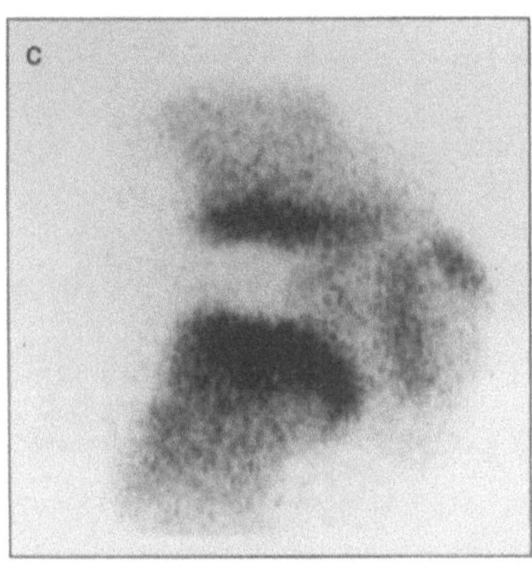

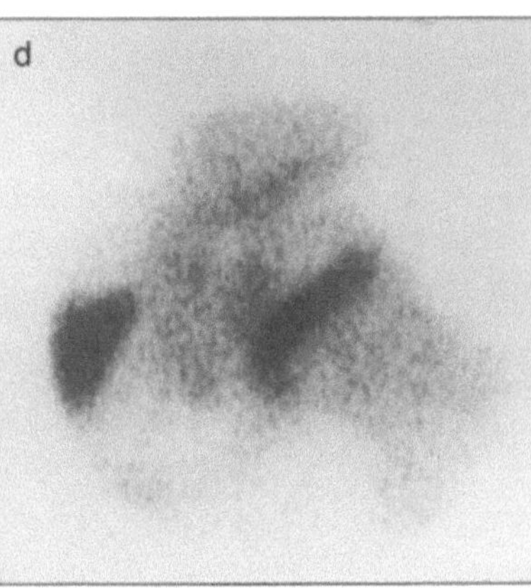

Fig. 6.5c. Pin hole view of the right hip shows total absence of activity laterally with slight activity seen medially

Fig. 6.5d. Pin hole view of the left hip is normal

Fig. 6.5e. Coronal single photon emission computed tomography (SPECT) images show total absence of activity in the right femoral head

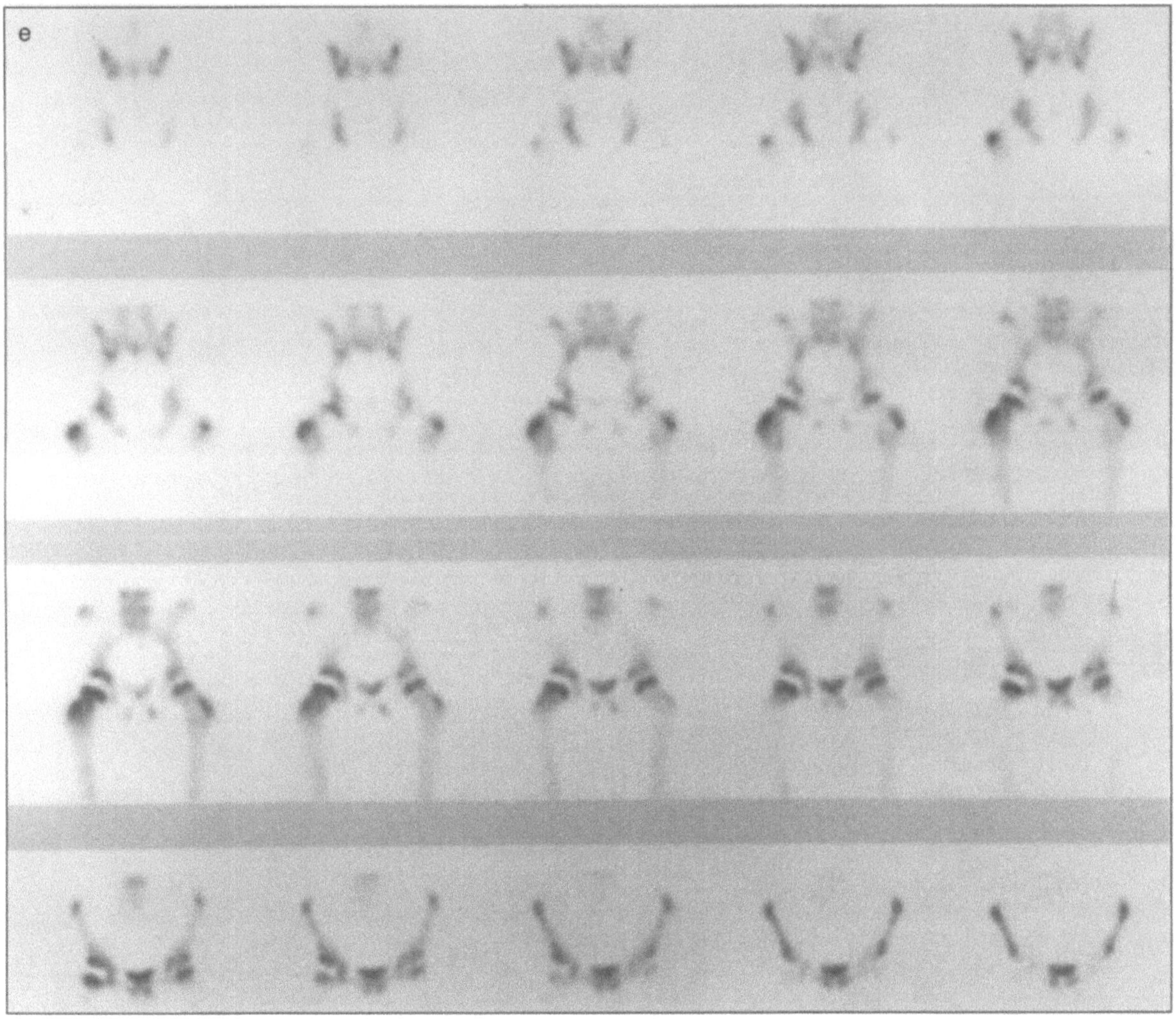

Teaching Point

Activity in the ischium may be seen on pin hole views and simulate slight activity on the medial aspect of a femoral head which is in fact totally devoid of activity.

**Case 6.6. A 6-year-old boy with
Legg-Perthes' disease of the left hip**

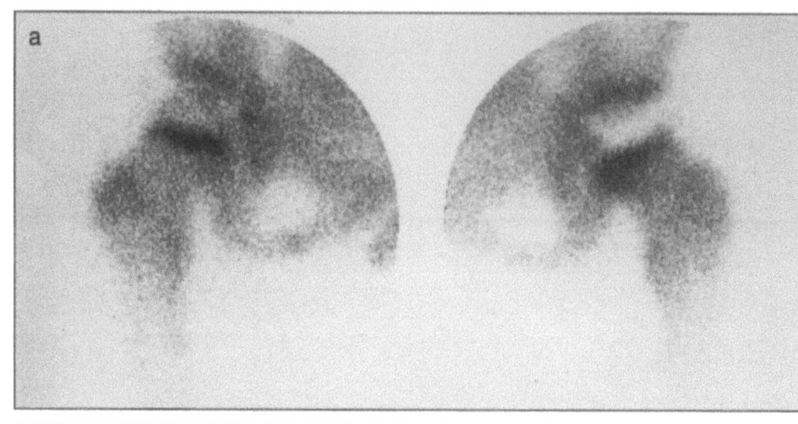

Fig. 6.6a. Pin hole images of the hips
show absence of activity in the lateral
four fifths of the left femoral head.
The right hip is normal.

A follow-up scan was performed
2 months later

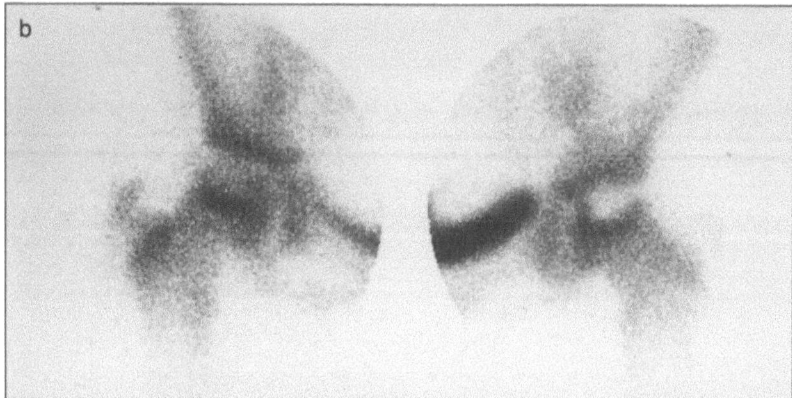

Fig. 6.6b. Pin hole images of both
hips show the healing phase on the left
with new activity now seen on the
lateral aspect of the femoral head and
also on the medial aspect

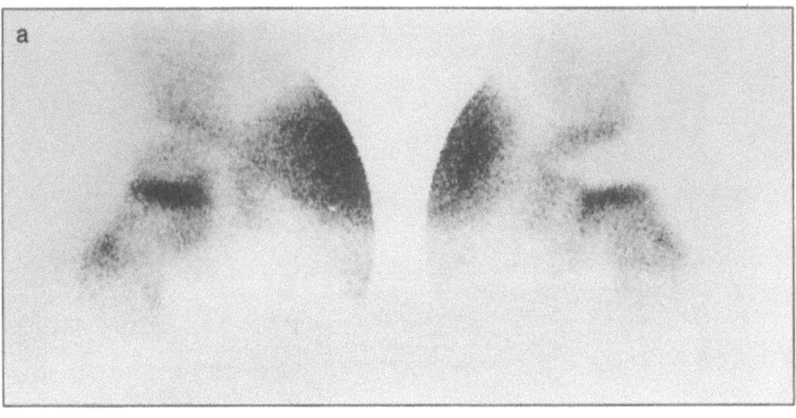

Case 6.7. A 4-year-old boy with Legg-Perthes' disease of the left hip

Fig. 6.7a. Pin hole images of both hips show total absence of activity in the left femoral head.

A follow-up bone scan was performed 5 months later

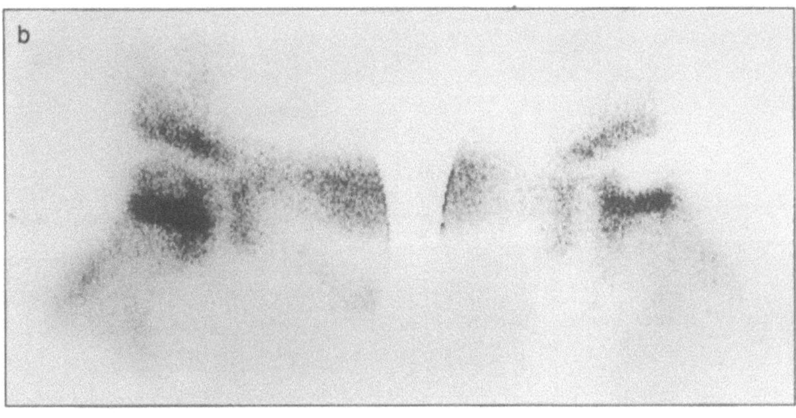

Fig. 6.7b. Pin hole images show new activity on the medial aspect of the left femoral head immediately above the epiphyseal plate

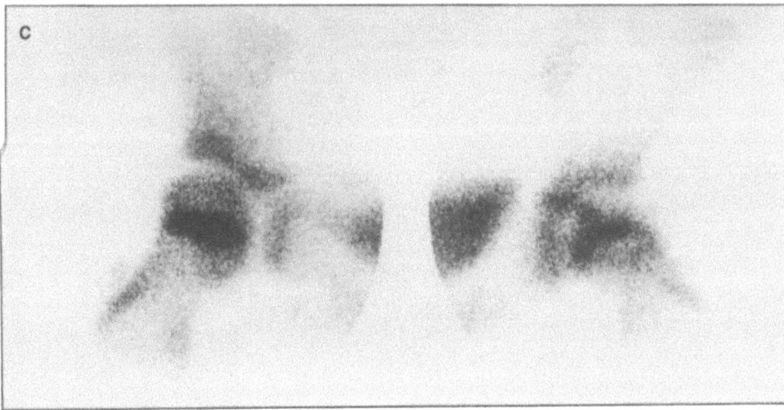

Fig. 6.7c. A second follow-up bone scan was obtained 15 months following the original scan where there is focal increased uptake of isotope in the mid portion of the left femoral head

Teaching Point

Notice the difference between the two joint spaces on Fig. 6.7c, suggesting that the flattened head has not yet re-expanded. Since this is 15 months following the original bone scan, the prognosis for a normal femoral head is poor.

**Case 6.8. A 7-year-old boy with
Legg-Perthes' disease of the right hip**

Fig. 6.8a. Pin hole images of the hips
show mainly a cold femoral head on
the right but a little activity is seen on
the lateral aspect immediately above
the epiphyseal plate. This area of
increased activity suggests that this is
not early Legg-Perthes' disease. Note
the preservation of the joint space.

A follow-up bone scan was performed
1 year later

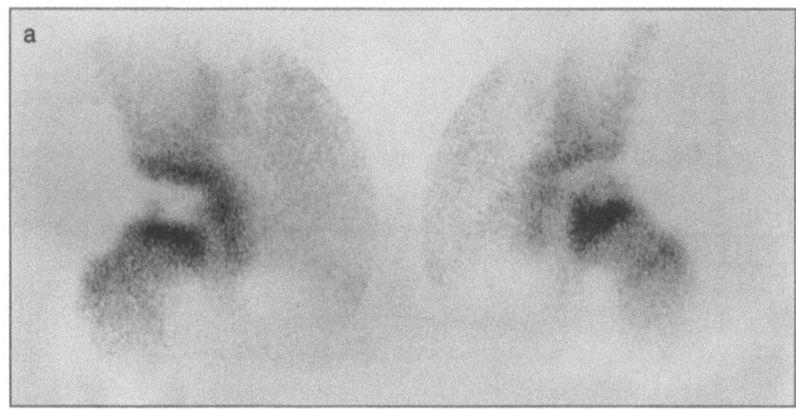

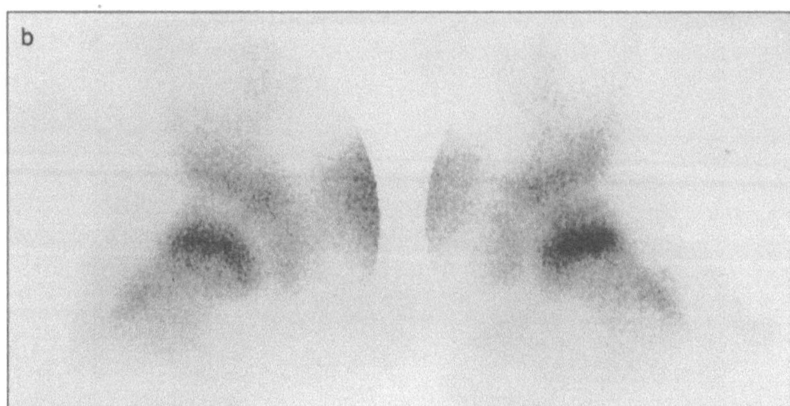

Fig. 6.8b. Anterior pin hole images
of both hips now reveal activity in the
lateral aspect of the right femoral
head. This shows the healing phase

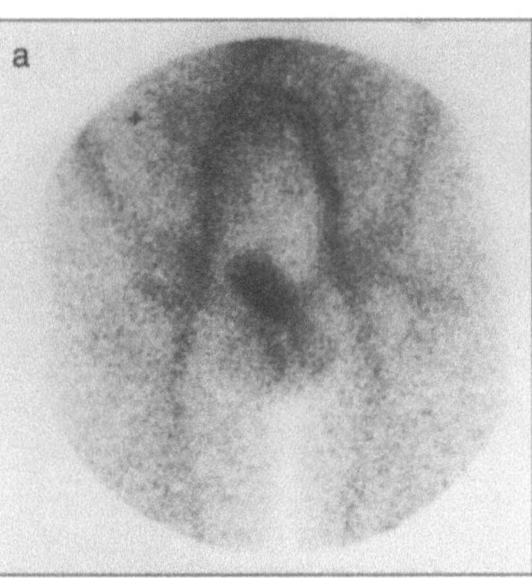

Case 6.9. A 14-year-old boy with pain in the left hip. The final diagnosis was atypical Legg-Perthes' disease. The child is a little old for Legg-Perthes' disease. The imaging features are atypical

Fig. 6.9a. Anterior blood pool image of the pelvis shows slight increased activity in the region of the left hip

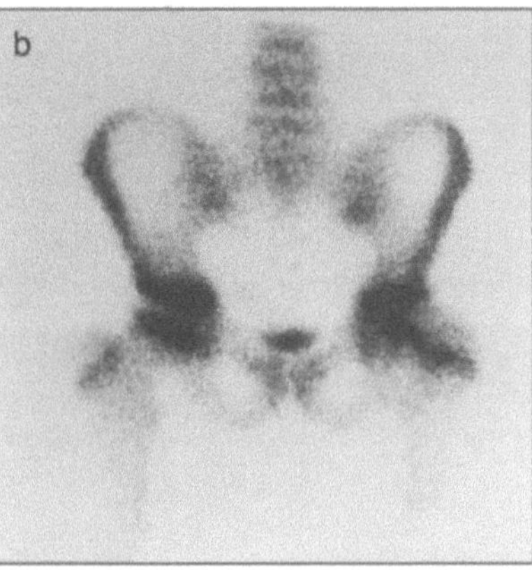

Fig. 6.9b. Anterior image of the lower lumbar spine, pelvis and upper femora shows abnormal increased activity in the left femoral neck extending to the greater trochanter. The normal epiphyseal plate is lost

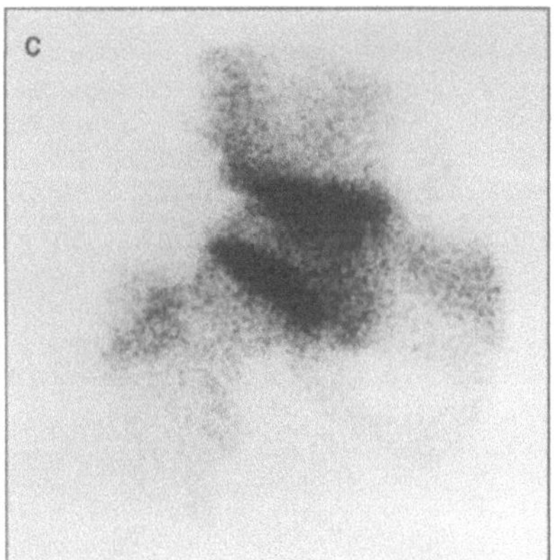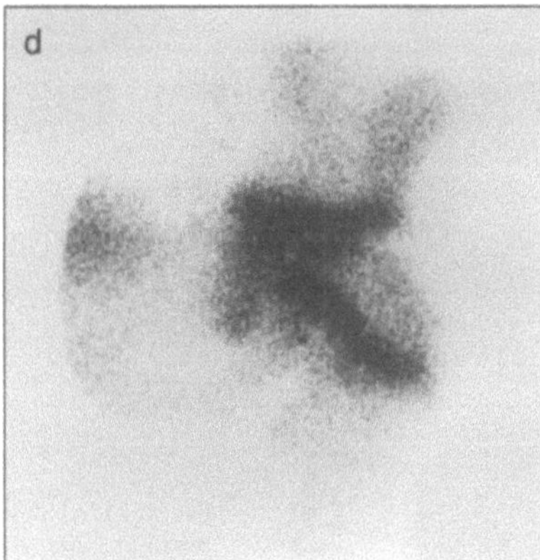

Fig. 6.9c. Pin hole image of the right hip is normal

Fig. 6.9d. Pin hole image of the left hip fails to show the normal architecture. There is loss of joint space and the capital epiphysis cannot be seen, but the increased activity in the upper femur suggests that there has been marked rotation of the femur and that the area of increased uptake represents the epiphyseal plate

Teaching Point

The femoral head had undergone necrosis and never recovered. This was an idiopathic avascular necrosis of the femoral head which has been classified as an atypical Legg-Perthes' disease. The isotope scan was undertaken at a late stage of the disease in the reparative phase.

6.2 Other Sites of Osteochondritis Dissecans
(3 Cases; Fig. 6.10–6.12)

Case 6.10. An 11-year-old girl with pain in the right knee due to osteochondritis dissecans

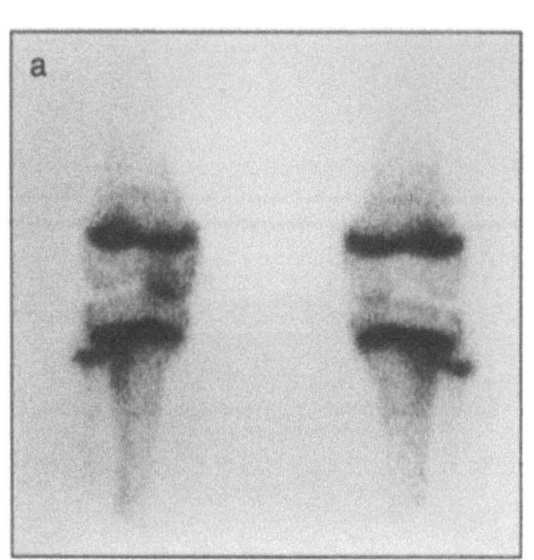

Fig. 6.10a. Anterior image of the knees (magnified view) shows focal abnormal increased uptake of isotope in the right medial femoral condyle. This was due to osteochondritis dissecans of the medial condyle of the right femur

Case 6.11. A 10-year-old boy with pain in the left foot due to Köhler's disease

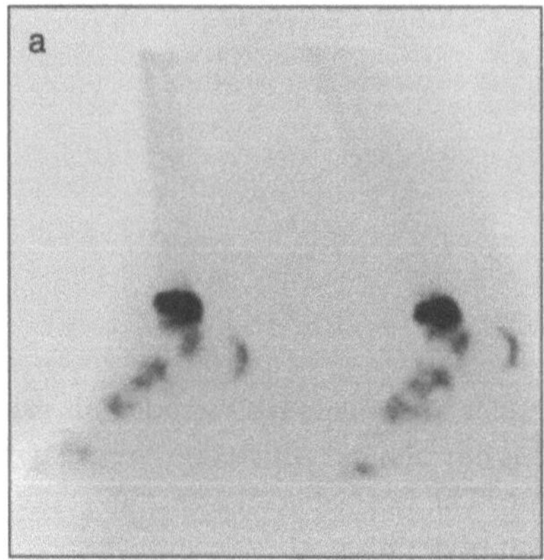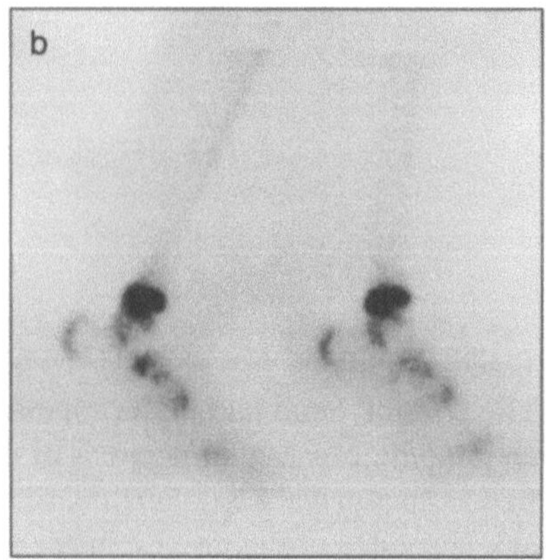

Fig. 6.11a,b. Lateral images of the feet from both the medial lateral and lateral lateral projections. There is abnormal increased uptake of isotope in the navicular bone on the left on both projections

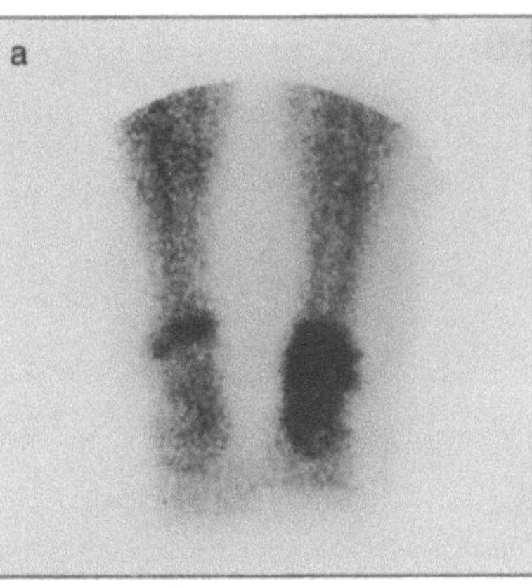

Case 6.12. An 8-year-old boy with pain in the right foot which was due to osteochondritis dissecans of the os naviculare (Köhler's disease)

Fig. 6.12a. Posterior blood pool image of the feet shows increased uptake of isotope in the right foot

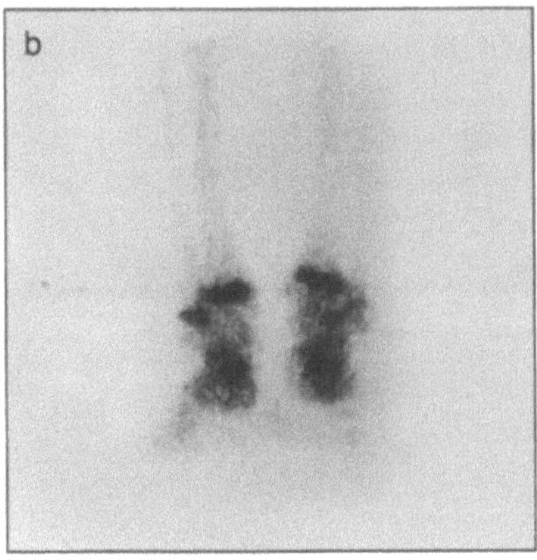

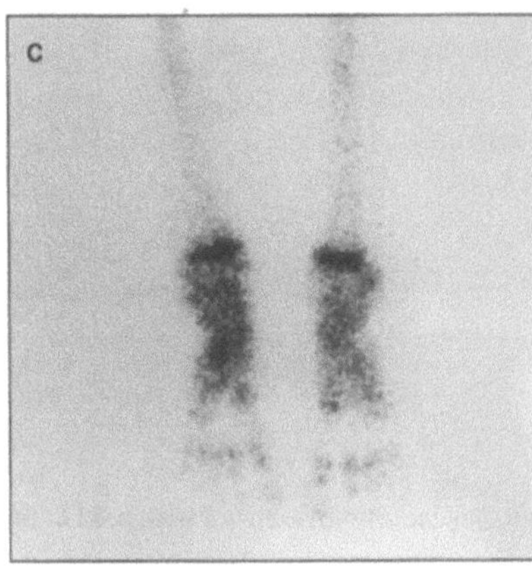

Fig. 6.12b. Posterior image of the ankles and feet shows increased activity in the region of the small bones of the right foot

Fig. 6.12c. Anterior image of the ankles and feet shows increased activity throughout the hind foot on the right

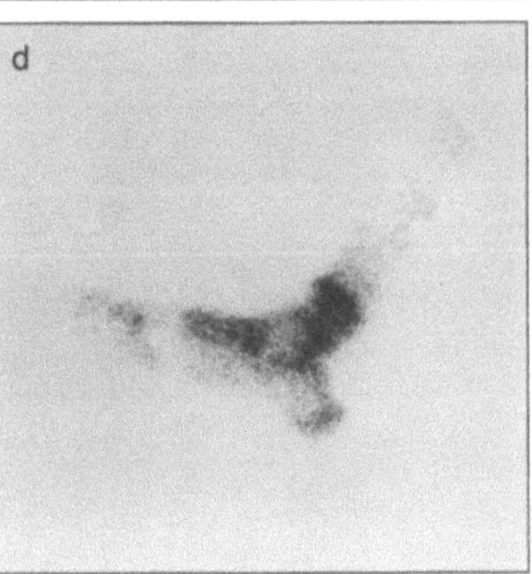

Fig. 6.12d. Lateral image of the right foot shows increased activity in the region of the os naviculare with normal activity in the talus and calcaneus

6.3 Sickle Cell Disease

(7 Cases; Figs. 6.13–6.19)

Teaching Point

The retention of isotope by the kidneys is very common in these children, but the explanation remains uncertain. These children have bone scans when they are acutely unwell. The loss of clarity of the epiphyseal plates due to increased activity in the metaphyses of the long bones is an important observation and does not reflect infection.

The differentiation between infection and recent infarction is not easy. Recent infarction is usually seen as a cold area if the bone scan is carried out within a few days. However, the presence of previous infarcts results in areas of increased uptake of isotope on bone scan. The appearances must be considered in conjunction with the full clinical and radiological picture.

Case 6.13. A 5-year-old boy with sickle cell disease who presented with pain in the hips and right shoulder

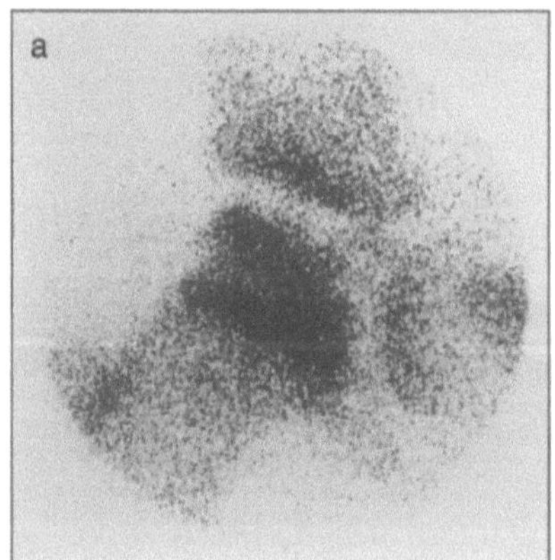

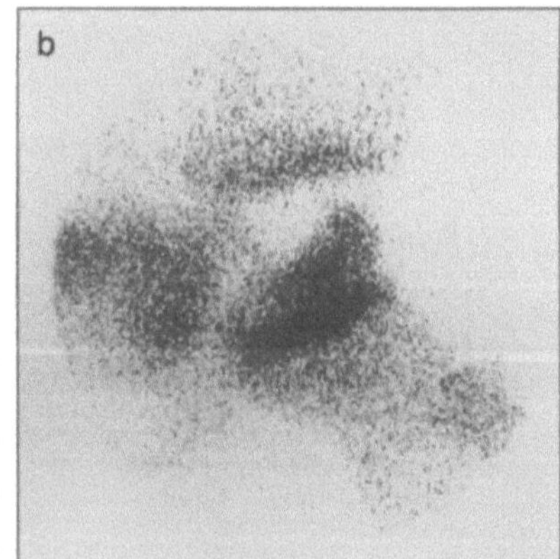

Fig. 6.13a. Anterior pin hole image of the right hip shows abnormal increased activity in the femoral head with some indistinctness of the epiphyseal plate

Fig. 6.13b. Anterior pin hole image of the left hip shows total absence of activity in the mid aspect of the femoral head with abnormal increased uptake of isotope in the distal and lateral aspect, making the epiphyseal plate somewhat indistinct

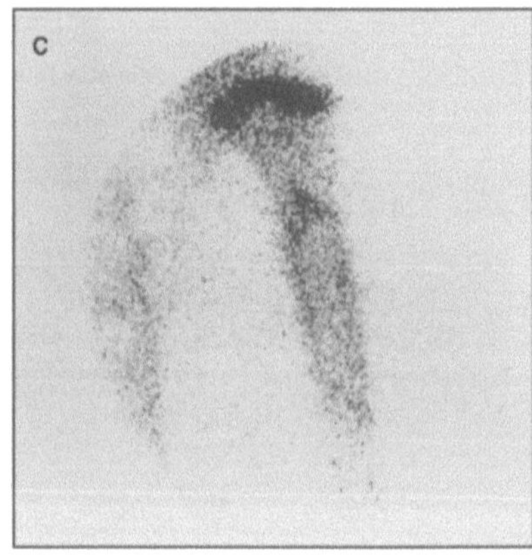

Fig. 6.13c. Posterior image of the right humerus shows focal abnormal increased uptake of isotope in the mid third of the shaft

Teaching Point

1. The appearances in the hips suggest that the child had previous acute episodes of infarction of the femoral heads. The appearances on the right suggest healing, whilst on the left there is a combination of recent infarction and also healing.
2. Similar appearances may be seen in Legg-Perthes' disease (Cases 6.1–6.9).

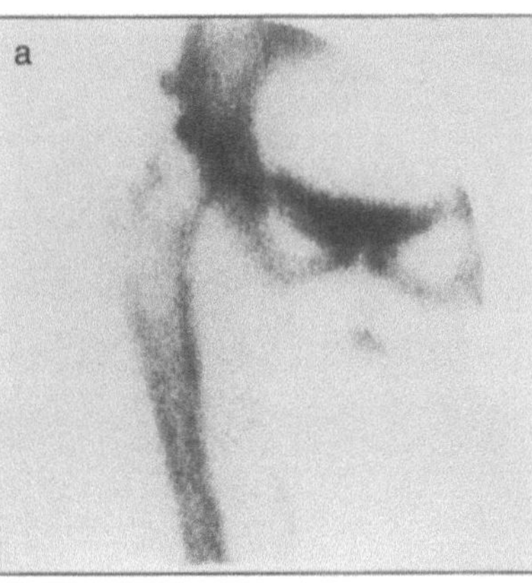

Case 6.14. A 14-year-old girl with known sickle cell disease presented with pain in the right hip

Fig. 6.14a. Anterior image of the right hemipelvis, hip and upper femur shows decreased activity in the femoral neck and upper femoral shaft with abnormal increase in activity in the remainder of the femoral shaft. Follow-up showed that there was no infection in the hip or femur, and this reflected the healing phase of previous infarcts

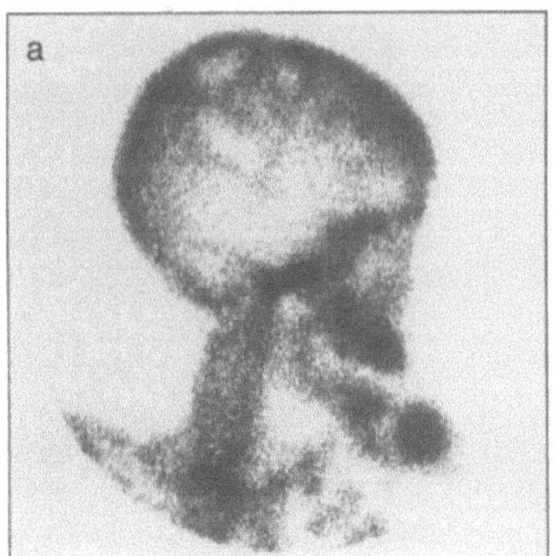

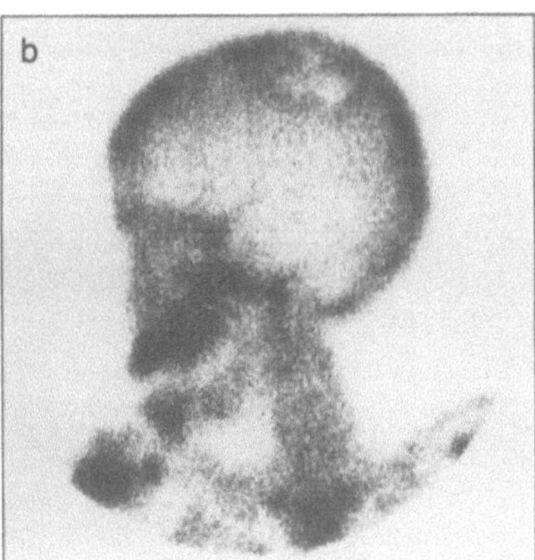

Case 6.15. A 9-year-old girl with known sickle cell disease presented with fever and oedema of the scalp. Follow-up showed that there was no infection in the skull vault, rather that infarction of part of the parietal bone had occurred

Fig. 6.15a. Right lateral image of the skull shows diffuse abnormal increased uptake of isotope in the frontal and posterior parietal bones with focal decreased uptake in the parietal bone. Note the epiphyseal plate of the left humerus overlying the tip of the mandible

Fig. 6.15b. Left lateral image of the skull shows the focal area of decreased uptake of isotope in the parietal bone to better advantage with surrounding increased activity which extends into the posterior parietal and occipital bones

Case 6.16. A 9-year-old boy with established sickle cell disease. He was shown to have multiple bony infarcts

Fig. 6.16a. Right lateral image of the skull and right arm is unremarkable

Fig. 6.16b. Left lateral image of the skull and left arm shows abnormal increased uptake of isotope in the left humerus; this is patchy and involves the entire humerus

Fig. 6.16c. Posterior image of the thorax, dorsal and lumbar spine shows decreased activity in the vertebral body at the level of D11 and L1. The posterior ribs bilaterally show patchy areas of increased and decreased uptake of isotope

Fig. 6.16d. Right posterior oblique image of the thorax and spine shows to better advantage the abnormalities in the ribs

Fig. 6.16e. Left posterior oblique image of the thorax, spine and upper pelvis shows the abnormalities in the ribs on the left. Both oblique projections show the abnormality in the vertebral bodies at D11 and L1

Fig. 6.16f. Anterior image of the spine, pelvis and upper femora shows increased activity in both femoral necks extending inferiorly

Fig. 6.16g. Posterior image of the lower femora and knees shows patchy abnormal increased uptake of isotope in both femoral shafts

Teaching Point
Similar appearances of the thorax may be seen in infection (see Cases 2.22, 2.30, 2.34, 2.35) and tumours (see Cases 4.28, 4.30, 4.53).

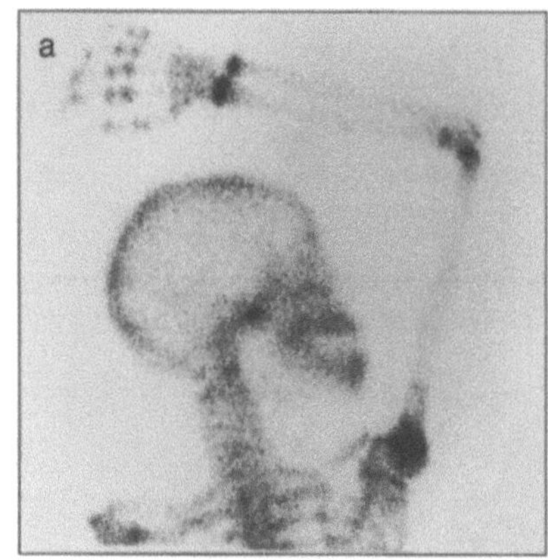
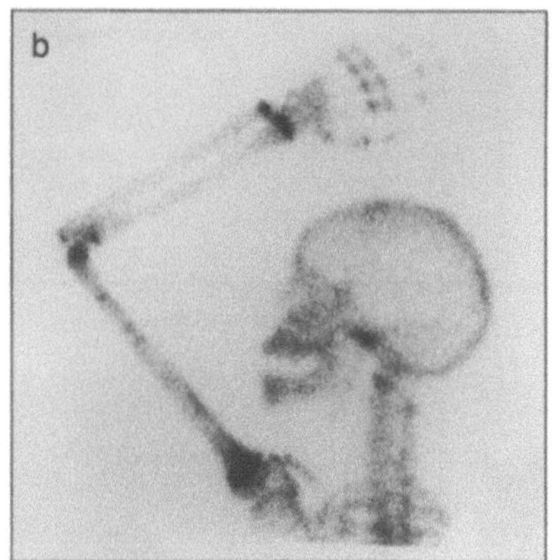
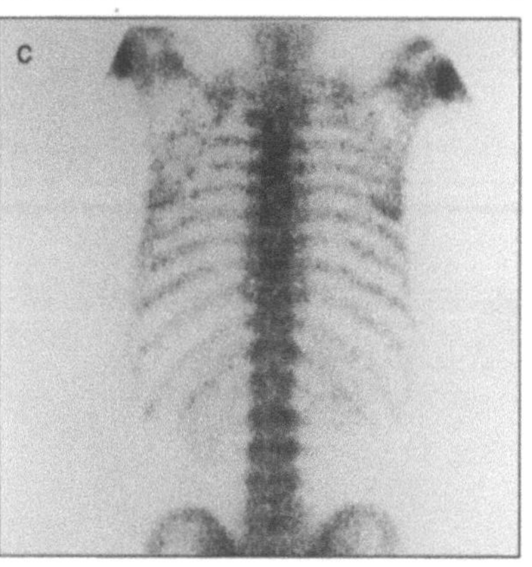
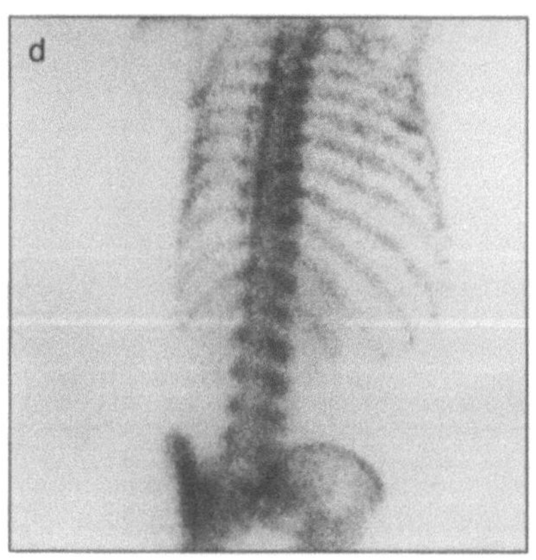
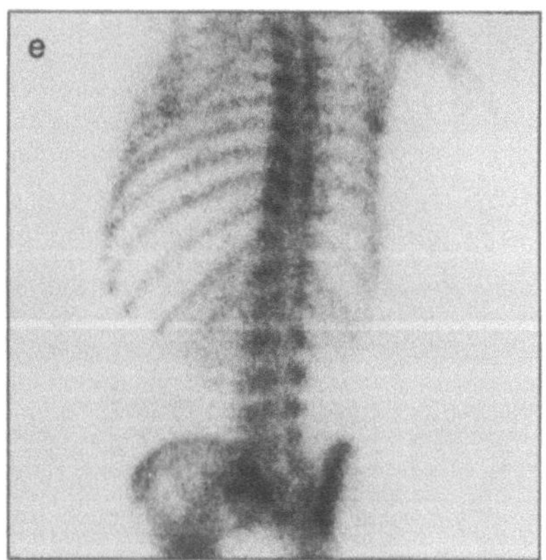
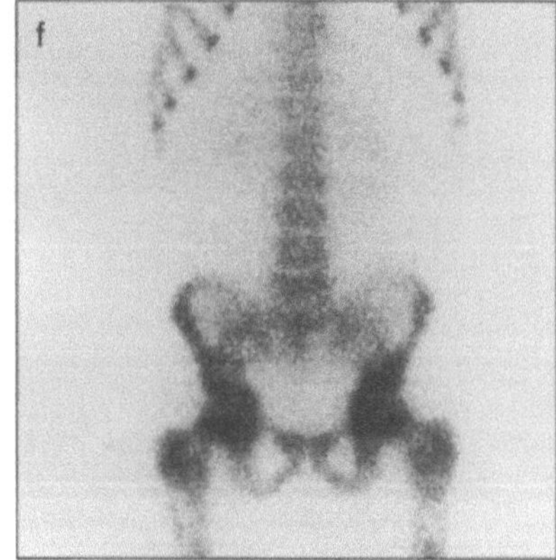
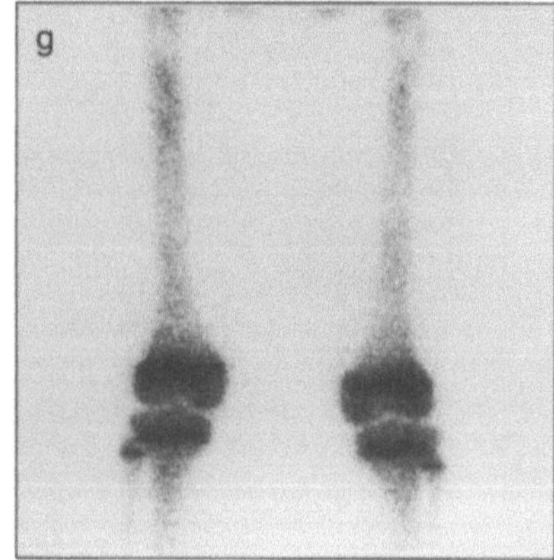

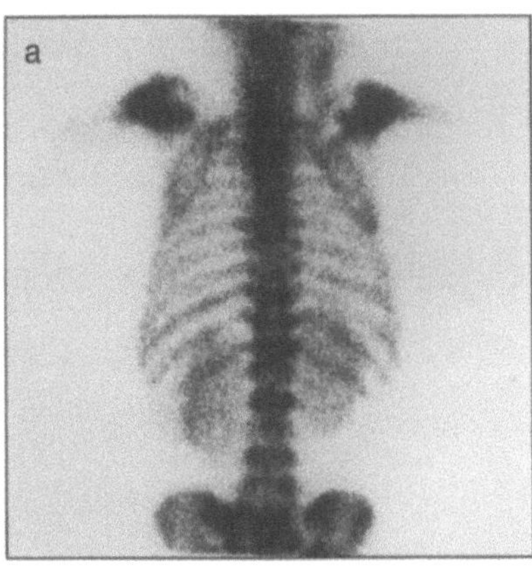

Case 6.17. A 5-year-old boy with sickle cell disease. He had been unwell and taken to his bed for 3 days prior to the scan. No infection was found. All the bony abnormalities were considered to be due to bone infarction

Fig. 6.17a. Posterior image of the thorax, dorsal and lumbar spine. Some vertebrae show areas of decreased activity in the mid dorsal and mid lumbar spine, while other vertebrae show areas of increased activity (e.g. D11 and D12). The ribs are not homogeneous, with some ribs showing increased activity, best seen in the left tenth and right ninth ribs, among others

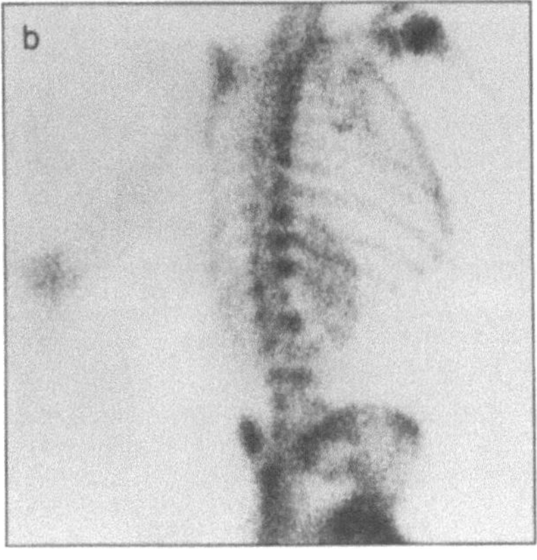

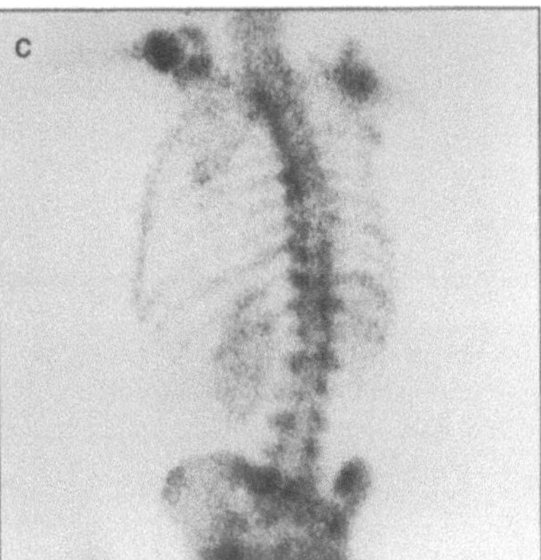

Fig. 6.17b. Right posterior oblique image of the thorax and spine shows the uneven distribution of isotope in the vertebral bodies. The patchy uptake in the ribs on the right is again noted

Fig. 6.17c. Left posterior oblique image of the thorax, spine and upper pelvis. The vertebral and rib abnormalities are again noted

Fig. 6.17d. Posterior magnification view of the knees shows lack of clarity of the epiphyseal plates throughout the knees, with slightly abnormal increased uptake of isotope in the distal left femoral metaphysis.

The child remained persistently unwell with pain especially around the knees, and a repeat bone scan was undertaken 3 weeks later

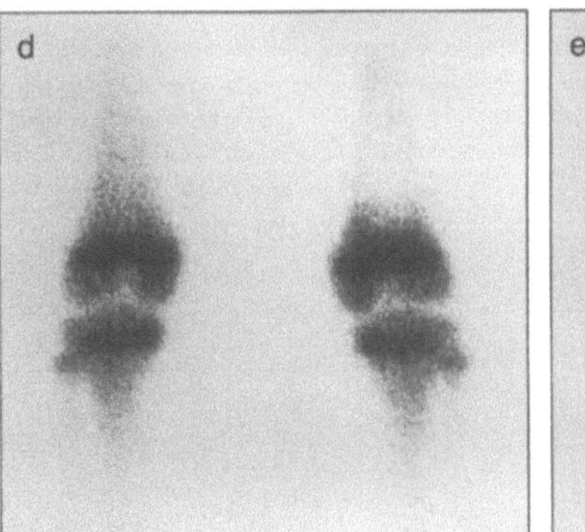

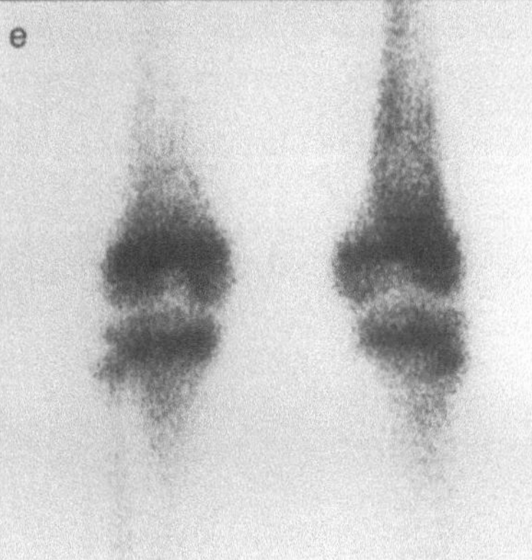

Fig. 6.17e. Posterior image of the knees (magnified view) shows new areas of focal increased activity of isotope in the distal right femoral metaphysis laterally but extending to the diaphysis medially. There is also abnormal uptake of isotope in the mid shaft of the left femur. Neither of these two areas were abnormal on the earlier scan.

Technical Comment

Note the retention of tracer in the kidneys in Fig. 6.17a–c.

Teaching Point

1. Similar appearances of the thorax may be seen in PNET tumours (see Case 4.53).
2. The child was unwell and the loss of clarity of the epiphyseal plates could have been simply due to acute immobilisation (also see Chap. 7.6, "Sick Child").

Case 6.18. A 2-year-old boy with sickle cell disease who presented with a severe crisis. Multiple bony infarcts throughout the skeleton were detected

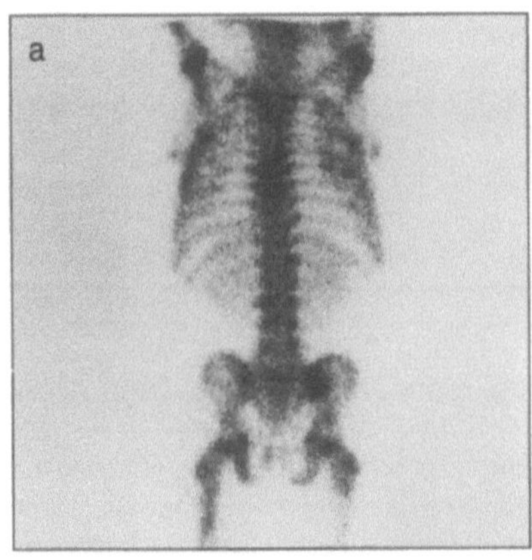

Fig. 6.18a. Posterior image of the thorax, spine, pelvis and upper femora shows abnormal uptake in the ribs, especially on the right. The vertebral bodies, especially in the lumbar spine, show areas of decreased and increased activity. There is increased activity in the right sacro-iliac joint as well as in the upper femora, more marked on the left than on the right

Fig. 6.18b. Right posterior oblique image of the thorax, spine, pelvis and upper femora reveals the extent of the abnormalities in the ribs with two ribs showing focal increased uptake of isotope. The vertebral bodies with decreased uptake in the lumbar spine are better seen

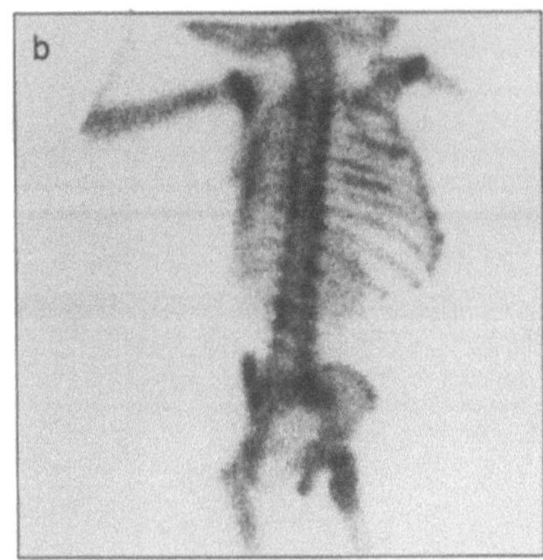

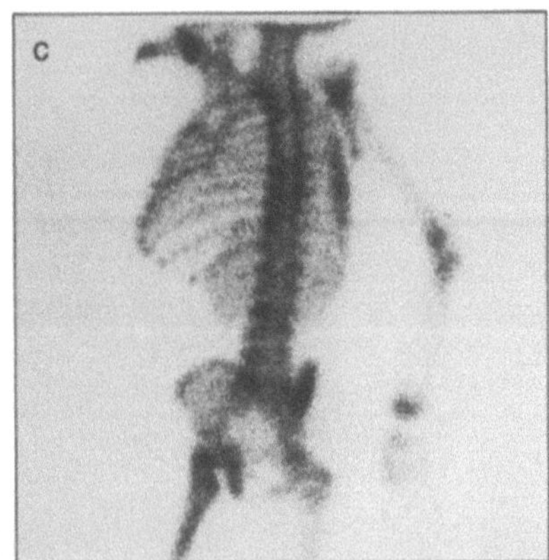

Fig. 6.18c. Left posterior oblique image of the thorax, spine, pelvis and upper femora shows that the ribs on the left are involved to a lesser extent than on the right. Increased uptake is noted in the left femoral shaft

Fig. 6.18d. Posterior view of the right arm is unremarkable

Fig. 6.18e. Posterior view of the left arm shows abnormal increased uptake throughout the left humerus and also in the proximal two thirds of the left radius

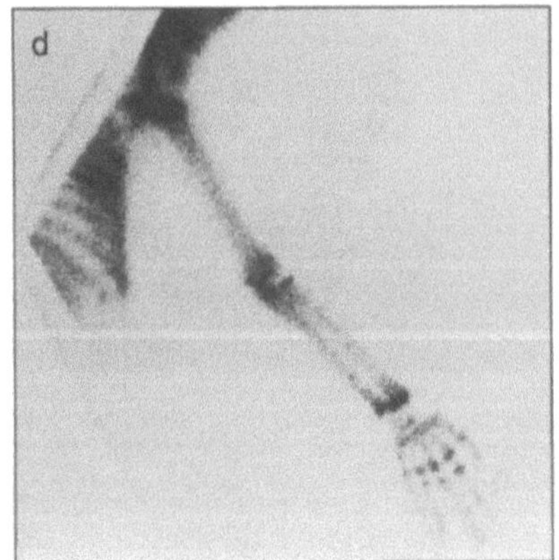

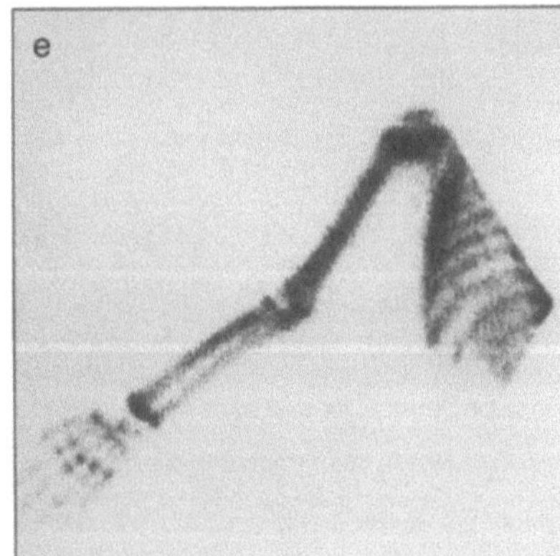

Technical Comment
Note the importance of positioning of the hand so that the radius and ulna can be clearly separated.

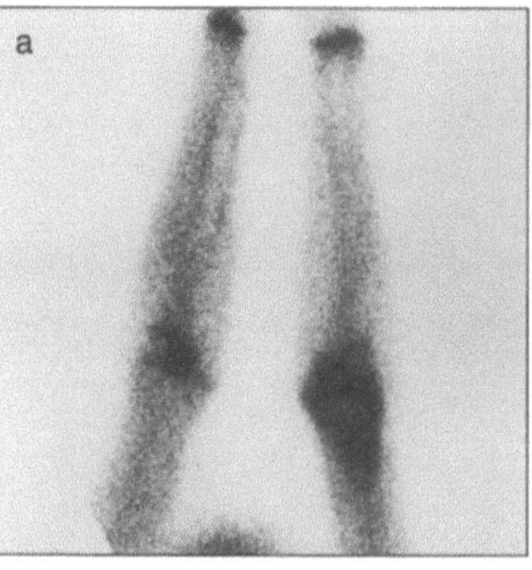

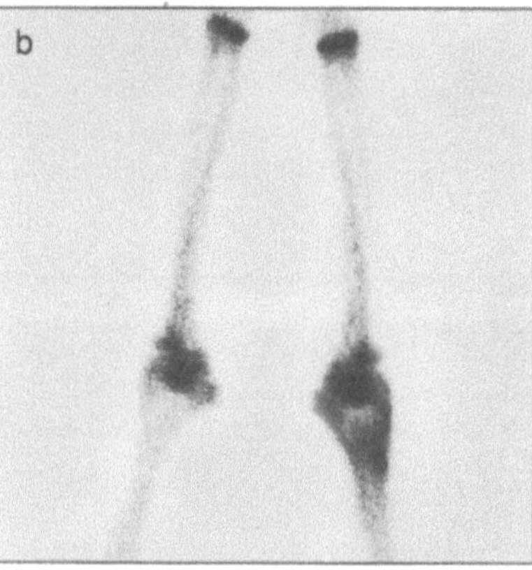

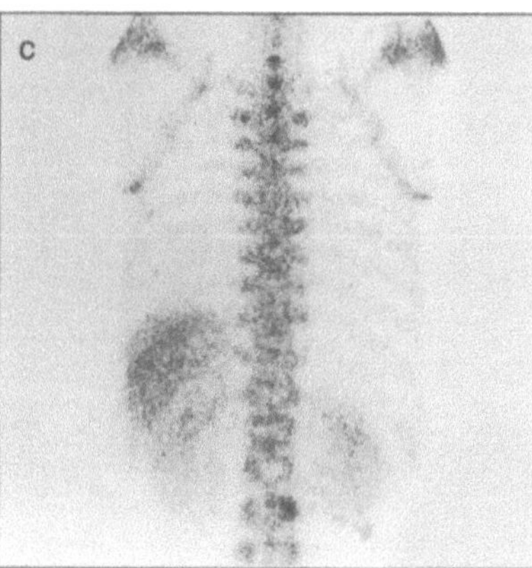

Case 6.19. A 13-year-old boy with known sickle cell disease who presented with an acute swollen painful left elbow and was found to have septicaemia. The final diagnosis was that of sepsis around the left elbow in addition to multiple infarcts in both the skeleton and spleen

Fig. 6.19a. Posterior blood pool image of the elbows and forearms shows abnormal increased uptake of isotope in the left distal humerus with reduction of isotope in the left forearm compared to the right

Fig. 6.19b. Posterior image of the elbows shows focal areas of increased uptake of isotope in the left distal humerus

Fig. 6.19c. Posterior image of the thorax, dorsal and lumbar spine shows focal abnormal increased uptake of isotope on the right side of the body of L3. There is retention of tracer by both kidneys. Splenic activity is also noted

7 Miscellaneous

7.1 Dysplasia

7.1.1 Fibrous Dysplasia
(5 Cases; Figs. 7.1–7.5)

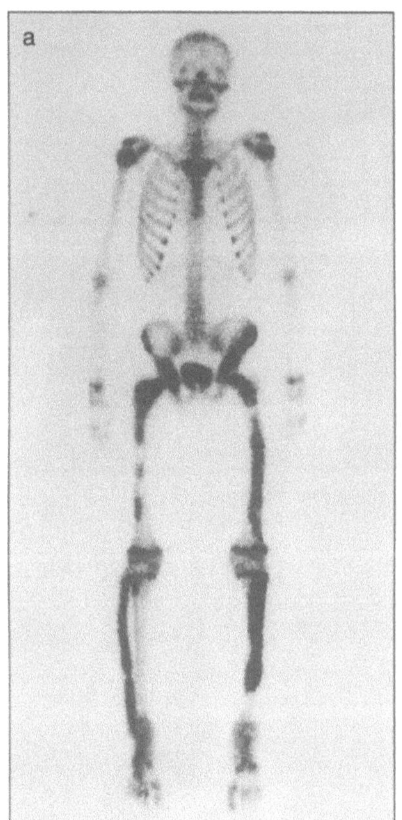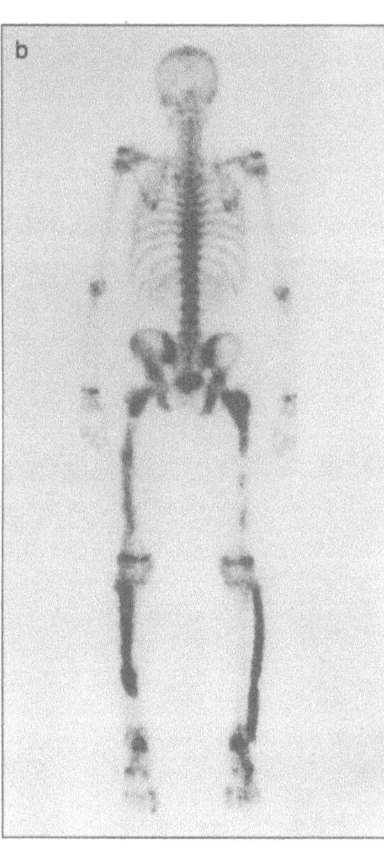

Case 7.1. A 16-year-old girl with known fibrous dysplasia

Fig. 7.1a,b. Whole body scans show abnormal increased uptake of isotope in both femora, the right acetabulum as well as in the left tibia and right fibula. The right foot also shows involvement mainly on the lateral aspect

**Case 7.2. A 6-year-old boy with
known fibrous dysplasia**

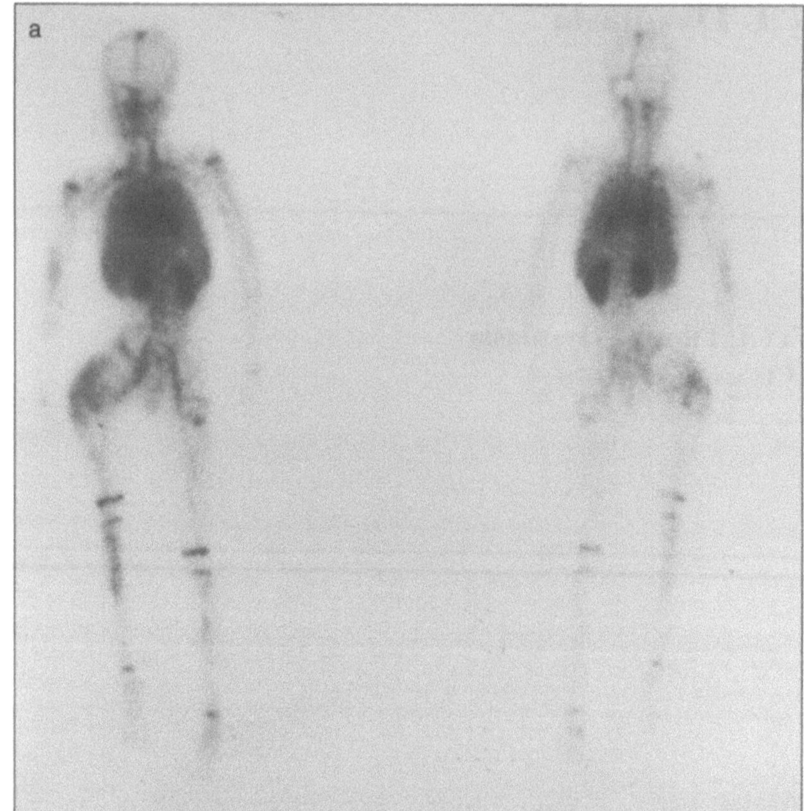

Fig. 7.2a. Blood pool whole body
images show abnormal increased
uptake of isotope in the region of the
right thigh, in the right upper calf and
the right distal humerus. The short
right lower limb is noted

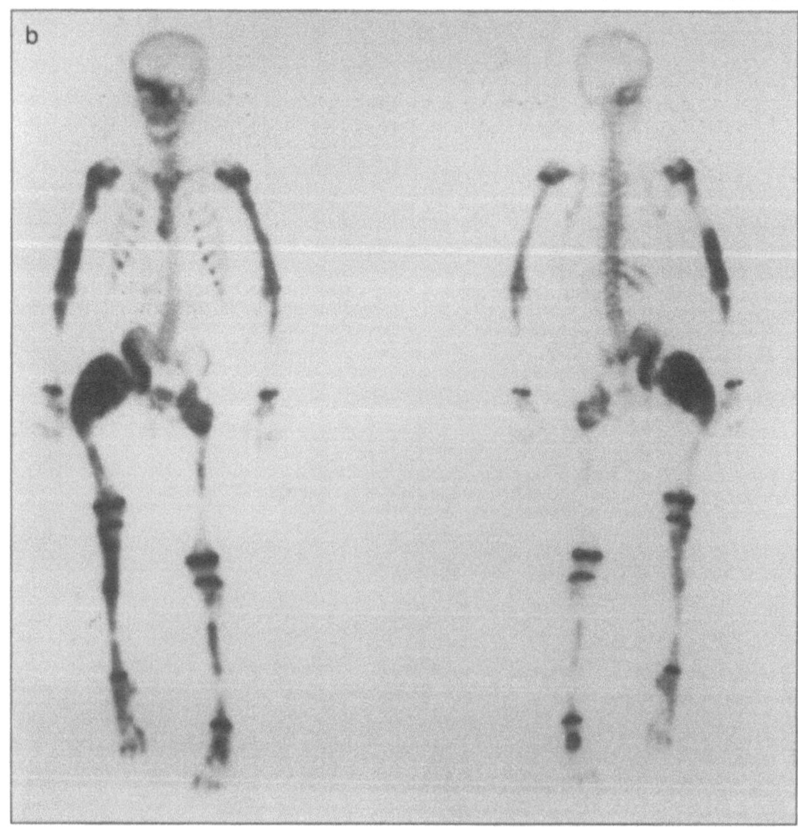

Fig. 7.2b. Whole body scans show
abnormal increased uptake of isotope
in the facial bones on the right, in
both humeri, more marked on the
right than on the left as well as in the
proximal right forearm. There is
abnormal increased uptake of isotope
in the right hemipelvis with intense
increased uptake in the shortened,
expanded and deformed right proximal femur. The left femoral neck and
shaft show areas of abnormal increased uptake of isotope. Similar features
are seen in both tibiae.

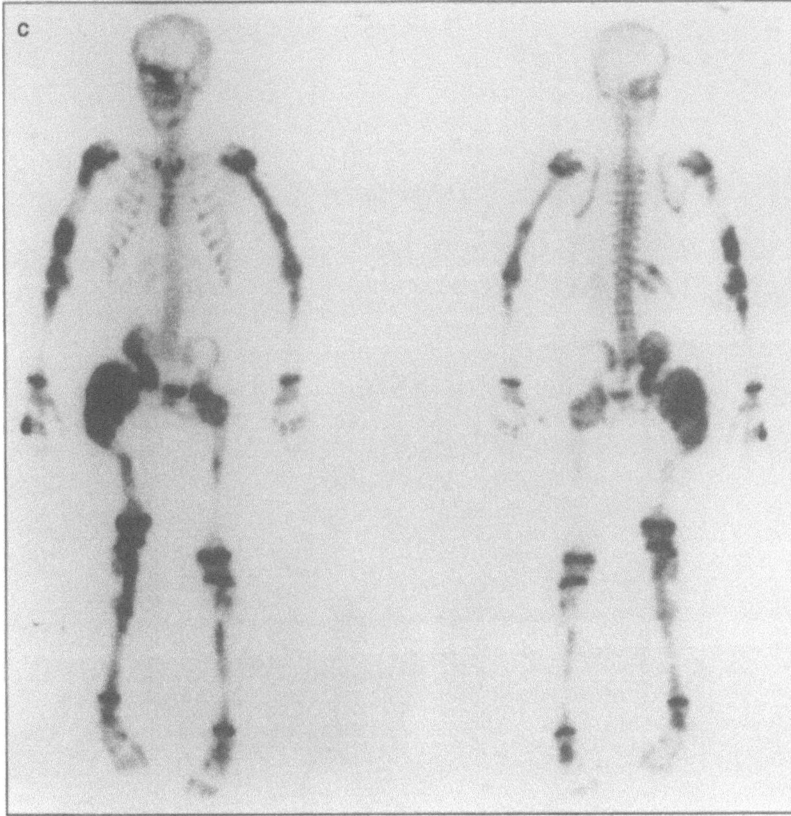

A follow-up bone scan was undertaken
4 years later

Fig. 7.2c. Whole body scans show
abnormal increased uptake of isotope
in the facial bones around the orbit on
the right. The shoulder girdle, both
humeri and forearms show abnormal
patchy increased uptake of isotope.
The posterior right 11th and 12th ribs
show abnormal increased uptake of
isotope which is also noted in the right
ilium. There has been little change in
the appearances of the femora. In the
tibiae areas of increased uptake of isotope are again seen. Note that especially in the upper and mid portions of
the right tibia, there appears to be
expansion. These were sites of fracture
with callus formation

Teaching Point
In order to detect fractures in pathological bones, radiographs of the bone
at the site of increased activity are required.

**Case 7.3. A 13-year-old boy with
known fibrous dysplasia**

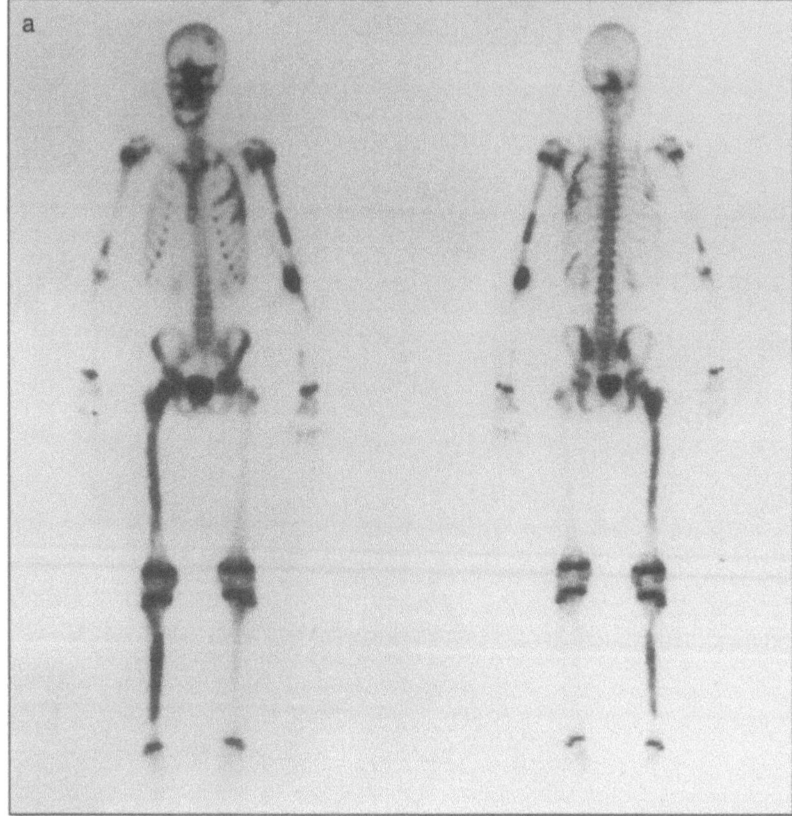

Fig. 7.3a. Whole body scans show
abnormal focal increased uptake of
isotope in the skull vault on the left.
Increased uptake of isotope is noted
in the facial bones and also in the
humeri, more marked on the left than
on the right. The distal left radius is
involved as are the ribs on the left,
both the upper ribs and one lower rib.
The right femur and tibia also show
abnormal increased uptake of isotope.
Note extravasation of isotope in the
left cubital fossa, the site of the intravenous injection.

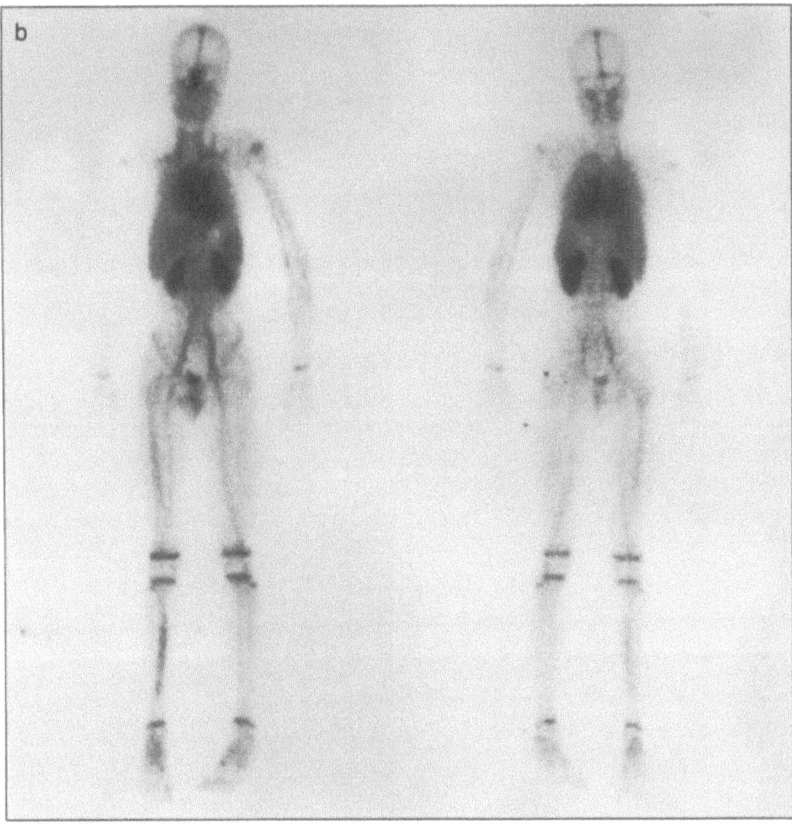

A follow-up bone scan was undertaken 14 months later

Fig. 7.3b. Whole body blood pool images show abnormal increased uptake of isotope in the left humerus and in the right femur and tibia

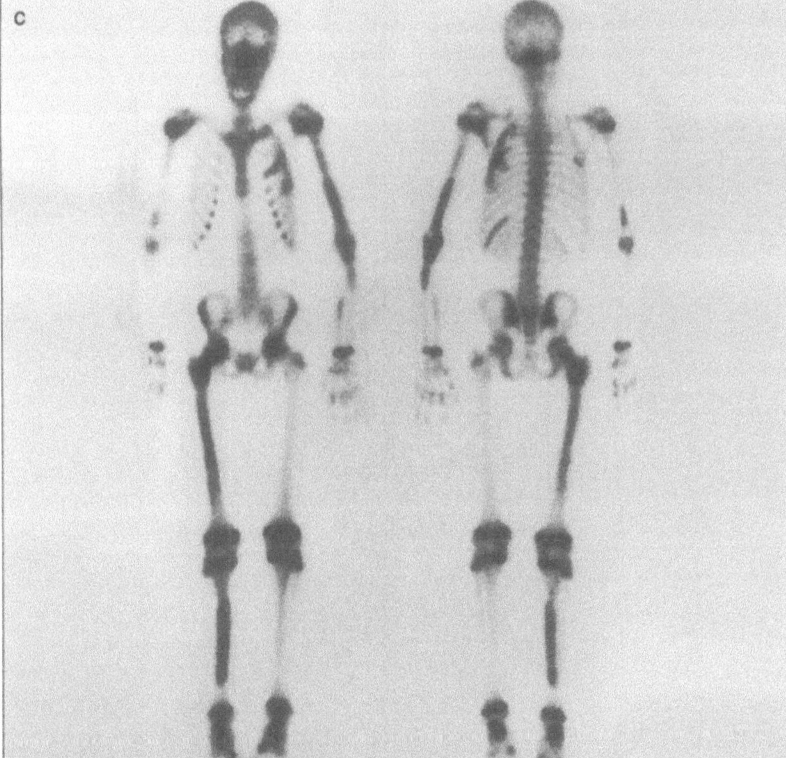

Fig. 7.3c. Whole body scans show abnormal increased uptake of isotope in the skull vault and facial bones. Both humeri as well as the left radius and ulna are also involved. There has been progression in the involvement of the radius and ulna when compared to the previous study. The right femur and tibia are abnormal but have not changed. There is little change in the appearances of the ribs on the left

Case 7.4. A 13-year-old boy with fibrous dysplasia

Fig. 7.4a. Right lateral image of the skull and right arm shows abnormal increased uptake of isotope in the parietal and occipital bones as well as in the region of the anterior cranial fossa. Note the deformity of the upper humeral shaft

Fig. 7.4b. Left lateral image of the skull and left arm shows abnormal uptake of isotope in the parietal and occipital bones as well as in the region of the floor of the anterior cranial fossa. The deformed left humerus with focal abnormal increased uptake of isotope is noted, and the bone is also expanded proximally. The left radius is also expanded, with abnormal increased uptake of isotope

Fig. 7.4c. Posterior view of the lower pelvis, femora and knees shows abnormal increased uptake of isotope in the upper left femoral shaft

Fig. 7.4d. Posterior view of the tibiae and fibulae shows patchy increased uptake of isotope in the left tibia

Case 7.5. A 4-year-old girl with known fibrous dysplasia who developed McCune-Albright syndrome

Fig. 7.5a. Blood pool whole body images show focal abnormal increased uptake of isotope on the right side of the face and also in the right femur and right tibia. Note extravasation of isotope in the right cubital fossa

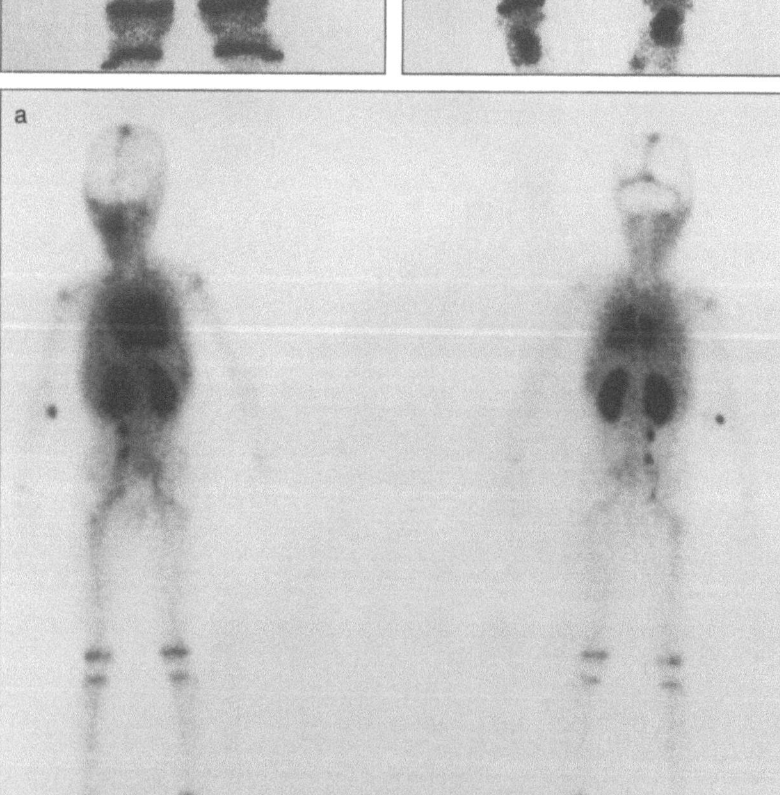

284

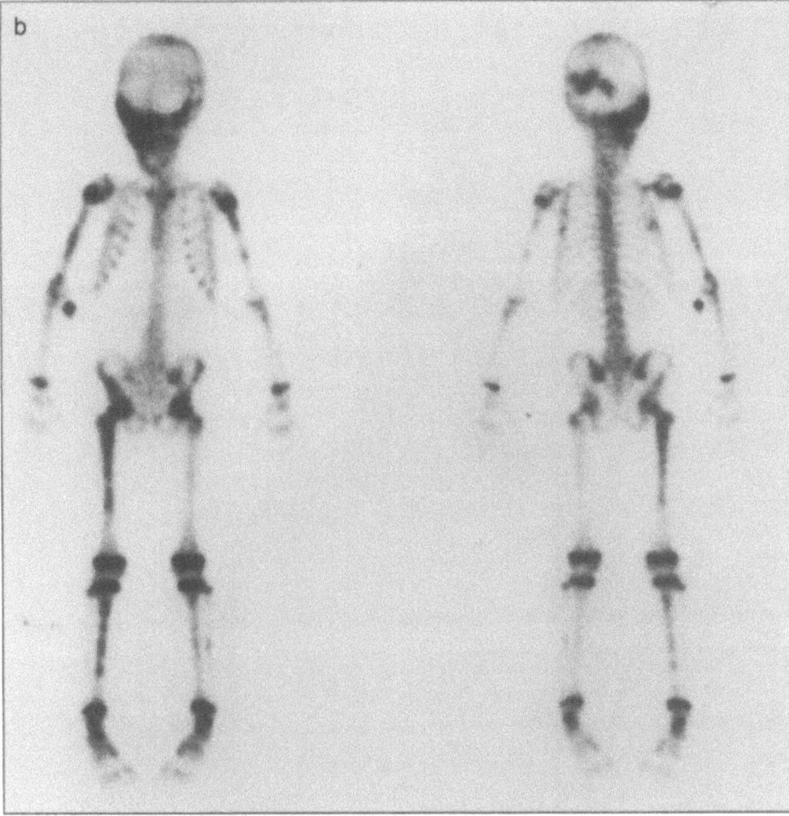

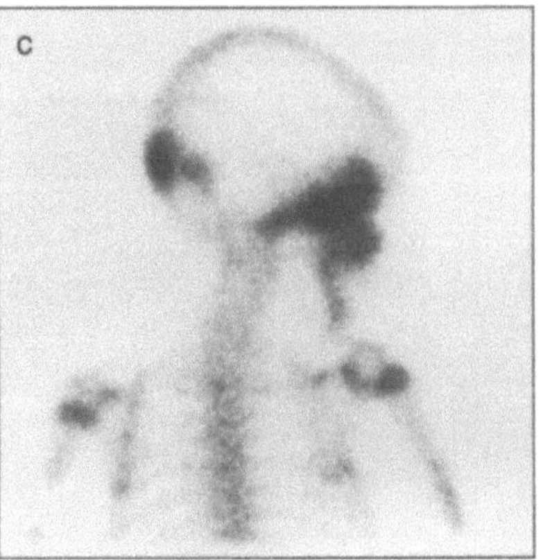

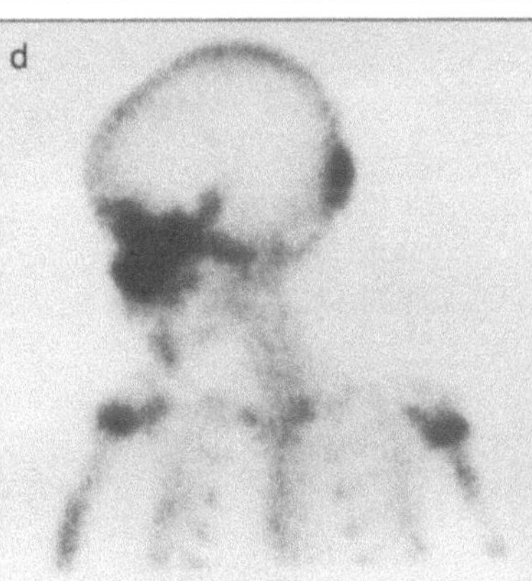

Fig. 7.5b. Whole body scans show abnormal uptake in the facial bones on the right as well as in the skull vault on the left. Abnormal uptake of isotope is noted in both humeri as well as in both forearms, more marked on the right than on the left and in the right anterior hemithorax and the left sacro-iliac joint. The upper two thirds of the right femur, both tibiae and the left fibula are also involved, but to different degrees. Note extravasation of isotope in the right cubital fossa

Fig. 7.5c. Right lateral image of the skull, upper thorax and both humeri shows focal abnormal increased uptake of isotope in the facial bones extending to involve the floor of the middle and anterior cranial fossae. The occipital bone is also involved. The abnormal activity in both humeri is again seen

Fig. 7.5d. Left lateral image of the skull and anterior view of thorax and humeri shows abnormal activity in the facial bones and floor of the anterior and middle cranial fossae as well as in the occipital bone. The abnormal thorax and humeri are again noted

7.1.2 Hemihypertrophy
(1 Case; Fig. 7.6)

Case 7.6. A 12-year-old boy with an abnormal gait who was found to have hemihypertrophy of the left side of his body

Fig. 7.6a. Posterior view of the dorsal and lumbar spine shows no significant asymmetry in the ribs

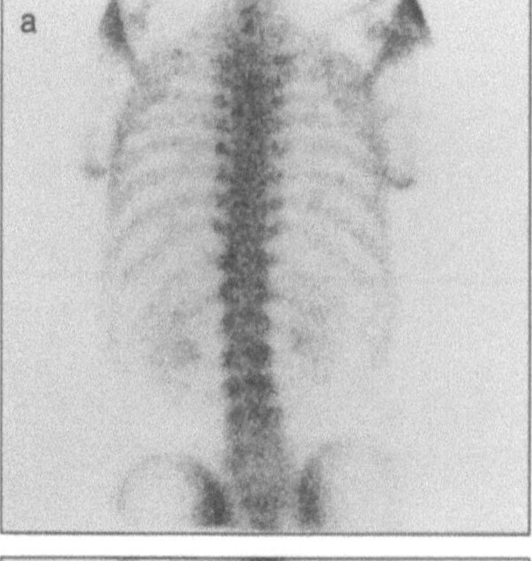

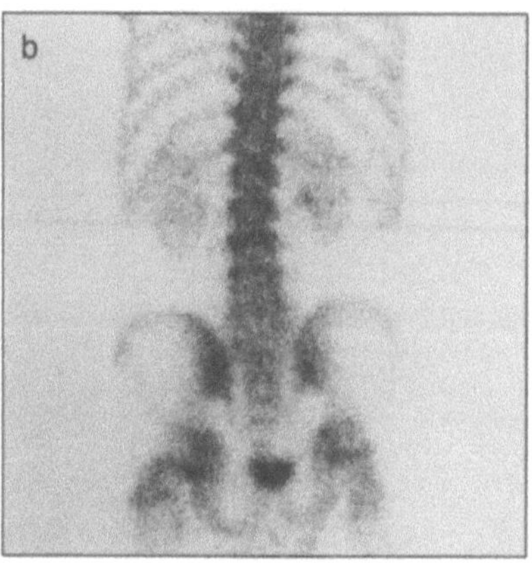

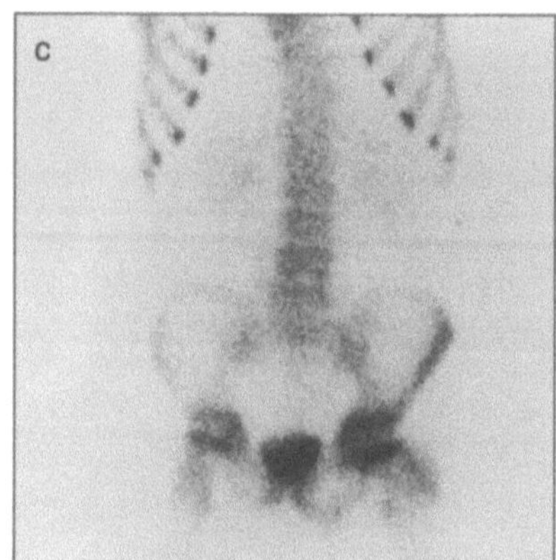

Fig. 7.6b. Posterior image of the lower dorsal and lumbar spine as well as pelvis and upper femora shows the larger left hemipelvis and left upper femur

Fig. 7.6c. Anterior image of the lumbar spine and pelvis shows the large left hemipelvis

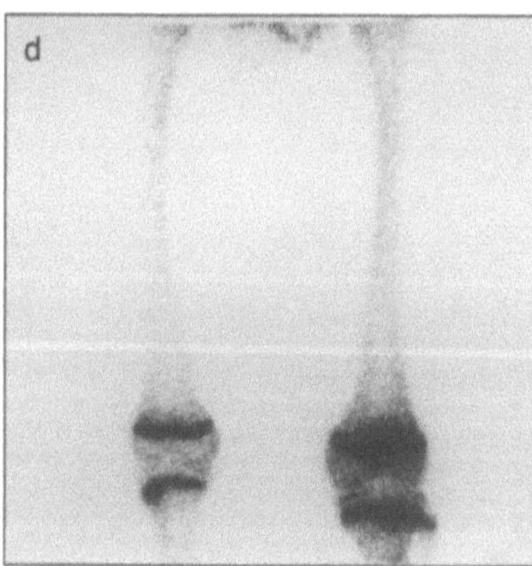

Fig. 7.6d. Anterior image of the femora and knees shows the larger left femur and knee

7.1.3 Osteogenesis Imperfecta
(1 Case; Fig. 7.7)

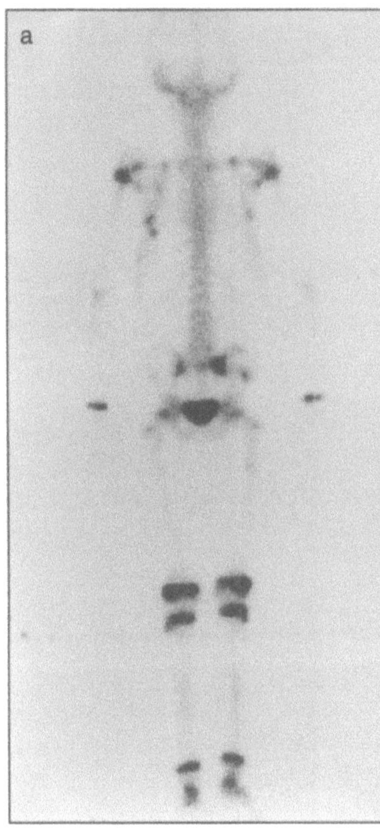

Case 7.7. A 6-year-old boy with known osteogenesis imperfecta in whom new fractures were suspected

Fig. 7.7a. Whole body posterior view shows abnormal increased uptake of isotope in the left shoulder, in the ribs on the left, the right sacro-iliac joint extending into the ilium as well as in the mid shaft of the right femur

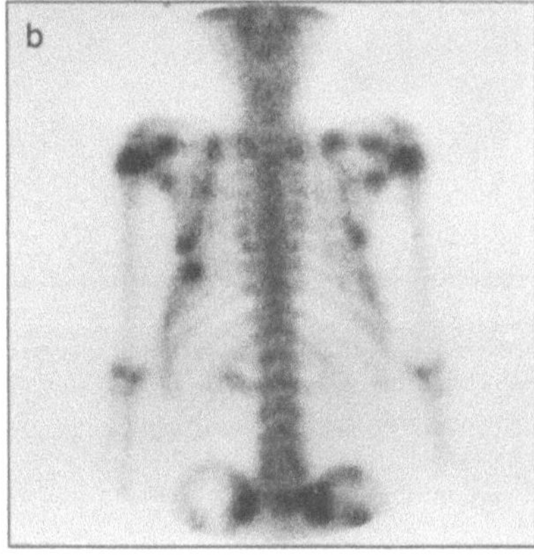

Fig. 7.7b. Posterior image of the thorax, humeri and dorsal spine shows the abnormal increase of isotope in one of the ribs on the left, suggesting a new fracture. Focal abnormalities are seen in both scapulae and the right sacro-iliac joint

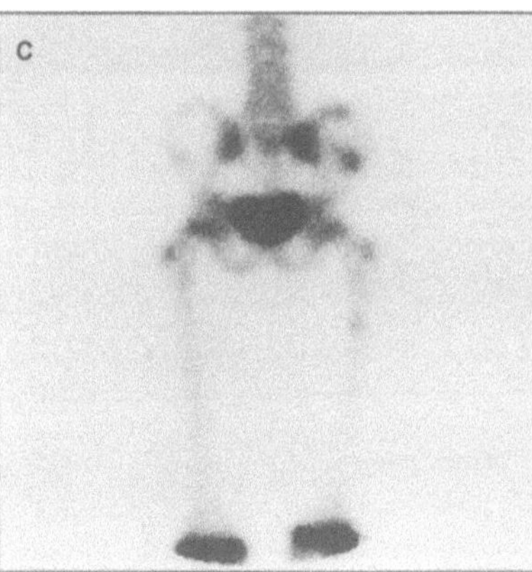

Fig. 7.7c. Posterior view of the lower lumbar spine, pelvis and femora shows abnormal increased activity in the right sacro-iliac joint extending into the right ilium. There is also abnormal increased uptake of isotope in the upper shaft of the right femur. The new fractures were confined to the right iliac bone, extending to and involving the right sacro-iliac joint

Teaching Point
Also see Case 5.45.

7.1.4 Neurofibromatosis
(2 Cases; Fig. 7.8, 7.9)

Case 7.8. A 10-year-old boy with known neurofibromatosis

Fig. 7.8a. Anterior image of part of the chest and left humerus shows abnormal increased uptake of isotope in both the upper and mid portions of the humerus

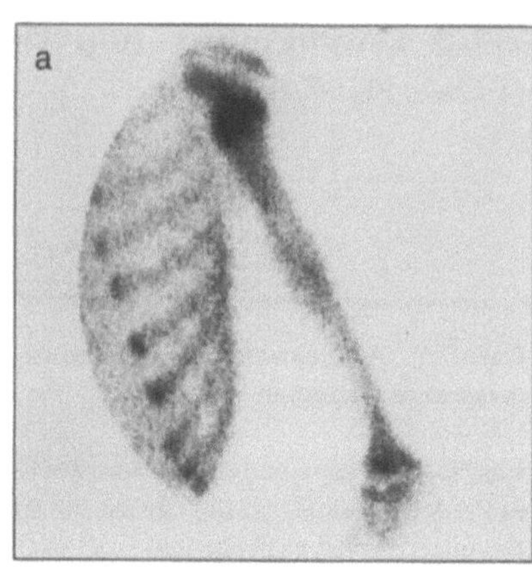

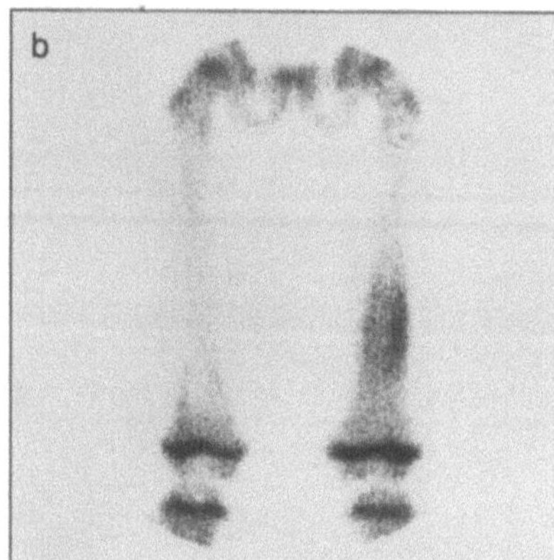

Fig. 7.8b. Posterior image of the femora shows abnormal increased uptake of isotope in the lower third of the right femur with abnormal modelling of the bones

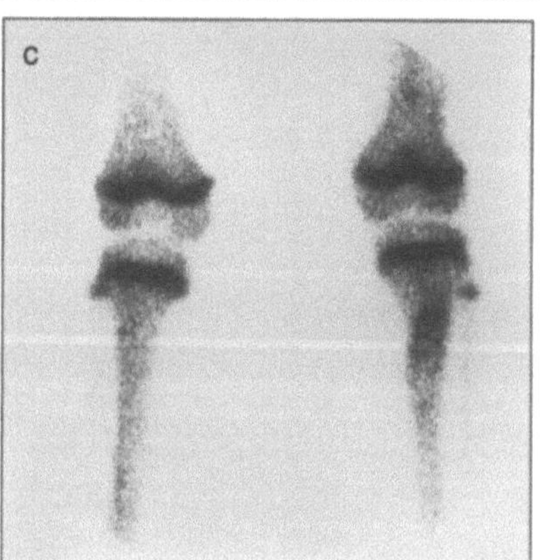

Fig. 7.8c. Posterior image of the knees shows abnormal increased uptake of isotope in the distal right femoral diaphysis as well as in the proximal right tibial diaphysis

Teaching Point
These radioisotope features are not specific to neurofibromatosis and the diagnosis cannot be made on radioisotope appearances.

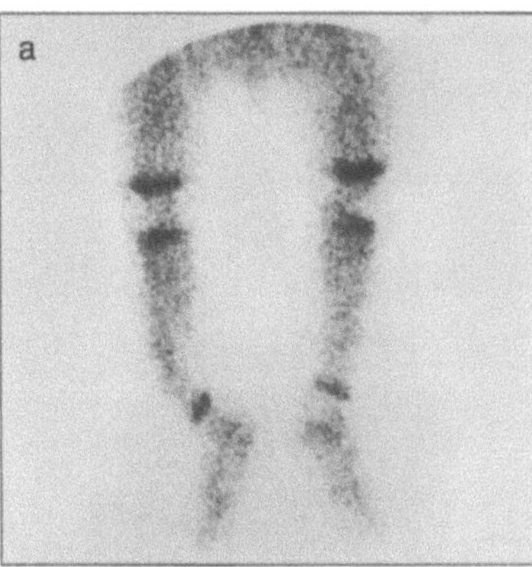

Case 7.9. A 13-month-old boy with neurofibromatosis and a deformity of the left tibia due to a pseudarthrosis

Fig. 7.9a. Posterior blood pool image of the lower limbs shows the deformity of the left tibia and fibula

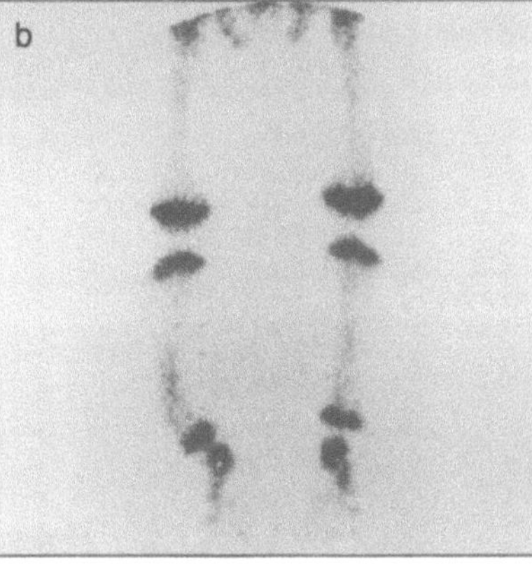

Fig. 7.9b. Posterior image of the lower limbs shows the deformity of the tibia and the abnormal increased uptake in the lower third of the tibia

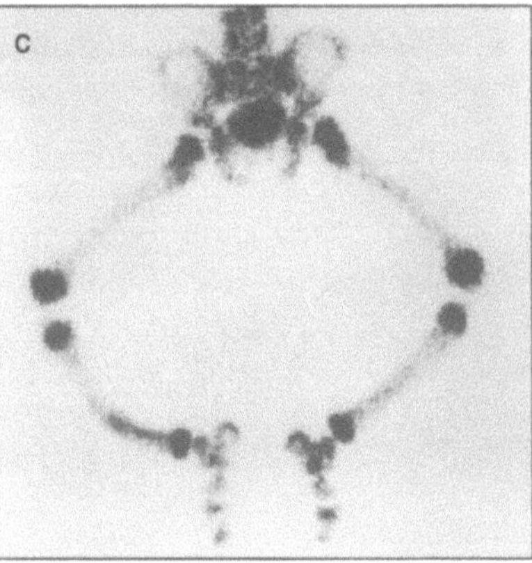

Fig. 7.9c. Posterior view of the pelvis and lateral views of the lower limbs and feet show the positional deformity of the left tibia and the abnormal increased uptake of isotope in the lower third

Teaching Point
See also Chap. 5.41, "Pseudarthrosis".

7.1.5 Craniodiaphyseal Dysplasia
(1 Case; Fig. 7.10)

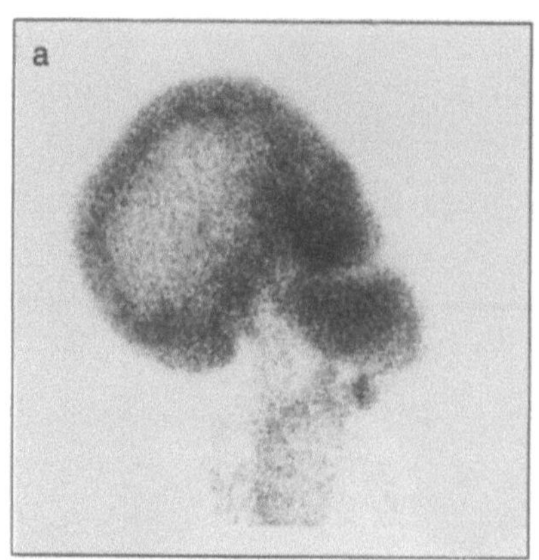

Case 7.10. An 11-year-old girl with craniodiaphyseal dysplasia

Fig. 7.10a. Right lateral image of the skull shows abnormal uptake of isotope in the enlarged mandible and also in the facial and vault bones

Fig. 7.10b. Left lateral image of the skull shows increased uptake of isotope in the facial and vault bones and mandible

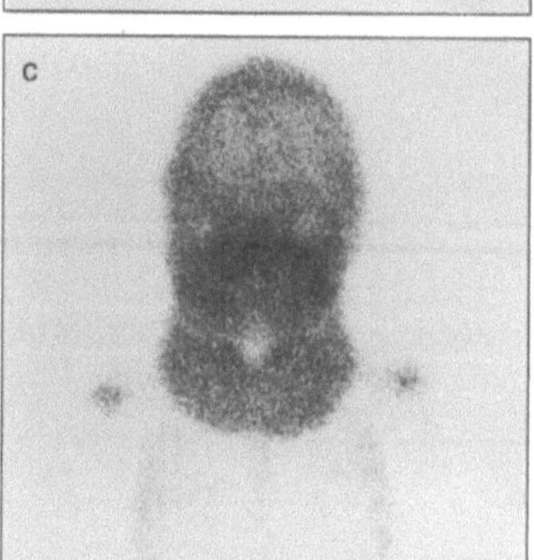

Fig. 7.10c. Anterior view of the skull and face shows symmetrical abnormal increased uptake of isotope in all the facial bones and also in the expanded mandible

Fig. 7.10d. Anterior image of the right arm shows increased uptake of isotope in the humerus with poor modelling

Fig. 7.10e. Anterior image of the left upper limb shows increased activity in the humerus with abnormal modelling

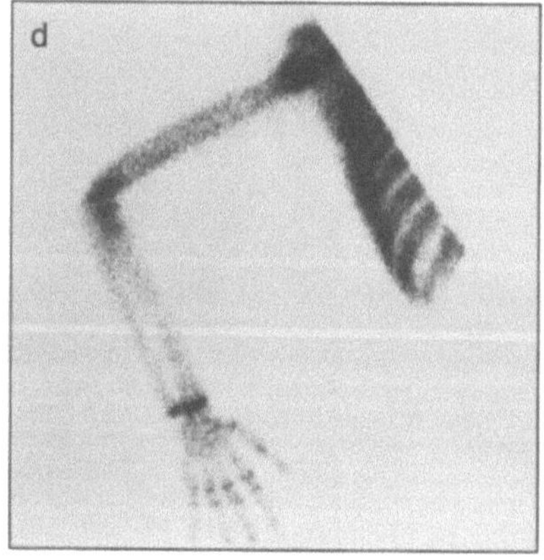

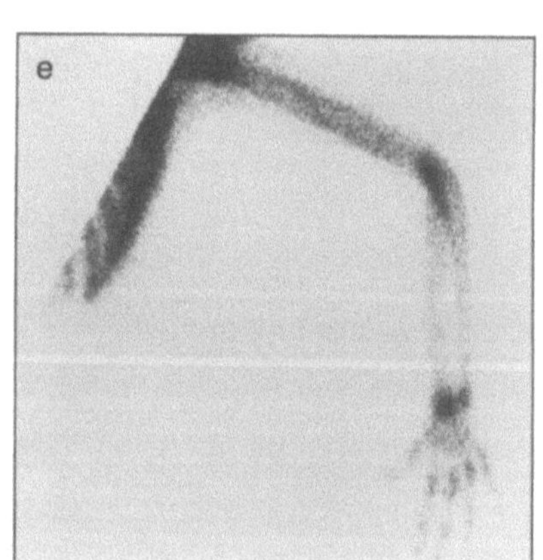

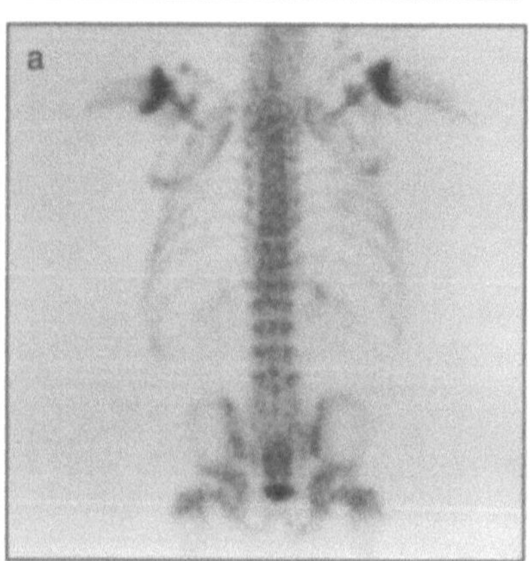

7.1.6 Spondyloepiphyseal Dysplasia
(1 Case; Fig. 7.11)

Case 7.11. A 9-year-old boy with spondyloepiphyseal dysplasia

Fig. 7.11a. Posterior image of the thorax, shoulder girdle, spine, pelvis and upper femora shows abnormal hips with foreshortening of both femoral necks. There is abnormal modelling of the upper humeri. The abnormalities in the spine cannot be identified on a bone scan

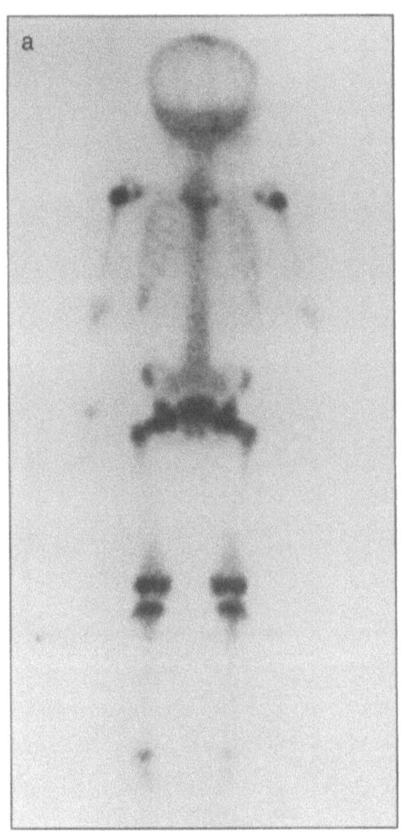
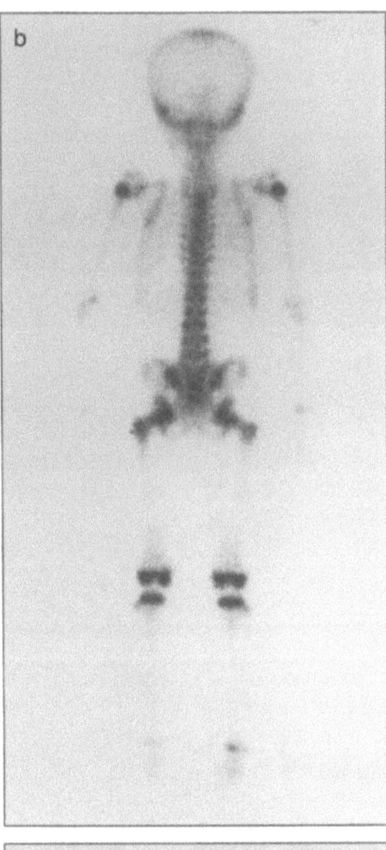
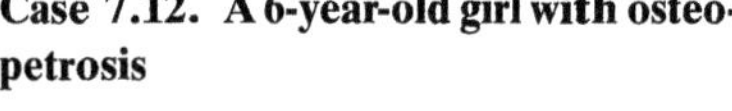
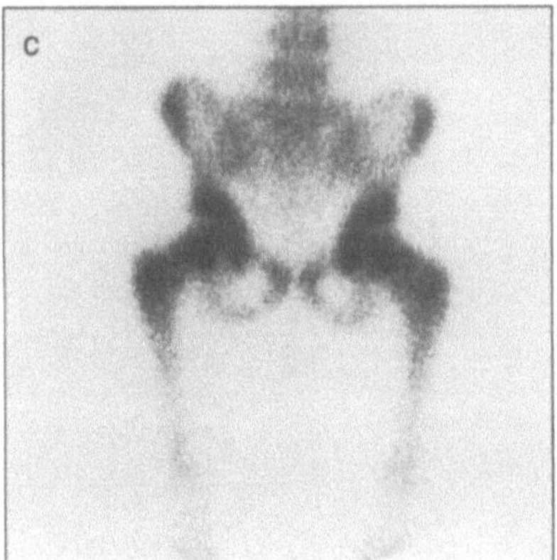
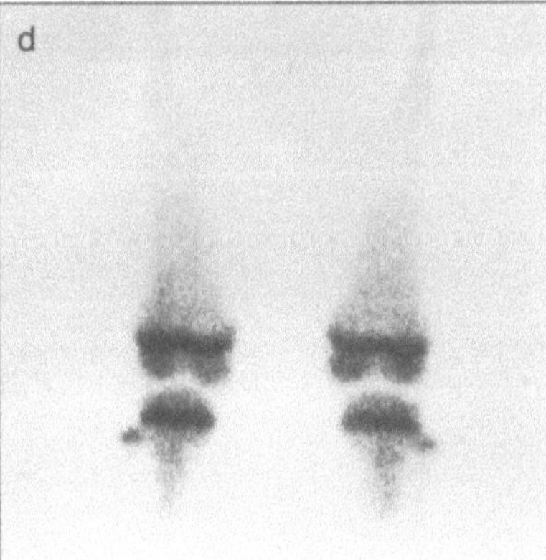

7.1.7 Osteopetrosis
(1 Case; Fig. 7.12)

Case 7.12. A 6-year-old girl with osteo-petrosis

Fig. 7.12a,b. Whole body anterior and posterior images show decreased uptake of isotope in the epiphyseal plates around the elbows, knees and ankles. The clarity of the epiphyseal growth plates in the upper femora is lost. The unusual configuration of the skull is noted

Fig. 7.12c. Anterior view of the lower lumbar spine, pelvis and upper femora shows abnormal increased uptake of isotope throughout the femoral necks extending into the proximal femoral shaft. There is lack of normal modelling of the femora

Fig. 7.12d. Posterior view of the lower femora and knees shows poor modelling of the lower femora with decreased uptake of isotope most marked in the growth plate of the head of the right fibula

7.1.8 Camurati-Engelmann Disease
(1 Case; Fig. 7.13)

Case 7.13. A 10-year-old girl with pain in the extremities over a prolonged period which was refractory to analgesics. The diagnosis of Camurati-Engelmann disease was based on the history, the radiographic imaging of the long bones and also the scintigraphic results. Confirmation of the diagnosis in the mother was made confirming the autosomal dominant nature of the disorder

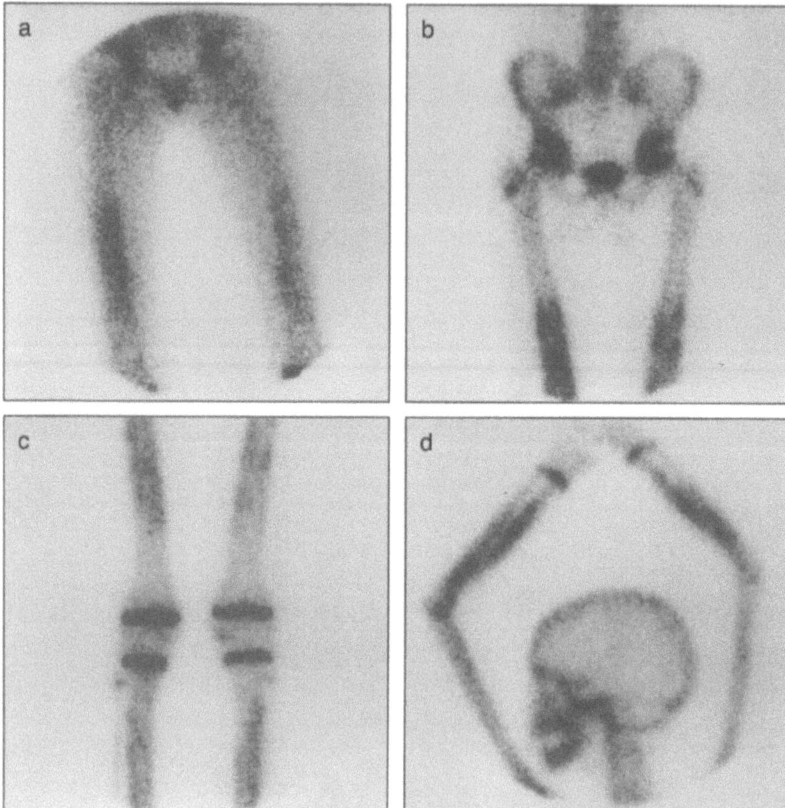

Fig. 7.13a. Anterior blood pool image of the pelvis and femora shows abnormal increased uptake of tracer in the mid portions of both femora

Fig. 7.13b. Anterior view of the pelvis and upper femora shows abnormal increased uptake of isotope in the shafts of the femora. This is of a patchy nature

Fig. 7.13c. Anterior view of the knees shows abnormal uptake in the shafts of both femora as well as the tibiae. There is loss of the normal modelling of the femora und tibiae

Fig. 7.13d. Left lateral view of the skull and dorsal view of the upper limbs shows abnormal increased uptake of isotope in the forearm bones bilaterally as well as in both humeri more marked on the left than on the right with failure of modelling in the humeri. There is also increased uptake of isotope in the base of the skull

7.1.9 Mucolipoidosis
(1 Case; Fig. 7.14)

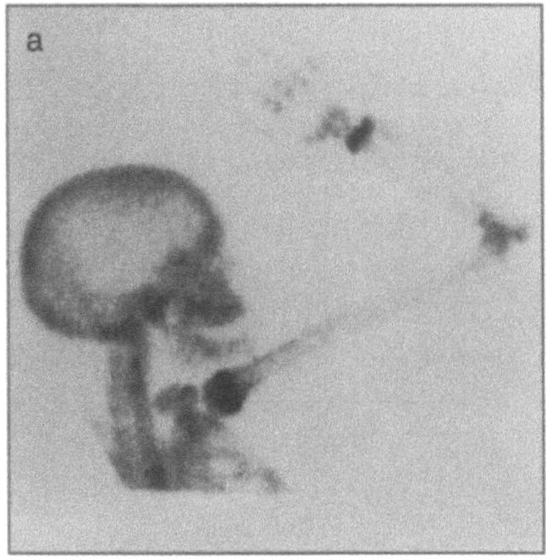

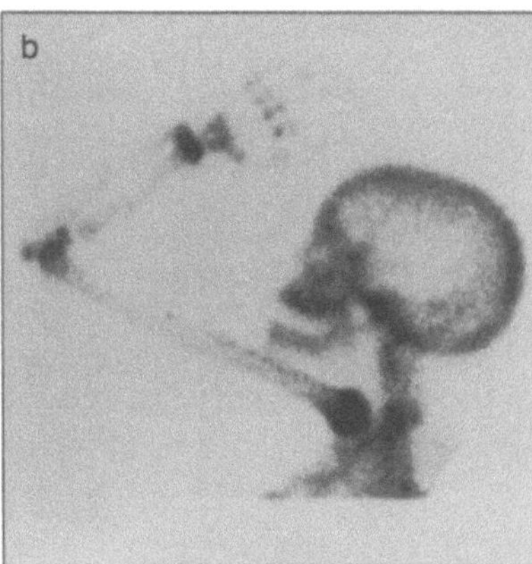

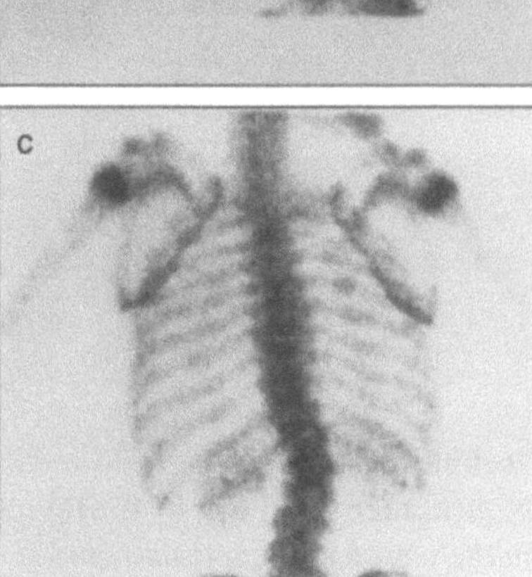

Case 7.14. **A girl with known mucolipoidosis who presented with pain in the foot with a differential diagnosis of avascular necrosis or infection. The bone scan was undertaken at the age of 14 years**

Fig. 7.14a. Right lateral view of the skull and right upper limb shows disparity in the length of the radius and ulna compared to the humerus

Fig. 7.14b. Left lateral skull and left upper limb shows similiar features to that seen on the right with a short radius and ulna compared to a normal length of the humerus. Note in both images the abnormal modelling of the humerus

Fig. 7.14c. Posterior view of the thorax, lumbar spine and upper pelvis shows an upper lumbar scoliosis concave to the left, a non-specific feature of this disease

Teaching Point
See also Chap. 7.5.5, "Scoliosis".

7.2 Chondromata

7.2.1 Enchondromata
(4 Cases; Figs. 7.15–7.18)

Case 7.15. A 13-year-old boy with an enchondroma in the upper right humerus

Fig. 7.15a. Posterior image of the thorax, upper limbs and left lateral skull shows abnormal increased uptake of isotope on the medial aspect of the right upper humerus running up to the epiphyseal plate

Fig. 7.15b. Anterior image of the upper limbs and thorax shows the abnormal increased uptake of isotope in the right humerus extending beyond the confines of the bone. The area of abnormality is not homogeneous with decreased uptake inferiorly compared to superiorly

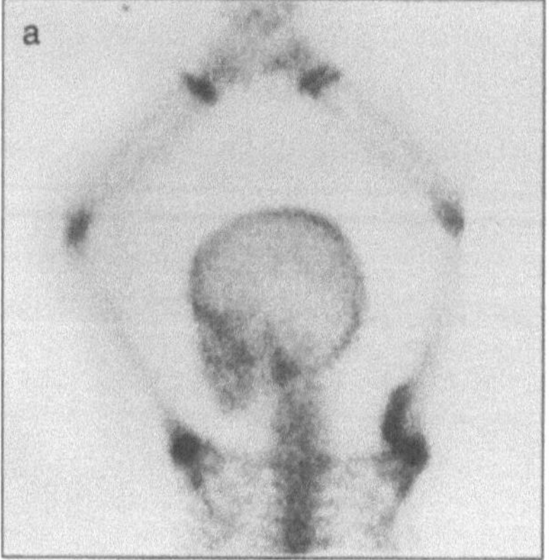
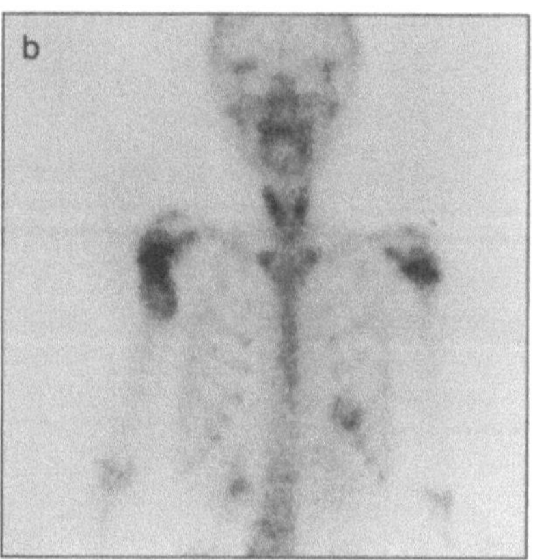

Technical Comment

Note uptake of isotope by the thyroid gland. There is also increased activity in the region of the left sixth and seventh ribs, which is presumably the free pertechnetate in the stomach. This could easily be confused with an enchondroma of the rib.

Case 7.16. A 16-year-old boy with swelling of the right upper humerus due to an enchondroma

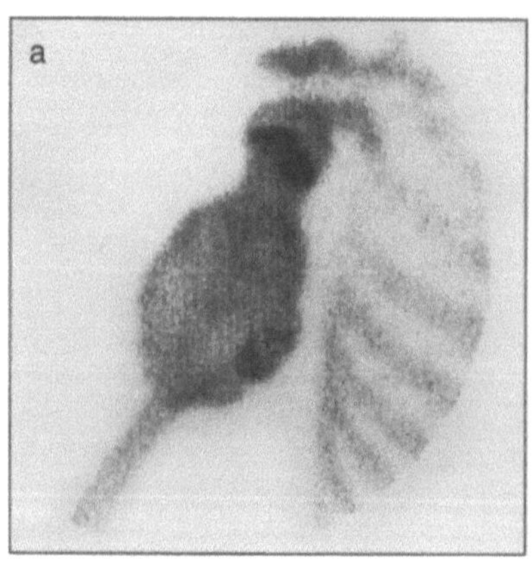

Fig. 7.16a. Anterior image of the right humerus and part of the thorax shows an expanding lesion of the upper third of the shaft of the right humerus with focal abnormal increased uptake of isotope in the medial aspect

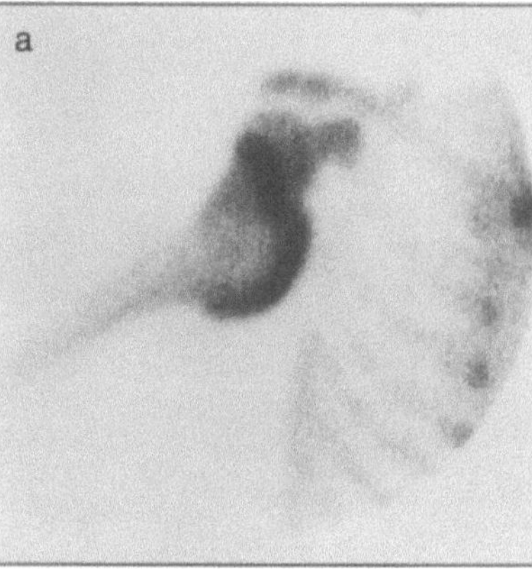

Case 7.17. A 13-year-old boy with slight limitation of movement of the upper right arm due to an enchondroma

Fig. 7.17a. Anterior image of the right shoulder and part of the thorax shows abnormal increased uptake of isotope in the medial aspect of the upper third of the humeral shaft. This appears contiguous with the growth plate of the upper humerus

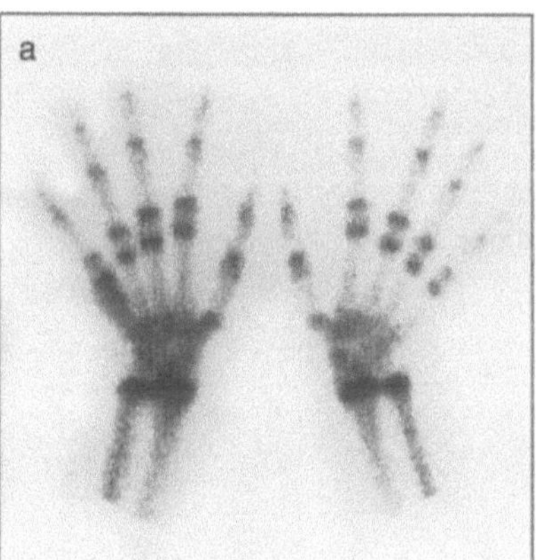

Case 7.18. An 8-year-old girl with a swelling of the medial aspect of the right hand due to an enchondroma

Fig. 7.18a. Palmar view of the hands shows increased uptake of isotope in the right fifth metacarpal with expansion of this bone, the features suggesting an enchondroma

Teaching Point
Similar appearances could be due to a bone cyst with a healing fracture (see Case 4.21).

7.2.2 Exostoses
(4 Cases; Fig. 7.19–7.22)

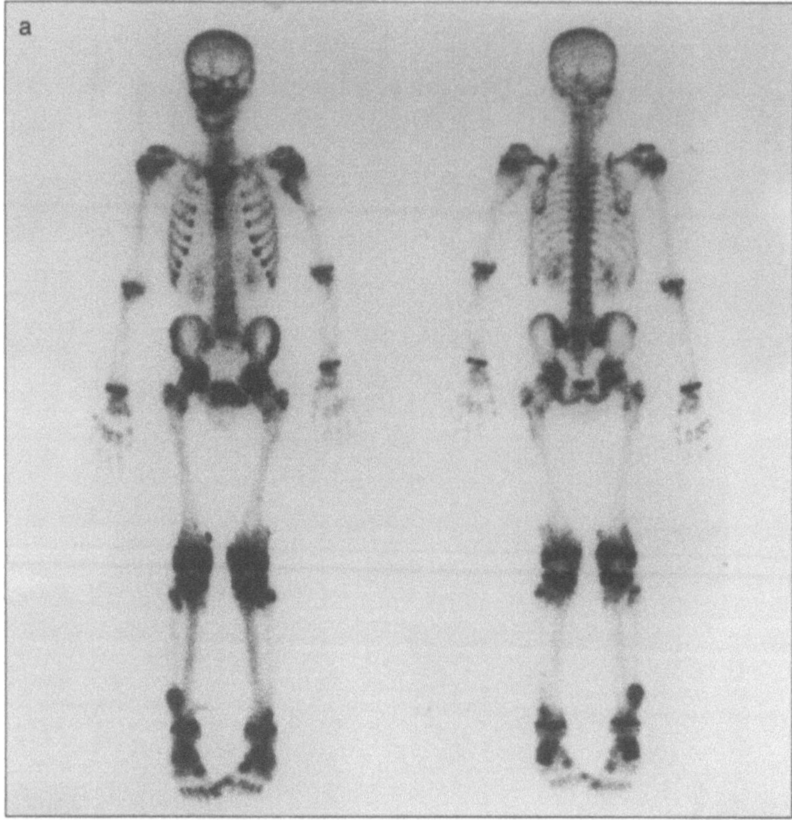

Case 7.19. A 13-year-old boy with multiple exostoses

Fig. 7.19a. Whole body scans show abnormal increased uptake of isotope in the upper left humerus seen on both the anterior and posterior views. There are also abnormal areas of uptake of isotope in the distal ends of both femora as well as in the proximal ends of both tibiae and fibulae. The distal right fibula and, to a lesser extent, the left fibula also show abnormal areas of increased uptake of isotope

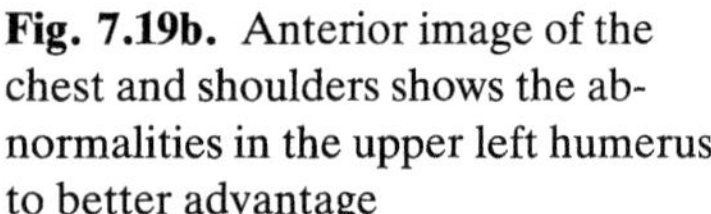

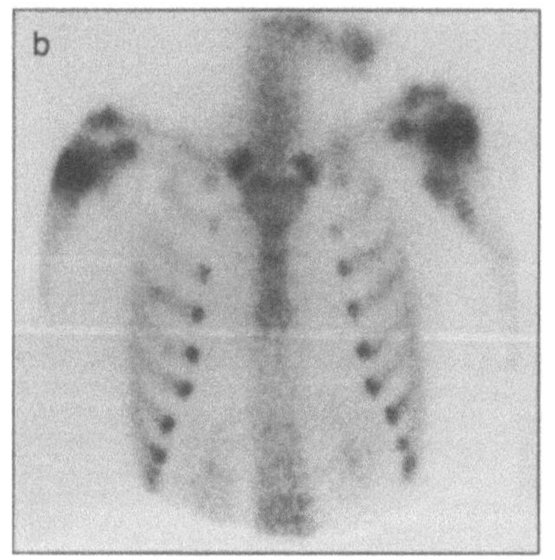

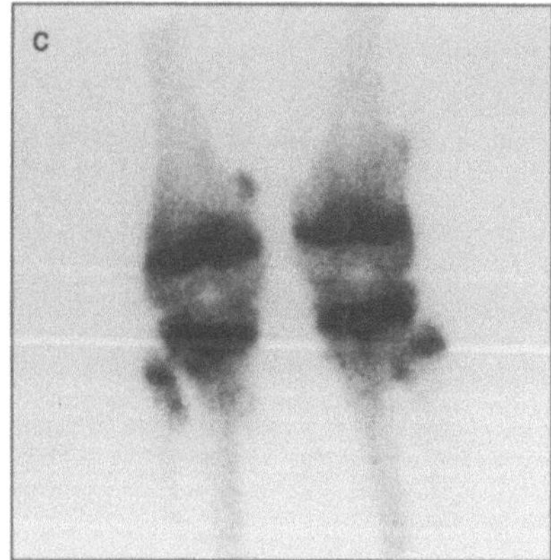

Fig. 7.19b. Anterior image of the chest and shoulders shows the abnormalities in the upper left humerus to better advantage

Fig. 7.19c. Anterior image of the knees shows abnormalities in the medial aspect of the right femur and the lateral aspect of the left femur. The exostoses of the fibulae are seen as is the one on the medial aspect of the right tibia

Fig. 7.19d. Anterior image of the ankles shows the exostoses of the fibulae. Note the difference in the appearances of the two fibulae

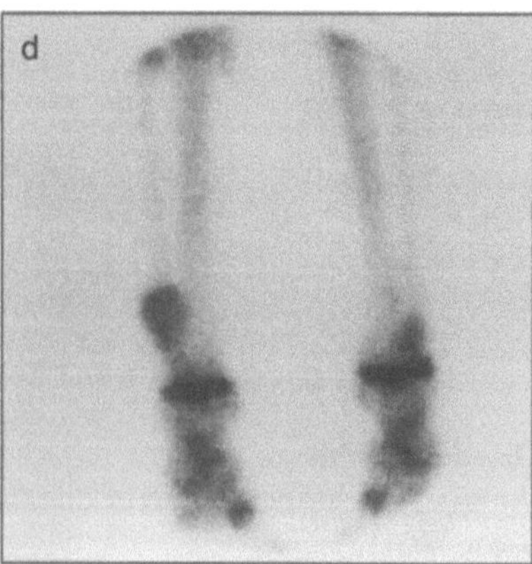

Technical Comment
Higher resolution is obtained using spot images with a high-resolution collimator than whole body images.

296

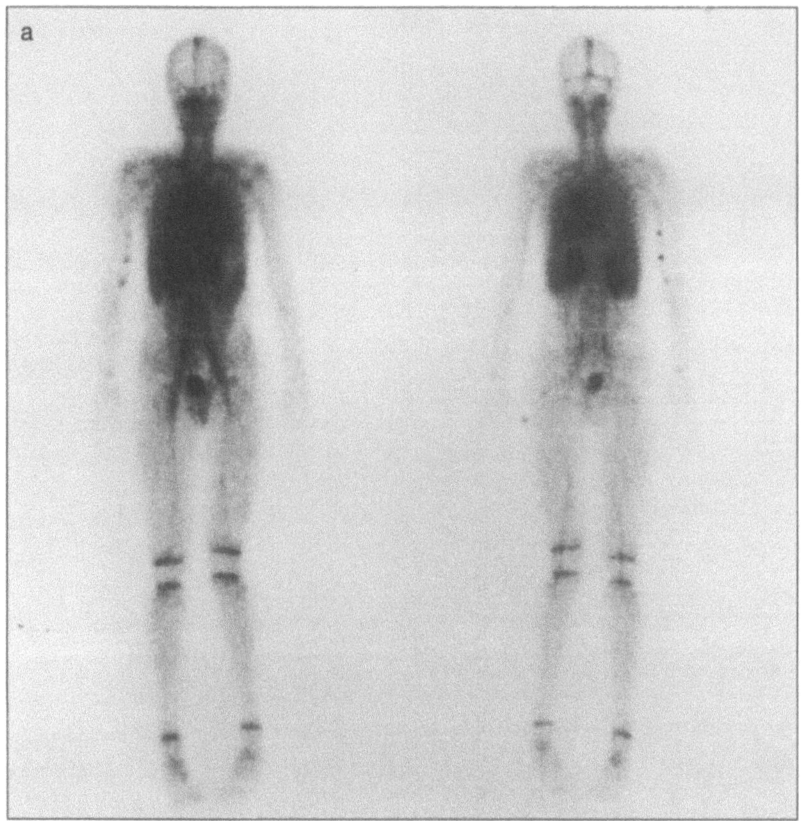

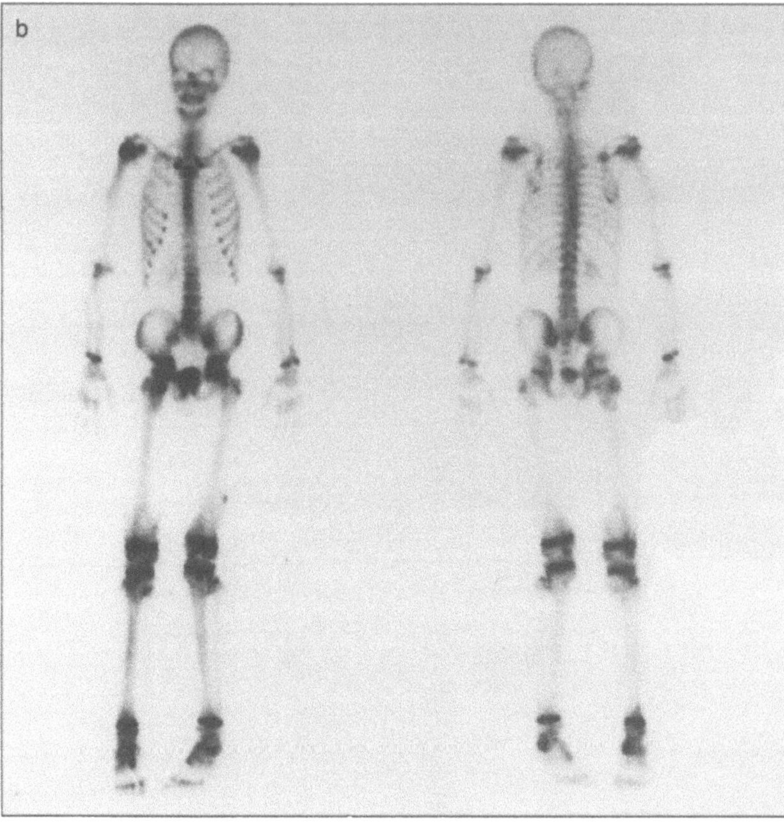

Case 27.20. A 12-year-old boy with multiple exostoses

Fig. 7.20a. Blood pool whole body images. No significant asymmetry is noted

Fig. 7.20b. Whole body scans show abnormal increased uptake of isotope in the upper right humerus, upper right femur, distal femora bilaterally, upper right tibia and upper fibulae bilaterally. The anterior right seventh rib also shows increased uptake of isotope due to an exostosis. Note the post-operative defect on the upper right anterior thorax

Technical Comment
The three focal hot spots seen in the upper right arm in Fig. 7.20a are due to isotope following the intravenous injection in the right elbow. This was due to venous stasis and not extravasation.

**Case 7.21. A 17-year-old boy with
multiple exostoses**

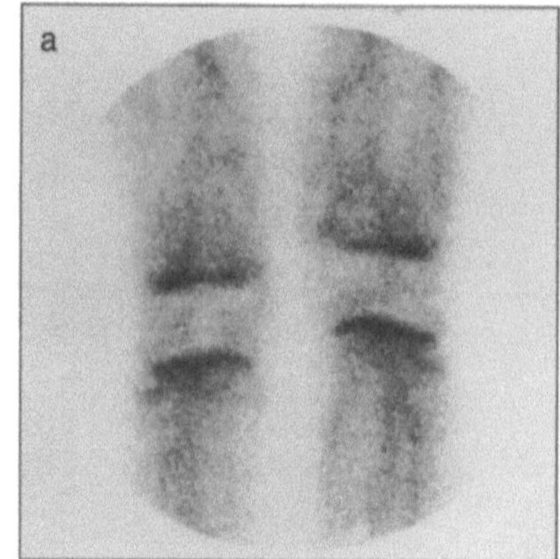

Fig. 7.21a. Blood pool anterior image
of the knees shows slightly decreased
uptake of isotope in the region of the
left medial femoral growth plate

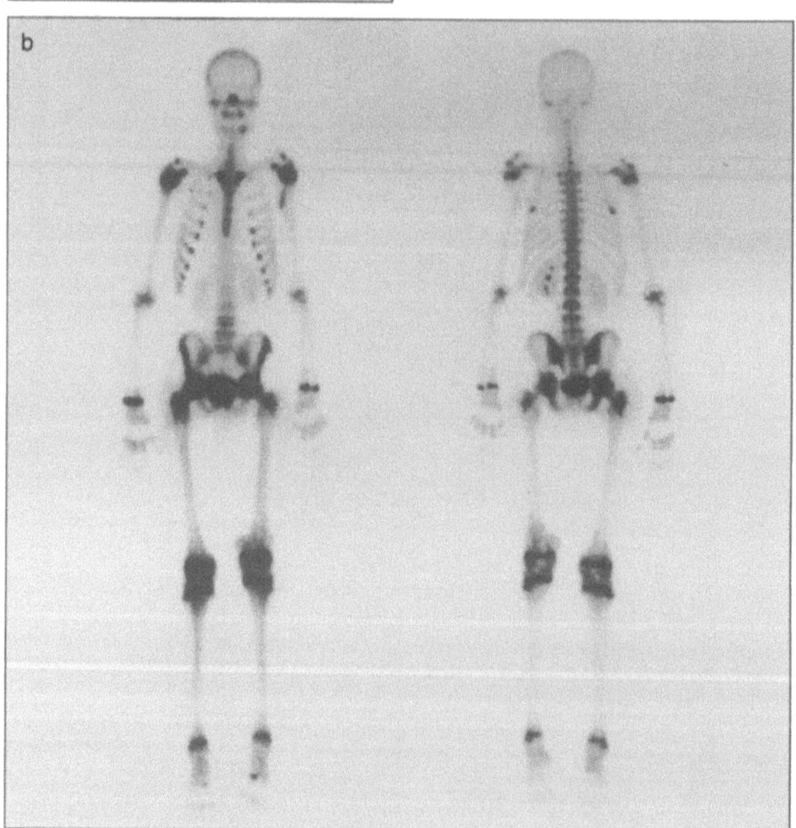

Fig. 7.21b. Whole body scans show
abnormal increased uptake of isotope
in the upper left humerus as well as in
the distal left femur and left foot

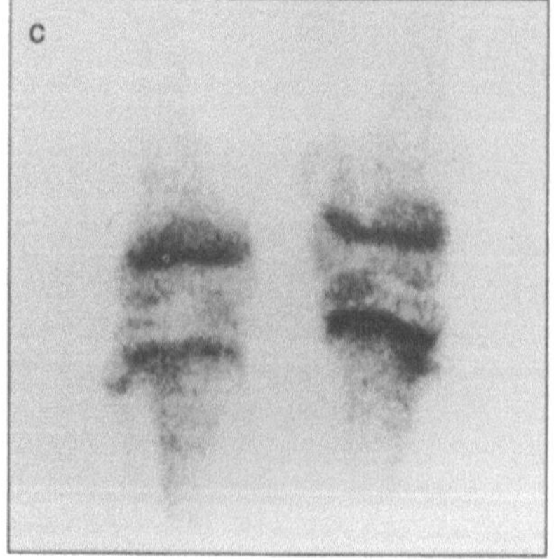

Fig. 7.21c. Anterior image of the
knees shows a slightly decreased
uptake in the medial aspect of the left
femoral growth plate and the exostosis
in the adjacent diaphysis. The difference between the growth plates in the
tibiae is probably related to the positioning of the feet since the head of
the fibula is not clearly seen on the
left side

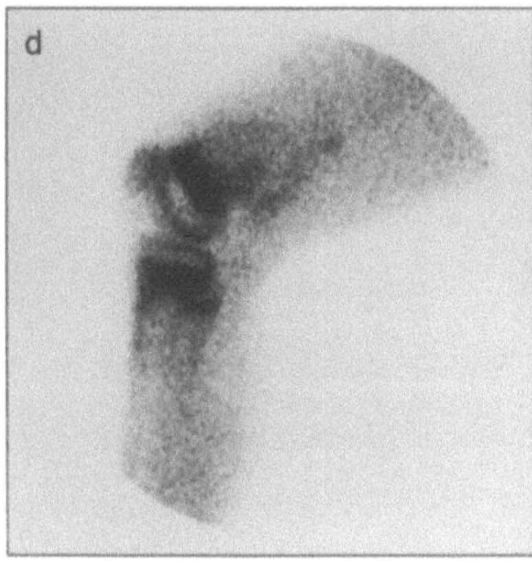

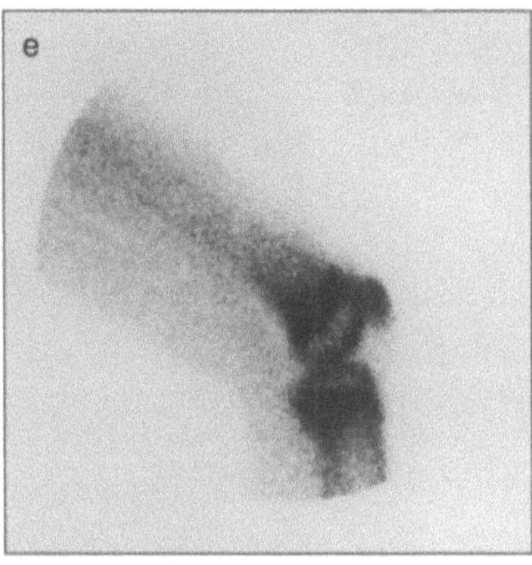

Fig. 7.21d. Lateral image of the left knee shows the abnormal accumulation of isotope extending into the soft tissue posteriorly

Fig. 7.21e. Lateral image of the right knee is normal

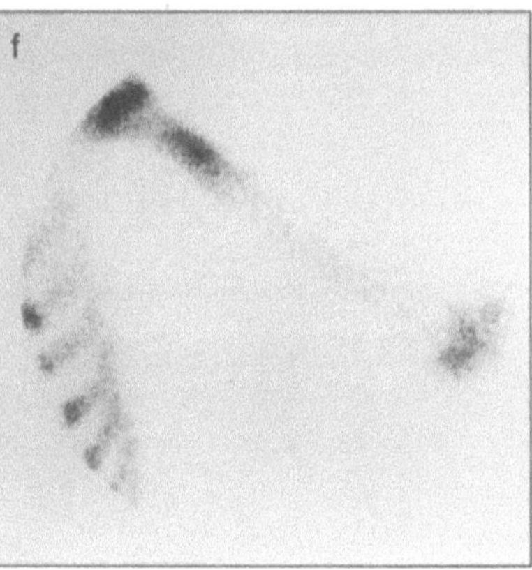

Fig. 7.21f. Anterior image of the left humerus and part of the left thorax shows the abnormal uptake in the proximal third of the humerus

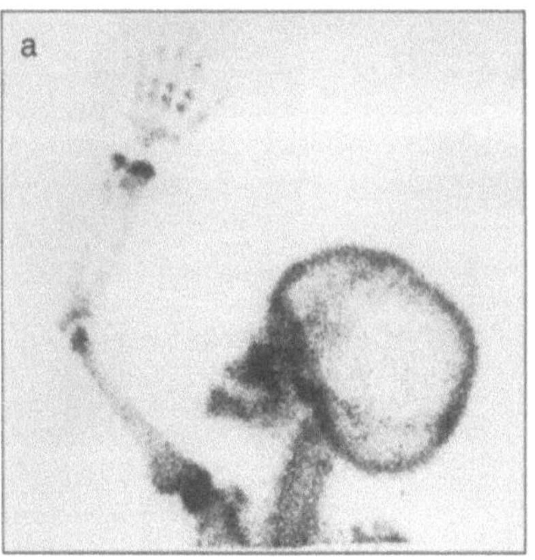

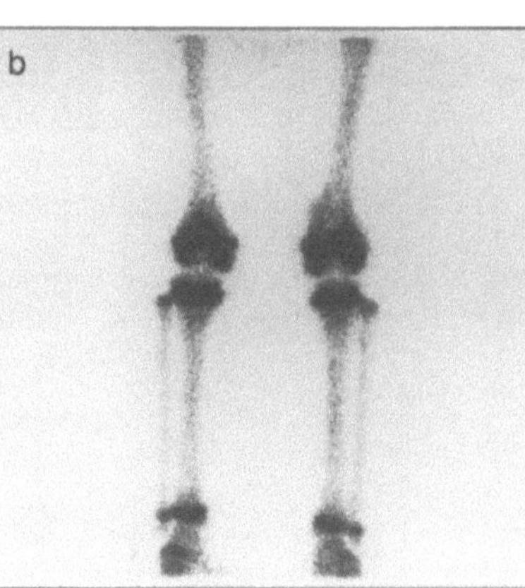

Case 7.22. A 4-year-old girl with multiple exostoses

Fig. 7.22a. Posterior image of the left arm and left lateral skull shows abnormal increased uptake of isotope in the proximal humerus as well as in the distal radius medially

Fig. 7.22b. Posterior image of the knees shows abnormal increased uptake of isotope in the distal right femur medially

Technical Comment

In the right tibia note the slight increased activity in the mid shaft. This is a variation of normality.

7.3 Blount's Disease

(1 Case; Fig. 7.23)

Case 7.23. A 10-year-old girl with deformity of the knees due to Blount's disease

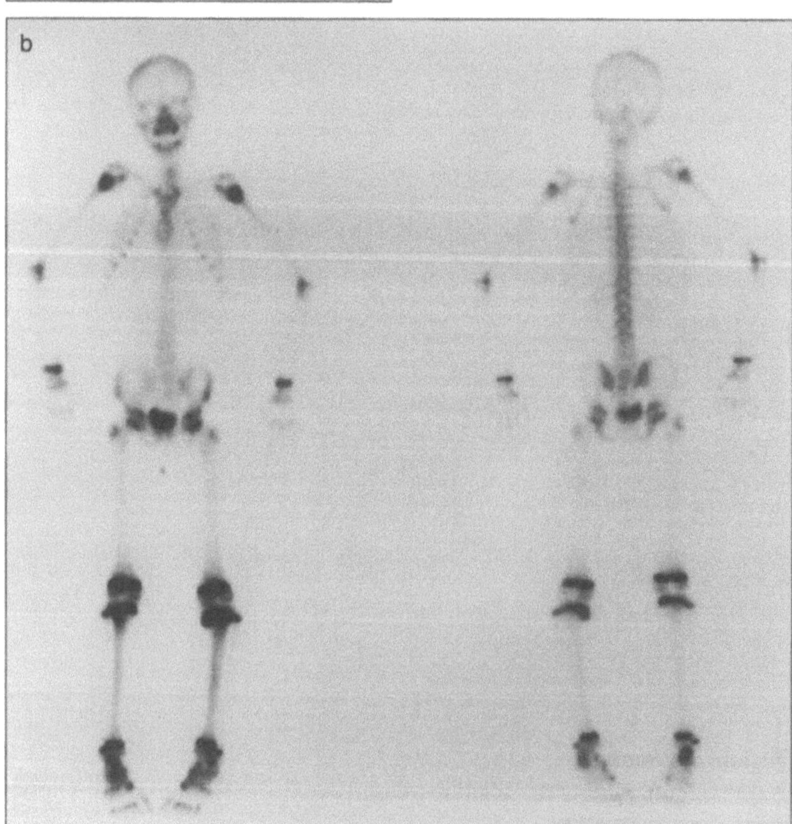

Fig. 7.23a. Posterior blood pool image of the knees shows slightly increased isotope in the medial left upper tibia

Fig. 7.23b. Whole body scans show abnormal positioning of the left knee with increased uptake of isotope seen in the upper left tibia where the epiphyseal plate shows expansion medially. This is better seen on the posterior than on the anterior scan

7.4 Gaucher's Disease

(2 Cases; Figs. 7.24, 7.25)

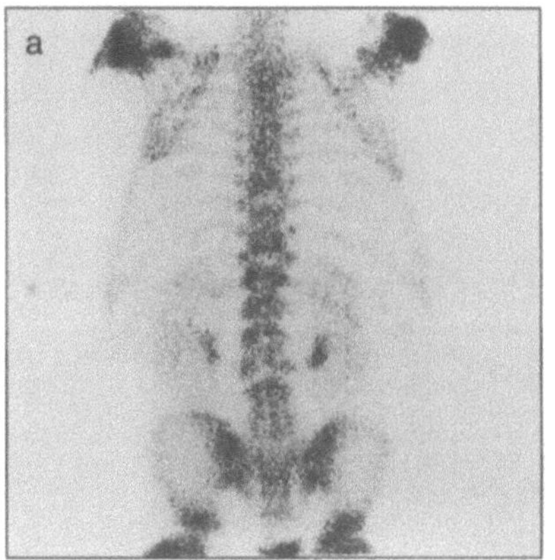

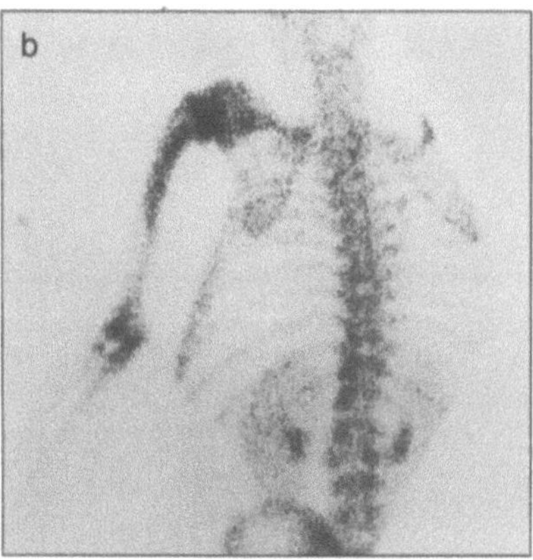

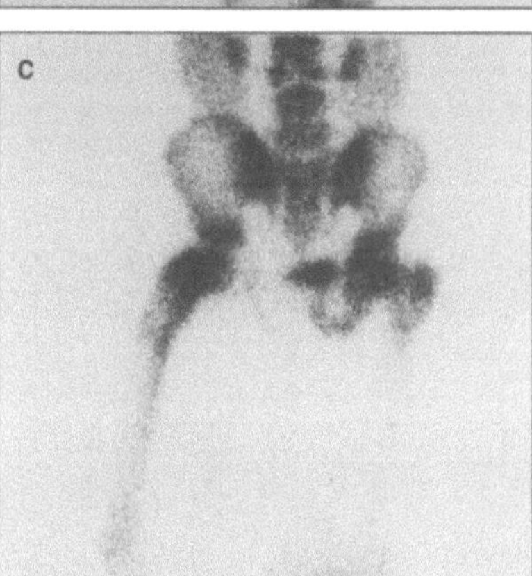

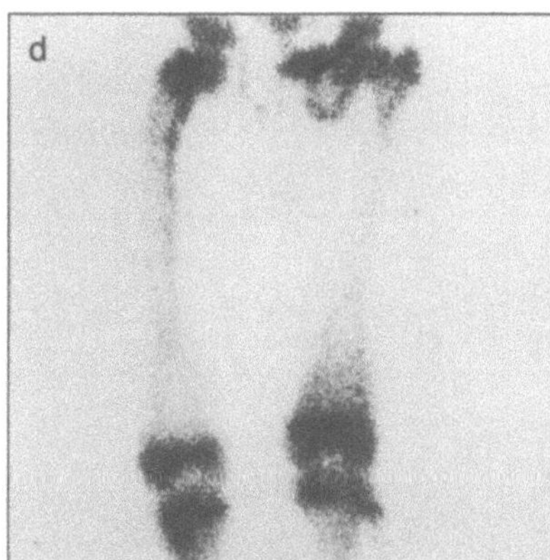

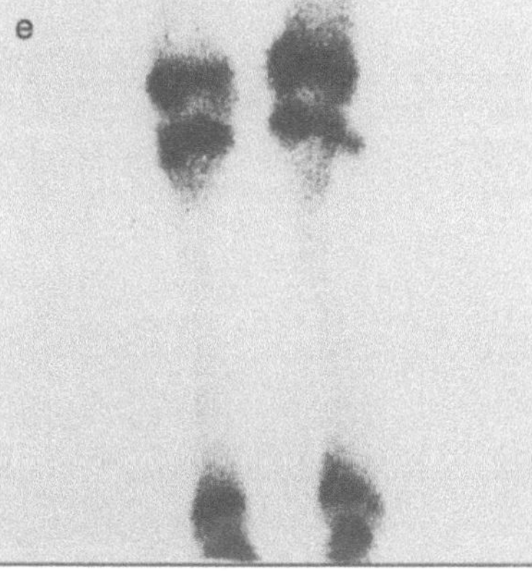

Case 7.24. A 13-year-old boy with Gaucher's disease

Fig. 7.24a. Posterior image of the spine and pelvis shows decreased activity in two dorsal vertebral bodies and one mid lumbar vertebral body

Fig. 7.24b. Posterior image of the left arm shows abnormal modelling with increased activity in the mid diaphysis extending to the proximal epiphyseal plate

Fig. 7.24c. Posterior image of the pelvis shows abnormal hips. There is total absence of activity in the pubic bones on the left

Fig. 7.24d. Posterior image of the femora and knees shows the abnormal hips. Total absence of activity is noted in the pubic bones on the left. The abnormal modelling of the femora is noted

Fig. 7.24e. Posterior image of the knees shows the abnormal modelling of the distal femora, more marked on the right than on the left

Teaching Point
Patients with Gaucher's disease are susceptible to avascular necrosis. It is unusual to see such extensive involvement especially of the pubic bones.

Case 7.25. An 18-year-old girl with established Gaucher's disease who was limping. Avascular necrosis of the right femoral head had occurred

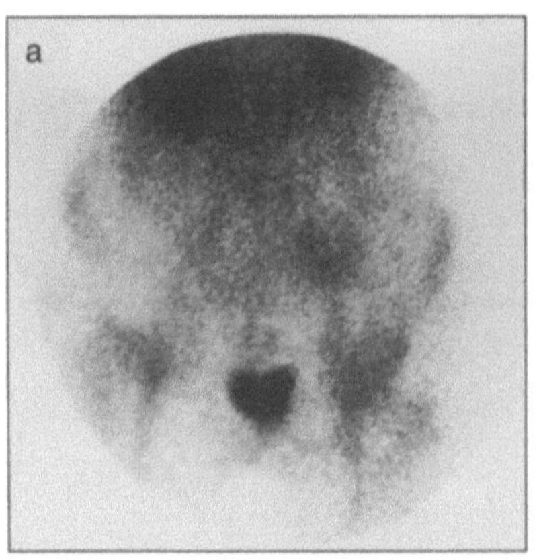

Fig. 7.25a. Anterior blood pool image of the pelvis shows decreased isotope in the region of the right hip. There is increased uptake of isotope in the left sacro-iliac joint

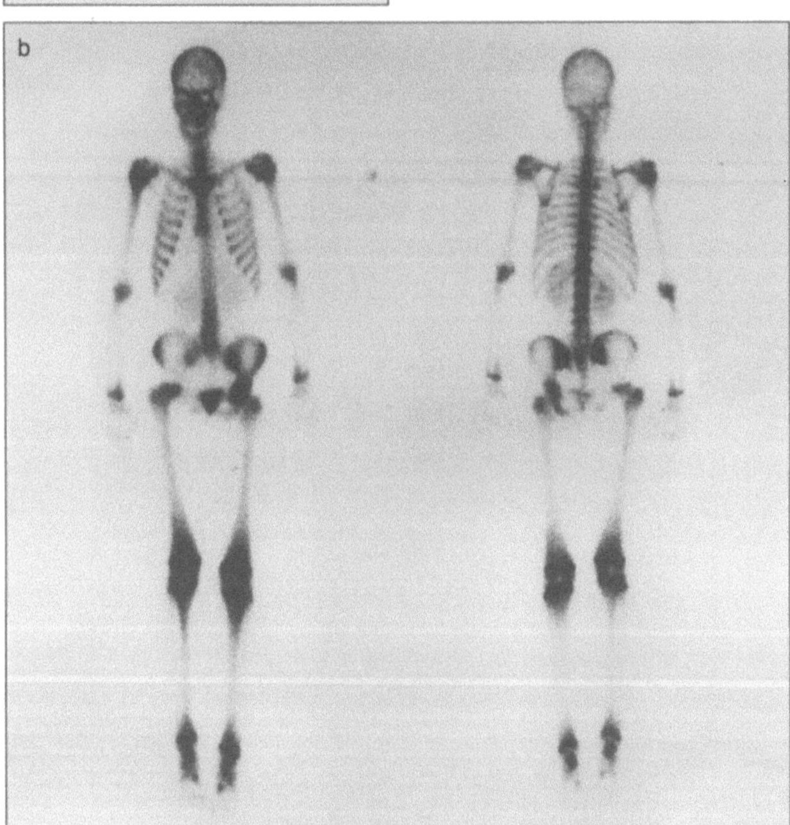

Fig. 7.25b. Whole body scans show abnormal positioning of the pelvis with decreased activity noted in the abnormal right hip, including the acetabulum, os ischium and os pubis. Note the failure of normal modelling of both lower femora bilaterally.

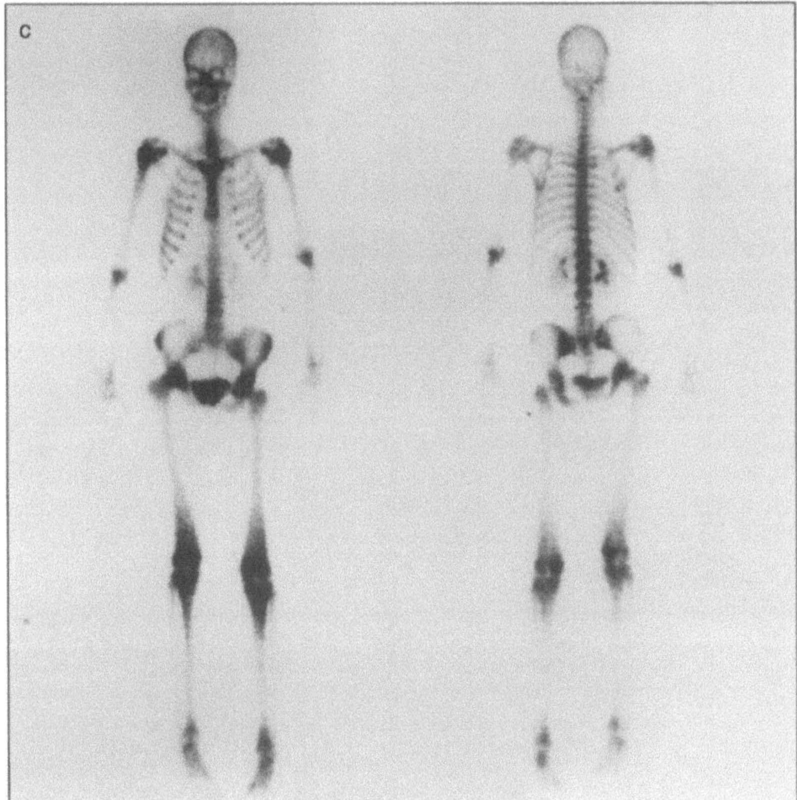

A follow-up scan was undertaken
2 years later

Fig. 7.25c. Whole body scans again
show tilting of the pelvis with decreased activity noted in the right hemipelvis. The abnormal modelling of the
femora is still present

Teaching Point
Similar appearances of the hips may be seen in Legg-Perthes' disease (see
Cases 6.1–6.9).

7.5 Scoliosis

(4 Cases; Fig. 7.26–7.29)

Case 7.26. A 13-year-old girl with a scoliosis who developed pain in her back which was considered to be due to a fractured upper left rib

Fig. 7.26a. Posterior image of the cervical, dorsal and upper lumbar spine shows the marked upper dorsal scoliosis concave to the left. There is focal abnormal increased uptake of isotope in one of the ribs in the upper left thorax

Fig. 7.26b. Left posterior oblique image of the thorax again shows the abnormal increased uptake of isotope in the ribs on the left. The spine curvature is again noted

Fig. 7.26c. Posterior image of the lower dorsal and lumbar spine and pelvis shows the scoliosis of the spine and also the abnormal left rib

Fig. 7.26d. Anterior image of the thorax and lumbar spine shows the abnormal activity in the upper ribs on the left

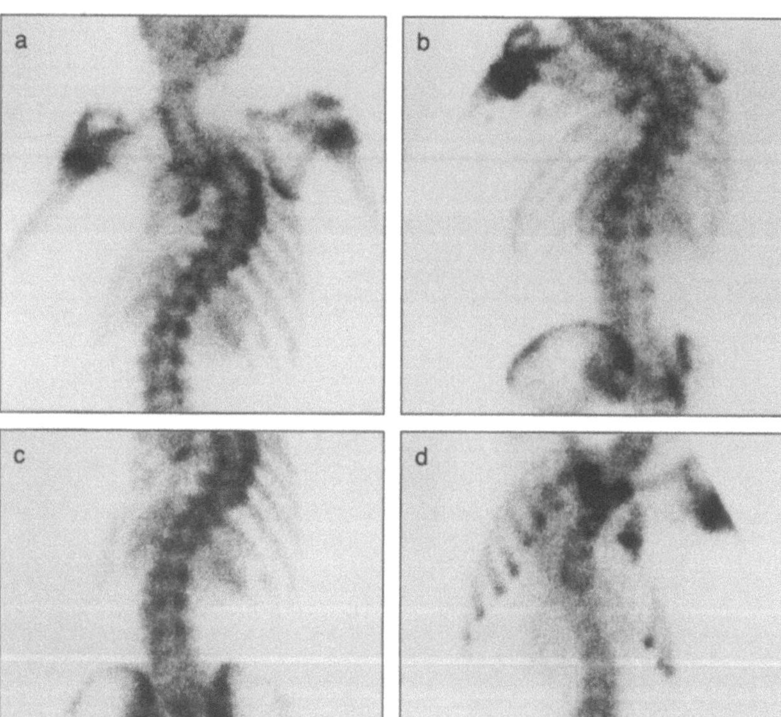

Teaching Point

The scoliosis was secondary to congenital deformities of the spine. The pain was due to the rib fracture.

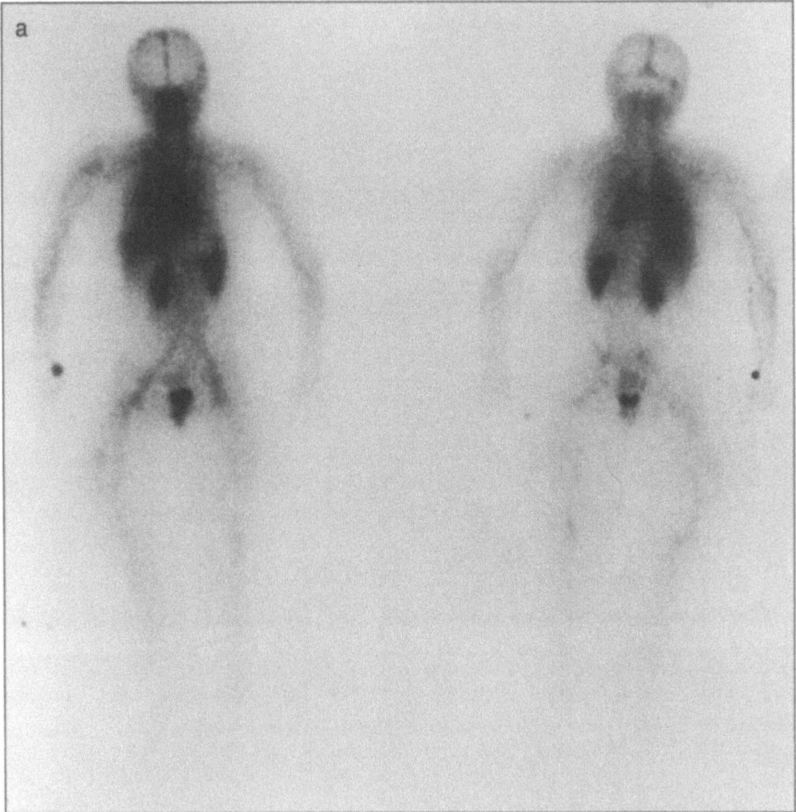

Case 7.27. An 18-year-old female with known osteogenesis imperfecta and a pseudarthrosis of the right femur. This is the same patient as in Case 5.45

Fig. 7.27a. Whole body blood pool scans show a positional deformity of the spine

Fig. 7.27b. Whole body scans show the marked scoliosis concave to the right centered on the dorsolumbar junction of the spine. A focal abnormal uptake of isotope is noted in the right femur, the site of pseudarthrosis. There is retention of isotope in the right renal pelvis, but this was due to a dilated non-obstructed pelvis

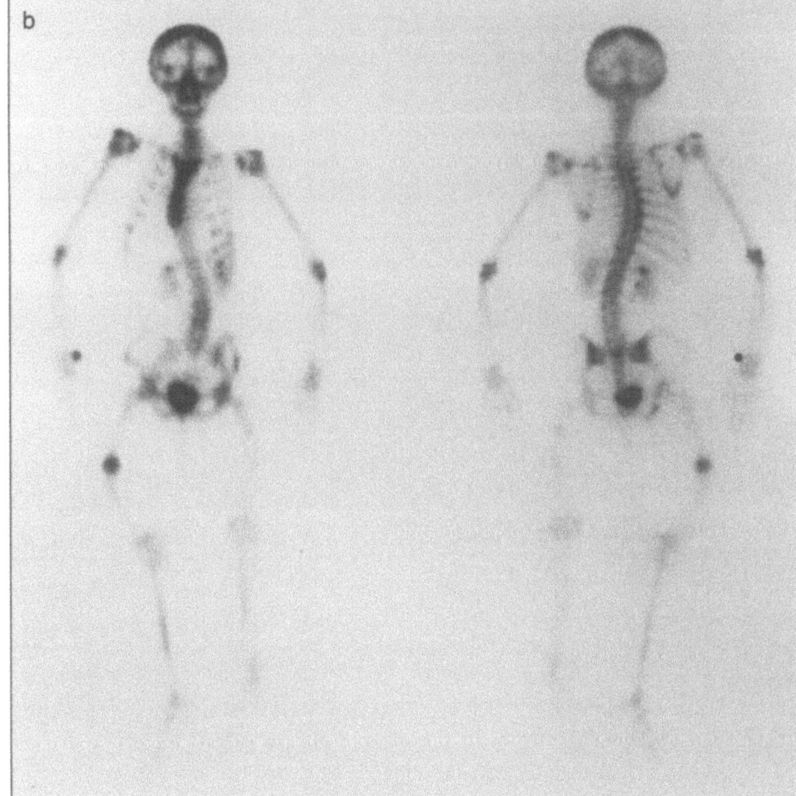

Technical Comment
Extravasation of isotope in noted in the right hand.

Teaching Point
Note how the epiphyses, especially of the lower limbs, are fusing and are therefore not clearly seen in this 18-year-old female.

Case 7.28. A 18-year-old male who presented with scoliosis after a spondylosyndesis

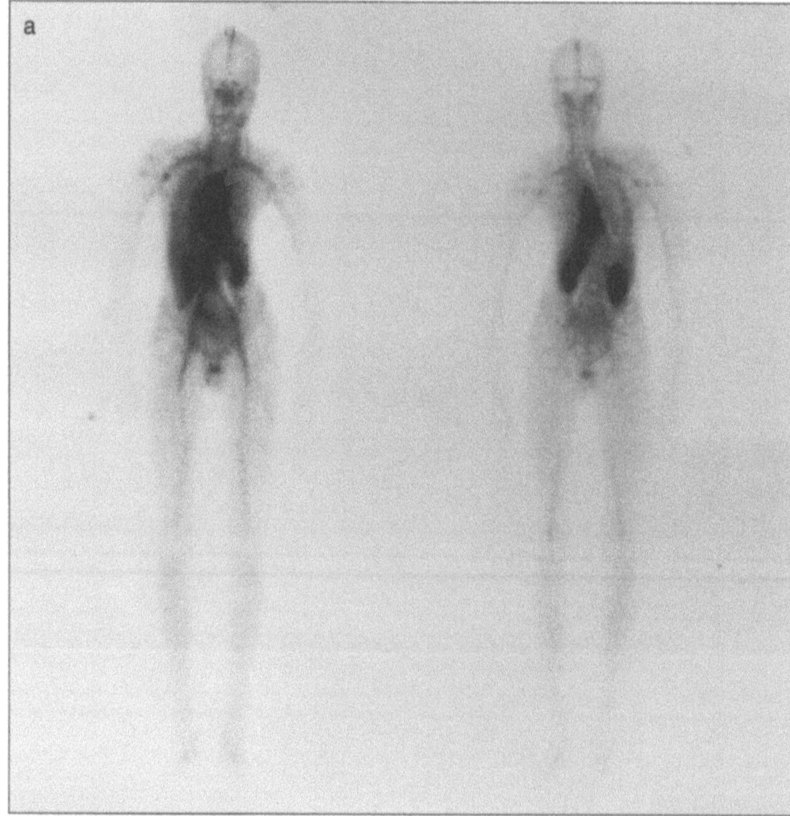

Fig. 7.28a. Blood pool whole body scans show the scoliosis to the right. Note the decreased blood pool activity beside the spine, due to the surgical prosthesis in the spine

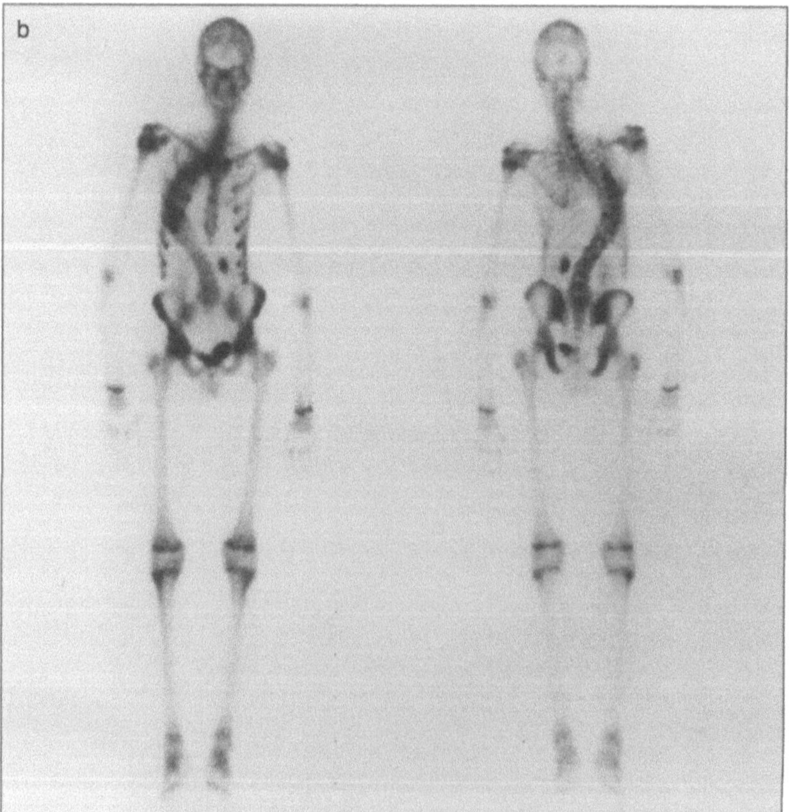

Fig. 7.28b. Whole body images show the scoliosis and patchy increased uptake in the whole spine. Note the focal increased uptake in the left kidney due to a dilated non-obstructed pelvis

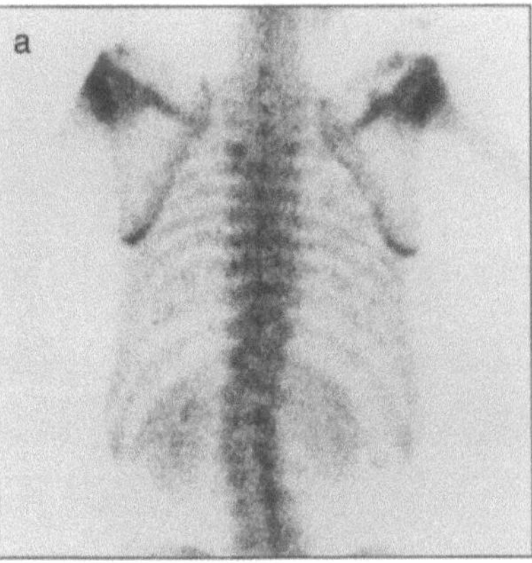

Case 7.29. A 15-year-old boy with a mild scoliosis

Fig. 7.29a. Posterior image of the thorax, dorsal and lumbar spine. There is a scoliosis concave to the right centered on the dorsolumbar junction. No focal abnormality is seen in the skeleton

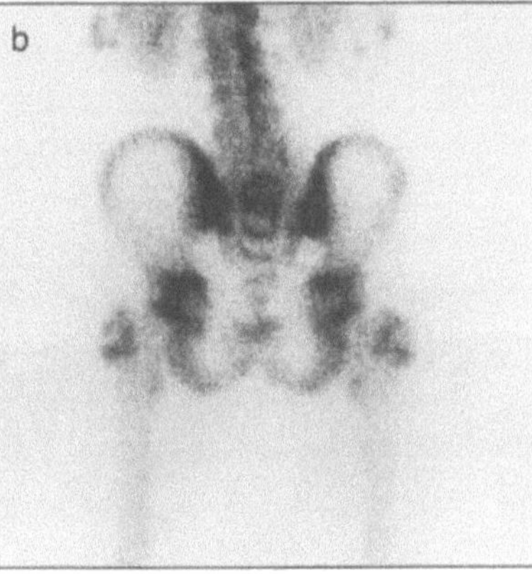

Fig. 7.29b. Posterior image of the lower lumbar spine and pelvis shows an apparent increase in the size of the left hemipelvis. This was secondary to the rotation of the pelvis consequent upon the scoliosis

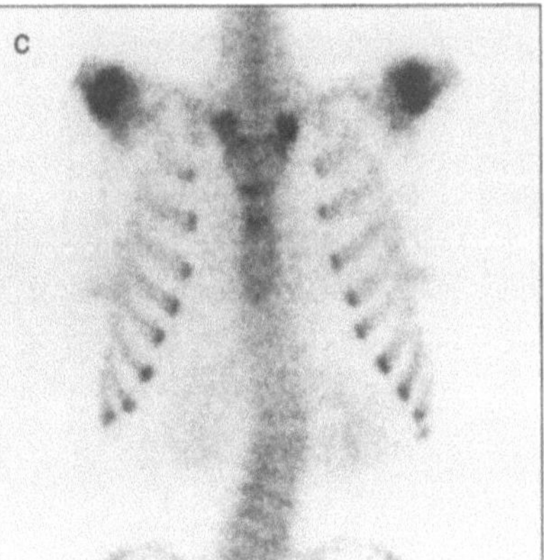

Fig. 7.29c. Anterior image of the thorax and lumbar spine shows the scoliosis of the dorsal and lumbar spine

Teaching Point
An acute scoliosis may be secondary to focal bone pathology especially a benign bone tumor (see Cases 4.9, 4.10).

7.6 The Sick Child

(3 Cases; Figs. 7.30–7.32)

Case 7.30. An 11-year-old girl who had a left Wilms' tumour removed. The bone scan was undertaken following the investigation of the mass and subsequent surgery. No deposits were seen in the skeleton, but the poor visualisation of the epiphyseal plates is due to the fact that the child was acutely immobilised

Fig. 7.30a. Posterior view of the femora and knees shows poor visualisation especially of the left tibial epiphyseal plate

Fig. 7.30b. Posterior image of the knees, tibiae and ankles shows poor uptake of isotope by the growth plates around the ankles

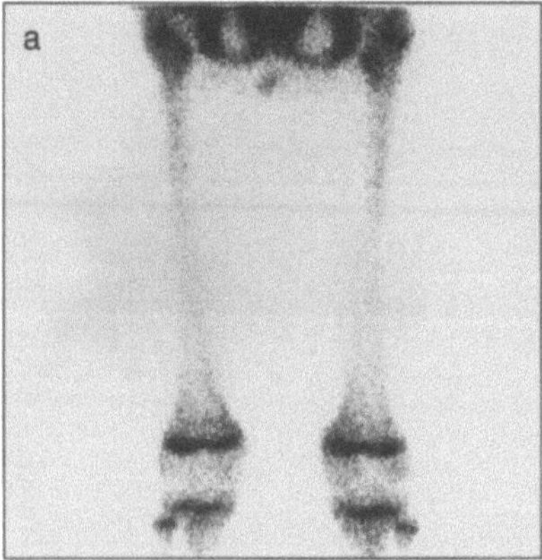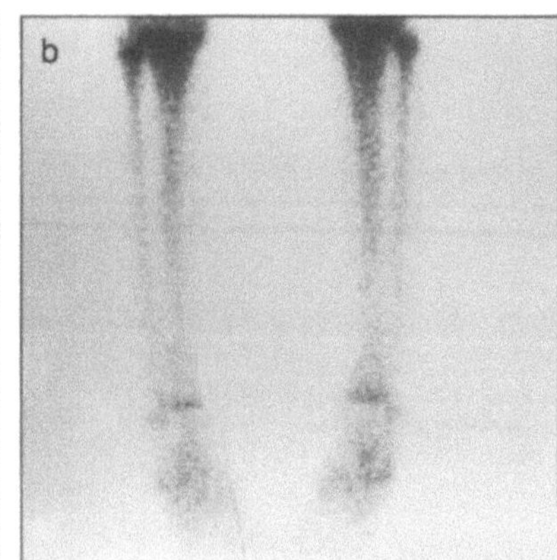

Case 7.31. A 7-year-old girl with a rhabdomyosarcoma of the soft tissue in the face. The bone scan was taken following investigation and surgical treatment of the rhabdomyosarcoma. No deposits are seen, but acute immobilisation caused indistinctness of the epiphyseal plates

Fig. 7.31a. Posterior image of the knees, tibiae and ankles. There is indistinctness of all the epiphyseal plates. This is so marked around the ankles that the epiphyseal plates of the distal ends of the fibulae cannot be made out at all

Fig. 7.31b. Posterior magnified image of the knees shows no clear epiphyseal plates

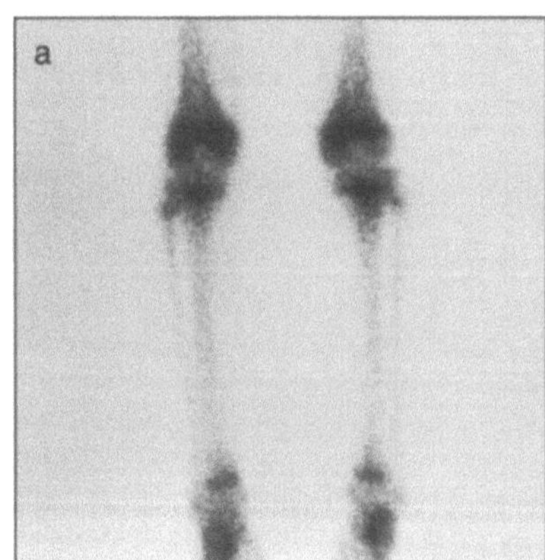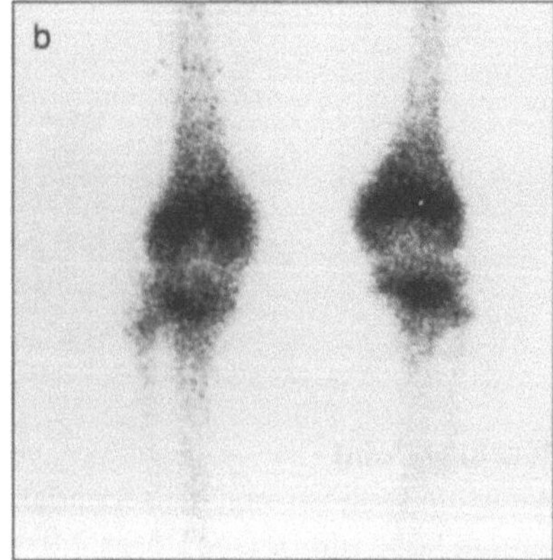

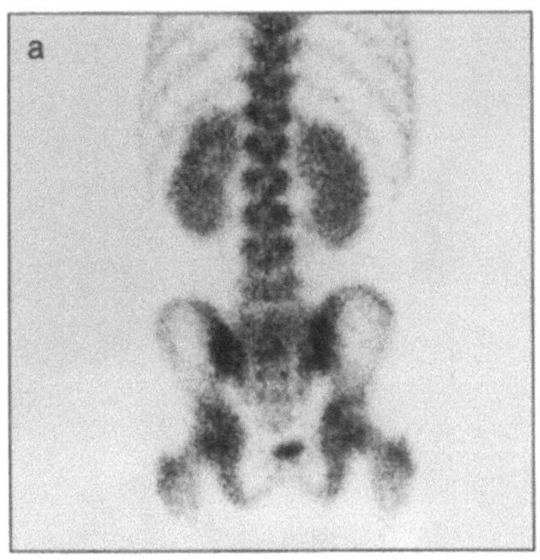 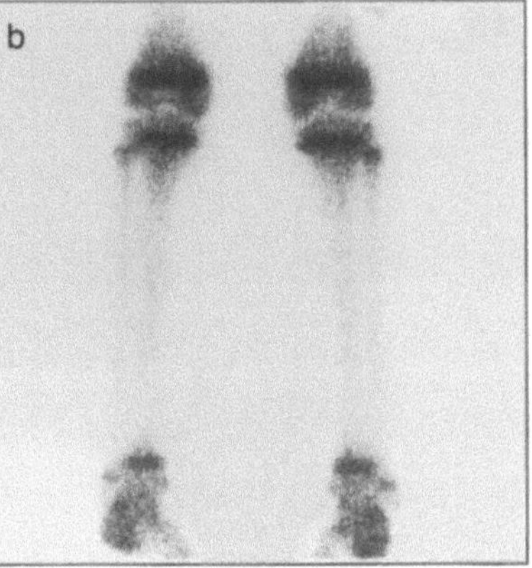

Case 7.32. A 10-year-old boy who was being investigated for pyrexia of unknown cause with a 3-week history. The child had hepatomegaly with a rash and the final diagnosis was that of vasculitis. The bone scan, undertaken 4 weeks into the illness, shows evidence of a sick child who had "gone off his feet"

Fig. 7.32a. Posterior image of the lower dorsal and lumbar spine, pelvis and upper femora. There is indistinctness of the epiphyseal plates of the femoral heads as well as the greater trochanters. Retention of isotope by both kidneys is noted

Fig. 7.32b. Posterior image of the knees, tibiae and ankles shows indistinctness of the epiphyseal plates; this is more marked in the ankles than around the knees and is typical of a child who has "gone off his feet"

Teaching Point

The retention of isotope by the kidneys has numerous causes. The exact mechanism is unknown in this child, especially since the dimercaptosuccinate (DMSA) scan undertaken 4 days prior to the bone scan was entirely normal, as was the ultrasound.

7.7 Disuse Arthropathy

(1 Case; Fig. 7.33)

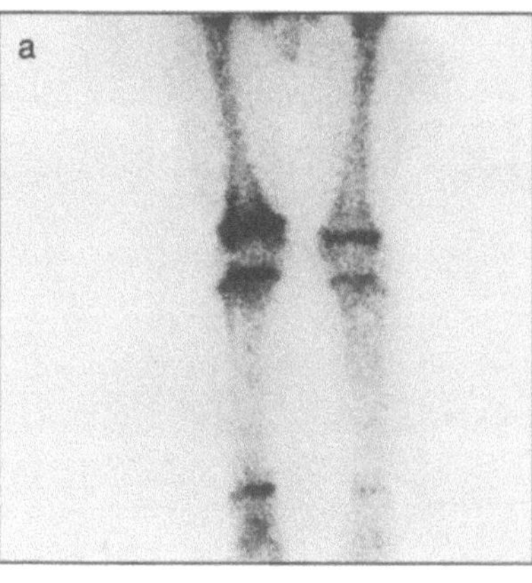

Case 7.33. A 3-year-old boy who was using crutches following surgery for a pelvic rhabdomyosarcoma. The boy was not bearing weight on the right leg

Fig. 7.33a. Posterior image of the femora, knees, tibiae and ankles shows reduced activity throughout the right leg. The epiphyseal plates around the knee have decreased activity but are still clearly seen, whilst those around the ankle joint cannot be seen at all

Teaching Point

1. Similar appearances may be seen in the late stage of reflex sympathetic dystrophy (see Chap. 5.4.4, "Reflex Sympathetic Dystrophy – Sudeck's Atrophy").
2. Also see Case 3.8.

7.8 Muscular Disorders

(1 Case; Fig. 7.34)

Case 7.34. A 4-year-old girl who was found to be suffering from dermato-myositis

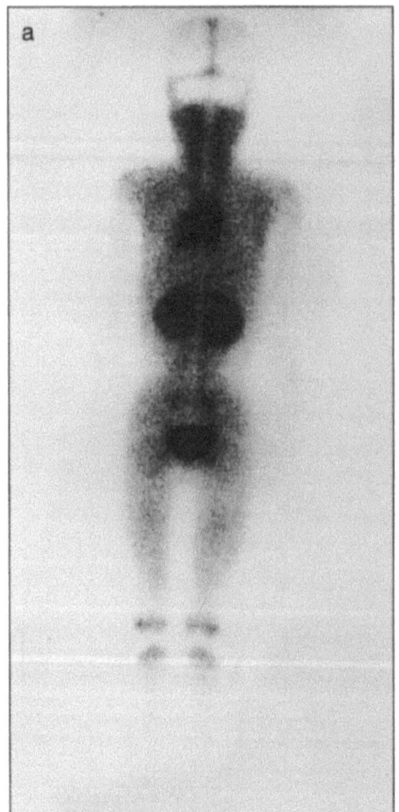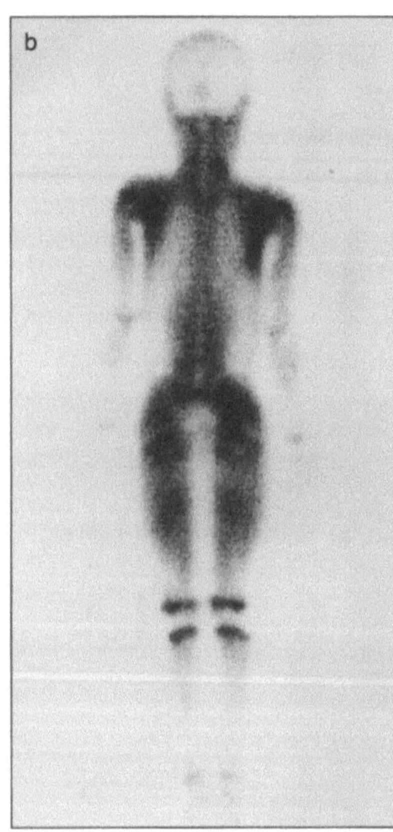

Fig. 7.34a. Posterior blood pool whole body image shows very little activity in the skeleton. The upper limbs and distal tibiae and ankles are barely visualised

Fig. 7.34b. Posterior whole body scan shows very little uptake of isotope in the skeleton. The epiphyseal plates around the knees are seen, but most of the activity is distributed within the soft tissues of the thighs, buttocks, shoulder girdle and back

7.9 Growth Arrest
(2 Cases; Figs. 7.35, 7.36)

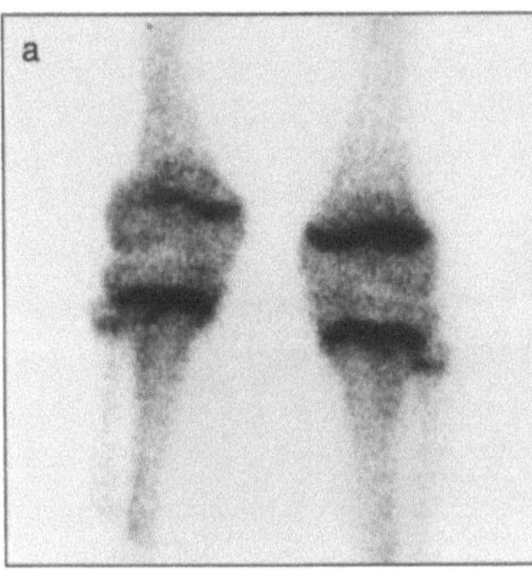

Case 7.35. An 11-year-old girl with genu valgum and discrepany between the lower limb length. There was no history of trauma

Fig. 7.35a. Anterior view of the knees shows poor uptake of isotope in the distal right femur. This is more marked laterally

Teaching Point
These are the features of partial epiphysiodesis.

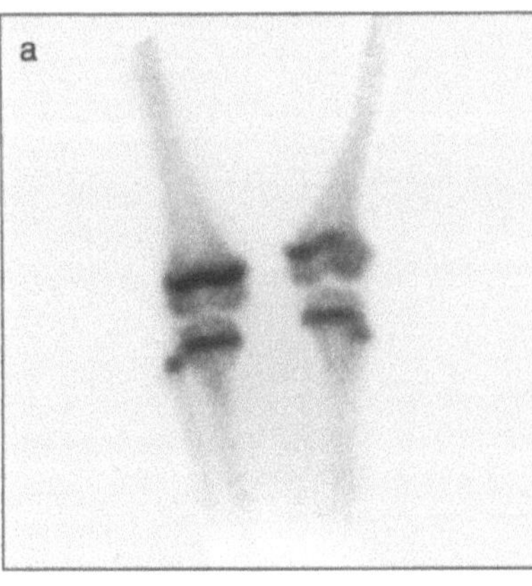

Case 7.36. A 5-year-old girl with genu valgum and partial epiphysiodesis of the left knee

Fig. 7.36a. Anterior image of the knees shows normal uptake by the medial aspect of the left distal femoral growth plate with no significant uptake laterally

Teaching Point
Since the knee is still symmetrical, the changes seen are probably of short duration.

8 Unusual Appearances of the Bone-Seeking Tracer

8.1 Kidney and Collecting System

8.1.1 Kidney Obstruction
(6 Cases; Figs. 8.1–8.6)

Teaching Point: Also see Cases 2.23 and 3.22.

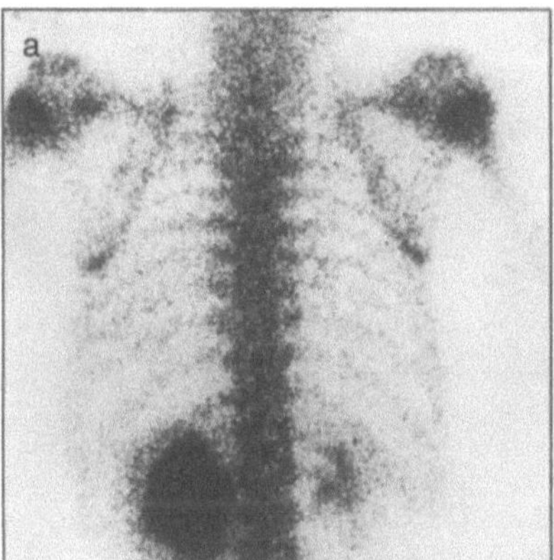

Case 8.1. A 5-year-old boy who was being investigated for backache thought to be due to a skeletal abnormality. Final diagnosis was a left pelviureteric junction obstruction as the cause for the pain

Fig. 8.1a. Posterior image of the dorsal and upper lumbar spine shows retention of tracer in a dilated left renal pelvis. The right kidney is normal. This was confirmed on dynamic renography

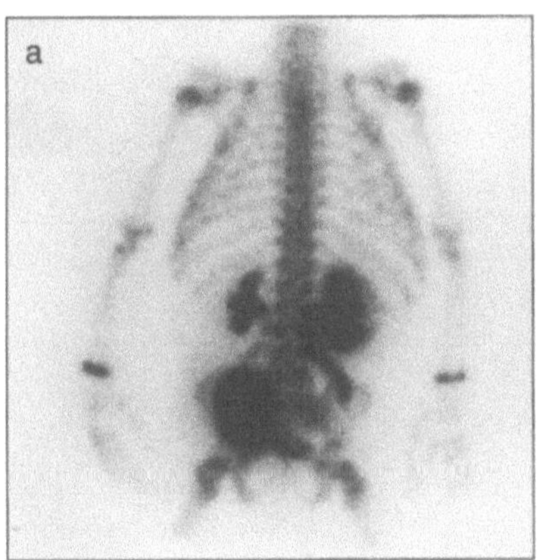

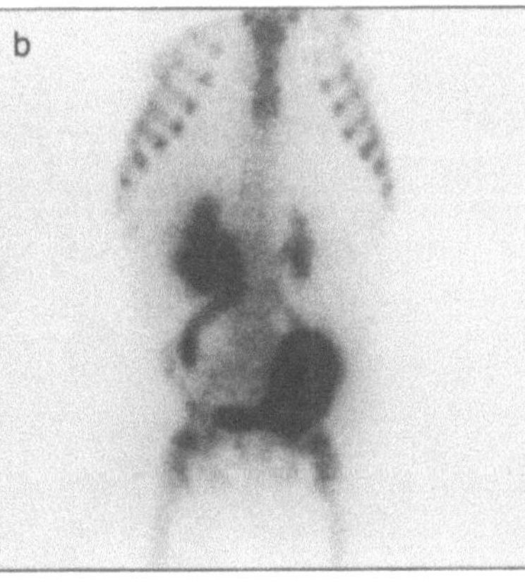

Case 8.2 A 2-year-old girl with a rhabdomyosarcoma of the pelvis causing obstruction to bladder outlet

Fig. 8.2a. Posterior image of the upper limbs, thorax, lumbar spine, pelvis and upper femora shows retention of isotope in the renal pelves and dilated ureters. The bladder is full and displaced to the left

Fig. 8.2b. Anterior image of the thorax, pelvis and femora shows the bilateral hydronephrosis, more marked on the right than on the left, as well as the large displaced bladder

Case 8.3. A 19-year-old male who presented with a prostatic rhabdomyosarcoma with acute urinary retention after chemotherapy. He was found to have disseminated disease at presentation and a urinary diversion was undertaken. (This is the same patient as in Case 4.78)

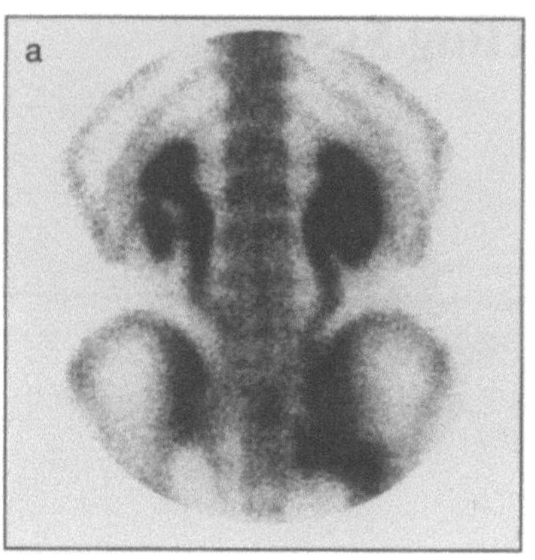

Fig. 8.3a. Posterior image of the spine and upper pelvis shows hydronephrotic kidneys and dilated ureters. Note the activity over the right sacroiliac joint due to a new formed bladder from bowel

Case 8.4. A 17-year-old girl with a Ewing's sarcoma of the distal left femur. (This is the same patient as in Case 4.35)

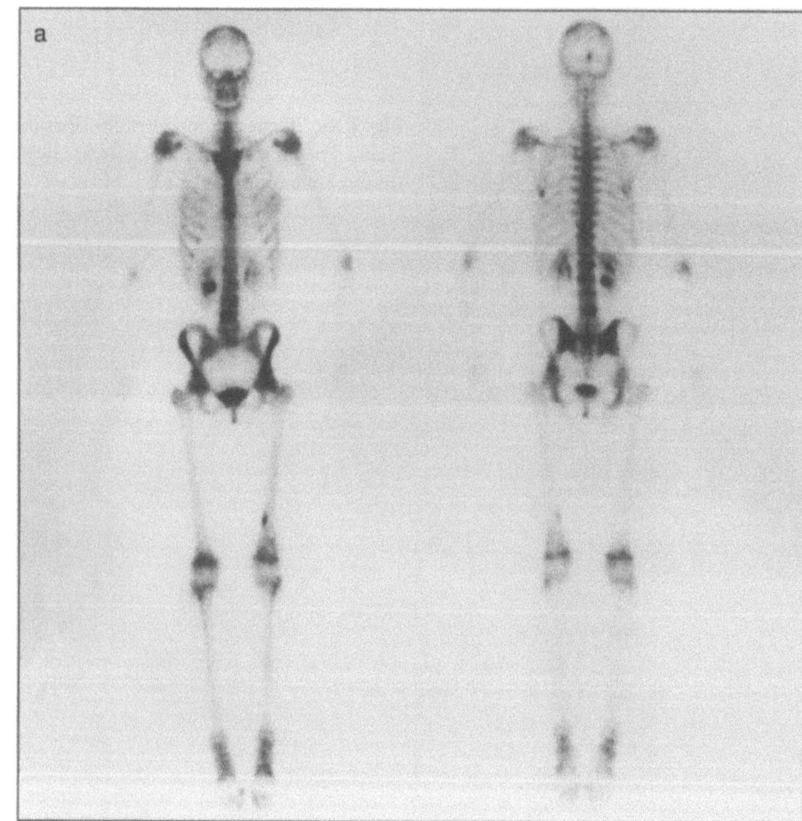

Fig. 8.4a. Whole body images show a dilated lower renal pelvis on the right following chemotherapy. Follow-up studies showed this to be non-obstructed. The abnomal uptake in the distal left femur was part of the malignant process

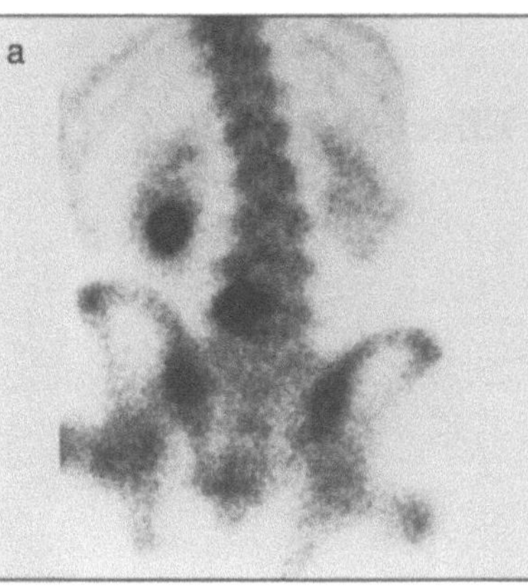

Case 8.5. An 8-year-old boy with back-ache. An osteoid osteoma was removed at surgery. The isotope in the renal pelvis was due to a pelviureteric junction obstruction. (This is the same patient as in Case 4.10)

Fig. 8.5a. Posterior image of the lumbar spine and pelvis. There is a scoliosis concave to the left. Focal abnormal uptake of isotope is noted at L5. There is increased activity in the left renal pelvis due to pelviureteric junction hold-up

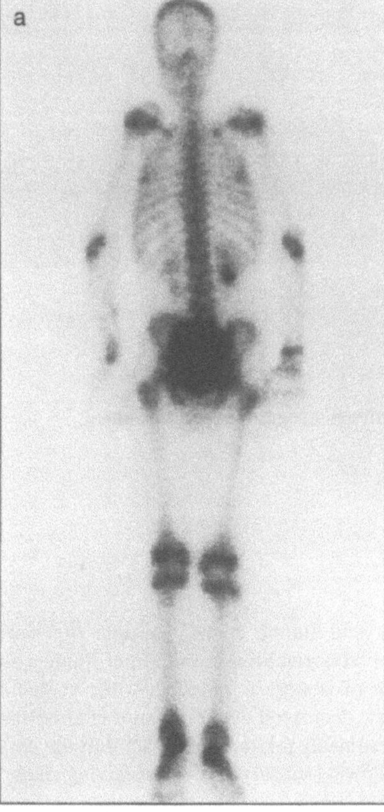

Case 8.6. A 10-year-old boy with septic osteomyelitis of the distal right tibia who presented unwell with a pyrexia and pain in the lower limb. Pseudo renal obstruction is seen. (This is the same patient as in Case 2.12)

Fig. 8.6a. Whole body scan on the day of presentation (posterior view). The skeleton appears normal. Note the full bladder since the child was too ill to co-operate and the retention of isotope in the pelvis of the right kidney

Teaching Point
A full bladder may simulate renal pelvic obstruction.

8.1.2 Retention of Tracer

8.1.2.1 Malignancy and / or Effect of Drugs
(4 Cases; Figs. 8.7–8.10)

Teaching Point
Also see Cases 4.55, 4.64, 5.74 and 8.31.

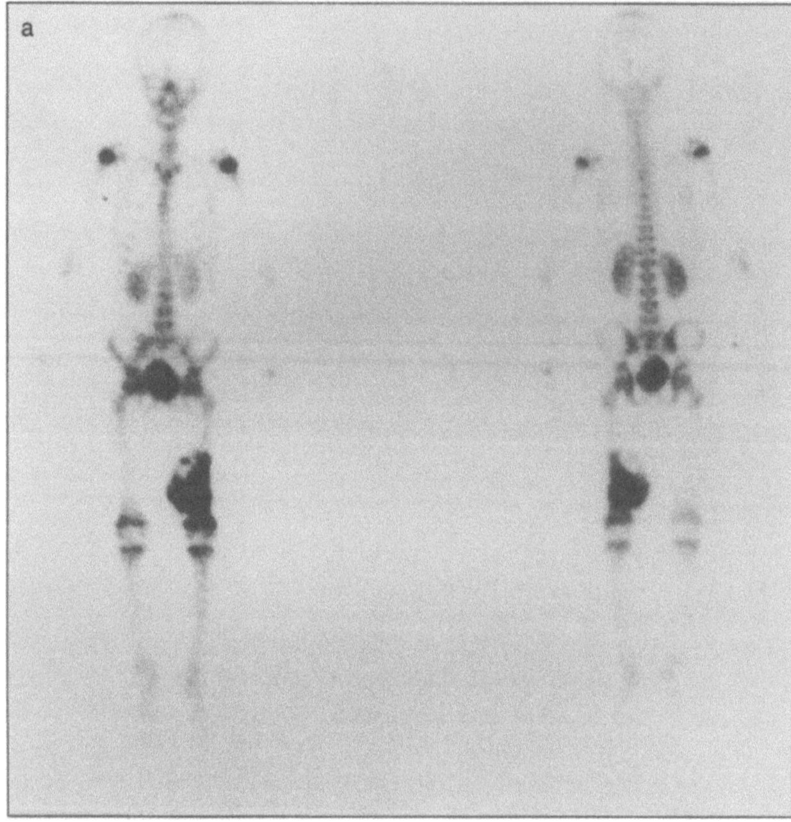

Case 8.7. An 8-year-old boy with a primary osteogenic sarcoma of the distal left femur. (This is the same patient as in Case 4.43)

Fig. 8.7a. Whole body scans show marked abnormal increased uptake of isotope in the lower half of the left femur, due to the osteogenic sarcoma. There is marked retention of radiotracer by both kidneys after chemotherapy

Case 8.8. A 13-year-old girl with a primitive neuroectodermal tumour. (Same patient as in Case 4.53)

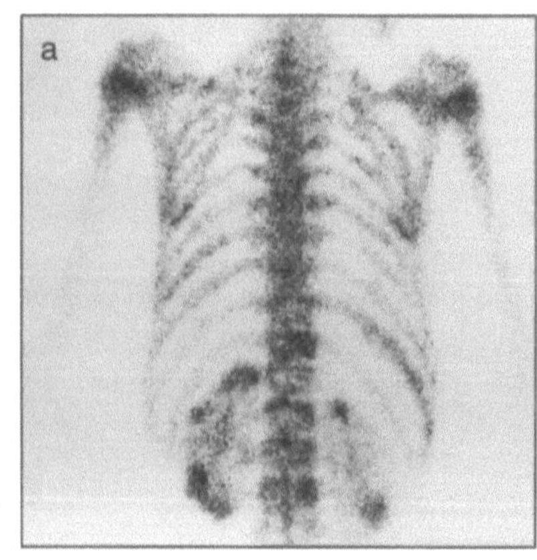

Fig. 8.8a. Posterior image of the thorax and lumbar spine. Multiple ribs show abnormal increased uptake of isotope and abnormalities in the upper humeri are seen. Patchy abnormal increased uptake of isotope is noted in some vertebral bodies, whilst other vertebral bodies show decreased activity. There is abnormal distribution of isotope in the kidneys, presumably related to the fact that the child was very ill and had been immobilised following surgery and was receiving chemotherapy

318

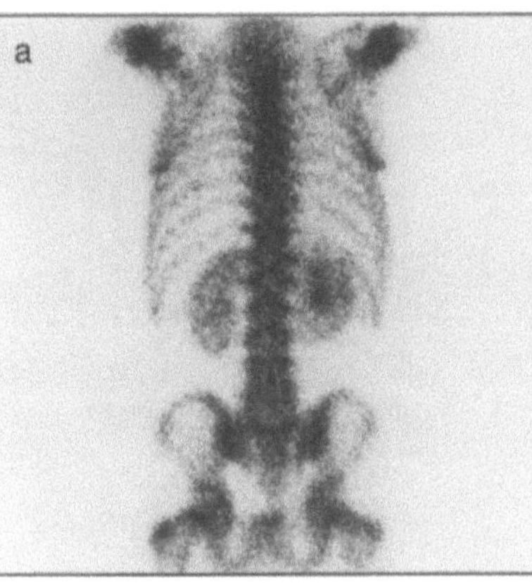

Case 8.9. A 5-year-old boy who was found to have a non-Hodgkin's lymphoma (B cell). (This is the same patient as in Case 4.67)

Fig. 8.9a. Posterior image of the spine and pelvis shows abnormal increased uptake of isotope in the femoral necks. Note the appearances of the kidneys, presumably due to a combination of renal involvement in the disease, acute immobilisation and chemotherapy

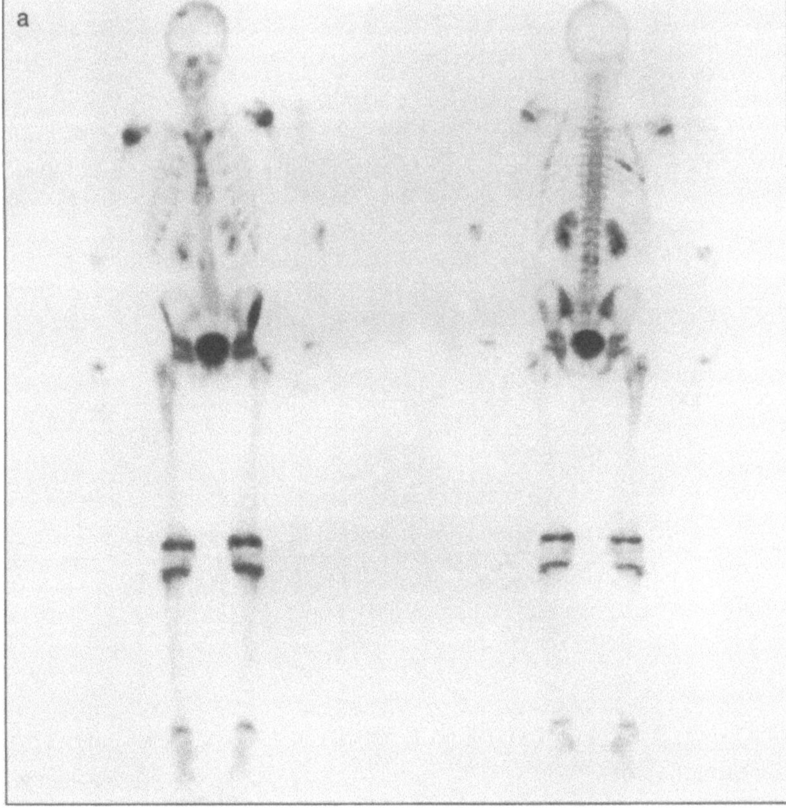

Case 8.10. A 14-year-old boy who was found to have secondary deposits from a malignant melanoma. (This is the same patient as in Case 4.80)

Fig. 8.10a. Whole body scans show areas of abnormal increased uptake of isotope in the skull vault, one rib on the right, the left iliac bone and right femur. There is increased uptake of isotope in the kidneys following chemotherapy

8.1.2.2 Sickle Cell Disease
(2 Cases; Figs. 8.11, 8.12)

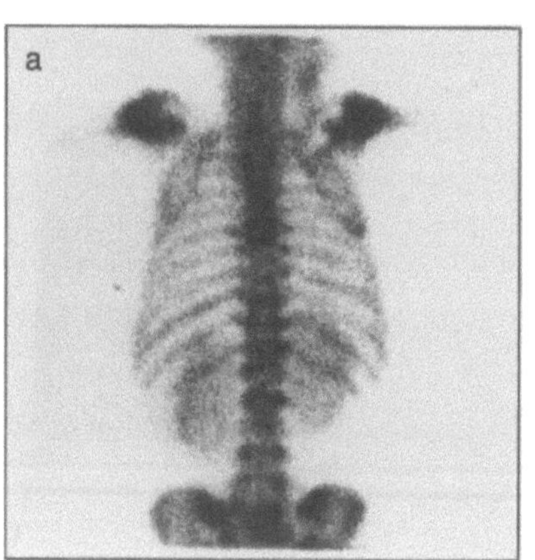

Case 8.11. A 5-year-old boy with sickle cell anaemia. (Same patient as in Case 6.17)

Fig. 8.11a. Posterior image of the thorax, spine and upper pelvis. Vertebral and rib abnormalities are noted. There is retention of tracer in the kidneys

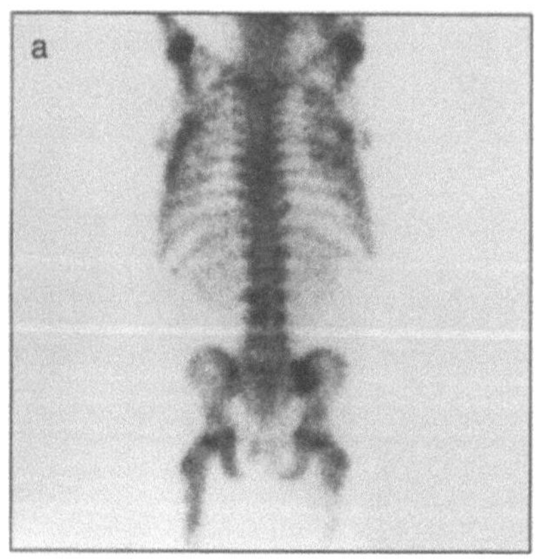

Case 8.12. A 2-year-old boy with sickle cell disease who presented with a severe crisis. (Same baby as in Case 6.18)

Fig. 8.12a. Posterior image of the thorax, spine, pelvis and upper femora shows abnormal uptake in the ribs especially on the right. The vertebral bodies especially in the lumbar spine show areas of decreased and increased activity. There is increased activity in the right sacro-iliac joint as well as in the upper femora, more marked on the left than on the right. There is retention of tracer in the kidneys

Teaching Point
See also Chap. 6.3, "Sickle Cell Disease".

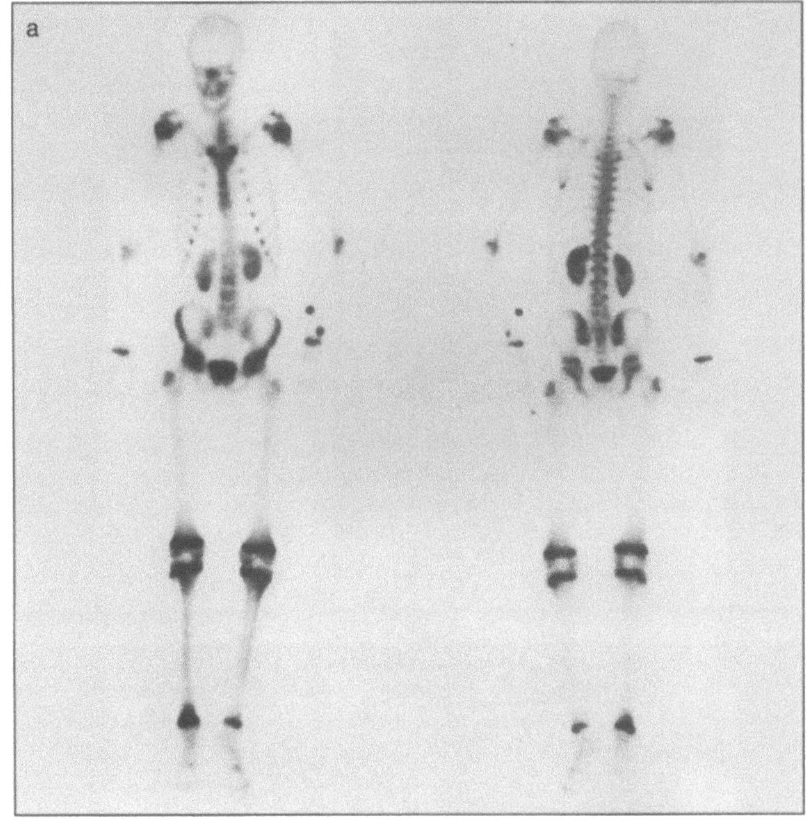

8.1.2.3 Septicaemia
(4 Cases; Figs. 8.13–8.16)

Case 8.13. A 13-year-old boy with osteomyelitis of the distal right tibia. (This is the same child as in Case 2.4)

Fig. 8.13a. Whole body images show marked increased uptake of isotope from the distal right tibial epiphysis extending proximally into the diaphysis. There is increased activity in the kidneys. The reason for this is unclear, but the child was septicaemic. There was no previous history of renal disease and the child was only on intravenous antibiotics at the time of the scan

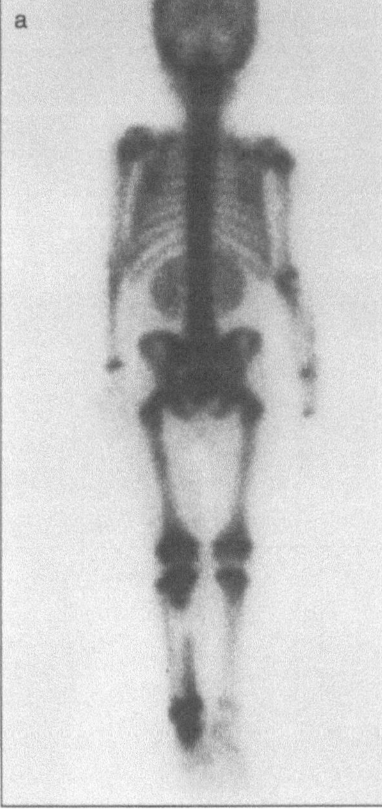

Case 8.14. A 3-year-old boy who had been treated for sepsis of the left leg. Final diagnosis was osteomyelitis of the tibia. (Same child as in Case 2.14)

Fig. 8.14a. Whole body scan (posterior view) shows abnormal increased uptake of isotope in the distal left tibial shaft with total absence of activity in the mid third of the tibia. Note the marked increased activity around the ankle joint (no pus was found in the ankle joint). There is increased uptake of isotope in both kidneys. This is presumably related to the chronic sepsis and antibiotic therapy

Case 8.15. A 4-year-old boy with osteomyelitis of the left scapula with possible involvement of the humerus. (This is the same child as in Case 2.36)

Fig. 8.15a. Posterior whole body scan shows abnormal increased uptake of isotope in the left scapula. The epiphysis of the proximal portion of the humerus also shows increased uptake of isotope, but this may well be secondary simply to hyperaemia. The kidneys are well seen. This finding is frequent in children who are ill and have septicaemia, but the cause is uncertain. Activity over the pelvis is due to a full bladder

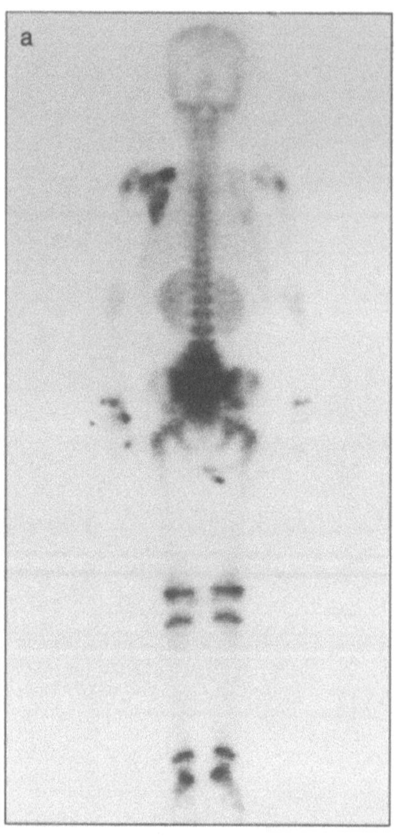

Case 8.16. An 11-year-old boy with septic arthritis of the right hip and right ankle. (This is the same patient as in Case 3.16)

Fig. 8.16a. Whole body scan (posterior view) shows virtually total absence of activity in the region of the right hip joint, whilst the right ankle shows increased activity. There is increased activity throughout both kidneys

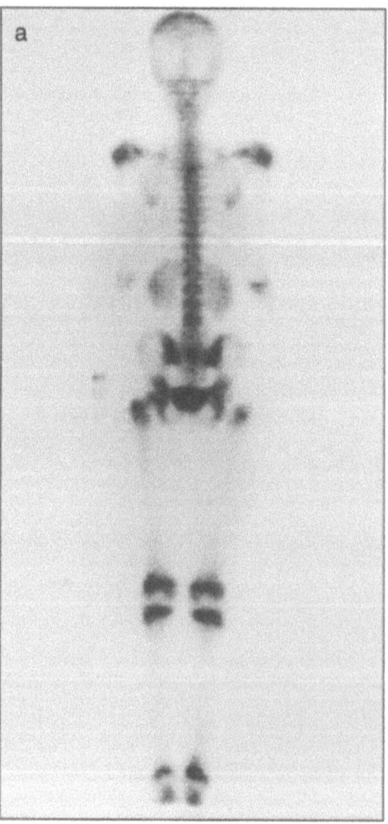

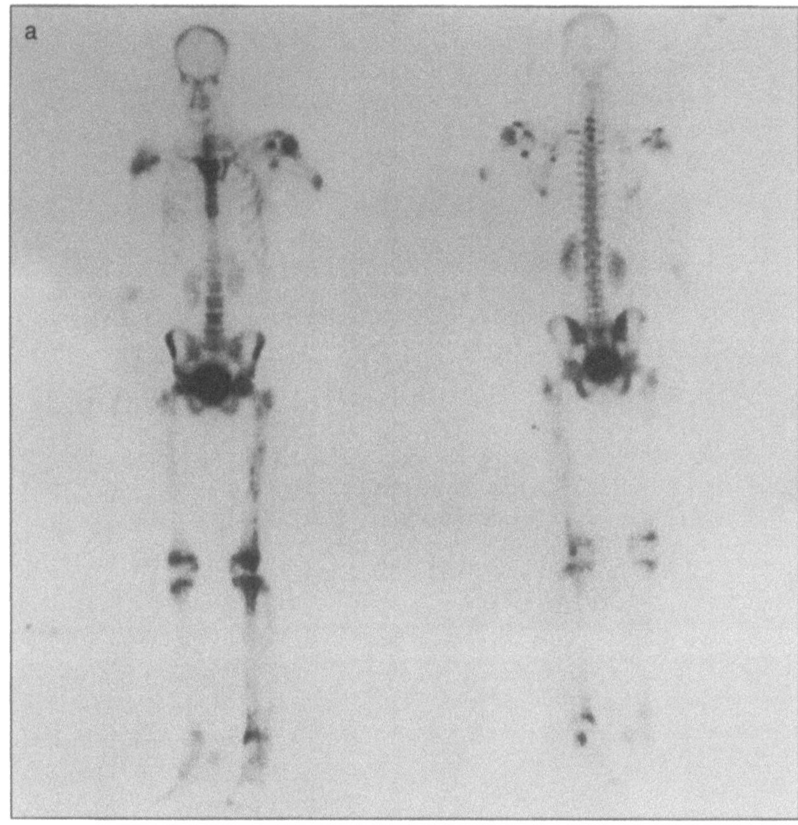

8.1.2.4 Post-trauma Retention
(4 Cases; Figs. 8.17–8.20)

Case 8.17. **A 16-year-old boy who had suffered a motor cycle accident and had undergone an amputation of the left arm. He was found to have a compound fracture of the left femur, left tibia and a fracture in the left foot as well as in the left scapula. (Same patient as in Case 5.33)**

Fig. 8.17a. Whole body images show abnormal uptake of isotope in the left femur as well as in the left tibia. The left calcaneous shows increased uptake of isotope, as does the left scapula and the upper dorsal spine. There is retention of tracer by the kidneys

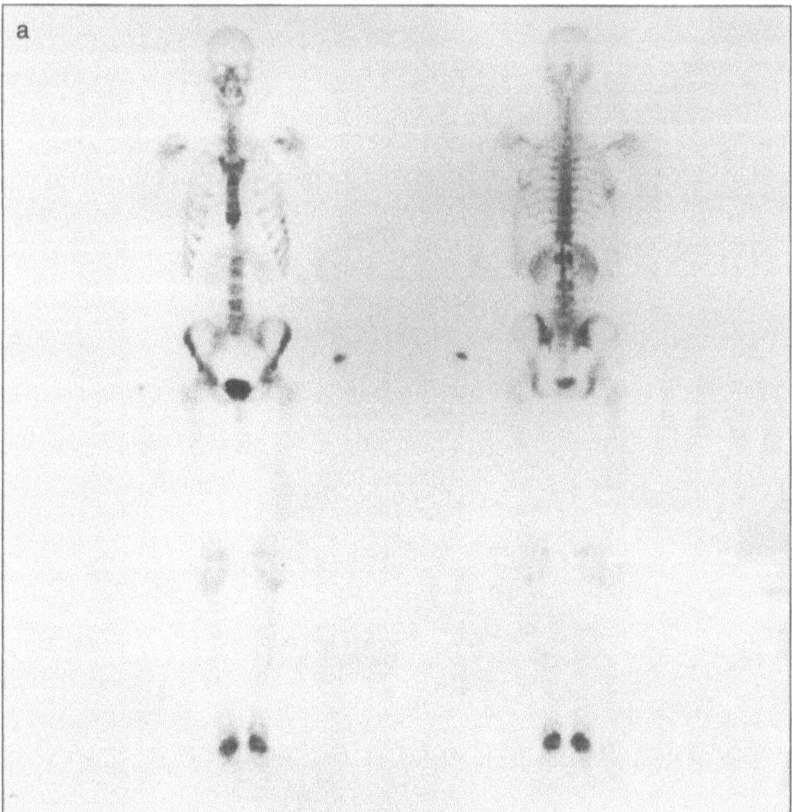

Case 8.18. **A 20-year-old female with fractures of the calcaneous and the cuboid as well as the radius. Prior to the bone scan, surgery with insertion of rods has been performed in the spine. (This is the same patient as in Case 5.34)**

Fig. 8.18a. Whole body images show absent activity in the mid lumbar spine. There is increased activity in the feet bilaterally. Retention of tracer by the kidneys is noted

Case 8.19. A 10-year-old boy following a road traffic accident who suffered fractures of the mid dorsal spine. (Same child as in Case 5.10)

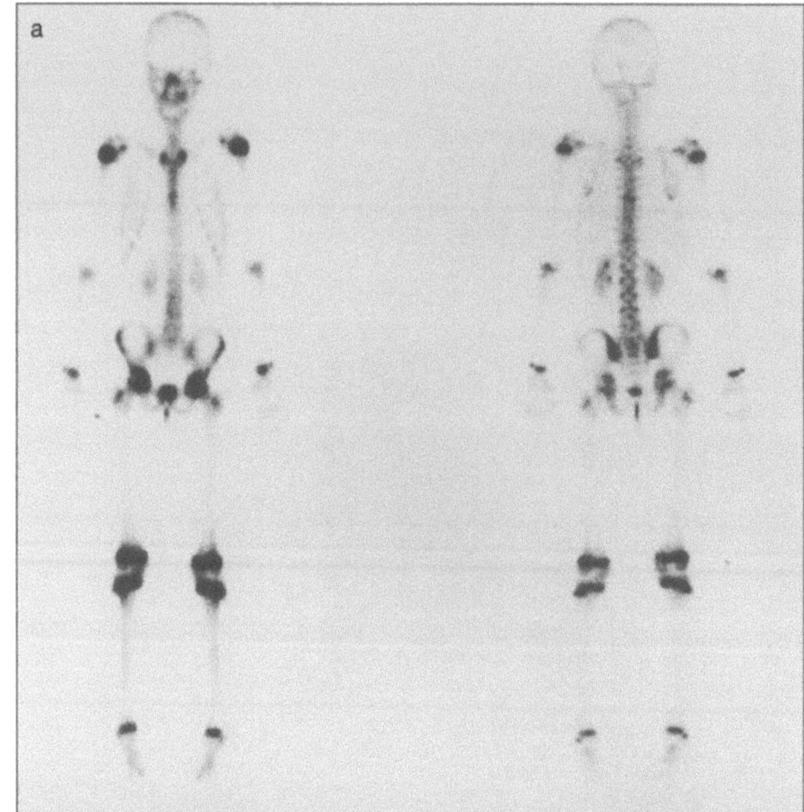

Fig. 8.19a. Whole body images show focal abnormal increased uptake of isotope in the mid dorsal spine. Note the unusual appearances of the kidneys, which have retained the tracer

Case 8.20. A 22-year-old male who had been involved in a road traffic accident. Fractures of the left femur and tibia were found as well as a fracture of the left clavicle and one upper left rib. There was occlusion of the right femoral artery. (This is the same patient as in Case 5.32)

Fig. 8.20a. Whole body images show intense abnormal uptake of isotope in the mid portion of the right femur as well as in the distal right tibia. The right knee is difficult to assess because of the positioning of the foot. Abnormal increased uptake of isotope is also noted in the left clavicle, best seen on the anterior view. Increased uptake of isotope is also noted in the right hand and one upper left rib. The kidneys retain the tracer. The reason for the abnormal retention of isotope by the kidneys is uncertain, but the possibility that the kidneys suffered ischaemia was highly likely

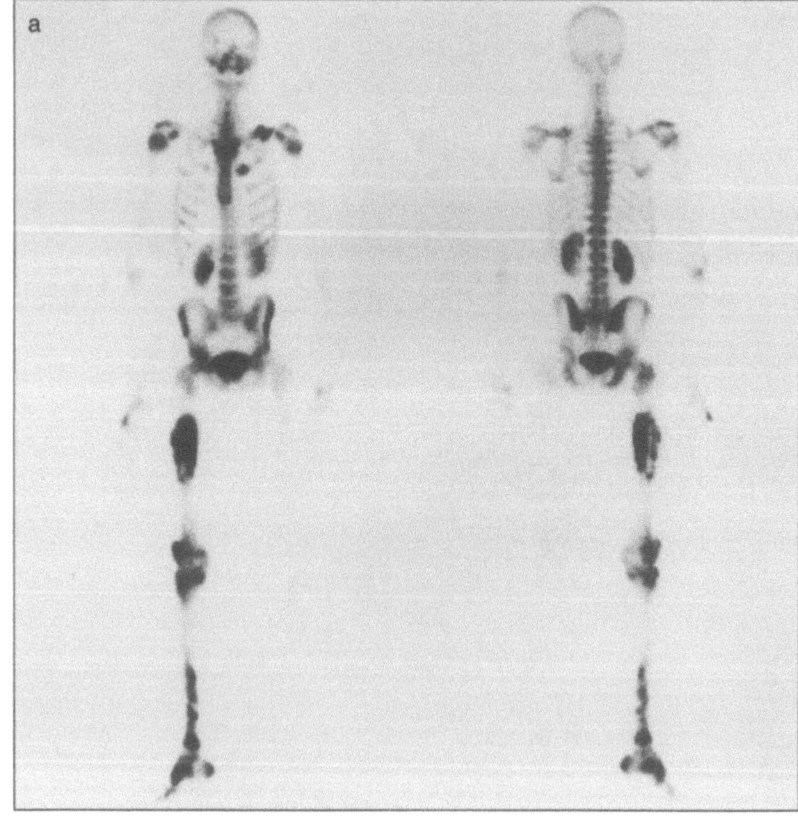

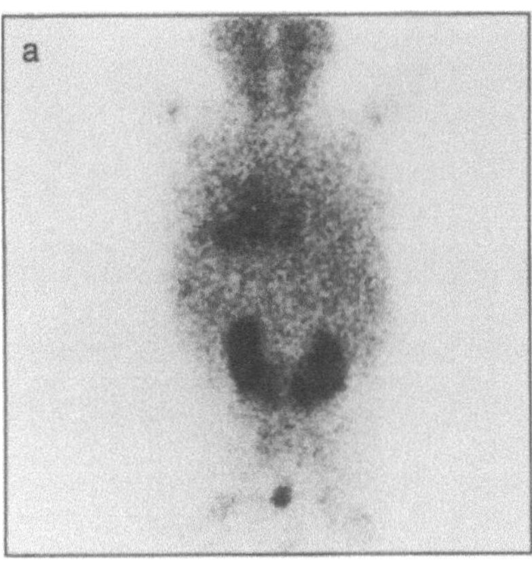

8.1.2.5 The Sick Child (1 Case; Fig. 8.21)

Case 8.21. A 10-year-old boy who was being investigated for pyrexia of unknown cause with a 3-week history. The child had hepatomegaly with a rash and the final diagnosis was that of vasculitis. The bone scan was undertaken 4 weeks into the illness. The bone scan shows evidence of an unwell child who had "gone off his feet". (This is the same patient as in Case 7.32)

Fig. 8.21a. Posterior image of the lower dorsal and lumbar spine, pelvis and upper femora. There is indistinctness of the epiphyseal plates of the femoral heads as well as the greater trochanters. Retention of isotope by both kidneys is noted. The retention of isotope by the kidneys has numerous causes, and the exact mechanism is unknown in this child, especially since the dimercaptosuccinate (DMSA) scan undertaken 4 days prior to the bone scan was entirely normal, as was the ultrasound

8.1.2.6 Isotope in Ureter

This may be seen in non-obstructed renal collecting systems, especially in the blood pool images. See Cases 2.50, 3.11, 3.12 and 4.55.

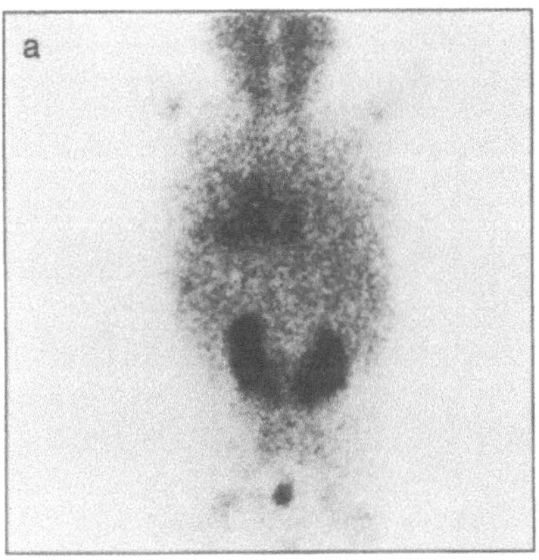

8.1.3 Positional Abnormality

(3 Cases; Figs. 8.22-8.24)

Case 8.22. A 10-month-old girl who had multiple fractures due to being battered. (Same baby as in Case 5.41)

Fig. 8.22a. Posterior blood pool image of the thorax and abdomen. The kidneys are clearly seen to be malrotated and joined in the centre due to a horseshoe kidney

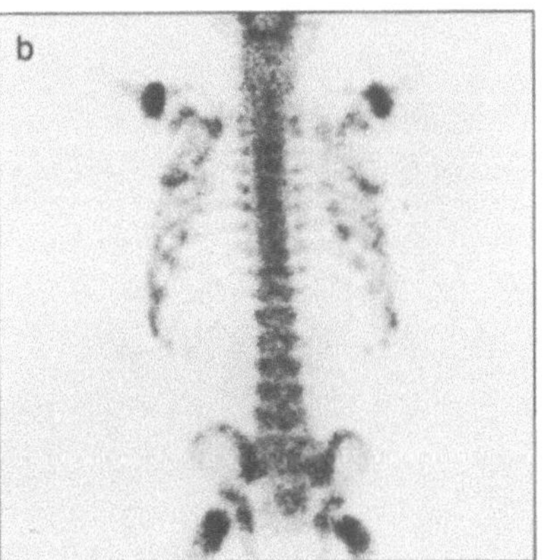

Fig. 8.22b. Posterior image of the dorsal and lumbar spine and pelvis shows abnormal uptake in the ribs on the right due to a trauma. The horseshoe kidney cannot be seen in this image

Case 8.23. A 15-year-old boy with pain around the knee due to a chondrosarcoma of the distal right femur. (This is the same patient as in Case 4.52)

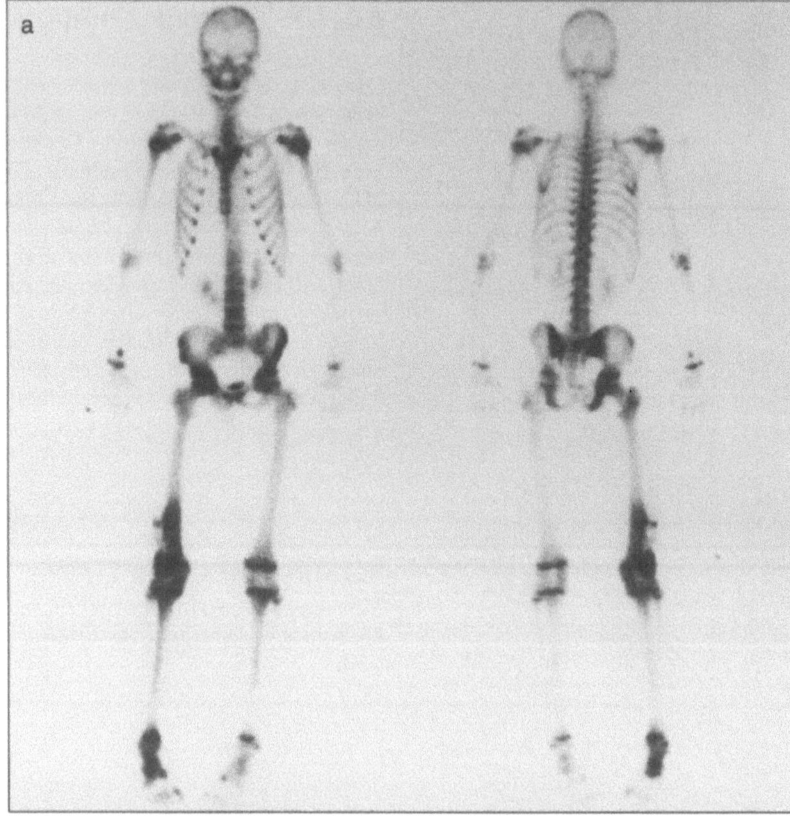

Fig. 8.23a. Whole body images show abnormal uptake of isotope in a non-homogeneous fashion in the lower right femur and right foot. The position of the right kidney is rather low, and the axes of the collecting systems of both kidneys are abnormal, suggesting a horseshoe kidney. The kidneys were not investigated, but the appearances on the whole body images strongly suggest a horseshoe kidney

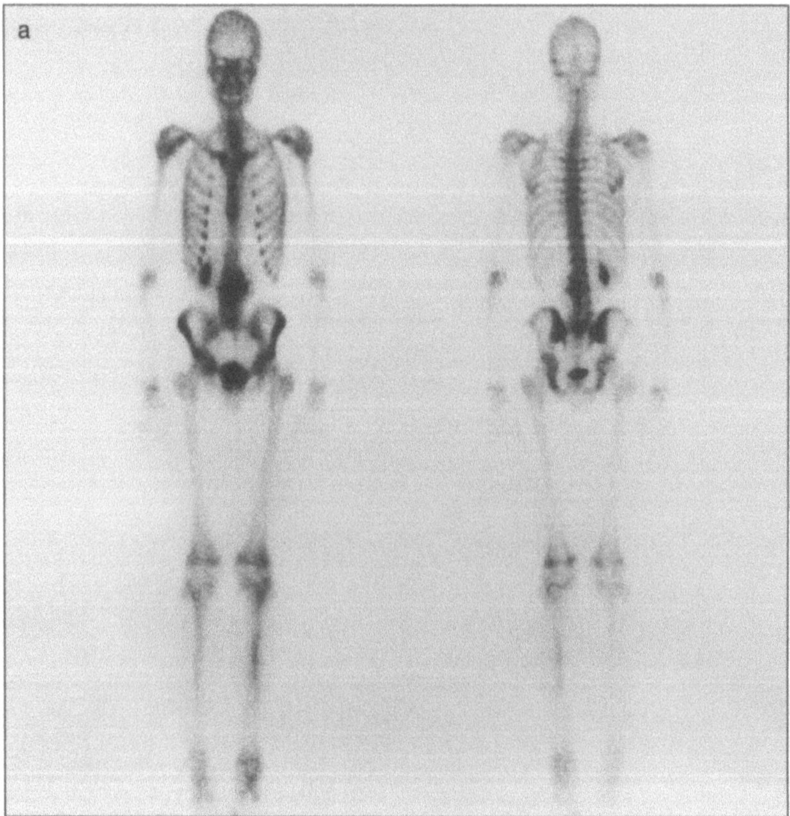

Case 8.24. A 16-year-old boy who had an accident on his bicycle 4 weeks prior to the bone scan. He had been immobilised and presented now with a swollen left foot

Fig. 8.24a. Whole body images show abnormal increased uptake of isotope in the distal left femur as well as in the upper and mid portions of the left tibia. The left foot also shows increased uptake of isotope. The left kidney is unusually situated and overlies the spine, strongly suggesting the diagnosis of crossed fused renal ectopia

8.1.4 Bladder
(5 Cases; Figs. 8.25–8.29)

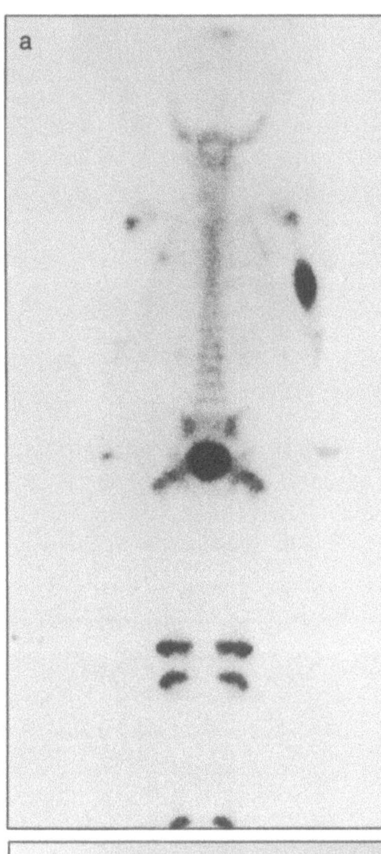

> **Teaching Point**
> A full bladder is not an uncommon finding; however, encouraging high fluid intake after the injection of the tracer decreases the frequency of a full bladder. If the child has been sedated for the bone scan images, the possibility of spontaneous voiding is very small and bladder catheterization may be required (this is another reason to try not to use sedation unless necessary). A full bladder in the blood pool phase may be seen as a photon-deficient area.

Case 8.25. A 13-year-old boy with active histiocytosis. (Same patient as in Case 4.87)

Fig. 8.25a. Whole body scan (posterior view) shows abnormal increased uptake of isotope in the right humerus. Highly specific activity is noted in the bladder. This child was unwell and refused to drink between the injection and the scan, so that the small volume of urine was highly radioactive

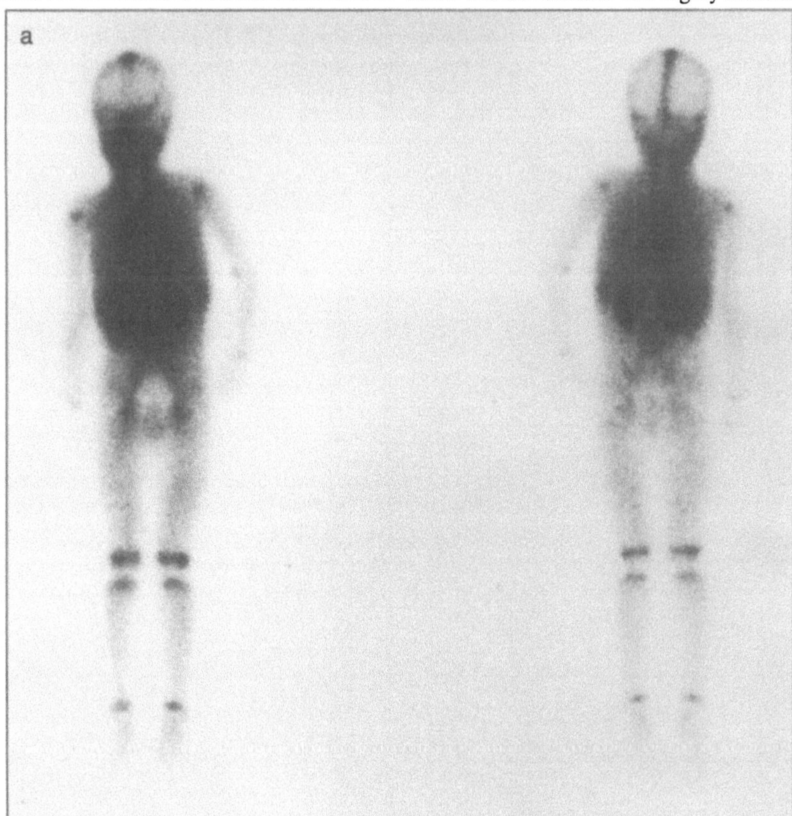

Case 8.26. A 3-year-old girl who had direct trauma to her back and was found to have a fracture of the lower lumbar vertebral bodies.

Fig. 8.26a. Blood pool whole body scan is unremarkable. Note the photon-deficient area on the anterior view in the region of the bladder. This is due to a full bladder at the time of the injection

Case 8.27. A 22-year-old male who had been involved in a road traffic accident. Fractures of the left femur and tibia were found as well as a fracture of the left clavicle. There was occlusion of the right femoral artery. (Same patient as in Case 5.32)

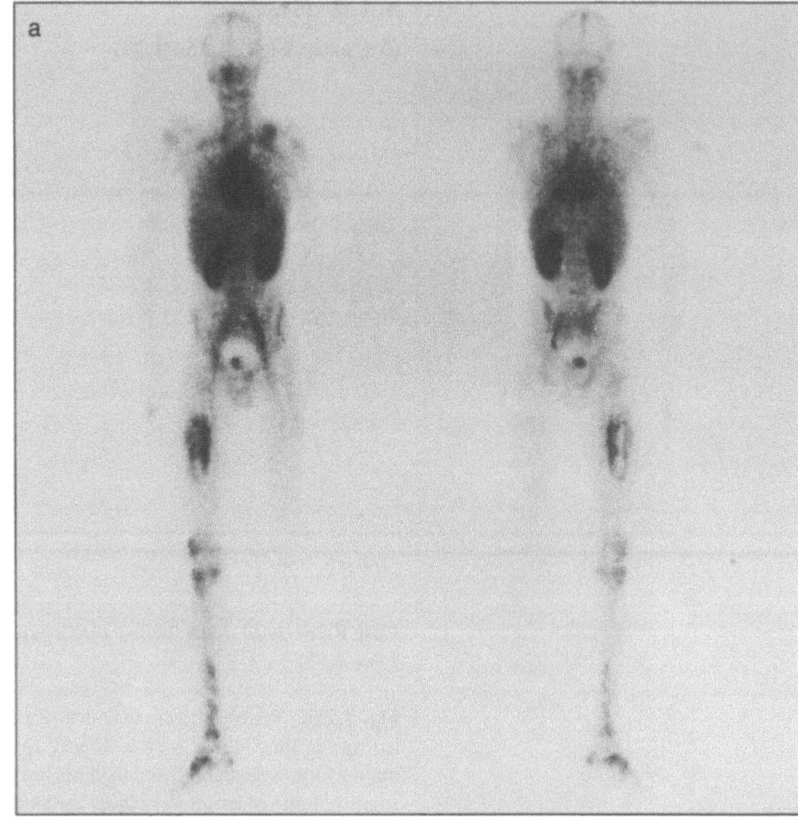

Fig. 8.27a. Whole body blood pool images show abnormal increased uptake of isotope in the left femur and left distal tibia as well as in the left foot. There is increased uptake of isotope in the left shoulder. Note the photon-deficient area in the region of the bladder. This is due to a full bladder at the time of injection

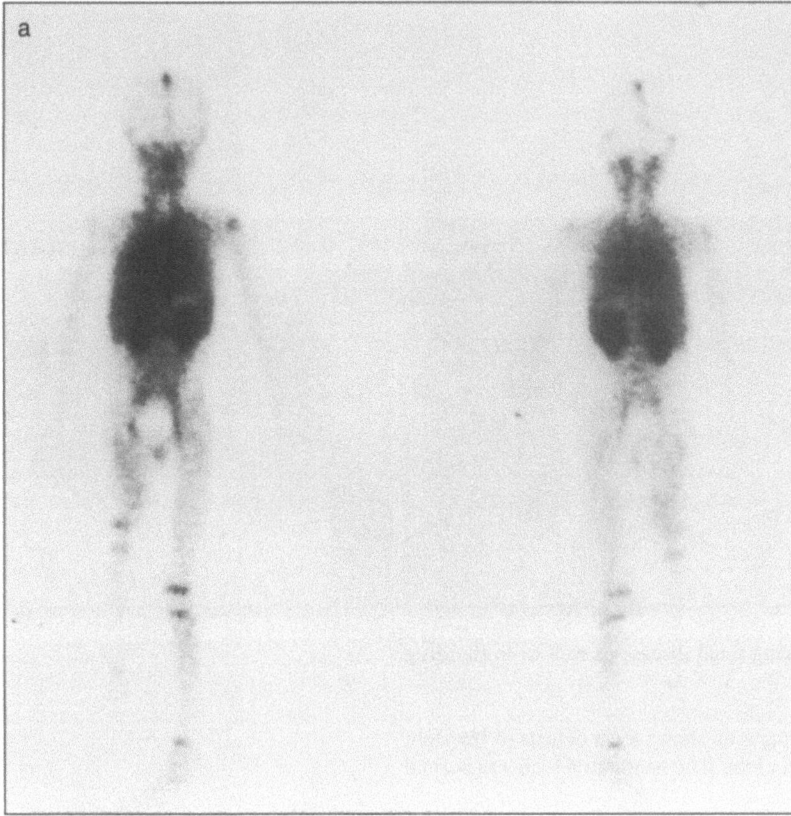

Case 8.28. A 6-year-old boy who had suffered trauma which required surgery for a fractured right femur. No union was noted at the site of the fracture. The clinical question now arose as to whether osteomyelitis existed within this femur. The result of the bone scan suggested that there was no infection within the bone. (Same child as in Case 5.44)

Fig. 8.28a. Blood pool whole body scans show abnormal increased uptake of isotope in the region of the right thigh. The right leg is shorter than the left. Note the photon-deficient area in the region of the bladder. This was due to a full bladder prior to the injection of the isotope

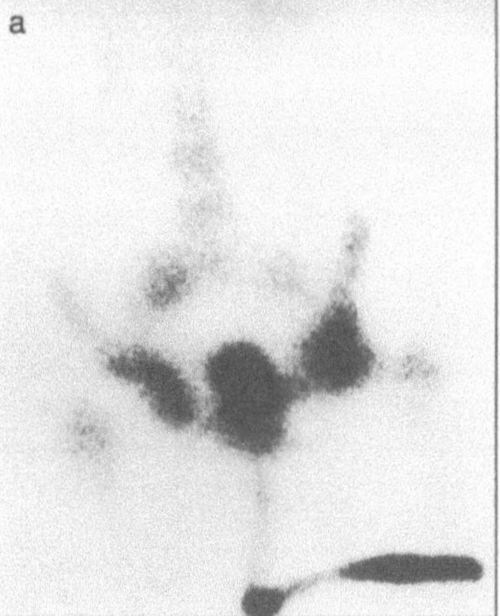

Case 8.29. A 12-year-old girl who suffered traumatic avascular necrosis of the head of the femur. (This is the same patient as in Case 5.53)

Fig. 8.29a. Anterior view of the pelvis shows a normal left hip. On the right there is total absence of activity of the femoral head and neck. Note the bladder is on catheter drainage with isotope seen in the bladder catheter

8.2 Lung Uptake
(2 Cases; Figs. 8.30, 8.31)

Case 8.30. A 12-year-old boy with a nephrotic syndrome who developed backache. He was found to be suffering from pulmonary embolism. These emboli took up isotope on the bone scan

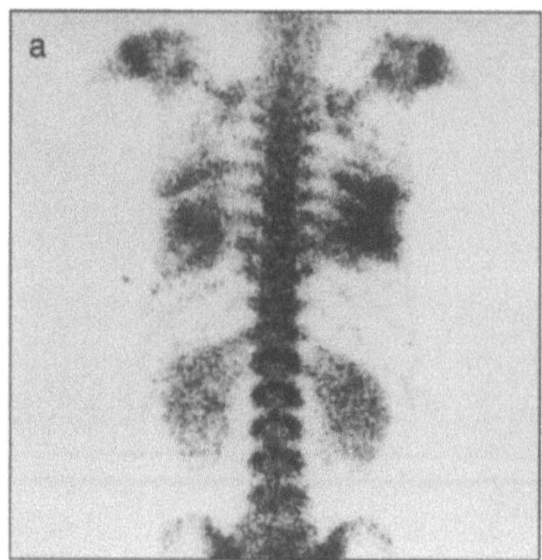
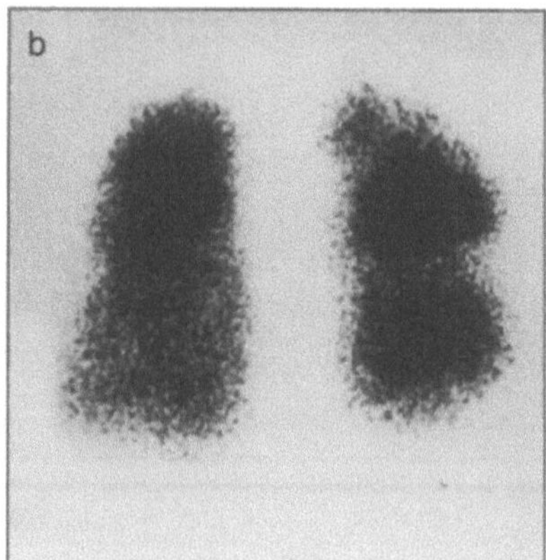

Fig. 8.30a. Posterior bone scan image of the thorax and lumbar spine fails to reveal any abnormality of the skeleton. Note the uptake of isotope by the lungs bilaterally. This is mainly basal. There is also retention of isotope by the renal parenchyma. The cause for the retention of isotope in the kidneys is presumably related both to the underlying renal disease as well as to the drug treatment of this condition

Fig. 8.30b. Posterior Tc 99m perfusion lung scan shows focal defects in the right lung and, to a lesser extent, in the left lower lobe. The ventilation scan was normal (not shown)

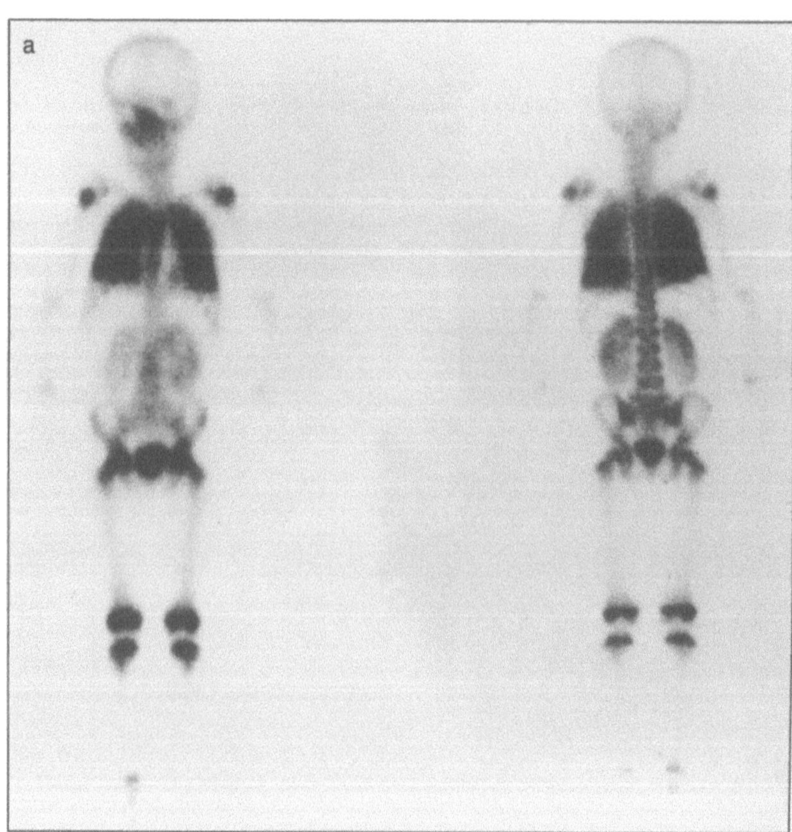

Case 8.31. A 5-year-old boy undergoing investigation for hypercalcaemia. The cause of the hypercalcaemia was never determined. The lung and kidney uptake was presumably secondary to the hypercalcaemia

Fig. 8.31a. Whole body scans show a normal skeleton. There is marked abnormal increased uptake of isotope throughout both lungs. Both kidneys are noted to be enlarged and retention of tracer in the renal parenchyma is noted

8.3 Splenic Uptake
(1 Case; Fig. 8.32)

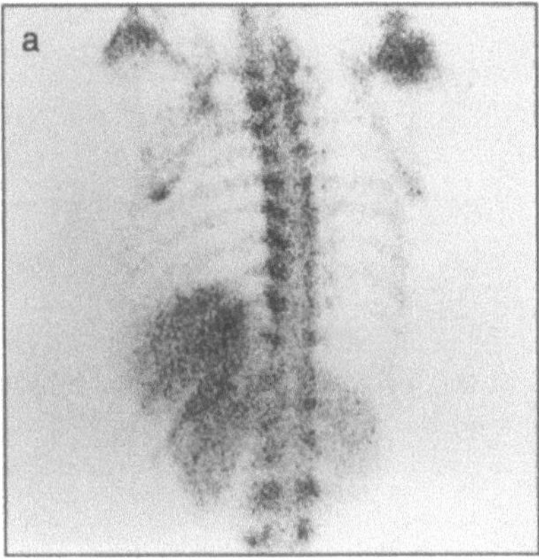

Case 8.32. A 13-year-old boy with known sickle cell disease who presented with an acute crisis. (This is the same child as in Case 6.19)

Fig. 8.32a. Left posterior oblique image of the thorax and spine shows multiple abnormalities in the skeleton. There is uptake of isotope in the spleen as well as in both kidneys. The uptake of isotope in the spleen may be due to the autosplenectomy which these children undergo during the repeated sickle cell crisis

8.4 Brain Uptake
(1 Case; Fig. 8.33)

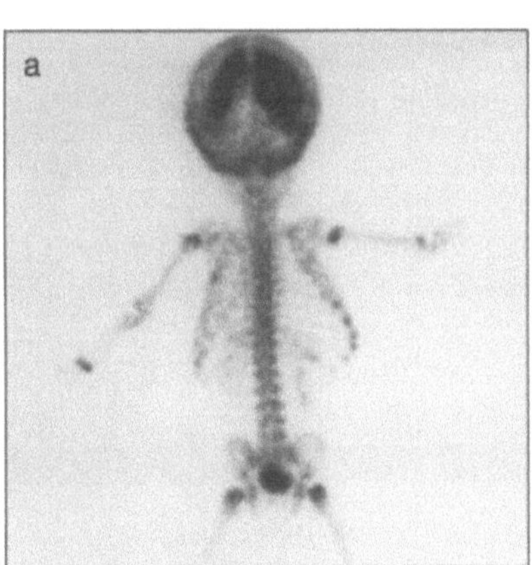

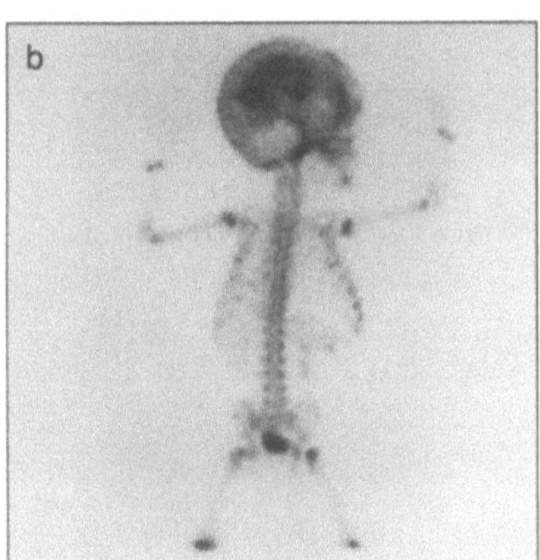

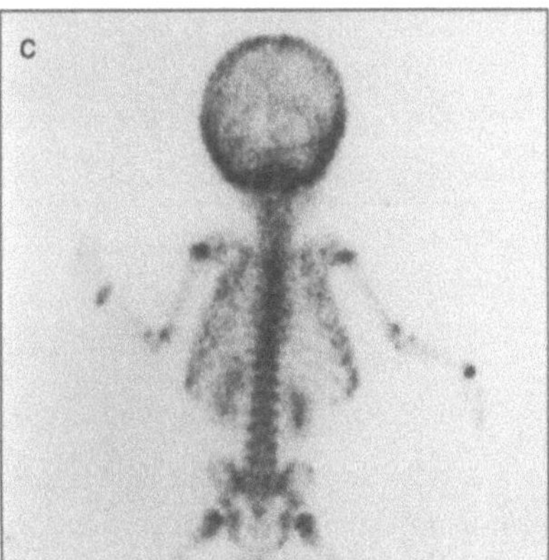

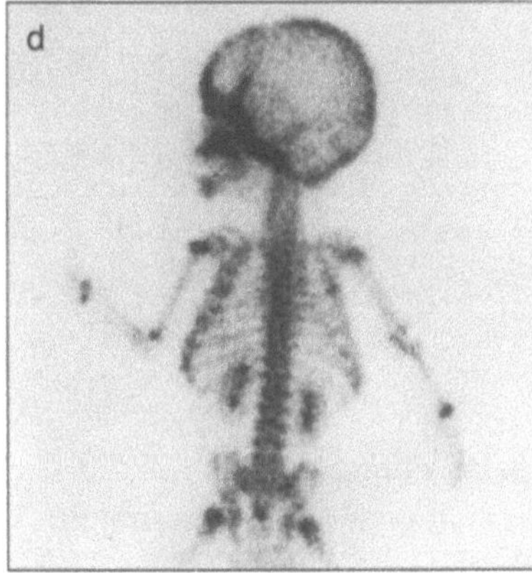

Case 8.33. A 6-month-old infant who had suffered a large acute subdural bleeding showed uptake of isotope in the brain during the acute phase, but this disappeared 1 week later

Fig. 8.33a Posterior image of the skull, upper limbs, body and pelvis shows abnormal increased uptake of isotope in the brain substance

Fig. 8.33b. Posterior image of the thorax and right lateral skull shows increased uptake of isotope in the brain.

The child underwent a follow-up scan 1 week later

Fig. 8.33c. Posterior image of the skull, axial skeleton and pelvis. No abnormality is seen in the skeleton. There is no uptake of isotope in the brain

Fig. 8.33d. Posterior image of the axial skeleton and left lateral skull fails to show any uptake of isotope in the brain

Teaching Point
For subdural uptake of isotope, see Case 5.37.

8.5 Soft Tissue Calcification

(1 Case; Fig. 8.34)

Case 8.34. A 1-month-old boy who had a drip for intravenous fluid inserted into the right foot. There was extravasation at the site of the intravenous drip and soft tissue calcification developed

Fig. 8.34a. Anterior image of the pelvis and lower limbs shows a marked abnormal increased uptake of isotope in the region of the right ankle as well as in the distal two thirds of the tibia and fibula

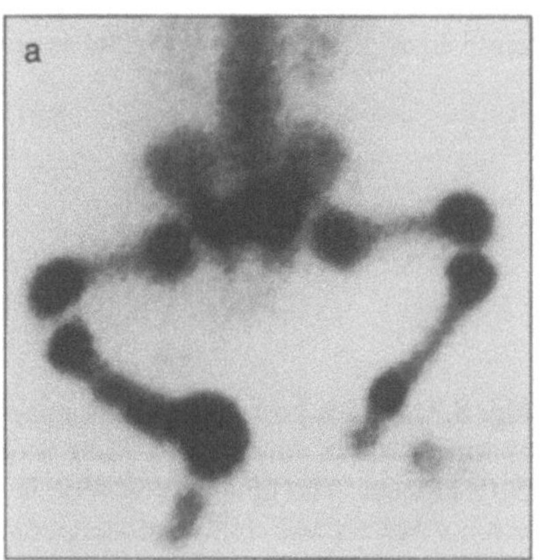

Fig. 8.34b. Radiograph in the lateral projection of both ankles and feet shows the extensive soft tissue calcification around the right tibia as well as in the hind foot

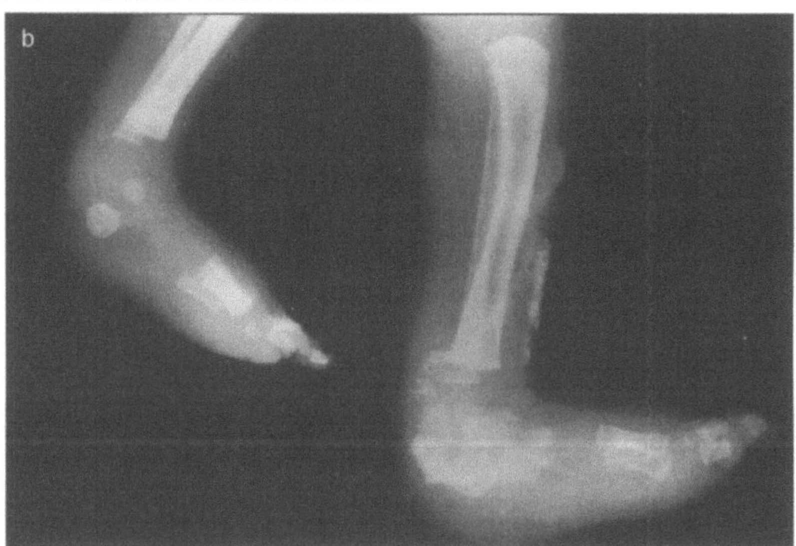

Teaching Point
The isotope is being taken up by the abnormal calcification following the trauma of extravasation.

8.6 Isotope Artefact

8.6.1 Injection Artefact
(3 Cases; Figs. 8.35–8.37)

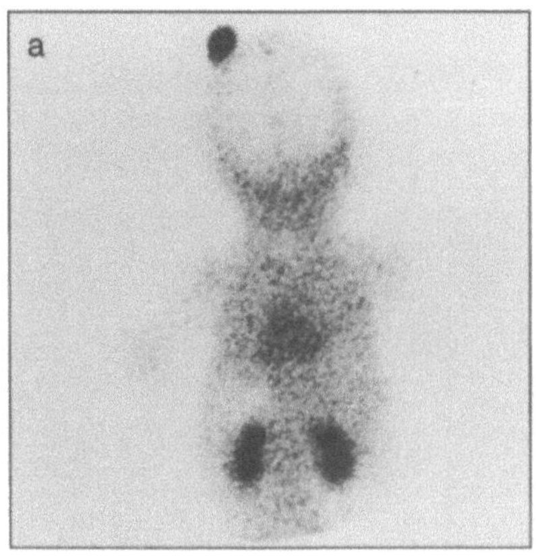

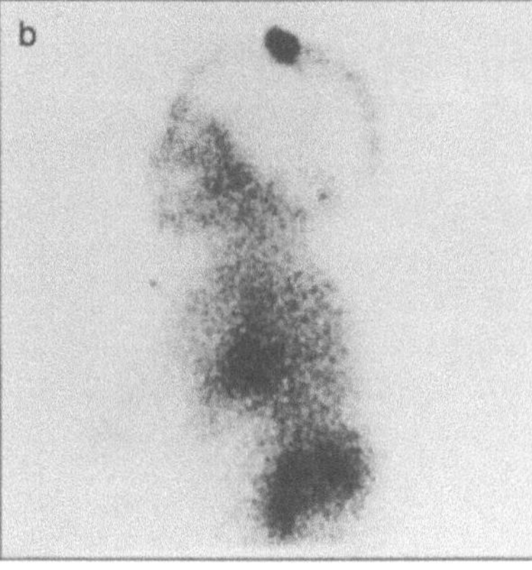

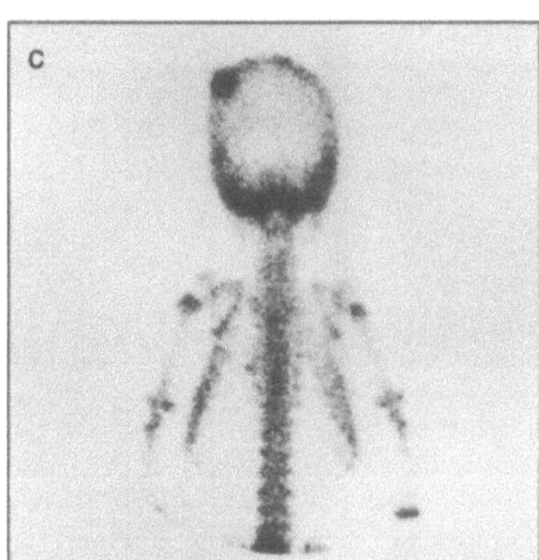

Case 8.35. A 2-month-old baby who had suffered from multiple repeated trauma (battered child). The skull radiograph showed a fracture, but no fracture was seen on the bone scan. (This is the same baby as in Case 5.1)

Fig. 8.35a. Posterior blood pool image of the skull shows intense focal increased uptake of isotope in the scalp

Fig. 8.35b. Left lateral blood pool phase shows abnormal uptake of isotope in the scalp

Fig. 8.35c. Posterior image of the skull, thorax and upper limbs. No fracture is seen. Abnormal uptake is noted in the skull vault

Technical Comment
The child was injected in the scalp and there was extravasation at the site of the injection.

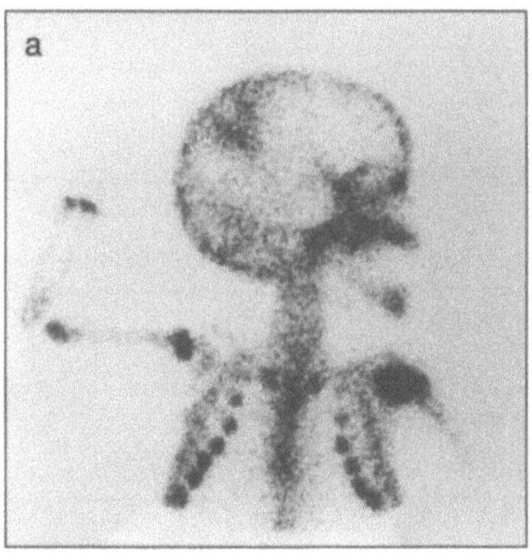

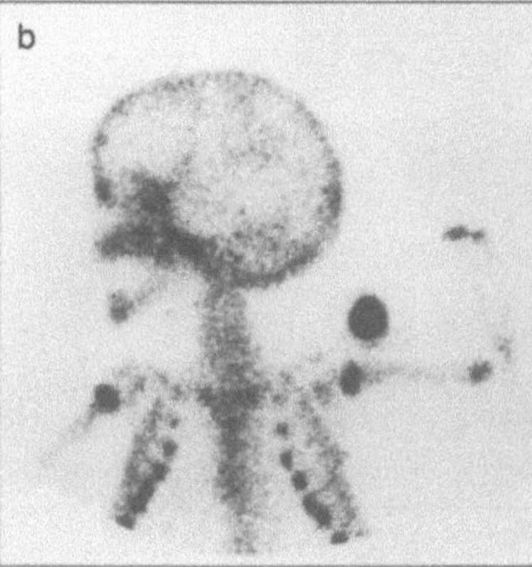

Case 8.36. A 5-month-old baby girl who was found to be battered. No fractures were identified at any stage. There was an epidural haematoma which took up the bone tracer. (Same patient as in Case 5.37)

Fig. 8.36a. Right lateral image of the skull and anterior chest shows abnormal increased uptake of isotope overlying the parietal bone

Fig. 8.36b. Left lateral image of the skull and anterior chest is normal

Technical Comment
In both images there is an artefact due to isotope on the side of the patient, caused by the injection system. In Fig. 8.36a it overlies the left shoulder.

Teaching Point
For other artefacts, see Case 2.17.

Case 8.37. A 19-year-old patient who was injected in the right cubital fossa. Isotope was held up in the right axilla

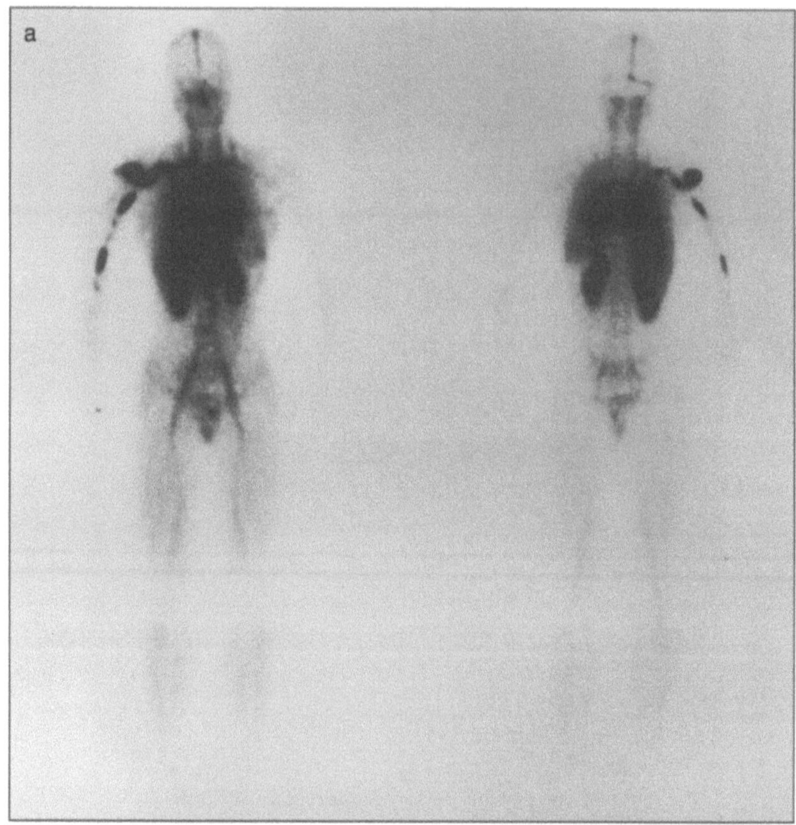

Fig. 8.37a. Whole body blood pool images show the isotope in the veins in the right upper arm as well as in the veins in the axilla

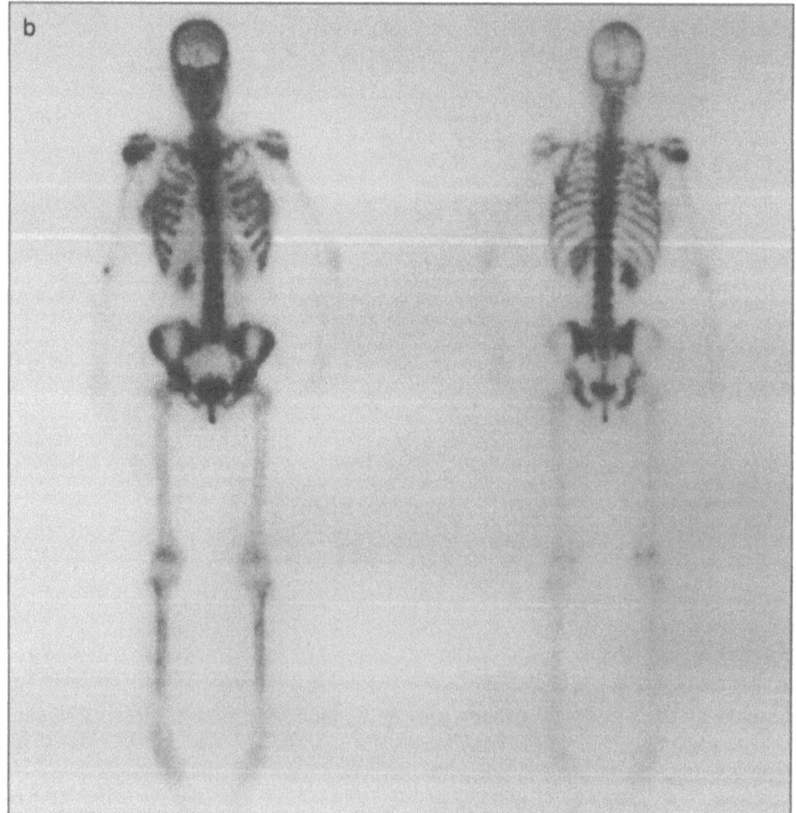

Fig. 8.37b. Whole body images fail to reveal any skeletal abnormality. Focal intensive increased uptake of isotope is noted in the region of the right humeral head. This was due to isotope in the venous system

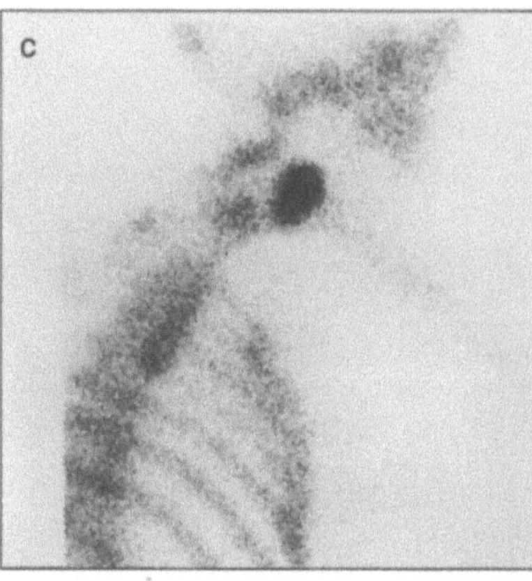

Fig. 8.37c. Right lateral image of the right shoulder shows focal intensive increased uptake of isotope in the region of the upper humerus.

The girl underwent a follow-up bone scan with injection in the left cubital fossa 1 week later

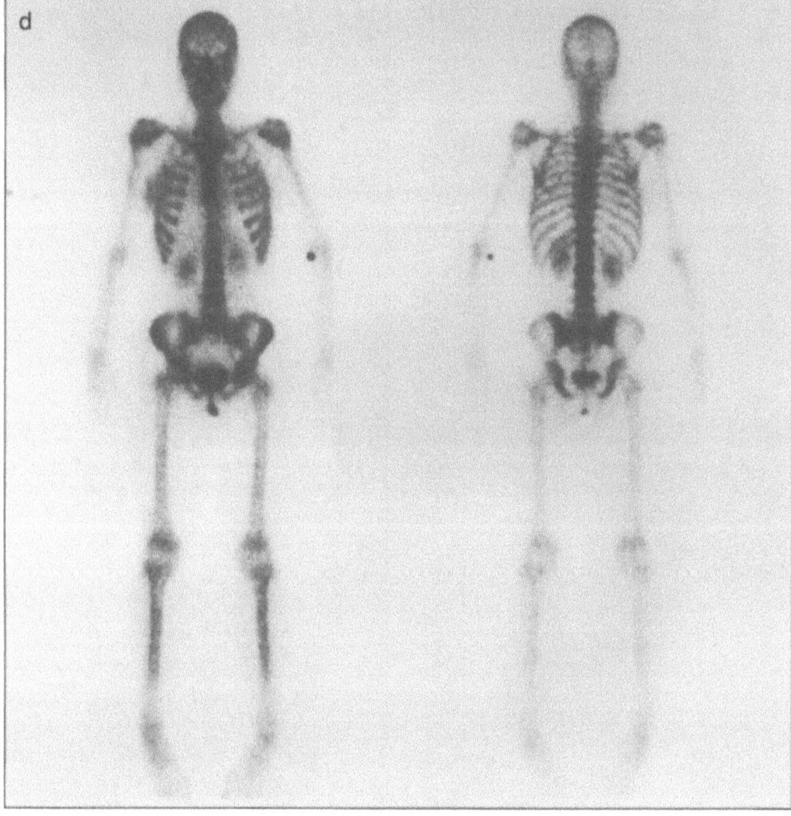

Fig. 8.37d. Whole body images fail to reveal any abnormality in the region of the humerus. Note extravasation of isotope in the left cubital fossa

8.6.2 Urine Contamination

(2 Cases; Figs. 8.38, 8.39)

Case 8.38. A 10-year-old boy with pain in the right femur. Urine contamination overlying the left side of the body of L5 is noted

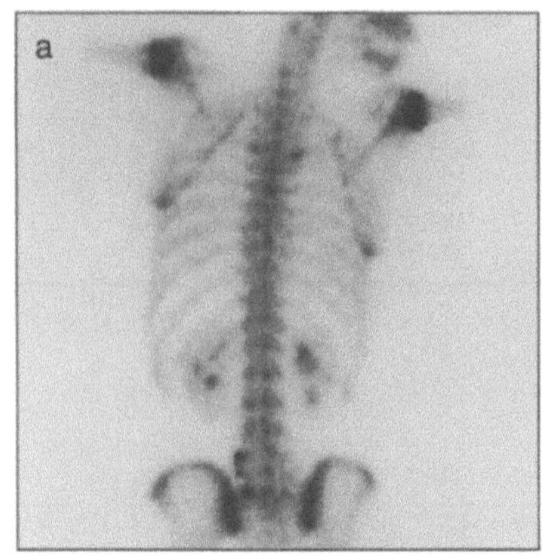

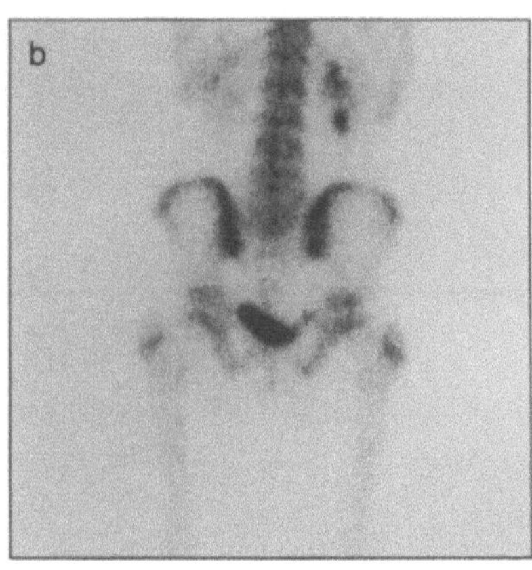

Fig. 8.38a. Posterior image of thorax, lumbar spine and upper pelvis shows abnormal increased uptake of isotope overlying the left lateral aspect of the body of L5. The skeleton appears normal

Fig. 8.38b. Repeat posterior image of the lumbar spine, pelvis and upper femora after a change of pyjama fails to reveal any abnormality

Case 8.39. A 10-year-old boy with a swelling of the face. An osteogenic sarcoma was arising from the maxilla. There is urine contamination over the thigh. (This is the same patient as in Case 4.37)

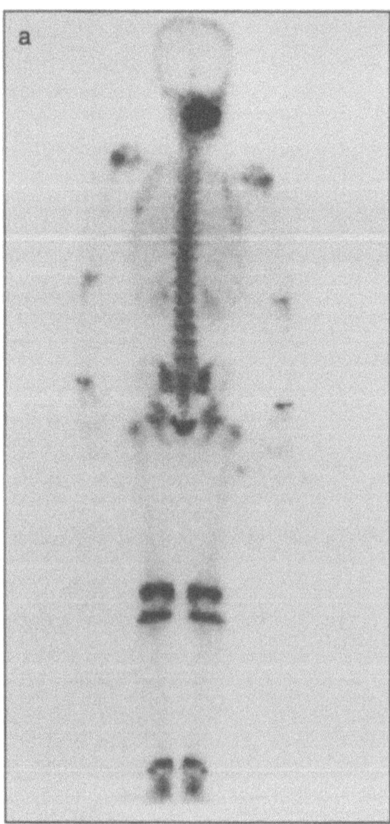

Fig. 8.39a. Whole body scan (posterior view) shows focal abnormal uptake of isotope in the mid face. Note activity in the region of the soft tissue of the upper aspect of the right femur. This was due to contamination and was not seen on the spot views (not shown)

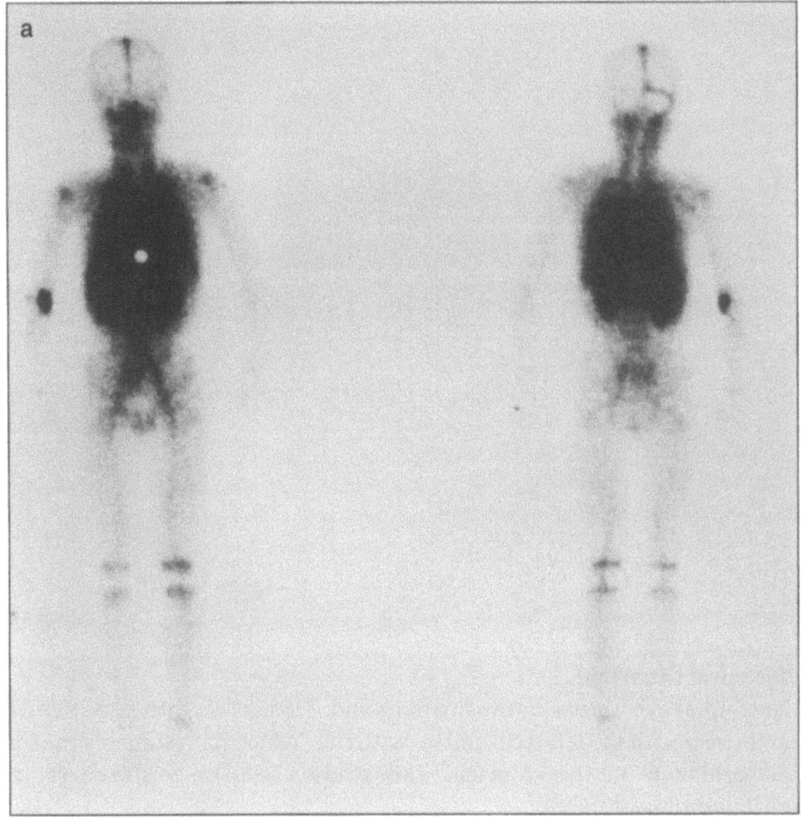

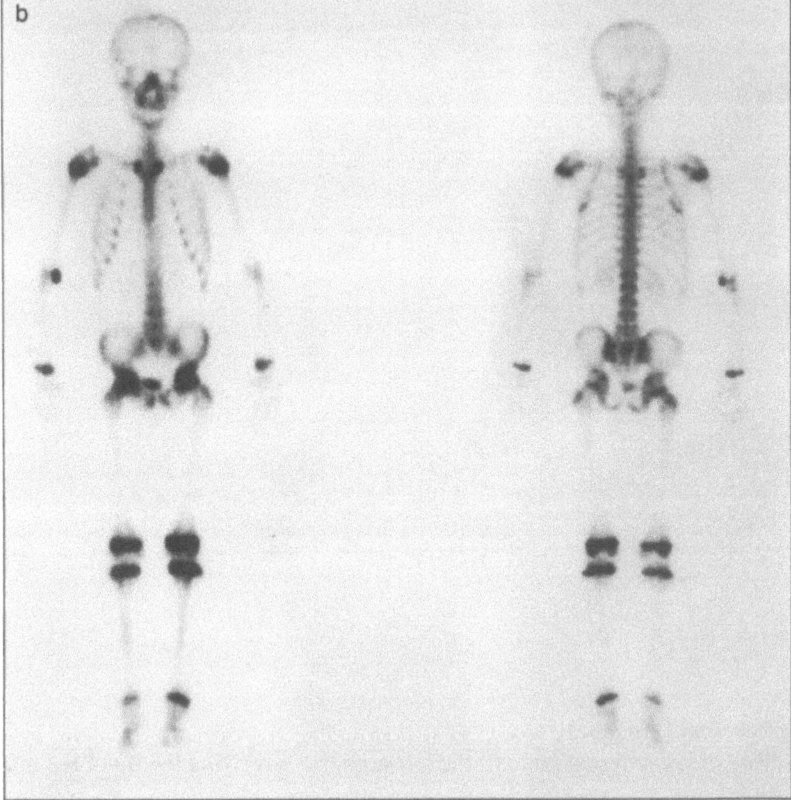

8.6.3 Foreign Body Artefact
(1 Case; Fig. 8.40)

Case 8.40. A 10-year-old boy who had a glass amulet necklace which he refused to take off for the blood pool images. (The bone scan was done for the diagnosis of a rheumatoid arthritis in the left foot)

Fig. 8.40a. Blood pool whole body scans show a photon-deficient area only seen on the anterior view in the mid line. Note extravasation at the site of the injection in the right cubital fossa

Fig. 8.40b. Whole body scans fail to show any abnormality in the region of the defect seen on the blood pool image. Extravasation at the site of the injection is noted in the left elbow

Teaching Point
Another example is seen in Case 4.2 in the blood pool image.

8.6.4 Free Pertechnetate
(1 Case; Fig. 8.41)

Case 8.41. A 13-year-old boy with an enchondroma in the upper right humerus. (This is the same patient as in Case 7.15)

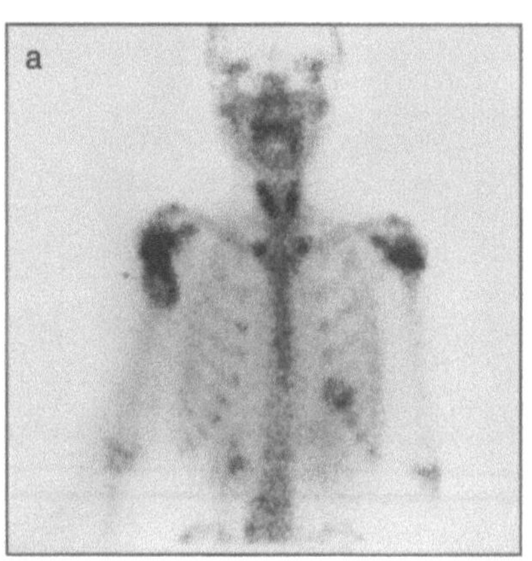

Fig. 8.41a. Anterior image of the upper limbs and thorax shows abnormal increased uptake of isotope on the right humerus extending beyond the confines of the bone. The area of abnormality is not homogeneous, with decreased uptake inferiorly compared to superiorly. Uptake of isotope by the tyroid gland is noted

Technical Comment

Note uptake of isotope by the thyroid gland. There is also increased activity in the region of the left sixth and seventh ribs, which is presumably the free pertechnetate in the stomach. This could easily be mistaken for an enchondroma of the rib.

8.6.5 Positional Abnormalities

Case 8.42. A 9-year-old girl with known sickle cell disease presented with fever and oedema of the scalp. Follow-up showed that there was no infection in the skull vault, rather that infarction of part of the parietal bone had occurred (This is the same patient as in Case 6.15)

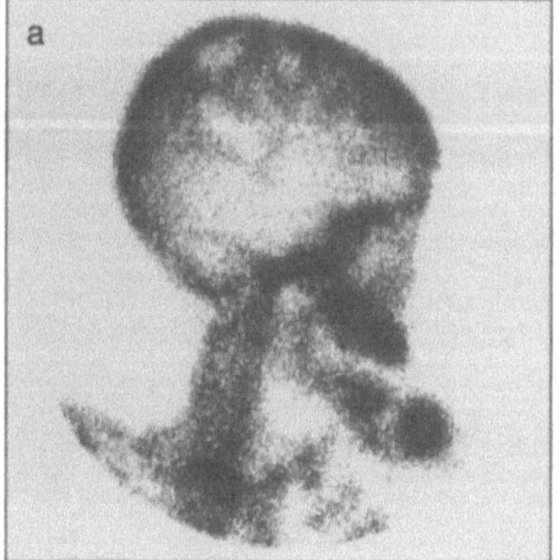

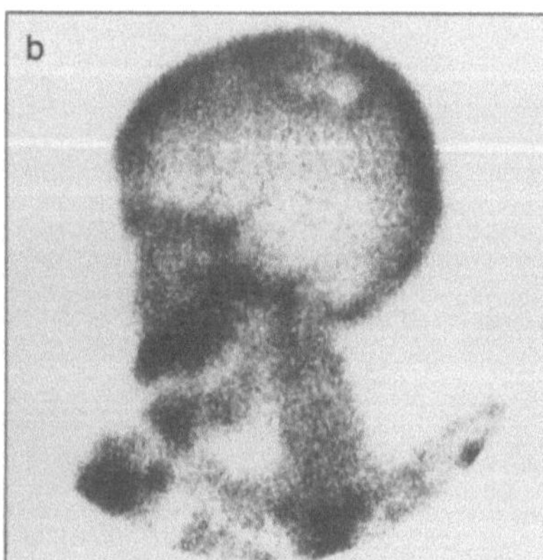

Fig. 8.42a. Right lateral image of the skull shows diffuse abnormal increased uptake of isotope in the frontal and posterior parietal bones with focal decreased uptake in the parietal bone.

Fig. 8.42b. Left lateral image of the skull shows the focal area of decreased uptake of isotope in the parietal bone to better advantage with surrounding increased activity which extends into the posterior parietal and occipital bones

Technical Comment

Note the epiphyseal plate of the left humerus overlying the tip of the mandible

Subject Index

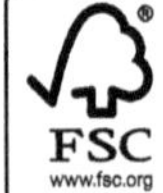